Endovascular Intervention
for
Vascular Disease

Endovascular Intervention
for
Vascular Disease
Principles and Practice

Edited by

Matt M. Thompson
St. George's Hospital
London, UK

Robert A. Morgan
St. George's Hospital
London, UK

Jon S. Matsumura
Northwestern University
Feinberg School of Medicine
Chicago, Illinois, USA

Marc Sapoval
Hôpital Européen Georges Pompidou
Paris, France

Ian M. Loftus
St. George's Hospital
London, UK

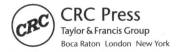

CRC Press
Taylor & Francis Group
Boca Raton London New York

CRC Press is an imprint of the
Taylor & Francis Group, an **informa** business

CRC Press
Taylor & Francis Group
6000 Broken Sound Parkway NW, Suite 300
Boca Raton, FL 33487-2742

First issued in paperback 2019

© 2008 by Taylor & Francis Group, LLC
CRC Press is an imprint of Taylor & Francis Group, an Informa business

No claim to original U.S. Government works

ISBN-13: 978-0-8493-3979-0 (hbk)
ISBN-13: 978-0-367-38790-7 (pbk)

This book contains information obtained from authentic and highly regarded sources. While all reasonable efforts have been made to publish reliable data and information, neither the author[s] nor the publisher can accept any legal responsibility or liability for any errors or omissions that may be made. The publishers wish to make clear that any views or opinions expressed in this book by individual editors, authors or contributors are personal to them and do not necessarily reflect the views/opinions of the publishers. The information or guidance contained in this book is intended for use by medical, scientific or health-care professionals and is provided strictly as a supplement to the medical or other professional's own judgement, their knowledge of the patient's medical history, relevant manufacturer's instructions and the appropriate best practice guidelines. Because of the rapid advances in medical science, any information or advice on dosages, procedures or diagnoses should be independently verified. The reader is strongly urged to consult the relevant national drug formulary and the drug companies' and device or material manufacturers' printed instructions, and their websites, before administering or utilizing any of the drugs, devices or materials mentioned in this book. This book does not indicate whether a particular treatment is appropriate or suitable for a particular individual. Ultimately it is the sole responsibility of the medical professional to make his or her own professional judgements, so as to advise and treat patients appropriately. The authors and publishers have also attempted to trace the copyright holders of all material reproduced in this publication and apologize to copyright holders if permission to publish in this form has not been obtained. If any copyright material has not been acknowledged please write and let us know so we may rectify in any future reprint.

Library of Congress Cataloging-in-Publication Data
Endovascular intervention for vascular disease : principles and practice / edited by Matt M. Thompson ... [et al.].   p. ; cm.   Includes bibliographical references and index.   ISBN-13: 978-0-8493-3979-0 (hardcover : alk. paper)   ISBN-10: 0-8493-3979-0 (hardcover : alk. paper) 1. Blood-vessels–Endoscopic surgery.   I. Thompson, M. M.   [DNLM: 1. Vascular Diseases–surgery. 2. Surgical Procedures, Minimally Invasive–methods. 3.   Vascular Surgical Procedures–methods. WG 170 E56115 2007]   RD598.5.E5245 2007   617.4'130597–dc22   2007025124

Visit the Informa Web site at
www.informa.com

and the Informa Healthcare Web site at
www.informahealthcare.com

Preface

Historically, vascular disease has been treated by a combination of open surgical procedures and medical management. Since the first description of a percutaneous procedure to dilate diseased lower limb arteries, the treatment of vascular disease has changed. In the last decade, it might be said that the slow evolution of endovascular techniques has become a revolution, and defining the place of medical, open, and endovascular therapies in the management of patients with peripheral vascular disease has become challenging.

In the last few years, endoluminal therapy of vascular disease has expanded from simple dilatation of atherosclerotic lesions to encompass treatment of arterial aneurysms, arteriovenous malformations, acute ischemia, and varicose veins. It has also assumed a significant role in the management of abdominal, thoracic, and extremity trauma. These broadened indications for endovascular therapy have been accompanied by technological improvements in the concept, design, and availability of endovascular devices, which have further expanded the spectrum of clinical conditions that may be managed using endoluminal techniques. Some of the most exciting advances have been observed when traditional surgical techniques have been combined with endovascular procedures to facilitate treatment of highly complex diseases—so-called "hybrid" procedures.

Endovascular therapy now draws inspiration from several inter-related disciplines, with vascular surgeons, interventional radiologists, angiologists, and cardiologists all contributing to this exciting and fast-moving field. As with all innovations, there are differences in opinion about the place of newer therapies in clinical practice. It is only by balancing the opinions of enthusiasts and skeptics that a realistic view emerges. This book has been written and edited to represent, as widely as possible, the views of experts in the field. The authors of individual chapters are drawn from a variety of specialities and also represent a global spectrum of opinion, since endovascular practice varies widely according to geographical location.

A book such as this can only represent opinion at a finite moment in time. The evidence to support endovascular techniques is as diverse as the techniques themselves. In some situations, such as endovascular repair of abdominal aortic aneurysms, endovascular therapy has been rigorously trialed against both open surgery and medical management. Several chapters describe these trials and offer comment on interpretation. This level of evidence is unfortunately rare in endovascular practice, as most therapies are supported by flawed, historical, or anecdotal evidence. In these situations, the evidence is discussed in detail with expert commentary on the significance of the findings and recommendations for practice.

This book offers a diverse and comprehensive review of the current status of endovascular therapy for peripheral vascular disease. In addition to summarizing the current techniques and available evidence, it discusses likely future advances in the field, and sets these against both the natural history of the disease and alternative therapies that may involve cell- or gene-based approaches.

Matt M. Thompson
Robert A. Morgan
Jon S. Matsumura
Marc Sapoval
Ian M. Loftus

Contents

PART II. ACUTE LOWER LIMB ISCHEMIA

PART III. CAROTID AND VERTEBRAL DISEASE

PART IV. VISCERAL ARTERY OCCLUSIVE DISEASE

PART V. THORACIC AORTA—ANEURYSMS AND DISSECTIONS

PART XII. ARTERIOVENOUS ACCESS

Contributors

Donald J. Adam   University Department of Vascular Surgery, Heart of England NHS Foundation Trust, Solihull, Birmingham, U.K.

Philippe Asseman   Cardiac Intensive Care Unit, Hôpital Cardiologique, Lille, France

Ali Azizzadeh   Department of Cardiothoracic and Vascular Surgery, University of Texas at Houston Medical School, Memorial Hermann Heart and Vascular Institute, Houston, Texas, U.S.A.

Carlos F. Bechara   Baylor College of Medicine, Houston, Texas, U.S.A.

J. P. Becquemin   Henri Mondor Hospital, University Paris XII, Creteil, France

Rachel Bell   Department of General and Vascular Surgery, Guy's and St. Thomas' Hospital, London, U.K.

Anna-Maria Belli   Department of Radiology, St. George's Hospital, London, U.K.

Jean-Paul Beregi   Cardio-Vascular Radiological and Imaging Unit, Service de Radiologie et d'Imageric Cardio-Vasculaire, Hôpital Cardiologique, Lille, France

P. Bergeron   Department of Thoracic and Cardiovascular Surgery, Hôpital Saint-Joseph, Marseille, France

J. D. Blankensteijn   Department of Surgery, Division of Vascular Surgery, Radboud University Nijmegen Medical Centre, Nijmegen, The Netherlands

Marc Bosiers   Department of Vascular Surgery, AZ St-Blasius, Dendermonde, Belgium

M. Boukhris   Department of Thoracic and Cardiovascular Surgery, Hôpital Saint-Joseph, Marseille, France

Matthew J. Bown   Department of Cardiovascular Sciences, University of Leicester, Vascular Surgery Research Group, Leicester Royal Infirmary, Leicester, U.K.

Andrew W. Bradbury   University Department of Vascular Surgery, Heart of England NHS Foundation Trust, Solihull, Birmingham, U.K.

Bruce D. Braithwaite   Department of Vascular and Endovascular Surgery, University Hospital, Nottingham, U.K.

J. A. Brennan   Royal Liverpool University Hospital, Liverpool, U.K.

Robert E. Brightwell   Division of Surgery, Oncology, Reproductive Biology and Anaesthetics, Imperial College London, St. Mary's Hospital, London, U.K.

Elias N. Brountzos   Second Department of Radiology, National and Kapodistrian University of Athens, Medical School, Attikon University Hospital, Haidari, Athens, Greece

Tim Buckenham   Radiology Services, Christchurch Hospital, Christchurch, New Zealand

Paul J. Burns   Department of Vascular Surgery, Royal Infirmary of Edinburgh, Edinburgh, U.K.

Manfred Cejna   Zentrales Radiologie Institut, LKH Feldkirch, Feldkirch, Austria

Nick Chalmers   Department of Radiology, Manchester Royal Infirmary, Manchester, U.K.

R. T. A. Chalmers   Department of Vascular Surgery, Royal Infirmary of Edinburgh, Edinburgh, U.K.

Y. C. Chan   Department of Vascular and Endovascular Surgery, Guy's and St. Thomas' NHS Foundation Trust, London, U.K.

Nicholas J. W. Cheshire   Division of Surgery, Oncology, Reproductive Biology and Anaesthetics, Imperial College London, St. Mary's Hospital, London, U.K.

Timothy A. M. Chuter   Division of Vascular Surgery, University of California San Francisco, San Francisco, California, U.S.A.

Trevor J. Cleveland   Sheffield Vascular Institute, Sheffield Teaching Hospitals NHSFT, Northern General Hospital, Sheffield, U.K.

Andrew G. Clifton   Department of Neuroradiology, St George's Hospital, London, U.K.

J. P. P. M. de Vries   Department of Vascular Surgery, St. Antonius Hospital, Nieuwegein, The Netherlands

Koen Deloose   Department of Vascular Surgery, AZ St-Blasius, Dendermonde, Belgium

Richard Donnelly   School of Medical and Surgical Sciences, University of Nottingham, Nottingham and Derby City General Hospital, Derby, U.K.

Anthony L. Estrera   Department of Cardiothoracic and Vascular Surgery, University of Texas at Houston Medical School, Memorial Hermann Heart and Vascular Institute, Houston, Texas, U.S.A.

Rossella Fattori   Cardiovascular Department, University Hospital S. Orsola, University of Bologna, Bologna, Italy

P. A. Gaines   Sheffield Vascular Institute, Northern General Hospital, Sheffield, U.K.

Virginia Gaxotte   Cardio-Vascular Radiological and Imaging Unit, Hôpital Cardiologique, Lille, France

J. Gay   Department of Thoracic and Cardiovascular Surgery, Hôpital Saint-Joseph, Marseille, France

Roy K. Greenberg   Department of Vascular Surgery, Cleveland Clinic, Cleveland, Ohio, U.S.A.

Mohamad Hamady   Department of Interventional Radiology, St. Mary's Hospital, London, U.K.

Peter Harris   University of Liverpool, Liverpool, U.K.

Andrew Edward Healey   Alder Hey Children's Hospital and Royal Liverpool University Hospital, Liverpool, U.K.

Johanna M. Hendriks Department of Vascular Surgery and Department of Radiology, Erasmus University Medical Center, Rotterdam, The Netherlands

Robert J. Hinchliffe Endovascular Department, University Hospital, Malmo, Sweden

R. Hissink Department of Vascular Surgery, University Medical Centre, Utrecht, The Netherlands

Peter Holt St. George's Vascular Institute, St. George's Hospital, London, U.K.

Adam Howard Department of Vascular and Endovascular Surgery, St. George's Healthcare NHS Trust, London, U.K.

Krassi Ivancev Endovascular Department, University Hospital, Malmo, Sweden

Thomas Jahnke Department of Radiology, University Clinics Schleswig-Holstein (UKSH), Campus Kiel, Kiel, Germany

Ravul Jindal Department of Vascular Surgery, St. Mary's Hospital, London, U.K.

David O. Kessel Department of Radiology, Leeds Teaching Hospitals, St. James's University Hospital, Leeds, U.K.

Mohamad Koussa Vascular Surgery Unit, Hôpital Cardiologique, Lille, France

Bernard Lee Vascular and Endovascular Surgery Unit, Belfast City Hospital, Belfast, Northern Ireland

Christophe Lions Cardio-Vascular Radiological and Imaging Unit, Hôpital Cardiologique, Lille, France

William Loan Vascular and Endovascular Surgery Unit, Belfast City Hospital, Belfast, Northern Ireland

Ian M. Loftus St. George's Vascular Institute, St. George's Hospital, London, U.K.

Alan B. Lumsden Methodist DeBakey Heart Center, Houston, Texas, U.S.A.

Hannu Manninen Department of Clinical Radiology, Kuopio University Hospital and Kuopio University, Kuopio, Finland

J. Marzelle Henri Mondor Hospital, University Paris XII, Creteil, France

Matthew Matson Department of Radiology, Royal London Hospital, Barts and the London NHS Trust, Whitechapel, London, U.K.

Jon S. Matsumura Division of Vascular Surgery, Department of Surgery, Northwestern University Feinberg School of Medicine, Chicago, Illinois, U.S.A.

Charles C. Miller III Department of Cardiothoracic and Vascular Surgery, University of Texas at Houston Medical School, Memorial Hermann Heart and Vascular Institute, Houston, Texas, U.S.A.

F. L. Moll Department of Vascular Surgery, University Medical Centre, Utrecht, The Netherlands

Robert A. Morgan Department of Radiology, St. George's Hospital, London, U.K.

Graham J. Munneke Department of Radiology, St. George's Hospital, London, U.K.

Ivan Murillo   Vascular Surgery, Thorax Institute, Hospital Clínic, University of Barcelona, Barcelona, Spain

A. Ross Naylor   Department of Vascular Surgery, Leicester Royal Infirmary, Leicester, U.K.

Ziad Negaiwi   Cardio-Vascular Radiological and Imaging Unit, Hôpital Cardiologique, Lille, France

Albert A. Nemcek   Section of Interventional Radiology, Northwestern University Feinberg School of Medicine, Chicago, Illinois, U.S.A.

Tony Nicholson   Leeds Teaching Hospitals NHS Trust, Leeds, U.K.

T. J. Parkinson   Northern Vascular Centre, Freeman Hospital, Newcastle, U.K.

Eric K. Peden   Methodist DeBakey Heart Center, Houston, Texas, U.S.A.

Patrick Peeters   Department of Cardiovascular and Thoracic Surgery, Imelda Hospital, Bonheiden, Belgium

Brian G. Peterson   Division of Vascular Surgery, Saint Louis University School of Medicine, St. Louis, Missouri, U.S.A.

Graham Plant   Department of Interventional Radiology, North Hampshire Hospital, Basingstoke, Hampshire, U.K.

E. D. Ponfoort   Department of Vascular Surgery, St. Antonius Hospital, Nieuwegein, The Netherlands

Janet T. Powell   Department of Vascular Surgery, Imperial College at Charing Cross, London, U.K.

Alain Prat   Cardiac and Thoracic Surgery Unit, Hôpital Cardiologique, Lille, France

Jowad Raja   Department of Radiology, St. George's Hospital, London, U.K.

Lakshmi A. Ratnam   Department of Radiology, St. George's Hospital, London, U.K.

Harjeet S. Rayt   Department of Cardiovascular Sciences, University of Leicester, Vascular Surgery Research Group, Leicester Royal Infirmary, Leicester, U.K.

Michael J. Reardon   Methodist DeBakey Heart Center, Houston, Texas, U.S.A.

Vincent Riambau   Vascular Surgery, Thorax Institute, Hospital Clínic, University of Barcelona, Barcelona, Spain

J. D. G. Rose   Northern Vascular Centre, Freeman Hospital, Newcastle, U.K.

Eric E. Roselli   Department of Thoracic and Cardiovascular Surgery, Cleveland Clinic, Cleveland, Ohio, U.S.A.

Peter Rowlands   Royal Liverpool University Hospital, Liverpool, U.K.

Timothy Rowlands   Derby Hospitals NHS Foundation Trust, Derby, U.K.

Hazim J. Safi   Department of Cardiothoracic and Vascular Surgery, University of Texas at Houston Medical School, Memorial Hermann Heart and Vascular Institute, Houston, Texas, U.S.A.

Robert D. Sayers   Department of Cardiovascular Sciences, University of Leicester, Vascular Surgery Research Group, Leicester Royal Infirmary, Leicester, U.K.

L. J. Schultze-Kool   Department of Radiology, Radboud University Nijmegen Medical Centre, Nijmegen, The Netherlands

Philip Coleridge Smith   UCL Medical School, Thames Valley Nuffield Hospital, London, U.K.

Chee V. Soong   Vascular and Endovascular Surgery Unit, Belfast City Hospital, Belfast, Northern Ireland

Andrew H. Stockland   Department of Radiology, Mayo Clinic, Jacksonville, Florida, U.S.A.

P. R. Taylor   Department of Vascular and Endovascular Surgery, Guy's and St. Thomas' NHS Foundation Trust, London, U.K.

Matt M. Thompson   St. George's Vascular Institute, St. George's Hospital, London, U.K.

Ignace Tielliu   Department of Surgery, Division of Vascular Surgery, University Medical Center Groningen, Groningen, The Netherlands

G. D. Treharne   Royal Liverpool University Hospital, Liverpool, U.K.

M. Truijers   Department of Surgery, Division of Vascular Surgery, Radboud University Nijmegen Medical Centre, Nijmegen, The Netherlands

G. B. Tshiombo   Department of Thoracic and Cardiovascular Surgery, Hôpital Saint-Joseph, Marseille, France

Luc Turmel-Rodrigues   Department of Vascular Radiology, Clinique St-Gatien, Tours, and Department of Vascular Radiology, Centre Médico-chirugical Ambroise Paré, Neuilly-sur-Seine, France

Renan Uflacker   Department of Radiology, Division of Vascular and Interventional Radiology, Medical University of South Carolina, Charleston, South Carolina, U.S.A.

Jan van den Dungen   Department of Surgery, Division of Vascular Surgery, University Medical Center Groningen, Groningen, The Netherlands

Lukas C. van Dijk   Department of Vascular Surgery and Department of Radiology, Erasmus University Medical Center, Rotterdam, The Netherlands

Marc R. H. M. van Sambeek   Department of Vascular Surgery and Department of Radiology, Erasmus University Medical Center, Rotterdam, The Netherlands

Jurgen Verbist   Department of Cardiovascular and Thoracic Surgery, Imelda Hospital, Bonheiden, Belgium

Eric Verhoeven   Department of Surgery, Division of Vascular Surgery, University Medical Center Groningen, Groningen, The Netherlands

Dierk Vorwerk   Department of Diagnostic and Interventional Radiology, Klinikum Ingolstadt, Krumenauerstrasse, Ingolstadt, Germany

Eric M. Walser   Department of Radiology, Mayo Clinic, Jacksonville, Florida, U.S.A.

M. L. Wang   Department of Thoracic and Cardiovascular Surgery, Hôpital Saint-Joseph, Marseille, France

Serge Willoteaux   Cardio-Vascular Radiological and Imaging Unit, Hôpital Cardiologique, Lille, France

M. G. Wyatt   Northern Vascular Centre, Freeman Hospital, Newcastle, U.K.

Clark Zeebregts   Department of Surgery, Division of Vascular Surgery, University Medical Center Groningen, Groningen, The Netherlands

Y. Y. Zhang   Department of Thoracic and Cardiovascular Surgery, Hôpital Saint-Joseph, Marseille, France

1 Occlusive Disease of the Aorta and Aortic Bifurcation

Ravul Jindal
Department of Vascular Surgery, St. Mary's Hospital, London, U.K.
Mohamad Hamady
Department of Interventional Radiology, St. Mary's Hospital, London, U.K.

INTRODUCTION

Many techniques for revascularization in aortoiliac occlusive disease are available, including surgical and endovascular procedures. However, few studies have directly compared these two types of reconstructive procedures. Aortoiliac atherosclerosis limited to the distal aorta and common iliac arteries occurs in approximately 10% of patients with symptomatic aortoiliac disease (1).

Aortobifemoral bypass or endarterectomy is the standard treatment of aortoiliac occlusive disease with five-year patency of approximately 90% to 95%. Despite the good patency rate and durability, surgery is associated with significant morbidity and mortality, 8% to 30% and 2% to 5%, respectively (2). Patients who are at high surgical risk and have extensive aortoiliac disease have been revascularized with extra-anatomical reconstructions such as axillofemoral bypass. There are potential disadvantages of extra-anatomical grafts such as infection and limited patency, making endovascular option an attractive alternative in this subset of patients.

Endovascular therapy including percutaneous transluminal angioplasty (PTA), with or without assisted stenting, and primary stenting has evolved as an attractive alternative. Endoluminal treatment provides potentially minimal invasiveness that obviates the need for general anesthesia, abdominal incision, requires shorter hospital stay with lower cost, as well as has lower mortality and morbidity rates (3–6). Moreover, endoluminal therapy was shown to improve or at least preserve sexual function in males (7,8).

AORTIC OCCLUSION OR STENOSIS AND AORTIC BIFURCATION DISEASE

Infrarenal aortic lesions are defined as atherosclerotic plaques located more than 2 cm above the aortic bifurcation whereas aortic bifurcation disease is that involving the distal 2 cm of the aorta and/or the proximal portions of the common iliac arteries (9,10).

The rationale for dividing these lesions is the difference in their pathogenesis. Isolated infrarenal aortic occlusive disease is relatively uncommon, affecting predominantly middle-aged females who are chronic smokers (1,11,12). Their exact pathogenesis remains unclear, even if several authors consider it a particular manifestation of aortic atherosclerosis. It has also been shown that this subgroup of patients may have high cholesterol levels in combination with a hypoplastic aorta. Life expectancy appears to be better in this group when compared with the group with diffuse atherosclerosis as the disease is more localized. However, some investigators do not support this hypothesis. In a retrospective study that involved 52 patients (35 aortic lesions and 17 aortoiliac) there was no difference in risk factors, gender prevalence or treatment outcome between the two groups (9).

Stenoses involving the aortic bifurcation are more common and represent a typical atherosclerotic presentation that involves the vessel bifurcation. This presentation is more common in elderly and male patients. Aortic lesions have been further subdivided based on the classification of the American Heart Association depending on the length of stenoses or occlusion (13).

CLINICAL PRESENTATION AND INDICATIONS FOR TREATMENT

The most common presenting symptom is intermittent claudication involving the buttock and calf. Less common presentations include critical limb ischemia (rest pain and foot ulcer) and blue toe syndrome secondary to micro embolization. The indications for endovascular intervention are no different from surgery and include all the above-mentioned presentations.

In a review of 586 patients by Yilmaz et al. (14), the mean age of the patients was reported to vary from 44 to 67 years and the symptoms were mainly claudication (90%), critical ischemia (7%), and blue toe syndrome (3%). However, in all the series, the majority of the lesions were found to be stenotic (96%) when compared with occlusions and were predominantly located in the aorta (75%).

TECHNICAL ASPECTS

Diagnostic angiography and/or computed tomography angiography are usually required to establish the diagnosis, assess the lesion/s (calcification, ulcerating plaque), and measure the exact diameter of the normal abdominal aorta above the lesion. This is required to avoid overdilation of the aorta and the potential danger of aortic rupture.

Following a secured arterial access, usually bilateral femoral approach, the aortic or iliac lesion is crossed with hydrophilic guidewire. This is followed by exchange for super stiff wire to support the balloon or stent. Depending on the technique used, the lesion is either dilated only or combined with stent deployment. Adequate ballooning of the aorta is achieved with either the single balloon or the kissing balloon technique. Primary technical success is defined as a residual stenosis of <30% and/or pressure gradient of <10 mmHg. Completion angiogram should pay particular attention to the status of the outflow to confirm the absence of significant distal embolization.

Type of Stent

Balloon-expandable steel stents or self-expanding nitinol stents may be used. For aortic lesions, self-expanding nitinol stents are the preferred option. Balloon expandable can also be used in aortic lesions when highly accurate placement is required or when the lesion involves high-grade calcification.

For aortic bifurcation disease self-expanding nitinol stents are preferred as they are flexible and can adapt to the angle between the aorta and the iliac arteries. Balloon-expandable stents are used when accuracy is required to place the stents in such a manner that the proximal end of the stent is flushed with the ostium of the common iliac artery.

Tips

In the common iliac arteries, stent and balloon diameter should be chosen through comparison with the normal distal reference segment, providing an optimal luminal gain and full expansion of the stent. The length of the stent is chosen to completely cover the entire lesion. This is especially critical for ostial lesions of the common iliac artery that extend into the aortic lumen.

The use of balloon-mounted stents to allow accurate positioning is important. Development of larger balloons decreases the chances of complications especially aortic rupture. Larger balloons need lower inflation pressures to achieve same radial force. The 10- to 15-mm balloons used for PTA of the aorta have normal dilation pressure of 4 atm, whereas the rated burst pressure is up to 6 atm. Usually inflation should not exceed 3 to 4 atm for more than one minute. This highlights the importance of using inflation device during those procedures. Increased care should be taken when treating calcified lesions because of higher risk of rupture.

Antiplatelet Therapy and Follow-Up

The patient usually receives antiplatelet therapy prior and after the procedure as well as unfractionated heparin during the procedure. If a stent is placed then patients are also given six weeks of clopidogrel along with aspirin.

CURRENT RESULTS FOR AORTIC STENOSIS AND OCCLUSION

Angioplasty With or Without Stenting

Angioplasty for aortic stenosis was first reported in the early 1980s (15). Since then several series have shown the safety and efficacy of aortic PTA (10).

Tegtmeyer et al. (3) used PTA to treat 200 patients with aortoiliac disease who were followed for 90 months (mean 28.7 months, median 23 months). The primary success rate was 93.0%. Follow-up was obtained in 176 patients. The long-term results were analyzed using life table methodology to determine cumulative patency. Fourteen patients were considered failures because of recurrent disease or symptoms. The projected 7.5-year cumulative patency rate was 85%. When the response to redilatation was considered, the projected 7.5-year cumulative patency rate was 92%.

Feugier et al. (16) also reported good long-term results following aortic PTA in 86 patients. Stents were placed in 22 patients with residual stenosis and in 4 with dissection. Primary actuarial patency was 94% at one year, 89% at three years, and 77% at five years.

Hedeman et al. (7) studied 38 patients aged 26 to 81 years (mean 50 years) who underwent PTA of the infrarenal aorta. All patients had symptomatic isolated stenotic lesions of the aorta located below the renal arteries and above the bifurcation. Initial clinical and angiographic success was achieved in 94% of cases. Mean follow-up was 34 months (range 1–92 months). Only five (13%) had clinically significant recurrent symptoms and were subsequently treated successfully with a second PTA. No major complications were reported.

Several investigators indicated that PTA should be considered the first-line treatment modality for localized aortic lesions (16). Though the result of the PTA appears to be good, the numbers of series in which these results are reported is small with short-to-midterm follow-up. In addition, most of the data are for short aortic occlusions and there is a lack of information on safety and efficacy of PTA for complex lesions like eccentric, heavily calcified, long, multiple or ulcerated stenoses.

Primary Aortic Stenting

Proponents of stenting have proposed various advantages of stenting over PTA. Primary stenting may decrease the incidence of distal embolization in complex plaques. However, the advantage of stent to PTA in terms of distal embolization is unproven. The risk of rupture is also thought to be low with stenting as it more evenly distributes the dilating forces against the arterial wall. Primary and secondary aortic patency rates reported with stent are 92% and 98%, respectively, with mean follow-up ranging from 3.6 to 19 months (17). A theoretical disadvantage of stent deployment is obstruction of the inferior mesenteric artery (IMA). However, mesenteric ischemia has not been reported following stent insertion to date.

Several studies with relatively small numbers of patients have established the safety and efficacy of primary stenting in focal aortic stenosis (4,14). Nyman et al. (17) reported primary stenting in 30 patients with 93% technical success, primary patency of 95% and primary assisted patency of 100% at a follow-up of median 19 months. Vallabhaneni et al. (18) also reported successful treatment of 6 occlusions and 15 stenosis of the aorta with primary aortic stenting with primary patency in 14 patients and secondary patency in the remaining patients at one-year follow-up. There was one death in postoperative period.

Sheeran et al. (4) reported on nine patients with focal mid-abdominal aortic stenoses treated with stent placement (Fig. 1). Of the 10 stenoses, seven were treated with primary stent

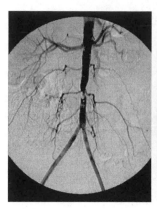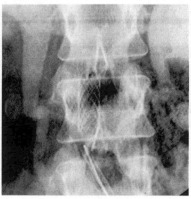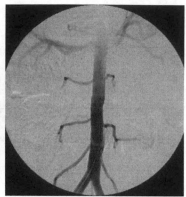

FIGURE 1   Mid-abdominal aortic stenosis treated by stenting.

placement, whereas three were treated with stent placement after suboptimal angioplasty. The technical success rate was 100%. Clinical success was achieved in 89% of patients with a mean follow-up of 1.6 years (range 0.2–3.0 years).

Yilmaz and colleagues (14) performed primary aortic stenting in 13 patients with a localized complex infrarenal aortic stenosis. The primary technical success rate was 100% without major complications or mortality. The angiographic patency was 100% during long-term follow-up of 96 months (mean 43 ± 23 months). However, clinical patency was 75% due to occlusive disease distal to the stented segments. The authors advocated that primary stenting should be considered the first-line treatment for selected patients with focal atherosclerotic infrarenal stenoses of the abdominal aorta.

Comparison of PTA and Primary Stenting of Aortic Lesions

No randomized trials have evaluated the significance of primary stent placement in aortic stenosis when compared with PTA. A few small series have reported a higher major complication rate with stenting than that with PTA (9.2% and 3.6%), but this may represent heterogenicity of the lesions treated. Technical success rates appear higher with stenting though there are no hard data to support this sentiment.

Stent Grafts

There is limited experience with the use of stent grafts in aortic occlusive lesions. Ahsan et al. (19) performed 22 stent grafts with an initial success rate of 95.2% with one technical failure. Primary patency at 24 months was $84.2\% \pm 8\%$ and limb salvage rate of $95.3\% \pm 5\%$. Maynar et al. (20) reported their experience with five cases of occlusive aortoiliac disease treated with bifurcated stent graft, but no reliable data are available to support the use of covered stent grafts at the present time.

CURRENT RESULTS FOR AORTIC BIFURCATION DISEASE

Angioplasty With or Without Stenting

Double-balloon PTA of localized stenotic and occlusive disease at the aortic bifurcation is an effective procedure. The potential of contralateral embolism or contralateral iliac artery occlusion due to dislodgement of atherosclerotic or thrombotic material during unilateral PTA has led to kissing balloon technique where simultaneous angioplasty of the common iliac arteries is performed.

Insall et al. (21) studied 79 patients who underwent kissing balloon angioplasty for aortoiliac atherosclerotic lesions of the aortic bifurcation. The procedure was technically successful in 94% of patients. However, there were significant procedure-related complications requiring surgical intervention (5%).

Kissing Stents for Aortic Bifurcation Disease

Despite the use of kissing balloon PTA, treatment of the aortic bifurcation has been reported to be associated with significant risks of dissection, thrombosis, and residual stenosis (3,22). For this purpose, the primary kissing stent technique has been advocated, which involves simultaneous deployment of stents to reconstruct the aortic bifurcation and avoid compromise of the contralateral common iliac artery.

The potential of stents to improve the results of angioplasty at the aortic bifurcation has not been systematically analyzed. Stent implantation at the ostia appears to be theoretically beneficial as the ostia are prone to severe atherosclerotic changes with extensive calcification (Fig. 2).

Scheinert et al. (23) primarily stented the aortic bifurcation in 48 patients with 85% clinical patency rate after 24 months and angiographic patency of 86% after 24 months. In this series laser was used to debulk the obstructive segment before placement of the stent. Predilatation with a kissing balloon technique was also used in 16 patients. Balloon-mounted stents were used and positioned such that they extended 3 to 5 mm into the distal aorta. Mohamad et al. (24) also showed primary assisted patency of 84% at two years and complication rate of 4%. Picquet et al. (25) reported recently good results in 20 patients, with primary and secondary patency rates at 12 and 36 months as 94.7%, 84.4% and 100%, 89%, respectively.

In contrast to these good results, Greiner et al. (26) reported a two-year patency of only 65% and Murphy et al. demonstrated a 82% secondary patency rate at two years, which is inferior to the two-year patency rates of 92% to 94% reported for surgical bypass. Similarly, Brittenden et al. (22) and Haulon et al. (27) also reported poor long-term patency rates.

Suboptimal patency rates obtained from kissing stents in bilateral iliac lesions is considered to result from thrombus formation in the dead space, between the stents and the rest of the aortic lumen, neointimal hyperplasia and disturbance of blood flow in the distal aorta (28–31).

PTA vs. Primary Stenting for Bifurcation Disease

PTA has become one of the favoured treatment options in patients with iliac bifurcation disease. Stents have been recommended to reduce the procedural complications (acute dissection and residual stenosis) and improve long-term patency. Many series also advocate routine stent placement in an attempt to prevent recurrent disease with a view to preventing immediate recoil and obstructive plaque dissection. However, there is a tendency for the development of intrastent hyperplasia, which may result in recurrent stenosis.

Although the Dutch randomized study (30) (primary stenting vs. selective stenting) showed that selective iliac stenting was as effective as primary stenting, most of the patients

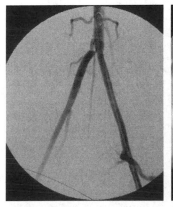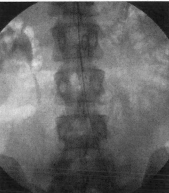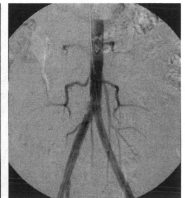

FIGURE 2 Aortic bifurcation disease treated with iliac stents.

included did not have disease affecting the aortic bifurcation. In the literature, the complication rates of iliac stenting are between 4% and 19% whereas rates with PTA vary between 3% and 8% (31).

There are no published randomized controlled trials between primary angioplasty and primary stenting. In meta-analysis of 2116 patients (1300 PTA and 816 stents), there was a statistically significant difference in the primary technical success rate between PTA and stenting, 96% and 100%, respectively. The primary and secondary patency rates were higher following stenting when compared with PTA (77% and 88% vs. 64% and 80%) (32).

COMPLICATIONS

Complications include aortic rupture, dissection, pseudoaneurysm and distal embolization. Many authors feel that aorta is at higher risk of rupture than the smaller arteries due to the Laplace's law [Wall stress = (Pressure × Radius)/(2 × Wall thickness)]. Surprisingly the reported incidence of aortic rupture is extremely low (4,9,33). Berger et al. (33) reviewed 606 cases of aortic PTA and found only one case of rupture. Some authors also believe that calcification is related to rupture and proper selection of patients should avoid this problem. Because of the low compliance of the large diameter balloons, inflation pressure should be < 4 atm in order to limit the risk of aortic rupture. The management of aortic rupture is either endovascular stent graft or urgent surgery. In case of aortic rupture, low-pressure inflation of the balloon can be used to control hemorrhage while definitive treatment is instituted.

Aortic dissection is an anticipated complication in aortic PTA. Significant aortic dissection is rarely reported in the literature (14). The clinical relevance is considered minor except in cases of major dissection or in cases where pseudoaneurysm develops on follow-up. The management of dissection is conservative or stenting if the dissection is flow limiting.

Distal embolization can be a limb-threatening condition. The reported incidence of distal embolization ranges between 2% and 4% (6,9). Significant emboli do not usually migrate beyond the level of the femoral arteries and treatment of this complication is usually successful with immediate thrombectomy or thrombolysis.

REFERENCES

1. De Vries JPPM, Van Den Heuvel DAF, Vos JA, et al. Freedom from secondary interventions to treat stenotic disease after percutaneous transluminal angioplasty of infrarenal aorta: long term results. J Vasc Surg 2004; 39:427–31.
2. Crawford ES, Bomberger RA, Glaeser DH, et al. Aortoiliac occlusive disease: factors influencing survival and function following reconstructive operation over a twenty-five-year period. Surgery 1981; 90(6):1055–67.
3. Tegtmeyer CJ, Hartwell GD, Selby JB, et al. Results and complications of angioplasty in aortoiliac disease. Circulation 1991; 83(2):153–60.
4. Sheeran SR, Hallisey MJ, Ferguson D. Percutaneous transluminal stent placement in the abdominal aorta. J Vasc Interv Radiol 1997; 8(1 Pt 1):55–60.
5. Morag B, Garniek A, Bass A, et al. Percutaneous transluminal aortic angioplasty: early and late results. Cardiovasc Intervent Radiol 1993; 16(1):37–42.
6. Ravimandalam K, Rao VR, Kumar S, et al. Obstruction of the infrarenal portion of the abdominal aorta: results of treatment with balloon angioplasty. AJR Am J Roentgenol 1991; 156(6):1257–60.
7. Hedeman Joosten PP, Ho GH, Breuking FA, Jr., et al. Percutaneous transluminal angioplasty of the infrarenal aorta: initial outcome and long-term clinical and angiographic results. Eur J Vasc Endovasc Surg 1996; 12(2):201–6.
8. Long AL, Gaux JC, Raynaud AC, et al. Infrarenal aortic stents: initial clinical experience and angiographic follow-up. Cardiovasc Intervent Radiol 1993; 16(4):203–8.
9. D'Othee BJ, Haulon S, Mounier-Vehier C, et al. Percutaneous endovascular treatment for stenoses and occlusions of infrarenal aorta and aortoiliac bifurcation: midterm results. Eur J Vasc Endovasc Surg 2002; 24(6):516–23.
10. Audet P, Therasse E, Oliva VL, et al. Infrarenal aortic stenosis: long-term clinical and hemodynamic results of percutaneous transluminal angioplasty. Radiology 1998; 209(2):357–63.
11. Charlebois N, Saint-Georges G, Hudon G. Percutaneous transluminal angioplasty of the lower abdominal aorta. AJR Am J Roentgenol 1986; 146(2):369–71.

12. Ingrisch H, Stiegler H, Rath M. Non-operative treatment of infrarenal aortic stenoses by catheter dilation. Rontgenpraxis 1983; 36(11):363–7.
13. Pentecost MJ, Criqui MH, Dorros G, et al. Guidelines for peripheral percutaneous transluminal angioplasty of the abdominal aorta and lower extremity vessels. Circulation 1994; 89:511–31.
14. Yilmaz S, Sindel T, Yegin A, et al. Primary stenting of focal atherosclerotic infrarenal aortic stenoses: long-term results in 13 patients and a literature review. Cardiovasc Intervent Radiol 2004; 27(2):121–8.
15. Grollman JH, Jr., Del Vicario M, Mittal AK. Percutaneous transluminal abdominal aortic angioplasty. AJR 1980; 134:1053–4.
16. Feugier P, Toursarkissian B, Chevalier JM, et al. Endovascular treatment of isolated atherosclerotic stenosis of the infrarenal abdominal aorta: long term outcome. Ann Vasc Surg 2003; 17(4):375–85.
17. Nyman U, Uher P, Lindh M, et al. Primary stenting in infrarenal aortic occlusive disease. Cardiovasc Intervent Radiol 2000; 23:97–108.
18. Vallabhaneni SR, Bjorses K, Malina M, et al. Endovascular management of isolated infrarenal aortic occlusive disease is safe and effective in selected patients. Eur J Vasc Endovasc Surg 2005; 30(3):307–10.
19. Ali AT, Modrall G, Lopez J, et al. Emerging role of endovascular grafs in complex aortoiliac disease. J Vasc Surg 2003; 38:486–91.
20. Maynar M, Baro M, Qian Z, et al. Endovascular repair of brachial artery transection associated with trauma. J Trauma 2004; 56(6):1336–41.
21. Insall RL, Loose HW, Chamberlain J. Long-term results of double-balloon percutaneous transluminal angioplasty of the aorta and iliac arteries. Eur J Vasc Surg 1993; 7(1):31–6.
22. Brittenden J, Beattie G, Bradbury AW. Outcome of iliac kissing stents. Eur J Vasc Endovasc Surg 2001; 22(5):466–8.
23. Scheinert D, Schroder M, Balzer JO, et al. Stent supported reconstruction of the aortoiliac bifurcation with the kissing balloon technique. Circulation 1999; 100:295–300.
24. Mohamad F, Sarkar B, Timmons G, et al. Outcome of kissing stent for aortoiliac atherosclerotic disease, including the effect on the non-diseased contralateral iliac limb. Cardiovasc Intervent Radiol 2002; 25:472–5.
25. Picquet J, Blin V, Bouye P, et al. Endovascular treatment for obstructive disease of the aortoiliac bifurcation by the kissing stent technique. J Mal Vasc 2005; 30(3):163–70.
26. Greiner A, Dessl A, Klein-Weigel P, et al. Kissing stents for treatment of complex aortoiliac disease. Eur J Vasc Endovasc Surg 2003; 26(2):161–5.
27. Haulon S, Mounier-Vehier C, Gaxotte V, et al. Percutaneous reconstruction of aorto iliac bifurcation with the kissing stents technique: long- term follow-up in 106 patients. J Endovasc Ther 2002; 9:363–8.
28. Saker MB, Oppat WF, Kent SA, et al. Early failure of aortoiliac kissing stents: histopathologic correlation. J Vasc Interv Radiol 2000; 11(3):333–6.
29. Reyes R, Maynar M, Lopera J, et al. Treatment of chronic iliac artery occlusions with guide wire recanalization and primary stent placement. J Vasc Interv Radiol 1997; 8(6):1049–55.
30. Klein WM, Graaf YVD, Seegers J, et al. Long-term cardiovascular morbidity, mortality, and reintervention after endovascular treatment in patients with Iliac artery disease: the Dutch iliac Stent Trial Study. Radiology 2004; 232:491–8.
31. Kudo T, Chandra FA, Ahn SS. Long-term outcomes and predictors of iliac angioplasty with selective shunting. J Vasc Surg 2005; 42:466–75.
32. Bosch JL, Hunink MG. Meta-analysis of the results of percutaneous transluminal angioplasty and stent placement for aortoiliac disease. Radiology 1997; 204(1):87–96.
33. Berger T, Sorensen R, Konrad J. Aortic rupture: a complication of transluminal angioplasty. AJR Am J Roentgenol 1986; 146(2):373–4.

2 | Iliac Occlusive Disease (Indications for Treatment, Technical Aspects, Current Results, and Troubleshooting Complications)

P. A. Gaines
Sheffield Vascular Institute, Northern General Hospital, Sheffield, U.K.

INTRODUCTION

Occlusive iliac disease is due to atherosclerosis in the vast majority of cases and is a common distribution of that pathology. Occasionally the lesion is restenotic (myointimal hyperplasia following previous intervention or trauma) and very rarely it may be due to pelvic irradiation, fibromuscular dysplasia, or follow exuberant protracted cycling. These rarities will not be discussed further here.

Iliac atherosclerosis may be asymptomatic, or cause acute ischemia, intermittent claudication, critical limb ischemia (CLI) or blue toe syndrome. Intermittent claudication is typically associated with iliac disease alone (single-level disease) whereas CLI is due to multilevel disease. Blue toe syndrome results from cholesterol crystals or microemboli of thrombus/atheroma embolizing into the foot vessels from proximal ulcerating disease.

This chapter will discuss technique and complications, progress through the data to support practice, and finish with proposed treatment strategies.

TECHNIQUE

Iliac Stenoses

With prior imaging available it is usually a simple matter to plan the endovascular management of an iliac stenosis:

1. An ipsilateral puncture of the common femoral artery (CFA) is required. This may be difficult by palpation because the pulse is likely to be weak or absent. Puncture of the superficial femoral artery (SFA) makes compression difficult resulting in a higher frequency of post-procedural hematomas and false aneurysm formation. Unfortunately the skin crease is not a useful guide as to the position of the CFA bifurcation. If a closure device is to complete the procedure, inadvertent placement into the SFA or profunda femoris artery has a significant risk of occlusion, and placement into a diseased CFA results in failure of hemostasis. In addition, if the lesion to be treated is low external iliac artery then the puncture needs to be well away from the treatment site. For all these reasons it is my practice to use ultrasound to guide arterial access for all interventional procedures.
2. Once access has been achieved a 6-F sheath is placed in the CFA. Whilst a 5-F sheath may accommodate modern balloon catheters required for iliac angioplasty it is not possible in this situation to inject contrast when a 5-F catheter is in the sheath and it will not easily accommodate most stent systems. Heparin 3500 IU is given immediately after arterial access and sheath placement has been achieved.
3. The iliac stenosis should now be imaged by retrograde injection of contrast and then crossed, preferably under road map conditions, with a guidewire. Whilst it is tempting to use a hydrophilic wire from the start (e.g., a Terumo) these wires can be difficult to control, easily dissect vessels in inexperienced hands, and become sticky and difficult to use when

allowed to dry. Most lesions can be crossed with a combination of conventional guidewire and curved catheter (e.g., cobra). If this fails then a hydrophilic wire should be used but replaced by a conventional wire once the lesion is crossed.

4. Whilst it would make sense to measure the diameter of the iliac artery before choosing an appropriate-sized balloon, most experienced interventionalists tends to eye the patient and angiogram and choose appropriately. In males the common iliac artery is approximately 7 to 9 mm and the external 6 to 7 mm in diameter. Vessels in women are approximately 1 mm smaller. The balloon is inflated for one minute, deflated and removed. The inflation pressure is entirely arbitrary. It makes no sense to keep inflating once the wasting has gone, nor to stop inflating if there is residual wasting of the balloon. Although it is sensible to stop before reaching the maximum recommended inflation pressure of the balloon, if the balloon were to burst the manufacturing ensures that the balloons tear longitudinally (in the majority of cases) and are therefore not too difficult to remove.

5. The "end point" at which to cease further intervention is debatable. Some would be happy with a residual stenosis diameter of less than 50%, others choose 30%. This end point is very subjective and non-reproducible. Other interventionists choose to measure residual pressure gradient and finish when there is less than either a 10 mmHg peak systolic or mean gradient. A very basic principle of any intervention is that the guidewire should not be pulled back across the treated lesion until the end point has been reached. This is because, should it be necessary to proceed with further intervention, it can be very difficult to recross the treated segment because of disruption and dissection of the arterial wall. So that a gradient can be measured using a pullback catheter, the standard 0.035-in. wire should be replaced by a fine-wire (e.g., 0.018 in.) that does not damp the pressure transmission within the catheter but does provide the option of safely recrossing the lesion with the catheter. The pull-back gradient is thought to be useful when deciding when to selectively place a stent but it is unclear as to whether a high-grade residual stenosis predicts outcome.

6. If a stent is to be placed then this is positioned over a 0.035-in. guidewire. It is conventional to re-dilate a self-expanding stent to the desired size. Balloon expandable stents are used for common iliac artery ostial lesions that require extra radial force and very precise placement so that they do not overhang the contralateral iliac artery (see chap. 1). Self-expanding stents are preferred elsewhere because of their ability to conform to the natural curve of the iliac artery.

7. Patients should be warned that they may experience pain during balloon inflation. This is particularly so when treating iliac occlusions. Pain should signify to the interventionist that the adventitia is being stretched and it is unwise to proceed further for fear of vessel rupture. If pain persists, or even worse intensifies following balloon deflation then angiography should be urgently undertaken to exclude arterial rupture.

8. When the chosen end point has been achieved it is probably good practice to document runoff to confirm that there has been no distal embolization before wires and catheters are removed. Pressure hemostasis is applied for five minutes or a closure device is placed. Day-case intervention can be safely undertaken (1,2) without reversal of anticoagulation at the end of the procedure.

Iliac Occlusions

It is normal practice to treat iliac occlusions with primary stent placement and there are some important variations to the basic technique:

1. For several reasons all interventions should begin with bilateral femoral artery sheath placement. Firstly this ensures that a catheter can be placed in the aorta that allows visualization of the proximal extent of the occlusion at all times to ensure correct stent placement. Secondly, approximately 40% of lesions will require to be crossed with a wire-loop (3) (through-and-through wire). Finally an aortic catheter facilitates both completion angiography and simultaneous pressure assessment between aorta and ipsilateral CFA.

2. 5000 IU of heparin are given as soon as arterial sheath placement is achieved. This is slightly more heparin than used for a stenosis because the procedure is likely to be more protracted and a potentially thrombogenic metallic foreign body will be placed in the arterial lumen (4).
3. The occlusion should initially be approached from the ipsilateral side using a combination of catheter with conventional or hydrophilic wire. This is successful in approximately 60% of cases.
4. If the ipsilateral approach fails then the lesion should be crossed from the contralateral side with a hydrophilic wire and either sidewinder catheter [common iliac artery (CIA) occlusion] or cobra catheter [external iliac artery (EIA) occlusion] with the intention of breaking back into the passage that the initial ipsilateral manipulation created (Fig. 1). There seems little sense in trying to place a stent from the contralateral side, therefore the wire is brought out through the ipsilateral sheath either by steering the wire into the sheath or grasping it with a snare from the ipsilateral groin (3).
5. Predilatation prior to stent placement should be avoided since this increases the risk of distal embolization (5). The majority of lesions should be managed by primary placement of a self-expanding stent and post-dilating to the required size.
6. Stent infection is rare (6) and therefore antibiotics are not routinely prescribed.

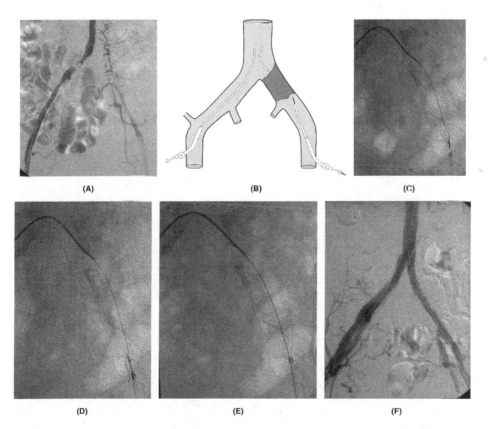

FIGURE 1 (**A**) Angiography shows bilateral common iliac occlusions (TransAtlantic Inter-Society Consensus C pattern). Bilateral 6-F sheaths are in place and heparin 5000 IU given. The right occlusion has been crossed from the ipsilateral side with a guidewire but the left occlusion could not be crossed from the left side. (**B**) The left common iliac occlusion is now crossed from above using a sidewinder catheter. (**C**) The hydrophilic guidewire has crossed the occlusion and a snare from the left side is open waiting to grasp the wire. (**D**) The guidewire has been caught and the snare is closed. (**E**) The wire has been pulled through the left sheath. From this position the guidewire can now be buckled up into the aorta and stents placed from the ipsilateral sides. (**F**) Final appearances after bilateral iliac stents have been placed.

COMPLICATIONS

Aorto-iliac intervention is a commonly performed endovascular procedure and yet the data to indicate the prevalence of complications are few. The problem is compounded by a lack in uniformity of the definition of a complication of endovascular intervention. Perhaps the best contemporary data comes from the second British Society of Interventional Radiology Second (BIAS) report (1) which prospectively looked at outcomes in 2152 patients from 46 hospitals in the U.K. That report detailed an overall peri-procedural complication rate of 5.7%. Complications were more likely to occur in patients with CLI compared to claudication (18% vs. 2.5%), but interestingly there was no significant difference between those patients treated with angioplasty or stents. In addition, there was a low rate (0%) of complications in patients treated as a day case, again reflecting good patient selection and an undoubted bias towards claudicants rather than patients with CLI.

The meta-analysis of aorto-iliac intervention performed by Bosch et al. (7) detailed a systemic complication rate of 1%, a local (access and treatment site and embolization) complication rate of 9%, a complication rate requiring intervention of 5.2%, and a mortality rate of 0.3%.

The Dutch iliac stent trial (8) had prospective assessment and recorded an overall complication rate of 5.7% in a group of patients who were predominantly claudicants.

Peri-procedural complications can be assessed as occurring (*i*) at the access site, (*ii*) at the treatment site, and (*iii*) systemic, away from the treated area.

Access Site Complications

Hematoma and False Aneurysms
The incidence of hematoma formation varies approximately between 2% and 6% and risk includes site of puncture, blood pressure, size of devices used, and anticoagulation status of the patient. In recent years, collagen plug devices and percutaneous suture-mediated arteriotomy closure devices have been developed to reduce time to hemostasis and ambulation, resulting in increased patient comfort and potentially earlier discharge from hospital. A meta-analysis (9) demonstrated that complications and success rates are not significantly different between mechanical compression and closure devices. In addition infrequent but significant complications such as arterial thrombosis, infection, dissection, and pseudoaneurysm have been described with use of percutaneous closure devices (see chap. 49).

The incidence of iatrogenic pseudoaneurysm of the femoral artery about 1% to 6% (10), is more common following interventional than diagnostic procedures (11), and the risk of increases with adjunctive usage of thrombolytic drugs, anticoagulation, obesity, compression time, and sheath size. Spontaneous thrombosis is related to size and is very unusual in lesions greater than 6 mL (2 cm in diameter) in size (12). Ultrasound-guided compression has a reported 100% technical success rate for aneurysms less than 2 cm or smaller in diameter and 67% for those 4 to 6 cm in diameter (13). However, compression is time-consuming and painful for both the patient and radiologist. Percutaneous ultrasound-guided injection of thrombin is now widely accepted as the treatment of choice with obliteration of the sac within seconds (14) (see chap. 48). A multicenter registry study reported 96% initial technical success rate after a single injection and negligible recurrence rates (15). Although the overall complication rate is low (0–4%) the risk of distal embolization can be as high as 2% and therefore the peripheral pulses should be checked before and after the procedure. Other rarer complications include anaphylaxis and infection.

Arteriovenous Fistula
This is an extremely rare complication with an estimated incidence of 0.1% to 0.2% (16). Most are asymptomatic and rarely require any intervention.

Access Vessel Thrombosis
Acute occlusion of the femoral artery may be due to extension of a treatment site thrombosis, failure to recognize access site dissection, access into a diseased femoral artery, or

a complication of the closure device. Any intervention will be dependent upon the degree of ischemia.

Target Site Complications

Acute Closure
The frequency of occlusion at the treatment site varies between 1% and 7% and is usually due to dissection. Acute thrombosis follows a primary mechanism that limits flow, and spasm sufficient to close a diseased iliac artery must be extremely rare. The patient should be sufficiently anticoagulated to limit thrombus formation and the dissection should be managed with a stent.

Rupture
Iliac artery rupture following endovascular interventions is uncommon but life threatening. The BIAS II dataset recorded rupture in 0.6% of procedures but limited entirely to patients receiving a stent (1.2%) (1). This is undoubtedly because stents are associated with the management of complex disease, in particular occlusions. Rupture is more common when treating the external rather than the common iliac artery because of the loose adventitial support and is possibly more common in patients taking steroids (17). Rupture is usually an acute event characterized by pain that persists after deflation of the balloon, associated with hypotension. The pulse rate normally increases but occasionally the clinical picture may mimic a vagal episode with initial bradycardia. It is commonly noted that the retroperitoneal blood displaces the contrast-filled bladder to the contralateral side and this can be clearly witnessed on fluoroscopy.

The diagnosis can be confirmed by angiography followed by resuscitation (Fig. 2) which should include: (*i*) rapid blood volume replacement, (*ii*) tamponade of the rupture by gently inflating a balloon across or proximal to the tear, (*iii*) reversal of anticoagulation, and (*iv*) analgesia. A stent graft is then placed across the tear (18,19).

Stent Infection
This is a very rare complication of simple stents placed in the iliac vessels (6).

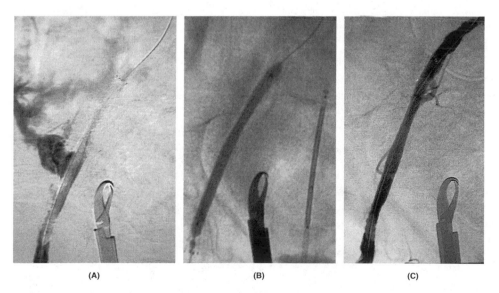

(A)   (B)   (C)

FIGURE 2 **(A)** An external iliac occlusion (TransAtlantic Inter-Society Consensus C) has been treated with a stent. The patient complained of pain and became hypotensive. **(B)** The rupture has been temporarily managed by balloon tamponade. **(C)** Definitive treatment with a stent graft.

Distal Complications

Embolization

Distal embolization following peripheral angioplasty occurs in approximately 1% to 5% of procedures and is more frequent when there is attempted revasularization of fully occluded segments (20). In BIAS II distal embolization complicated 0.4% of angioplasty and 1% of stent procedures (1). The nature of intervention will depend upon the site of the embolus and local expertise. A common femoral embolus is best removed surgically. We would treat more distal embolization by percutaneous aspiration thromboembolectomy which has a 90% success rate (21). Alternatively, surgical embolectomy or thrombolysis may be needed.

Cholesterol Embolization

Prolonged catheter manipulation in a diseased aorta can cause cholesterol plaques to gain entry to the peripheral or visceral circulation. This complication is associated with a mortality rate of about 80% with poorly described and inadequate treatment options (22). Its development is heralded by leg pain with livedo reticularis despite palpable pulses. Outcome is poor despite any active intervention often resulting in confusion, renal failure, and death (23).

OUTCOMES

Clinical Outcomes

The limb salvage rate for CLI is highly dependent on a number of factors including distribution of disease, severity of ischemia, and runoff. Unsurprisingly therefore the outcomes of intervention are usually reported as patency rates, as described below, rather than clinical improvement.

The change in quality of life after iliac intervention for claudication has been reported following the Dutch Iliac Stent Trial (24). All measures showed a significant and durable improvement following intervention, persisting to last follow-up at two years. Similar results had previously been demonstrated by other studies (25–27).

Upon the premise that the distribution and morphology of the iliac disease may affect outcomes the TransAtlantic Inter-Society Consensus (TASC) document (28) developed the type A–D classification. Currently there is little literature that separates the outcomes according to that classification but this will be highlighted where appropriate.

Patency

Stenoses

Iliac artery stenoses are included as part of TASC A and B lesions. In general they are treated by simple balloon angioplasty with a primary success rate which exceeds 90% for all reported series, and long-term patencies of 75% to 95% at one year, 60% to 90% at three years, and 60% to 80% at five years (28–32). The use of stents for iliac stenoses has continued despite the lack of data to support this activity. In general, stents are used when the lesion is thought to be at high risk from primary failure and embolization (e.g., eccentric stenosis) or when angioplasty fails (usually defined as residual stenosis of greater than 50%, a residual pressure gradient or an extensive dissection). Large series of stents, used mainly for iliac stenoses, have shown a primary technical success 95% to 100% and long-term patencies of 78% to 95% at one year, 53% to 81% at three years, and 54% to 72% at five years (33–35). These results appear to be similar to angioplasty alone but the studies are all non-randomized. The long-awaited randomized trial by Richter has yet to be published although abstracts have appeared (36). In this study, stenoses were randomized between angioplasty and stent placement with a significantly improved primary success rate in the stent group and a better five-year angiographic patency (64.6% vs. 93.6%). Similarly, the five-year clinical success rates rose from 69.7% to 92.7% in the stent group. The Dutch Iliac Stent Trial Group have published a randomized trial of primary stent placement versus selective stent placement in patients with iliac artery occlusive disease (8). In this study, 279 patients with intermittent claudication (including only 12 iliac occlusions) were randomized to either primary stent placement or stent placement after angioplasty if there was a residual mean gradient of greater than 10 mm or mercury. They found no difference in the two strategies at short- and long-term follow-up but the policy of selective stent placement was cheaper. However, the trial was based on the premise that a residual gradient following angioplasty predicts poor outcome, something for which there is no good scientific base. A meta-analysis of the results of angioplasty and stent placement for aorta iliac occlusive disease (7) concluded that compared to angioplasty, stents have:

- An improved technical success rate
- A similar complication rate
- A 39% reduction in the risk of long-term failure

In the majority of units, because of the generally good outcome of stenoses treated by simple balloon angioplasty and the extra cost of stents, most lesions are managed by angioplasty with stents being reserved for a poor result or complication following percutaneous transluminal angioplasty (PTA). In addition, considering that there is 25% to 47% recoil following simple angioplasty (37), I think it reasonable to consider stent placement when a maximal hemodynamic result is required instantly (e.g., when iliac intervention is immediately combined with a distal graft).

Occlusions
Chronic iliac occlusions are generally managed by primary stent placement (Fig. 3). The primary success rate for treating occlusions with stents is now 92% to 97% with two- and five-year primary patency rates of as 75% to 87% and 75% to 65% respectively (38–40). Until recently there was no good data to compare the outcomes of angioplasty and stenting, and what there was indicated that the outcomes were very similar (41–43). Why then treat occlusions primarily by stent placement? The advantage was suggested by the Gupta paper which documented a peripheral embolization rate of 8% when managing occlusions with angioplasty alone. A U.K. trial (the stents versus angioplasty (STAG) trial), as yet unpublished, randomized 114 patients with an iliac occlusion to angioplasty or primary stent placement.

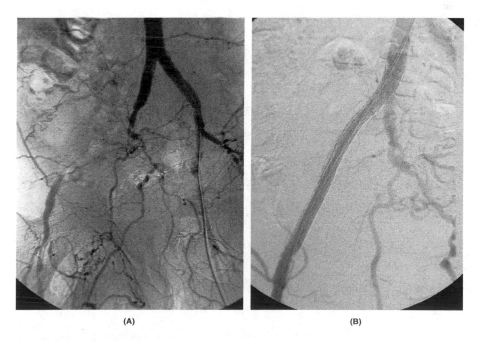

(A) (B)

FIGURE 3 **(A)** Chronic external iliac artery occlusion. **(B)** Excellent morphological result following stent placement with no residual pressure gradient.

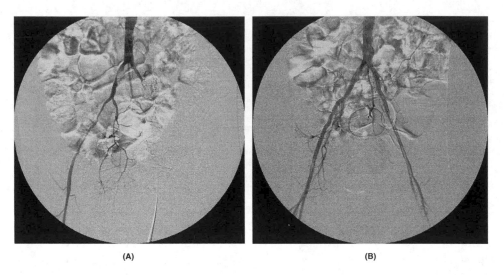

(A)   (B)

FIGURE 4   (**A**) Right common and external iliac artery stenoses and full length left common and external iliac artery occlusions. As is common with extensive iliac disease, the left common femoral artery, although patent, was not demonstrated on angiography. (**B**) Excellent morphological appearance following bilateral iliac stent placement.

There was no difference in patency at two years but there was a significantly higher complication rate following angioplasty, particularly distal embolization.

Complex Disease

Increasing confidence combined with the ready availability of excellent vascular stents and a willingness to combine endovascular therapy with conventional open surgery has led to these techniques being used to manage extensive complex iliac disease (Figs. 4 and 5). The results indicate one-, three- and five-year patencies of 61% to 85%, 43% to 76%, and 64% (44–46).

PREDICTING THE OUTCOME OF ENDOVASCULAR INTERVENTION

The factors adversely affecting long-term patency of iliac intervention have been variably reported to be occlusions, poor runoff, female sex, hormone replacement therapy, external iliac disease, critical ischemia, and elevated cholesterol (38,45,47–53). My own experience concurs

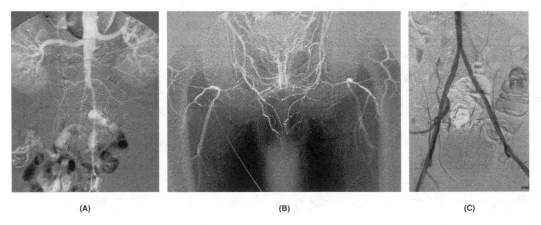

(A)   (B)   (C)

FIGURE 5   (**A**) The aorta is occluded below the inferior mesenteric artery. (**B**) Both common and external iliac arteries are occluded. Once again the common femoral arteries were not visualized on angiography but were shown to be patent on ultrasound. (**C**) The distal aorta and both iliac systems have been reconstructed with stents.

with those (48,52,53) who feel that external iliac disease in women, probably because of the small size of vessel, adversely affects outcome.

INTERVENTIONAL STRATEGY

Although conventional surgery is more durable than endovascular intervention in iliac disease it is associated with a significant burden of mortality and morbidity as well as a reduction in quality of life in the post-operative period (37). For many clinicians, endovascular intervention is now the treatment of choice for occlusive iliac disease. There remains debate as to the use of angioplasty or stents to manage iliac disease. With the available data it appears reasonable to treat simple stenoses using angioplasty and reserve stents for angioplasty failure (residual stenosis or gradient, and flow limiting dissection) and occlusions.

Claudication

All patients with peripheral vascular disease have their risk factors modified to prevent death from myocardial infarction and stroke, and limit new disease formation. It is well recognized that a significant number of patients with claudication improve with time without active intervention. It is sensible therefore to limit intervention to stable claudicants.

When intermittent claudication is due to iliac disease alone then the results from intervention are often dramatic and durable as described earlier. Since (*i*) exercise therapy may not be durable, and in patients with iliac disease may not be as effective as in patients with infrainguinal and (*ii*) endovascular intervention is associated with low-level risk, endovascular intervention is often recommended as first-line therapy after risk factor modification. When claudication is due to two-level arterial disease (e.g., iliac and SFA disease) then the results are often less dramatic and the patients should be advised as such.

Critical Limb Ischemia

Iliac disease is common in this fragile group of patients for whom endovascular intervention is an attractive option. The disease distribution is frequently complex for which we now have demonstrable good outcomes (44,46,51), but the treatment strategies often requires imagination. For example, bilateral iliac disease and ipsilateral common femoral disease can be treated at the same sitting by common femoral endarterectomy (with more distal grafting if required) combined with either an ipsilateral or contralateral recannalisation plus extra-anatomic femoro-femoral bypass. Careful planning of resource and skills is required. Whilst angioplasty is still preferred as the first option for simple stenoses, primary stent placement for complex stenoses as well as occlusions may be reasonable since it is important to optimize flow as soon as possible, particularly if this is being used to support a distal graft.

Blue Toe Syndrome

Patients with blue toe syndrome require increased perfusion to the foot and treatment to the source of emboli. It is our practice to (*i*) prescribe maximum antiplatelet therapy and (*ii*) convert the fragile stenosis to a smooth wide lumen using PTA or stent placement.

REFERENCES

1. Gaines P, Moss JG, Kinsman R. The British Society of Interventional Radiology Second BIAS Report. Henley-on-Thames, Oxfordshire: Dendrite Clinical Systems Ltd, 2005.
2. Macdonald S, Thomas SM, Cleveland TJ, Gaines PA. Outpatient vascular intervention: a two-year experience. Cardiovasc Intervent Radiol 2002; 25(5):403–12.
3. Gaines PA, Cumberland DC. Wire-loop technique for angioplasty of total iliac artery occlusions. Radiology 1988; 168(1):275–6.
4. Zaman SM, de Vroos Meiring P, Gandhi MR, Gaines PA. The pharmacokinetics and U.K. usage of heparin in vascular intervention. Clin Radiol 1996; 51(2):113–6.
5. Dyet JF, Gaines PA, Nicholson AA, et al. Treatment of chronic iliac artery occlusions by means of percutaneous endovascular stent placement. J Vasc Interv Radiol 1997; 8(3):349–53.

6. Chalmers N, Eadington DW, Gandanhamo D, Gillespie IN, Ruckley CV. Case report: infected false aneurysm at the site of an iliac stent. Br J Radiol 1993; 66(790):946–8.
7. Bosch JL, Hunink MG. Meta-analysis of the results of percutaneous transluminal angioplasty and stent placement for aortoiliac occlusive disease. Radiology 1997; 204(1):87–96.
8. Tetteroo E, van der Graaf Y, Bosch JL, et al. Randomised comparison of primary stent placement versus primary angioplasty followed by selective stent placement in patients with iliac-artery occlusive disease. Dutch Iliac Stent Trial Study Group. Lancet 1998; 351(9110):1153–9.
9. Nikolsky E, Mehran R, Halkin A, et al. Vascular complications associated with arteriotomy closure devices in patients undergoing percutaneous coronary procedures: a meta-analysis. J Am Coll Cardiol 2004; 44(6):1200–9.
10. Kresowik TF, Khoury MD, Miller BV, et al. A prospective study of the incidence and natural history of femoral vascular complications after percutaneous transluminal coronary angioplasty. J Vasc Surg 1991; 13(2):328–33 (discussion 333–5).
11. Katzenschlager R, Ugurluoglu A, Ahmadi A, et al. Incidence of pseudoaneurysm after diagnostic and therapeutic angiography. Radiology 1995; 195(2):463–6.
12. Kent KC, McArdle CR, Kennedy B, Baim DS, Anninos E, Skillman JJ. A prospective study of the clinical outcome of femoral pseudoaneurysms and arteriovenous fistulas induced by arterial puncture. J Vasc Surg 1993; 17(1):125–31 (discussion 131–3).
13. Fellmeth BD, Roberts AC, Bookstein JJ, et al. Postangiographic femoral artery injuries: nonsurgical repair with U.S.-guided compression. Radiology 1991; 178(3):671–5.
14. Brophy DP, Sheiman RG, Amatulle P, Akbari CM. Iatrogenic femoral pseudoaneurysms: thrombin injection after failed U.S.-guided compression. Radiology 2000; 214(1):278–82.
15. Mohler ER, III, Mitchell ME, Carpenter JP, et al. Therapeutic thrombin injection of pseudoaneurysms: a multicenter experience. Vasc Med 2001; 6(4):241–4.
16. Muller DW, Shamir KJ, Ellis SG, Topol EJ. Peripheral vascular complications after conventional and complex percutaneous coronary interventional procedures. Am J Cardiol 1992; 69(1):63–8.
17. Lois JF, Takiff H, Schechter MS, Gomes AS, Machleder HI. Vessel rupture by balloon catheters complicating chronic steroid therapy. AJR Am J Roentgenol 1985; 144(5):1073–4.
18. Allaire E, Melliere D, Poussier B, Kobeiter H, Desranges P, Becquemin J. Iliac artery rupture during balloon dilatation: what treatment? Ann Vasc Surg 2003; 17(3):306–14.
19. Formichi M, Raybaud G, Benichou H, Ciosi G. Rupture of the external iliac artery during balloon angioplasty: endovascular treatment using a covered stent. J Endovasc Surg 1998; 5(1):37–41.
20. Belli AM, Cumberland DC, Knox AM, Procter AE, Welsh CL. The complication rate of percutaneous peripheral balloon angioplasty. Clin Radiol 1990; 41(6):380–3.
21. Cleveland TJ, Cumberland DC, Gaines PA. Percutaneous aspiration thromboembolectomy to manage the embolic complications of angioplasty and as an adjunct to thrombolysis. Clin Radiol 1994; 49(8):549–52.
22. Hawthorn IE, Rochester J, Gaines PA, Morris-Jones W. Severe lower limb ischaemia with pulses: cholesterol embolisation—a little known complication of aortic surgery. Eur J Vasc Surg 1993; 7(4):470–4.
23. Gaines PA, Cumberland DC, Kennedy A, Welsh CL, Moorhead P, Rutley MS. Cholesterol embolisation: a lethal complication of vascular catheterisation. Lancet 1988; 1(8578):168–70.
24. Bosch JL, van der Graaf Y, Hunink MG. Health-related quality of life after angioplasty and stent placement in patients with iliac artery occlusive disease: results of a randomized controlled clinical trial. The Dutch Iliac Stent Trial Study Group. Circulation 1999; 99(24):3155–60.
25. Whyman M, Fowkes F, Kerracher E, et al. Randomised controlled trial of percutaneous transluminal angioplasty for claudication. Eur J Vasc Endovasc Surg 1996; 12:167–72.
26. Cook T, O'Regan M, Galland R. Quality of life following percutaneous angioplasty for claudication. Eur J Vasc Endovasc Surg 1996; 11:191–4.
27. Currie I, Wilson Y, Bairdd R, Lamont P. Treatment of intermittent claudication: the impact on quality of life. Eur J Vasc Endovasc Surg 1995; 10:356–61.
28. TASC Working Group. Management of peripheral arterial disease. TransAtlantic Inter-Society Consensus. Eur J Vasc Endovasc Surg 2000; 19(Suppl. A):S144–243.
29. Jeans W, Armstrong S, Cole S, Horrocks M, Baird RN. Fate of patients undergoing transluminal angioplasty for lower limb ischaemia. Radiology 1990; 177:559–64.
30. Tegtmeyer C, Hartwell C, Selby J, Robertson R, Kron I, Tribbloe C. Results and complications of angioplasty in aortoiliac disease. Circulation 1991; 83(2):207–18.
31. Johnston K. Iliac arteries: reanalysis of results of balloon angioplasty. Radiology 1993; 186:382–6.
32. Jorgensen K, Skovgaard N, Norgard J, Holstein P. Percutaneous transluminal angioplasty in 226 iliac aretry stenoses: role of superficial femoral artery for clinical success. Vasa 1992; 21:382–6.
33. Murphy KD, Encarnacion CE, Le VA, Palmaz JC. Iliac artery stent placement with the Palmaz stent: follow-up study. J Vasc Interv Radiol 1995; 6(3):321–9.
34. Martin EC, Katzen BT, Benenati JF, et al. Multicenter trial of the wallstent in the iliac and femoral arteries. J Vasc Interv Radiol 1995; 6(6):843–9.

35. Murphy TP, Webb MS, Lambiase RE, et al. Percutaneous revascularization of complex iliac artery stenoses and occlusions with use of Wallstents: three-year experience. J Vasc Interv Radiol 1996; 7(1):21–7.
36. Richter G, Roeren T, Brado M. Further udate on the randomised trial. Iliac stent placement versus PTA—morphology, clinical success rates, and failure analysis. J Vasc Interv Radiol 1993; 4:30–1 (Absract).
37. Brewster D. Current controversies in the management of aorto-iliac occlusive disease. J Vasc Surg 1997; 25:365–79.
38. Funovics MA, Lackner B, Cejna M, et al. Predictors of long-term results after treatment of iliac artery obliteration by transluminal angioplasty and stent deployment. Cardiovasc Intervent Radiol 2002; 25(5):397–402.
39. Carnevale FC, De Blas M, Merino S, Egana JM, Caldas JG. Percutaneous endovascular treatment of chronic iliac artery occlusion. Cardiovasc Intervent Radiol 2004; 27(5):447–52.
40. Reyes R, Maynar M, Lopera J, et al. Treatment of chronic iliac artery occlusions with guide wire recanalization and primary stent placement. J Vasc Interv Radiol 1997; 8(6):1049–55.
41. Colapinto R, Stronell R, Johnston W. Transluminal angioplasty of complete iliac obstructions. AJR Am J Roentgenol 1986; 146:859–62.
42. Leu AJ, Schneider E, Canova CR, Hoffmann U. Long-term results after recanalisation of chronic iliac artery occlusions by combined catheter therapy without stent placement. Eur J Vasc Endovasc Surg 1999; 18(6):499–505.
43. Gupta AK, Ravimandalam K, Rao VR, et al. Total occlusion of iliac arteries: results of balloon angioplasty. Cardiovasc Intervent Radiol 1993; 16(3):165–77.
44. Leville C, Kashyap V, Clair D, et al. Endovascular management of iliac artery occlusions: extending treatment to TransAtlantic Inter-Society Consensus class C and D patients. J Vasc Surg 2006; 43:32–9.
45. Powell RJ, Fillinger M, Walsh DB, Zwolak R, Cronenwett JL. Predicting outcome of angioplasty and selective stenting of multisegment iliac artery occlusive disease. J Vasc Surg 2000; 32(3):564–9.
46. Timaran CH, Prault TL, Stevens SL, Freeman MB, Goldman MH. Iliac artery stenting versus surgical reconstruction for TASC (TransAtlantic Inter-Society Consensus) type B and type C iliac lesions. J Vasc Surg 2003; 38(2):272–8.
47. Timaran CH, Ohki T, Gargiulo NJ, III, et al. Iliac artery stenting in patients with poor distal runoff: influence of concomitant infrainguinal arterial reconstruction. J Vasc Surg 2003; 38(3):479–84 (discussion 484–5).
48. Timaran CH, Stevens SL, Freeman MB, Goldman MH. External iliac and common iliac artery angioplasty and stenting in men and women. J Vasc Surg 2001; 34(3):440–6.
49. Timaran CH, Stevens SL, Grandas OH, Freeman MB, Goldman MH. Influence of hormone replacement therapy on the outcome of iliac angioplasty and stenting. J Vasc Surg 2001; 33(Suppl. 2):S85–92.
50. Ballard JL, Bergan JJ, Singh P, Yonemoto H, Killeen JD. Aortoiliac stent deployment versus surgical reconstruction: analysis of outcome and cost. J Vasc Surg 1998; 28(1):94–101 (discussion 101–3).
51. Powell RJ, Fillinger M, Bettmann M, et al. The durability of endovascular treatment of multisegment iliac occlusive disease. J Vasc Surg 2000; 31(6):1178–84.
52. Murphy TP, Ariaratnam NS, Carney WI, Jr., et al. Aortoiliac insufficiency: long-term experience with stent placement for treatment. Radiology 2004; 231(1):243–9.
53. Sullivan TM, Childs MB, Bacharach JM, Gray BH, Piedmonte MR. Percutaneous transluminal angioplasty and primary stenting of the iliac arteries in 288 patients. J Vasc Surg 1997; 25(5):829–38 (discussion 838–9).

3 | Femoropopliteal Occlusive Disease (Indications for Treatment, Technical Aspects, Current Results, and Troubleshooting Complications)

Hannu Manninen
Department of Clinical Radiology, Kuopio University Hospital and Kuopio University, Kuopio, Finland

CHRONIC LIMB ISCHEMIA: FEMOROPOPLITEAL OCCLUSIVE DISEASE

This chapter focuses on the role of percutaneous transluminal angioplasty (PTA) in the treatment of femoropopliteal disease, and includes a discussion on the use of stents and stent-grafts. The use of laser (1,2) and catheter-directed atherectomy (3,4) are discussed elsewhere.

Indications for Endovascular Treatment

Claudication

The management of most claudicants is conservative. According to recently published ACC/AHH practice guidelines, endovascular procedures are indicated for individuals with a vocational or lifestyle-limiting disability due to intermittent claudication, when clinical features suggest a reasonable likelihood of symptomatic improvement from endovascular intervention. Furthermore, there should be evidence of an inadequate response to exercise or pharmaceutical therapy and/or a very favorable risk–benefit ratio (5). Usually, intervention is only indicated after an unsuccessful trial of at least six months in an exercise program. In the TransAtlantic Inter-Society Consensus (TASC) recommendations of 2000, occlusive femoropopliteal disease is divided into four classes (A–D; Table 1). These definitions are currently under revision regarding lesion length. Endovascular procedures are suggested to be the treatment of choice for type A and B lesions, and surgery for type D lesions. For type C lesions the treatment decision between surgical and endovascular therapy should be performed on an individual basis after considering the risks, benefits, durability and therapeutic goals.

Critical Limb Ischemia

To avoid amputation in patients with critical limb ischemia (CLI), revascularization should be considered unless life expectancy is very limited, tissue necrosis or flexion contracture limit the likelihood of independent ambulation, or the patient's general medical condition is poor (5). Endovascular treatment, with lower complication rates than surgery, should often be considered as the first-line option. Multiple, patient- and lesion-related factors should be considered when deciding between endovascular and open surgical treatment options. Furthermore, local variations may exist due to the availability of advanced endovascular intervention and/or surgical facilities. While TASC recommendations for morphologic stratification of lesions can be considered as a basis for therapy selection in CLI, advanced age and associated comorbidity must also be considered, and would tend to favor endovascular therapy in type C, and often in type D lesions.

Technical Aspects of Femoropopliteal Interventions

The basic techniques of femoropopliteal angioplasty rely on antegrade puncture of the common femoral artery. On occasions, especially in obese patients, contralateral access with flexible 45 to 90 cm long introducers is a useful option (Fig. 1). This technique is associated with a lower rate

TABLE 1 Morphologic Stratification of Femoropopliteal Lesions

TASC type A femoropopliteal lesions
  1. Single stenosis or occlusion <3 cm (<10 cm, not involving trifurcation)

TASC type B femoropopliteal lesions
  2. Single stenosis or occlusion 3 to 10 cm in length, not involving the distal popliteal artery (10–15 cm)
  3. Heavily calcified stenoses up to 3 cm in length
  4. Multiple lesions, each less than 3 cm (stenoses or occlusions) (<5 cm)
  5. Single or multiple lesions in the absence of continuous tibial runoff to improve inflow for distal surgical bypass

TASC type C femoropopliteal lesions
  6. Single stenosis or occlusion longer than 5 cm (>15 cm)
  7. Multiple stenoses or occlusions, each 3–5 cm, with or without heavy calcification (heavily calcified common femoral artery stenoses, heavily calcified stenoses or occlusions >15 cm)

TASC type D femoropopliteal lesions
  8. Complete common femoral artery or superficial femoral artery occlusions or complete popliteal and proximal trifurcation occlusions

Abbreviation: TASC, TransAtlantic Inter-Society Consensus.

of puncture site complications, facilitates effective treatment of proximal femoral lesions, and can be used for stent placement (6). Traversing of lesions is usually performed using a hydrophilic guide wire with the aid of a rigid angled, torsion resistant, diagnostic catheter.

For proximal superficial femoral artery (SFA) disease or after failure to antegradely traverse an occlusion, popliteal access is a useful alternative. For this technique, the patient is positioned prone and the popliteal artery is punctured under ultrasound guidance, carefully avoiding venous puncture which could predispose to arteriovenous fistula (AV fistula) creation. In one study of angioplasty for femoropopliteal disease, 24% (28/117) of interventions were performed via the popliteal artery approach, one-third of which were preceded by unsuccessful antegrade puncture (7). Some authors now favor the popliteal approach for subintimal recanalization of femoral artery occlusions (8).

Residual stenoses, elastic recoil or flow-limiting dissection can present a major problem after balloon angioplasty. For long diseased segments where stent placement is not preferable, prolonged balloon inflation up to 10 to 15 minutes may effectively improve the angiographic result (9), although this technique does not improve long-term patency (10).

Recanalization of Occlusions
Intraluminal or Subintimal Recanalization
The basic technique for recanalization of a chronic occlusion is to navigate a hydrophilic 0.035-inch guide wire with the aid of torsion resistant, slightly angled (multipurpose type) diagnostic catheter through the occlusion while trying to remain within the vessel lumen. Often, in long occlusions, the recanalization route is partly subintimal. While this may be unintentional,

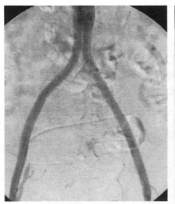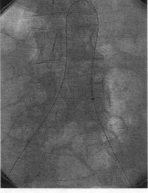

FIGURE 1 Contralateral approach: a 6 French, 45 cm long introducer sheath is advanced from right femoral artery puncture into the left limb of the Y-prosthesis to facilitate left femoropopliteal artery intervention.

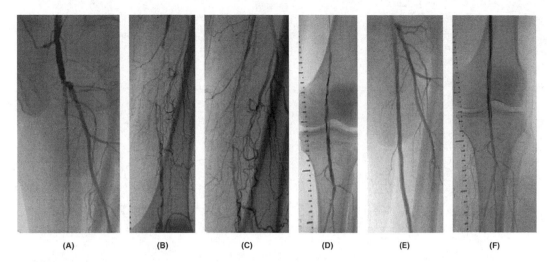

(A) (B) (C) (D) (E) (F)

FIGURE 2 (**A,B**) Subintimal recanalization of a chronic occlusion. Diffusely diseased left femoral artery with a 6 cm long total occlusion. (**C**) From a contralateral approach a hydrophilic guide wire was advanced as a loop at the subintimal space over the occlusion. (**D**) Because of difficulty re-entering the vascular lumen the subintimal recanalization channel continues to the popliteal artery (**E,F**) and in order to obtain adequate hemodynamical result a segment of about 30 cm in length has to be covered with self-expanding nitinol stents.

the technique of subintimal angioplasty relies on intentionally traversing the occlusion in the subintimal channel to exit downstream in the natural lumen (Fig. 2). Subintimally, the lesion is traversed after manipulation of the guide wire as a loop pushed with the aid of the catheter to the distal end of the occlusion and back into the true lumen. Access back into the lumen can be performed by active navigation of the angled tip of the guide wire or simply by pushing the guide wire loop until it enters the lumen. The most common reason for failure is inability to re-enter the vessel lumen distal to the occlusion. Special catheters have recently been introduced to facilitate successful re-entry (11,12), but the clinical experience of these devices is still very limited. Some authors have used subintimal arterial flossing with antegrade–retrograde intervention in cases of difficult luminal re-entry (13). The main drawback of subintimal recanalization is that important collaterals or run-off vessels may sometimes be compromised. In case of inadequate angiographic patency adjunctive stent placement has been found useful (8).

There is no firm evidence supporting thrombolysis during recanalization of femoropopliteal occlusions (14). However, thrombus removal by thrombectomy catheters may be useful as an adjunctive technique for treatment of acute, and some subacute, occlusions (Fig. 3) (15).

Current Results

Percutaneous Transluminal Angioplasty
Complications
After infrainguinal PTA, the reported rate of all complications is approximately 10%, with major complication rates of between 2.2% and 6.4% (10,16,17). Complications are more often encountered during recanalization of total occlusions than stenoses (16). The complication rate of stent placement following angioplasty is similar to PTA alone. Most problems are puncture site-related complications (hematoma, pseudoaneurysm or AV-fistula), peripheral embolization, thrombosis, and renal failure. Distal embolization following subintimal recanalization has been reported in 6.0% to 7.3% of cases (18,19), and after 3% following intraluminal recanalization (7). Thromboembolic complications are effectively treated by local fibrinolysis or manual percutaneous aspiration. Regarding puncture site complications, these are less frequent after contralateral puncture. Closure devices should be used with caution following antegrade puncture. Most pseudoaneurysms can be effectively treated percutaneously by

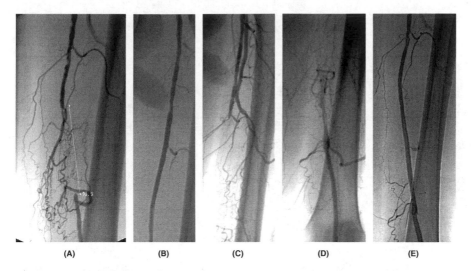

(A)   (B)   (C)   (D)   (E)

FIGURE 3   Long-term failure of femoral artery stent-graft. (**A**) A 9 cm long chronic occlusion was treated with a 15 cm long polytetrafluoroethylene-covered stent-graft. (**B**) Note the dissection proximal to the stent-graft due to balloon angioplasty. (**C,D**) Four months later the vascular segment occluded. (**E**) After thrombus removal with a Rotarex device and additional stent placement proximal to the stent-graft, the angiographic result is exact.

ultrasound-guided thrombin injection (20). Non-procedure related complications are rarely reported but are predominantly cardiopulmonary in nature (21).

Primary Success
The technical success rate of femoropopliteal PTA is high, ranging in the literature from 84% to 91% (Table 2) (7,22,26,30,32). The technical and hemodynamic success has been shown to be higher for stenoses than occlusions (86–100% and 74–85% respectively). Other predictors of poor primary success include the length of the lesion and calcification (26). These results are predominantly for intraluminal recanalization techniques. There are no direct comparative studies between intraluminal and subintimal recanalization of chronic occlusions but the reported technical success rates for the subintimal technique range from 86% to 100%

TABLE 2   Primary Results of Femoropopliteal Percutaneous Transluminal Angioplasty

Reference	Patients/limbs (*n*)	Mean lesion length (range)	Total occlusion (%)	Primary success[a]
Krepel (22)	129/164	NA	23	138/164 = 84%
Murray (23)	162/193	NA	40	157/193 = 81%
Capek (24)	152/217	0–2 cm, 45%	32	93%[b]
		2–5 cm, 29%		82%[c]
		>5 cm, 26%		
Johnston (25)	236/254	NA	NA	89%, 1 month
Matsi (26)	106/140	8.0 cm (1–31)	49	125/40 = 89%
Vroegindeweij (27)	62/62	4.7 cm (0.5–15)	100	51/62 = 82%
Murray (28)	42/44	24.3 cm (10–40)	159	41/44 = 93%
Stanley (29)	176/200	NA	41	146/200 = 73%
Golledge (30)	74/74	1 cm (0.1–10)	26	67/74 = 91%
Karch (31)	85/112 (lesions)	<2 cm, 72%[b]	7	Six technical failures
		2–5 cm, 20%[b]		
		5–10 cm, 8%[b]		
Soder (10)	97/112	7.2 cm	34	82/112 = 73% (no technical failures)
Jamsen (17)	173/218	8.8 cm	55	182/18 = 83.5%

Variable criteria in: [a] individual publications, [b] stenosis, and [c] occlusion respectively
Abbreviation: NA, not available.

TABLE 3 Long-Term Outcome of Femoropopliteal Percutaneous Transluminal Angioplasty

Reference	Year	Study type	Claudication (%)	Limbs	Cumulative primary patency ($\pm$SE%)				Mean lesion length (cm)
					3 Years	4 Years	5 Years	6 Years	
Gallino (36)	1984	R S	61	280	–	–	58	–	ND
Johnston (25)	1992	P S	80	254	51	44	38	36	ND
Hunink (21)	1993	P S	58	131	–	–	45	–	Mainly <5
Matsi (26)	1994	P S	100	140	42	–	–	–	5.1
Stanley (29)	1996	R S	74	200	38	30	26	–	ND
Martin (37)	1999	R S	74	88	57	44	37	29	Mainly <3
Karch (31)	2000	R S	59	112	57	52	–	–	2.3
Clark (38)	2001	P M	61	219	69	–	55	–	4
Löfberg (39)	2001	R S	0	121	27	–	27	–	ND
Soder (10)	2002	P S	96	112	39	–	25	–	7.2
Jamsen (17)	2002	P S	100	173	31	27		23*	8.8

Abbreviations: M, multicenter; ND, not detectable; P, prospective; R, retrospective; S, single center; SE, standard error.

(8,18,19,33–35). Comparison between studies is difficult because variable criteria for technical success are used.

Long-Term Results

The reported long-term patency rates of infrainguinal PTA are variable. At one, three and six years, primary patency rates range from 47% to 86%, 27% to 69%, and 23% to 36% respectively (Table 3). In one prospective, single center study of 218 claudicants who underwent femoropopliteal PTA, the primary patency at 10 years was only 14% and reinterventions were required in one-third of limbs, including surgical revascularization in 35 cases (17). On the other hand, only 14 (6.4%) limbs developed CLI, resulting in a 0.8% incidence per year; that implies significant long-term benefits of treatment.

There are no comparative studies between the long-term results of intraluminal and subintimal recanalization for the treatment of chronic occlusions, though the subintimal technique seems to have a similar reocclusion rate. Primary patency rates of 22% to 62% at one year have been reported in recent studies (Table 4).

There are few comparative studies to compare patency rates of femoropopliteal PTA and bypass surgery. Meta-analysis of observational cohort studies showed a pooled one-year primary patency of PTA for 85% (83–86%), and 95% (94–97%) for vein bypass surgery (40). In a randomized, controlled multicenter trial with only 54 patients, an absolute risk reduction for reocclusion of 31% was identified in favor of bypass surgery at one year (41).

Predictors of Patency

Lesion- and Procedure-Related Factors. Although the primary technical success rate is better for stenotic lesions, many studies show no difference in long-term patency between stenoses and occlusions (22,24,26,32,38). In one study, stenoses had a better long-term outcome than occlusions (25) and a meta-analysis of 19 claudication studies revealed combined three-year patency rates of 61% and 48% for stenoses and occlusions respectively (42).

Lesion length has been observed by many authors to be an important determinant of long-term patency (24,26,28,32,38). Shorter lesions (<2 and 2–5 cm) fare better than lesions

TABLE 4 Primary Success and Long-Term Results of Subintimal Percutaneous Transluminal Angioplasty of Femoropopliteal Artery in Recent Publications

Reference	Limbs	Occlusion length (cm)	Technical success (%)	Primary patency (%)		
				1 Year	2 Years	3 Years
Yilmaz (8)	67	20 (average)	88	22		
Laxdal (18)	124	NA	90	37		
Lipsitz (33)	39	8 (median)	87	64	51	
Florenes (19)	116	16	87	62		57
Desgranges (34)	100	12	88		61	

greater than 10 cm (24). Results from the SCVIR transluminal angioplasty and revascularization (STAR) registry demonstrated that lesions longer than 10 cm have a 2.8-fold relative risk of occlusion compared to lesions less than 10 cm (38).

Poor peripheral runoff is also associated with poorer long-term results. Long-term patency rates of 30% in limbs with poor runoff, versus 52% with good runoff, were reported by Johnston et al. (25), and this was identified as the strongest determinant for lower long-term patency rates in the STAR registry (38).

Other features which improve long-term results include concentric morphology, regular stenosis surface, absence of residual stenosis after angioplasty and single angioplasty site (22,24,26,38).

Patient-Related Factors. The influence of diabetes in outcome is controversial with some studies suggesting poorer long-term patency (24,32,38). However, other reports have identified no statistically significant differences in long-term results between diabetics or non-diabetics if lesion-related parameters are taken into account (25,43). The deleterious effect of renal failure has been clearly identified in a univariate analysis (38).

The clinical presentation is also a predictive factor, claudicants demonstrating better long-term patency than those with critical ischemia (25,29,44,45). In a meta-analysis, the combined three-year patency rates for patients with critical ischemia were worse than claudication for both stenoses (43% vs. 61%) and occlusions (30% and 48%) (42).

Clinical Results of Femoropopliteal PTA vs. Conservative Treatment in Claudicant Patients
There are only a few small randomized trials comparing PTA and conservative treatment of claudication, and no trials of PTA versus surgery (chap. 9). In one study 66 claudicants were randomized to PTA plus medical treatment (daily aspirin, stop smoking and exercise) or medical treatment only. At six months follow-up, significantly more patients in the PTA group reported no claudication and were asymptomatic on a treadmill exercise test compared to the control group. The ankle brachial pressure index was significantly higher and patients reported a lower pain score in the PTA group (46). However, after two years follow-up, the groups had comparable clinical outcomes (47). Another trial (48) demonstrated a greater improvement in claudication and maximal walking distance at up to six years follow-up from exercise training than from PTA, especially in patients with disease confined to the SFA.

Effect of Femoropopliteal PTA on Quality of Life in Claudicant Patients
In a prospective observational study 39 claudicant patients with unilateral femoral lesions undergoing PTA showed some short-term quality of life (QoL) benefit but, 12 months later, QoL scores failed to meet those of an age-matched population (49). A recent review identified seven prospective trials investigating the effect of PTA on QoL in claudication (49). The authors concluded that PTA may result in some QoL improvement, although level I evidence to support this is lacking.

Clinical Results of Femoropopliteal PTA in Chronic Critical Ischemia
Limb salvage rates following femoropopliteal PTA in CLI vary from 75% to over 90% (39,50,51), favoring the role of endovascular therapy over surgery. In the U.K. multicenter Bypass versus Angioplasty in Severe Ischaemia of the Leg trial, 452 patients with CLI and infrainguinal diseases were randomized to surgery ($n=228$) or angioplasty ($n=224$, 80% localized to SFA and 62% distal vessel PTA) (52). At six months, there was no difference in amputation-free survival or health-related QoL, but for the first year the hospital costs associated with surgery were one-third higher.

Patency of Femoropopliteal Stents
For femoropopliteal disease, highly variable one-year primary patency rates have been reported for stents, ranging from 22% to 81% (53–57). In three randomized studies, though the primary success rate following stent placement was higher than after balloon angioplasty alone, long-term patency was similar (58–60), confirmed by a meta-analysis (42). From the largest randomized trial of 154 patients, it was concluded that stents should be reserved for

rescue of PTA failures (59). However, Schllinger recently reported a randomized trial of 104 patients and demonstrated that patients undergoing placement of nitinol stents had lower rates of restenosis and better exercise capacity than those treated with PTA alone (61).

Currently, there is a tendency to favor self-expanding nitinol stents for infrainguinal angioplasty. A three-year primary patency rate of 76% has been demonstrated after primary stenting of relatively short (<6 cm) lesions (62). However, mid-term restenosis after long-segment femoropopliteal stenting remains a problem. In a recent single-center observational study in which long segments (median length 16 cm) were covered by nitinol stents after initial PTA failure, the primary patency was only 54% at one year. Results were particularly poor in diabetic patients (22% at one-year patency) (63). There are some data suggesting that intermediate-term results of nitinol stents are better than self-expanding steel stents (64).

Drug eluting stents have shown great promise in coronary artery interventions. The sirolimus-eluting self-expanding nitinol shape memory alloy recoverable technology stent was compared in a small (57 patients) randomized, double-blind multicenter study with a bare-metal stent (Sirolimus-coated Cordis Self-expandable Stent II trial) for femoral lesions (average length 8 cm) (65). No significant differences were identified between the groups.

Long-term stress predisposes to stent fractures in up to 50% of nitinol stents one year after placement (66) and in 19% of Wallstents 43 months after placement (67).

Patency of Stent-Grafts
The clinical experience of stent-grafts in atherosclerotic femoral artery disease is still very limited. In early studies a high incidence of complications were identified, associated with intense perivascular inflammation and early thrombosis. Restenosis at the uncovered ends of the endograft seems to be a particular problem (Fig. 3) (68,69). The short- and mid-term term results of Dacron-covered stent-grafts have been disappointing, with up to 17% reocclusion during the first 24 hours and only 23% primary patency at 12 months (70). However, more promising results have been published with use of polytetrafluoroethylene-covered stent-grafts. Two prospective, single-center, observational studies reported 58% to 78% primary patency at 12 months (71,72). There are also some prospective multicenter evaluations with limited number of patients. In a prospective multicenter trial of 80 limbs (mean lesion length 13 cm) a 79% primary patency at 12 months was identified (73). The cordis covered nitinol stent (COVENT) trialists recently reported an 89% primary patency rate at 12 months for short SFA (mean 5 cm) lesions (74). In a small prospective, randomized trial of 28 patients, stent-grafts resulted in better primary patency at 12 months than PTA (87% vs. 25% respectively, $p=0.02$) (75).

Current Role of Various Endovascular Techniques in Femoropopliteal Interventions of Chronic Ischemia

There are limited data available to support routine use of techniques other than PTA and stent placement for femoropopliteal disease. There is consensus that balloon angioplasty is the first-line treatment with other techniques reserved for PTA failure. Residual diameter stenosis greater than 30% is usually considered as an indication for stent placement, though a meta-analysis has suggested that primary stenting might be better for total occlusions in CLI (42). In extensive disease, the long-term patency of stents is poor and prolonged balloon inflation is an alternative to obtain hemodynamically acceptable primary results. The subintimal technique seems to be preferable for long lesions in CLI, particularly in unfit patients at high risk from bypass surgery.

REFERENCES

1. Belli AM, Cumberland DC, Procter AE, et al. Follow-up of conventional angioplasty versus laser thermal angioplasty for total femoropopliteal artery occlusions: results of a randomized trial. J Vasc Interv Radiol 1991; 2(4):458–85.
2. Fisher CM, Fletcher JP, May J, et al. No additional benefit from laser in balloon angioplasty of the superficial femoral artery. Eur J Vasc Endovasc Surg 1996; 11(3):349–52.

3. Nakamura S, Conroy RM, Gordon IL, et al. A randomized trial of transcutaneous extraction atherectomy in femoral arteries: intravascular ultrasound observations. J Clin Ultrasound 1995; 23(8):461–71.

4. Vroegindeweij D, Tielbeek AV, Buth J, et al. Directional atherectomy versus balloon angioplasty in segmental femoropopliteal artery disease: two-year follow-up with color-flow duplex scanning. J Vasc Surg 1995; 21(2):255–68 (discussion 268–269).

5. Hirsch AT, Haskal ZJ, Hertzer NR, et al. ACC/AHA 2005 Practice Guidelines for the management of patients with peripheral arterial disease (lower extremity, renal, mesenteric, and abdominal aortic). Circulation 2006; 113(11):e463–654.

6. Kashdan BJ, Trost DW, Jagust MB, et al. Retrograde approach for contralateral iliac and infrainguinal percutaneous transluminal angioplasty: experience in 100 patients. J Vasc Interv Radiol 1992; 3(3):515–21.

7. Matsi PJ, Manninen HI, Soder HK, et al. Percutaneous transluminal angioplasty in femoral artery occlusions: primary and long-term results in 107 claudicant patients using femoral and popliteal catheterization techniques. Clin Radiol 1995; 50(4):2344–72.

8. Yilmaz S, Sindel T, Yegin A, et al. Subintimal angioplasty of long superficial femoral artery occlusions. J Vasc Interv Radiol 2003; 14(8):997–1010.

9. Manninen HI, Soder HK, Matsi PJ, et al. Prolonged dilation improves an unsatisfactory primary result of femoropopliteal artery angioplasty: usefulness of a perfusion balloon catheter. J Vasc Interv Radiol 1997; 8(4):627–32.

10. Soder HK, Manninen HI, Rasanen HT, et al. Failure of prolonged dilation to improve long-term patency of femoropopliteal artery angioplasty: results of a prospective trial. J Vasc Interv Radiol 2002; 13(4):361–9.

11. Hausegger KA, Georgieva B, Portugaller H, et al. The outback catheter: a new device for true lumen re-entry after dissection during recanalization of arterial occlusions. Cardiovasc Intervent Radiol 2004; 27(1):26–30.

12. Saketkhoo RR, Razavi MK, Padidar A, et al. Percutaneous bypass: subintimal recanalization of peripheral occlusive disease with IVUS guided luminal re-entry. Tech Vasc Interv Radiol 2004; 7(1):23–7.

13. Spinosa DJ, Harthun NL, Bissonette EA, et al. Subintimal arterial flossing with antegrade-retrograde intervention (SAFARI) for subintimal recanalization to treat chronic critical limb ischemia. J Vasc Interv Radiol 2005; 16(1):37–44.

14. Nicholson T. Percutaneous transluminal angioplasty and enclosed thrombolysis versus percutaneous transluminal angioplasty in the treatment of femoropopliteal occlusions: results of a prospective randomized trial. Cardiovasc Intervent Radiol 1998; 21(6):470–4.

15. Duc SR, Schoch E, Pfyffer M, et al. Recanalization of acute and subacute femoropopliteal artery occlusions with the rotarex catheter: one year follow-up, single center experience. Cardiovasc Intervent Radiol 2005; 28(5):603–10.

16. Matsi PJ, Manninen HI. Complications of lower-limb percutaneous transluminal angioplasty: a prospective analysis of 410 procedures on 295 consecutive patients. Cardiovasc Intervent Radiol 1998; 21(5):361–6.

17. Jamsen TS, Manninen HI, Jaakkola PA, et al. Long-term outcome of patients with claudication after balloon angioplasty of the femoropopliteal arteries. Radiology 2002; 225(2):345–52.

18. Laxdal E, Jenssen GL, Pedersen G, et al. Subintimal angioplasty as a treatment of femoropopliteal artery occlusions. Eur J Vasc Endovasc Surg 2003; 25(6):578–82.

19. Florenes T, Bay D, Sandbaek G, et al. Subintimal angioplasty in the treatment of patients with intermittent claudication: long term results. Eur J Vasc Endovasc Surg 2004; 28(6):645–50.

20. Tisi P, Callam M. Surgery versus non-surgical treatment for femoral pseudoaneurysms. Cochrane Database Syst Rev 2006;(1):CD004981.

21. Hunink MG, Donaldson MC, Meyerovitz MF, et al. Risks and benefits of femoropopliteal percutaneous balloon angioplasty. J Vasc Surg 1993; 17(1):183–92 (discussion 192–194).

22. Krepel VM, van Andel GJ, van Erp WF, et al. Percutaneous transluminal angioplasty of the femoropopliteal artery: initial and long-term results. Radiology 1985; 156(2):325–8.

23. Murray RR, Jr., Hewes RC, White RI, Jr., et al. Long-segment femoropopliteal stenoses: is angioplasty a boon or a bust? Radiology 1987; 162(2):473–6.

24. Capek P, McLean GK, Berkowitz HD. Femoropopliteal angioplasty. Factors influencing long-term success. Circulation 1991; 83(2 Suppl.):I70–80.

25. Johnston KW. Femoral and popliteal arteries: reanalysis of results of balloon angioplasty. Radiology 1992; 183(3):767–71.

26. Matsi PJ, Manninen HI, Vanninen RL, et al. Femoropopliteal angioplasty in patients with claudication: primary and secondary patency in 140 limbs with 1–3-year follow-up. Radiology 1994; 191(3):727–33.

27. Vroegindeweij D, Tielbeek AV, Buth J, et al. Recanalization of femoropopliteal occlusive lesions: a comparison of long-term clinical, color duplex US, and arteriographic follow-up. J Vasc Interv Radiol 1995; 6(3):331–7.

28. Murray JG, Apthorp LA, Wilkins RA. Long-segment (> or =10 cm) femoropopliteal angioplasty: improved technical success and long-term patency. Radiology 1995; 195(1):1562–81.
29. Stanley B, Teague B, Raptis S, et al. Efficacy of balloon angioplasty of the superficial femoral artery and popliteal artery in the relief of leg ischemia. J Vasc Surg 1996; 23(4):679–85.
30. Golledge J, Ferguson K, Ellis M, et al. Outcome of femoropopliteal angioplasty. Ann Surg 1999; 229(1):146–53.
31. Karch LA, Mattos MA, Henretta JP, et al. Clinical failure after percutaneous transluminal angioplasty of the superficial femoral and popliteal arteries. J Vasc Surg 2000; 31(5):880–7.
32. Hewes RC, White RI, Jr., Murray RR, et al. Long-term results of superficial femoral artery angioplasty. AJR Am J Roentgenol 1986; 146(5):1025–9.
33. Lipsitz EC, Ohki T, Veith FJ, et al. Does subintimal angioplasty have a role in the treatment of severe lower extremity ischemia? J Vasc Surg 2003; 37(2):386–91.
34. Desgranges P, Boufi M, Lapeyre M, et al. Subintimal angioplasty: feasible and durable. Eur J Vasc Endovasc Surg 2004; 28(2):138–41.
35. Hynes N, Akhtar Y, Manning B, et al. Subintimal angioplasty as a primary modality in the management of critical limb ischemia: comparison to bypass grafting for aortoiliac and femoropopliteal occlusive disease. J Endovasc Ther 2004; 11(4):460–71.
36. Gallino A, Mahler F, Probst P, et al. Percutaneous transluminal angioplasty of the arteries of the lower limbs: a 5 year follow-up. Circulation 1984; 70(4):619–23.
37. Martin DR, Katz SG, Kohl RD, et al. Percutaneous transluminal angioplasty of infrainguinal vessels. Ann Vasc Surg 1999; 13(2):184–7.
38. Clark TW, Groffsky JL, Soulen MC. Predictors of long-term patency after femoropopliteal angioplasty: results from the star registry. J Vasc Interv Radiol 2001; 12(8):923–33.
39. Lofberg AM, Karacagil S, Ljungman C, et al. Percutaneous transluminal angioplasty of the femoropopliteal arteries in limbs with chronic critical lower limb ischemia. J Vasc Surg 2001; 34(1):114–21.
40. Hunink MG, Wong JB, Donaldson MC, et al. Patency results of percutaneous and surgical revascularization for femoropopliteal arterial disease. Med Decis Making 1994; 14(1):71–81.
41. van der Zaag ES, Legemate DA, Prins MH, et al. Angioplasty or bypass for superficial femoral artery disease? A randomised controlled trial. Eur J Vasc Endovasc Surg 2004; 28(2):132–7.
42. Muradin GS, Bosch JL, Stijnen T, et al. Balloon dilation and stent implantation for treatment of femoropopliteal arterial disease: meta-analysis. Radiology 2001; 221(1):137–45.
43. Stokes KR, Strunk HM, Campbell DR, et al. Five-year results of iliac and femoropopliteal angioplasty in diabetic patients. Radiology 1990; 174(3 Pt 2):977–82.
44. Adar R, Critchfield GC, Eddy DM. A confidence profile analysis of the results of femoropopliteal percutaneous transluminal angioplasty in the treatment of lower-extremity ischemia. J Vasc Surg 1989; 10(1):57–67.
45. Trocciola SM, Chaer R, Dayal R, et al. Comparison of results in endovascular interventions for infrainguinal lesions: claudication versus critical limb ischemia. Am Surg 2005; 71(6).474–9 (discussion 479–480).
46. Whyman MR, Fowkes FG, Kerracher EM, et al. Randomised controlled trial of percutaneous transluminal angioplasty for intermittent claudication. Eur J Vasc Endovasc Surg 1996; 12(2):167–72.
47. Whyman MR, Fowkes FG, Kerracher EM, et al. Is intermittent claudication improved by percutaneous transluminal angioplasty? A randomized controlled trial. J Vasc Surg 1997; 26(4):551–7.
48. Perkins JM, Collin J, Creasy TS, et al. Exercise training versus angioplasty for stable claudication. Long and medium term results of a prospective, randomised trial. Eur J Vasc Endovasc Surg 1996; 11(4):409–13.
49. Chetter IC, Spark JI, Kent PJ, et al. Percutaneous transluminal angioplasty for intermittent claudication: evidence on which to base the medicine. Eur J Vasc Endovasc Surg 1998; 16(6):477–84.
50. Kudo T, Chandra FA, Ahn SS. The effectiveness of percutaneous transluminal angioplasty for the treatment of critical limb ischemia: a 10-year experience. J Vasc Surg 2005; 41(3):423–35 (discussion 435).
51. Black JH, III, LaMuraglia GM, Kwolek CJ, et al. Contemporary results of angioplasty-based infrainguinal percutaneous interventions. J Vasc Surg 2005; 42(5):932–9.
52. Adam DJ, Beard JD, Cleveland T, et al. Bypass versus angioplasty in severe ischaemia of the leg (BASIL): multicentre, randomised controlled trial. Lancet 2005; 366(9501):1925–34.
53. Do dai D, Triller J, Walpoth BH, et al. A comparison study of self-expandable stents vs. balloon angioplasty alone in femoropopliteal artery occlusions. Cardiovasc Intervent Radiol 1992; 15(5):306–12.
54. Sapoval MR, Long AL, Raynaud AC, et al. Femoropopliteal stent placement: long-term results. Radiology 1992; 184(3):833–9.
55. Henry M, Amor M, Ethevenot G, et al. Palmaz stent placement in iliac and femoropopliteal arteries: primary and secondary patency in 310 patients with 2–4-year follow-up. Radiology 1995; 197(1):167–74.

56. Martin EC, Katzen BT, Benenati JF, et al. Multicenter trial of the wallstent in the iliac and femoral arteries. J Vasc Interv Radiol 1995; 6(6):843–9.
57. Gray BH, Olin JW. Limitations of percutaneous transluminal angioplasty with stenting for femoropopliteal arterial occlusive disease. Semin Vasc Surg 1997; 10(1):8–16.
58. Vroegindeweij D, Vos LD, Tielbeek AV, et al. Balloon angioplasty combined with primary stenting versus balloon angioplasty alone in femoropopliteal obstructions: a comparative randomized study. Cardiovasc Intervent Radiol 1997; 20(6):420–5.
59. Cejna M, Thurnher S, Illiasch H, et al. PTA versus Palmaz stent placement in femoropopliteal artery obstructions: a multicenter prospective randomized study. J Vasc Interv Radiol 2001; 12(1):23–31.
60. Grimm J, Muller-Hulsbeck S, Jahnke T, et al. Randomized study to compare PTA alone versus PTA with Palmaz stent placement for femoropopliteal lesions. J Vasc Interv Radiol 2001; 12(8):935–42.
61. Schillinger M, Sabeti S, Loewe C, et al. Balloon angioplasty versus implantation of nitinol stents in the superficial femoral artery. N Engl J Med 2006; 354(18):1879–88.
62. Lugmayr HF, Holzer H, Kastner M, et al. Treatment of complex arteriosclerotic lesions with nitinol stents in the superficial femoral and popliteal arteries: a midterm follow-up. Radiology 2002; 222(1):37–43.
63. Sabeti S, Mlekusch W, Amighi J, et al. Primary patency of long-segment self-expanding nitinol stents in the femoropopliteal arteries. J Endovasc Ther 2005; 12(1):6–12.
64. Sabeti S, Schillinger M, Amighi J, et al. Primary patency of femoropopliteal arteries treated with nitinol versus stainless steel self-expanding stents: propensity score-adjusted analysis. Radiology 2004; 232(2):516–21.
65. Duda SH, Bosiers M, Lammer J, et al. Sirolimus-eluting versus bare nitinol stent for obstructive superficial femoral artery disease: the SIROCCO II trial. J Vasc Interv Radiol 2005; 16(3):331–8.
66. Scheinert D, Scheinert S, Sax J, et al. Prevalence and clinical impact of stent fractures after femoropopliteal stenting. J Am Coll Cardiol 2005; 45(2):312–5.
67. Schlager O, Dick P, Sabeti S, et al. Long-segment SFA stenting—the dark sides: in-stent restenosis, clinical deterioration, and stent fractures. J Endovasc Ther 2005; 12(6):676–84.
68. Lukito G, Vandergoten P, Jaspers L, et al. Six months clinical, angiographic, and IVUS follow-up after PTFE graft stent implantation in native coronary arteries. Acta Cardiol 2000; 55(4):255–60.
69. Deutschmann HA, Schedlbauer P, Berczi V, et al. Placement of hemobahn stent-grafts in femoropopliteal arteries: early experience and midterm results in 18 patients. J Vasc Interv Radiol 2001; 12(8):943–50.
70. Ahmadi R, Schillinger M, Maca T, et al. Femoropopliteal arteries: immediate and long-term results with a Dacron-covered stent-graft. Radiology 2002; 223(2):345–50.
71. Bray PJ, Robson WJ, Bray AE. Percutaneous treatment of long superficial femoral artery occlusive disease: efficacy of the Hemobahn stent-graft. J Endovasc Ther 2003; 10(3):619–28.
72. Jahnke T, Andresen R, Muller-Hulsbeck S, et al. Hemobahn stent-grafts for treatment of femoropopliteal arterial obstructions: midterm results of a prospective trial. J Vasc Interv Radiol 2003; 14(1):41–51.
73. Lammer J, Dake MD, Bleyn J, et al. Peripheral arterial obstruction: prospective study of treatment with a transluminally placed self-expanding stent-graft. International Trial Study Group. Radiology 2000; 217(1):95–104.
74. Wiesinger B, Beregi JP, Oliva VL, et al. PTFE-covered self-expanding nitinol stents for the treatment of severe iliac and femoral artery stenoses and occlusions: final results from a prospective study. J Endovasc Ther 2005; 12(2):240–6.
75. Saxon RR, Coffman JM, Gooding JM, et al. Long-term results of ePTFE stent-graft versus angioplasty in the femoropopliteal artery: single center experience from a prospective, randomized trial. J Vasc Interv Radiol 2003; 14(3):303–11.

4 | Tibial Occlusive Disease

Marc Bosiers and Koen Deloose
Department of Vascular Surgery, AZ St-Blasius, Dendermonde, Belgium
Patrick Peeters and Jurgen Verbist
Department of Cardiovascular and Thoracic Surgery, Imelda Hospital, Bonheiden, Belgium

INTRODUCTION

The treatment of critical limb ischemia (CLI) consumes a significant amount of health care resources (1). Amputation remains a common procedure and is likely to increase due to an aging population, increasing recognition of CLI and a recognized trend toward a higher occurrence of diabetes (2). Patients requiring major amputation face a diminished quality of life, an unfavorable natural history and require extensive resources for their postamputation rehabilitation and course (3). Such resources would be better deployed in an aggressive approach to salvage affected limbs in those suffering from CLI in order to prevent progression to more serious complications.

Distal bypass for limb salvage with autogenous conduit is an excellent option for patients who are good candidates for surgical revascularization. However, prohibitive comorbidities, inadequate conduits, and lack of suitable distal targets for revascularization all conspire to erode the pool of good surgical bypass candidates. Moreover, with the advent of feasible techniques for endovascular therapy for tibial occlusive disease causing CLI, there may be a need to reevaluate current reporting standards for lower extremity revascularization. Morbidity following infrageniculate bypass surgery (IBS) is relatively underweighted in our present strategy of assessing postbypass surgery outcomes. Markers of perioperative morbidity such as index limb reoperation in three months, hospital readmission following IBS, or wound healing time exceeding three months have all been reported in approximately 50% and are examples of factors which may favor endovascular therapeutic strategies (4).

Thus, although surgery remains a good option for some patients with CLI, endovascular therapy offers the advantages of local anesthesia, potentially reduced costs (even anticipating the need for reintervention in many patients), shorter hospital stays as well as other benefits when compared with IBS (5–31). Efforts to extend the range of endovascular approaches to CLI are presently focused on several fronts. One of the most challenging of these frontiers is the treatment of tibial occlusive disease, alone or in combination with more proximal disease, for the purpose of limb salvage. The current chapter provides an overview of the diagnosis and endovascular treatment strategies for infrapopliteal lesions in patients with CLI.

INDICATIONS FOR TREATMENT

The indications for endovascular intervention for tibial occlusive disease should be primarily based on symptomatology, rather than on diagnostic images. The different diagnostic tools have an important value in the overall treatment, but should not be the deciding factor when intervention is considered.

Most patients with a diagnosis of tibial occlusive disease by color flow doppler ultrasound (CFDU) or magnetic resonance angiography are asymptomatic. When the pedal arch is intact, isolated lesions in one of the trifurcation vessels (anterior tibial, posterior tibial, or peroneal) are rarely significant. However, when the pedal arch is incomplete, regional ischemic signs or symptoms may develop. In addition, multiple diseased infrapopliteal vessels, often combined with above-knee segmental disease, may manifest as CLI (Fig. 1).

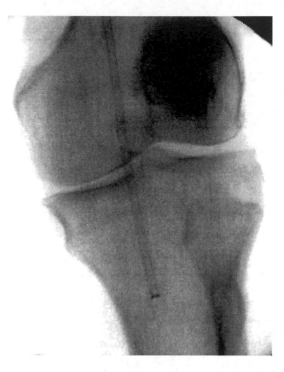

FIGURE 1 Crossover placement of 6-F, 90-cm-long arrow sheath into popliteal region to assist and protect catheter delivery for infrapopliteal treatment.

Only patients suffering from CLI, as defined by Rutherford classes 4 to 6, are candidates for infrapopliteal revascularization. Asymptomatic patients and claudicants found to have severe infrapopliteal lesions are closely monitored, but intervention only becomes mandatory if ischemic rest pain or ulceration develops.

Almost all CLI patients are threatened by other comorbidities (e.g., cerebral, coronary and pulmonary) related to the generalized atherosclerotic process. The general poor health status is key in the authors' opinion and supports the idea that endovascular intervention may be considered the primary treatment modality for CLI caused by infrapopliteal occlusive disease. This is also the opinion of the TransAtlantic Inter-Society Consensus.

ENDOVASCULAR TREATMENT STRATEGY

The clinical success of an infrapopliteal intervention for occlusive disease often depends on patient optimization with medical control of life-threatening comorbidities. Adequate inflow into the infragenicular region must be secured by either an endovascular or a surgical approach.

The primary goal of any endovascular approach is aimed at restoring straight in-line blood flow to the foot in at least one vessel (5). Procedural technical success cannot be declared with static angiographic images (Figs. 2 and 3). Rather improvement in the pattern of blood flow and hemodynamics of the treated lesion are the decisive factor for determining immediate technical success. In cases where this is not achievable, therapy is targeted at maximizing flow to the trifurcation vessels and geniculate collaterals. This is often the situation in diabetic patients who have a tendency to develop severe tibioperoneal trunk calcification.

Technical Details

Crossing the Lesion

Once access is obtained, multiplanar angiography with magnified views of the region of interest is performed and the details of the lesion are assessed.

The guidewire of choice for standard lesion passage is a stiff 0.014- or 0.018-in. hydrophilic wire. Often a 4- to 5-F multipurpose or glide catheter can provide extra support to the guidewire and facilitate lesion passage. A number of factors can make lesion passage difficult. However

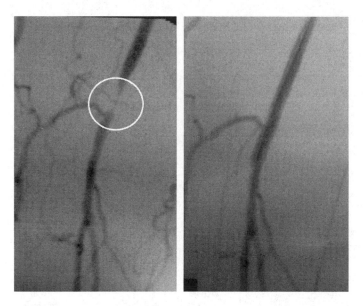

FIGURE 2 Preoperative (*left*) and postoperative (*right*) angiographic control after PTA of short focal infrapopliteal stenosis.

with advanced endovascular skills and experience in this region, three quarters of the lesions in our vascular center can be passed. If the lesion cannot be passed it must be remembered that alternative techniques can be used.

Subintimal lesion passage (6–8) offers an effective alternative to the intraluminal approach. In this technique, a wire is intentionally passed into the subintimal space proximal

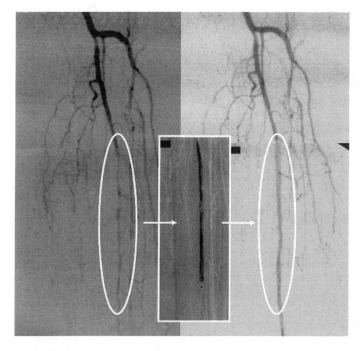

FIGURE 3 Preoperative (*left*) and postoperative (*right*) angiographic control of PTA (*inset*) of long diffuse infrapopliteal stenosis.

to the lesion, a false subintimal lumen is created and the true lumen is reentered distal to the occluded area.

An alternate intraluminal recanalization strategy is the step-by-step laser ablation with a 0.9 to 1.4-mm pulsed excimer lasercatheter. First the 0.014-in. guidewire is advanced into the origin of the occlusion, followed by the excimer laser catheter. The laser catheter is then advanced maximally 5 mm more distal into the occlusion, its tip unguided by the wire. This short ablation allows the guidewire to be advanced deeper into the occlusion. We continue alternating the laser catheter with guidewire advancement up to the distal 1 to 2 cm of the occlusion. From here the lesion is best crossed with the guidewire in order to prevent dissection (9,10).

Lesion Treatment

Percutaneous Transluminal Angioplasty

Infrapopliteal percutaneous transluminal angioplasty (PTA) became feasible with the introduction of low-profile peripheral balloon systems and the use of coronary balloons. In our center, after successful lesion passage, we insert a 4- to 5-F multipurpose guiding catheter into the popliteal artery. This provides sufficient support for the balloon catheter to pass the lesion and is particularly important with rapid exchange catheters. The diameter of the native infrapopliteal vessel and/or the dimension of the proximal and distal reference segment determines the selection of the PTA balloon. Oversizing should be avoided to prevent dissection. Mostly we opt for a hydrophilic-coated balloon catheter with a diameter range from 2.5 to 4.0 mm and a length chosen according to the lesion length. To avoid any further vessel wall damage, we preferably select a balloon which is shorter than the target lesion.

The bypass versus angioplasty in severe ischemia of the leg (BASIL) trial participants recently published the outcome of their randomized controlled trial comparing the outcome of PTA versus bypass surgery in patients presenting with CLI. They found that in the short term PTA was cheaper than surgery and that there were similar outcomes in terms of 12-month amputation-free survival for bypass surgery first and a balloon angioplasty first strategy being 68% and 71%, respectively (see chap. 9) (11).

This excellent limb salvage rate after PTA is confirmed by other earlier publications giving limb salvage rates of above 90% (12–14). The published primary patency rates are less uniform and vary from 15% up to 70% (12,15).

The treatment of longer lesions is often more complex and has a worse prognosis than the treatment of short lesions. A long-segment stenosis is best treated with a gentle PTA using a low-pressure balloon with sizes ranging from 8 to 10 cm in length and 2.5 to 3.5 mm in diameter. A perfect angiographic result is rarely achievable in this circumstance and an arteriographic evaluation of the flow through the vessel is extremely important.

Cutting or Scoring Balloon

The mechanism of action of peripheral cutting or scoring balloons has been referred to as atherotomy. With these advanced PTA technique, atherotomes are mounted on the surface of a noncompliant balloon (Peripheral Cutting Balloon, Boston Scientific Interventional Technologies, San Diego, California, U.S.A.) or a nitinol scoring element encircles a minimally compliant balloon (AngioSculpt, AngioScore, Inc., Fremont, California, U.S.A.) (Fig. 4). This technique is believed to decrease vessel elastic recoil and perivascular injury by a focal concentration of the dilating force. Preliminary data (16,17) described that these devices appear to lower the need for infrapopliteal stents.

Subintimal Angioplasty

In some centers subintimal angioplasty is gaining popularity for long-segment occlusions below the knee. The concept of passing a wire into the subintimal space and inflating a balloon to create a channel for blood flow violates many of the traditional endovascular principles and is somewhat counterintuitive. However, Bolia et al. (6–8) has reported their technical and clinical success rates of respectively 86% and 80% in a consecutive series of 67 patients. Limb salvage rates of 94% and freedom of CLI of 84% were reported after 36 months. Nydahl et al.

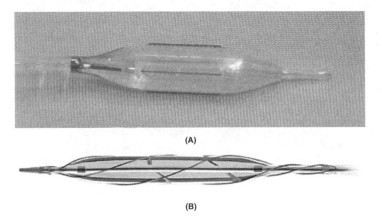

(A)

(B)

FIGURE 4 (**A**) Inflated Peripheral Cutting Balloon (Boston Scientific Interventional Technologies, San Diego, California, U.S.A.). (**B**) Inflated AngioSculpt (AngioScore, Inc., Fremont, California, U.S.A.).

(18) investigated the use of subintimal PTA for restoring blood flow in the infrapopliteal vessels. This paper reported a one-year limb salvage rate of 85%, even though the subintimal canal was hemodynamically patent in only 53% of the cases. Vraux et al. (19) found comparably low 12-month primary patency rates (56%) with an 81% limb salvage rate.

Stenting
To date, only limited evidence is available to support the need for stenting in tibial occlusive disease (Fig. 5). Therefore, stent implantation is generally reserved for cases with a suboptimal outcome after PTA (i.e., >50% residual stenosis, flow-limiting dissection). With the recent publication of two randomized controlled trials, data are available to support the use of stenting in the tibial area. The Vienna group (20) were the first to prove that the angiographic

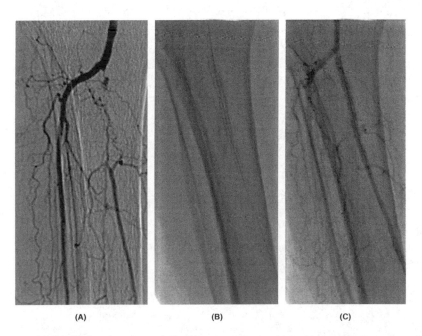

(A)   (B)   (C)

FIGURE 5 (**A**) Preoperative and (**B, C**) postoperative angiographic control of stenting with a sirolimus-eluting stent (Cypher®, Cordis, J & J Company, Waterloo, Belgium) of a short focal infrapopliteal occlusion.

outcome after stenting was superior to PTA alone in infrapopliteal vessels. For the stent group the cumulative primary patency at six months was 83.7% at the 70% restenosis threshold, and 79.7% at the 50% restenosis threshold. For PTA, the primary patency at six months was 61.1% at the 70% restenosis threshold and 45.6% at the 50% restenosis threshold. Both results were statistically significant ($p < 0.05$).

This important new evidence is further supported by the promising data on tibial stent use as presented in earlier publications on nonrandomized trials and case observations using different stent types: uncoated stainless steel (21) or nitinol stents (22), stainless steel stents with a passive (23) or active coating (24,25) and bioabsorbable magnesium alloy stents (26–29).

In our recent publication describing our personal results on endovascular techniques for tibial occlusive disease using all these different stent types in 300 consecutive tibial stenting cases, we reported a one-year primary patency of 75.5% and a limb salvage rate of 98.6% (12).

Excimer Laser

As mentioned earlier, a laser can be used to cross complex tibial lesions (Figs. 6 and 7). Using a wavelength of 308 nm for peripheral procedures, a cold-tipped, pulsed laser often opens occlusions when other interventional endovascular techniques fail, although severe calcification is a contraindication for excimer laser–assisted treatment of the infrageniculate arteries (30,31). A conventional mechanical guidewire is used to cross the entire occlusion up to the distal vessel beyond the target lesion. Next, the occlusion or stenosis can be treated with two different techniques: (*i*) a 0.9 or 1.4 laser catheter is used to debulk the vessel in order to ease PTA catheter delivery and to improve PTA results, (*ii*) a 1.7 or 2.0 laser catheter is used to ablate enough tissue so that the sole use of the laser results in an acceptable intraluminal diameter and flow.

Our own experience with 64 consecutive excimer laser cases for tibial occlusive disease results in a one-year primary patency of 75.4% and a limb salvage rate of 87.9% (12).

POSTPROCEDURAL SURVEILLANCE

Endovascular interventions in patients with CLI are designed to relieve symptoms and preserve the limb. Postoperatively, our regimen utilizes lifelong clopidogrel (75 mg daily).

Close surveillance of all revascularized below the knee (BTK) vessels is mandatory in our practice. Standard follow-up visits are planned at 1, 3, 6 and 12 months. Beside duplex

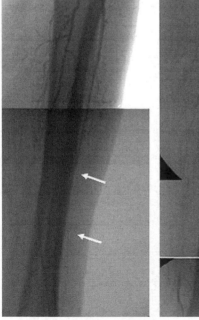
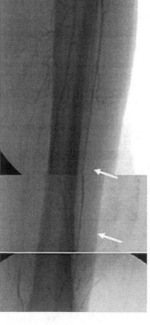

FIGURE 6 Preoperative (*left*) and post-operative (*right*) angiographic control of excimer laser for diffuse "outflow limiting" lesions of the anterior tibial artery (Excimer®, Spectranetics, Colorado Springs, Colorado, U.S.A.).

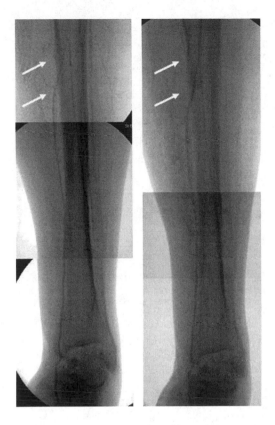

FIGURE 7 Preoperative (*left*) and postoperative (*right*) angiographic control of excimer laser for diffuse "inflow limiting" infrapopliteal disease (Excimer®, Spectranetics, Colorado Springs, Colorado, U.S.A.).

investigation for restenosis and flow assessment, careful attention is paid to pain and wound evolution. Recurrent complaints, such as healing deterioration despite intravenous antibiotic administration in ulcerated lesion and recurrence of rest pain, prompt immediate investigation and often necessitate aggressive reintervention to reestablish one open artery to the foot in order to prevent amputation. In contradiction with surgery, recurrent intervention is not complicated by previous endovascular treatment.

CONCLUSIONS

Limb preservation should be the goal in patients with CLI due to tibial occlusive disease. With a prompt diagnosis, treatment can be started early and serious consequences may be avoided. Any type of revascularization that can prevent amputation must be applied to the overall treatment strategy (1).

Morbidity and mortality rates associated with an endovascular revascularization are lower than with surgical bypass. Endovascular interventions do not prohibit future bypass or additional treatments. Moreover, the BASIL-investigator participants (11), concluded in their recent publication of their randomized controlled trail (RCT), that the PTA first strategy gave as good clinical results as the surgery first approach in CLI and that PTA is cheaper in the short turn. Patients require lifelong follow-up to repeatedly assess the status of the limb after intervention to maximize limb salvage rates. Recurrent symptoms warrant an immediate investigation and an aggressive reintervention strategy is indicated.

ACKNOWLEDGMENTS

The authors take great pleasure in thanking the staff of Flanders Medical Research Program (www.fmrp.be), with special regards to Koen De Meester and Erwin Vinck, for performing the systematic review of the literature and providing substantial support to the data analysis and the writing of the article.

REFERENCES

1. Allie DE, Hebert C, Lirtzman MD, et al. Critical limb ischemia: a global epidemic. A critical analysis of current treatment unmasks the clinical and economic costs of CLI. Eurointervention 2005; 1:75–84.
2. Jaff MR, Biamino G. An overview of critical limb ischemia: today's therapeutic advances are changing the way we evaluate and treat this common and often fatal disorder. Endovascular Today 2004; 3(2):45–8.
3. Wolfe JH, Wyatt MG. Critical and subcritical ischemia. Eur J Vasc Endovasc Surg 1997; 13:578–82.
4. Goshima KR, Mills JL, Sr, Hughes JD. A new look at outcomes after infrainguinal bypass surgery: traditional reporting standards systematically underestimate the expenditure of effort required to attain limb salvage. J Vasc Surg 2004; 39:330–5.
5. Horvath W, Oertl M, Haldinger D. Percutaneous transluminal angioplasty of crural arteries. Radiology 1990; 177:565–9.
6. Bolia A, Sayers RD, Thompson MM, Bell PR. Subintimal and intraluminal recanalisation of occluded crural arteries by percutaneous balloon angioplasty. Eur J Vasc Surg 1994; 8:214–9.
7. Ingle H, Nasim A, Bolia A, et al. Subintimal angioplasty of isolated infragenicular vessels in lower limb ischemia: long-term results. J Endovasc Ther 2002; 9(4):411–6.
8. Bolia A. Subintimal angioplasty in lower limb ischaemia. J Cardiovasc Surg (Torino) 2005; 46:385–94.
9. Biamino GM, Scheinert D. Excimer laser treatment of SFA occlusions. Endovascular Today 2003; 2(4):45–8.
10. Scheinert D, Laird JR, Schroder M, Steinkamp H, Balzer J, Biamino G. Excimer laser-assisted recanalization of long, chronic superficial femoral artery occlusions. J Endovasc Ther 2001; 8:156–66.
11. Adam DJ, Beard JD, Cleveland T, et al. BASIL trial participants. Bypass versus angioplasty in severe ischaemia of the leg (BASIL): multicentre, randomised controlled trial. Lancet 2005; 366(9501):1925–34.
12. Bosiers M, Hart JP, Deloose K, Verbist J, Peeters P. Endovascular therapy as the primary approach for limb salvage in patients with critical limb ischemia: experience with 443 infrapopliteal procedures. Vascular 2006;14:63–9.
13. Dorros G, Jaff MR, Dorros AM, Mathiak LM, He T. Tibioperoneal (outflow lesion) angioplasty can be used as primary treatment in 235 patients with critical limb ischemia: five year follow-up. Circulation 2001; 104:2057–62.
14. Hanna GP, Fujise K, Kjellgren O, et al. Infrapopliteal transcatheter interventions for limb salvage in diabetic patients: importance of aggressive interventional approach and role of transcutaneous oximetry. J Am Coll Cardiol 1997; 30:664–9.
15. Parsons RE, Suggs WD, Lee JJ, Sanchez LA, Lyon RT, Veith FJ. Percutaneous transluminal angioplasty for the treatment of limb threatening ischemia: do the results justify an attempt before bypass grafting? J Vasc Surg 1998; 28:1066–71.
16. Ansel GM, George BS, Botti CF, Jr., Silver MJ. Infrapopliteal endovascular techniques: indications, techniques, and results. Curr Interv Cardiol Rep 2001; 3:100–8.
17. Scheinert D, Graziani L, Peeters P, et al. Results from the multi-center registry of the novel angiosculpt scoring balloon catheter for the treatment of infra-popliteal disease. Cardiovasc Revasc Med 2006; 17(2):113.
18. Nydahl S, Hartshorne T, Bell PR, Bolia A, London NJ. Subintimal angioplasty of infrapopliteal occlusions in critically ischaemic limbs. Eur J Vasc Endovasc Surg 1997; 14:212–6.
19. Vraux H, Hammer F, Verhelst R, Goffette P, Vandeleene B. Subintimal angioplasty of tibial vessel occlusions in the treatment of critical limb ischaemia: mid-term results. Eur J Vasc Endovasc Surg 2000; 20:441–6.
20. Rand T, Basile A, Cejna M, et al. PTA versus carbofilm-coated stents in infrapopliteal arteries: pilot study. Cardiovasc Intervent Radiol 2006; 29(1):29–38.
21. Feiring AJ, Wesolowski AA, Lade S. Primary stent-supported angioplasty for treatment of below-knee critical limb ischemia and severe claudication: early and one-year outcomes. J Am Coll Cardiol 2004; 44(12):2307–14.
22. Bosiers M, Deloose K, Verbist J, Peeters P. Clinical application of the Xpert Stent: new data show effectiveness in the treatment of CLI caused by infrapopliteal lesions. Endovascular Today 2006; 5(2):24–6.
23. Peeters P, Bosiers M, Verbist J, Deloose K. Is there a role for the silicon carbide coated stent below the groin? TCT 2003 (personal communication).
24. Siablis D, Kraniotis P, Karnabatidis D, Kagadis GC, Katsanos K, Tsolakis J. Sirolimus-eluting versus bare stents for bailout after suboptimal infrapopliteal angioplasty for critical limb ischemia: 6-month angiographic results from a nonrandomized prospective single-center study. J Endovasc Ther 2005; 12(6):685–95.
25. Bosiers M, Deloose K, Verbist J, Peeters P. Percutaneous transluminal angioplasty for treatment of "below-the-knee" critical limb ischemia: early outcomes following the use of sirolimus-eluting stents. J Cardiovasc Surg (Torino) 2006; 47(2):171–6.

26. Peeters P, Bosiers M, Verbist J, Deloose K, Heublein B. Preliminary results after application of absorbable metal stents in patients with critical limb ischemia. J Endovasc Ther 2005; 12:1–5.
27. Di Mario C, Griffiths H, Goktekin O. Drug-eluting bioabsorbable magnesium stent. J Interv Cardiol 2004; 17:391–5.
28. Bosiers M, Deloose K, Verbist J, Peeters P. First clinical application of absorbable metal stents in the treatment of critical limb ischemia: 12-month results. Vasc Dis Manag 2005; 2:86–91.
29. Bosiers M, Deloose K, Verbist J, Peeters P. Will absorbable metal stent technology change our practice?. J Cardiovasc Surg (Torino) 2006;47:393–7.
30. Das TS. Percutaneous peripheral revascularisation with excimer laser: equipment, technique and results. Lasers Med Sci 2001; 16:101–7.
31. Bosiers M, Peeters P, Deloose K, et al. Excimer laser revascularization for critical limb ischemia: has a solution been found? Bus Brief: Glob Surg 2003; 37:1–4.

5 | Debulking Procedures for Long Occlusions of the Superficial Femoral Arteries

E. D. Ponfoort and J. P. P. M. de Vries
Department of Vascular Surgery, St. Antonius Hospital, Nieuwegein, The Netherlands
R. Hissink and F. L. Moll
Department of Vascular Surgery, University Medical Centre, Utrecht, The Netherlands

INTRODUCTION

Peripheral artery disease (PAD) affects 10% of the adult population and is particularly prevalent in the superficial femoral artery (SFA), where it may cause intermittent claudication or critical limb ischemia (1–5). This chapter will review the potential role of debulking procedures for long femoral occlusions and focus on the role of directional atherectomy, laser, and remote endarterectomy.

The SFA is one of the most frequent sites for atherosclerotic lesions and is involved in 70% of all PAD patients. SFA lesions are predominantly found at the hiatus of the adductor canal, with relative proximal and distal sparing (6). Although the SFA is almost uniformly involved in symptomatic patients, the clinical presentation is dependent on the extent of atherosclerosis throughout the affected limb. Because the SFA is so frequently involved in symptomatic PAD, this artery is a prime target for therapeutic action. A useful classification of SFA lesions was formulated by the 2000 TransAtlantic Inter-Society Consensus Commission (7) (chap. 3).

PERCUTANEOUS DEBULKING

Infrainguinal occlusive lesions are often characterized by a high calcium content, which predisposes to residual hemodynamic stenosis following angioplasty or stenting. To overcome this problem, percutaneous plaque debulking techniques have been developed.

DIRECTIONAL ATHERECTOMY

Directional atherectomy employs a specially developed catheter with a container in the tip, in which atheroma is collected and subsequently removed (Silverhawk®, FoxHollow Technologies). The lesion is crossed with a guidewire and catheter, after which the atherectomy catheter is advanced, a cutting blade engaged and debris collected. In a series of 52 patients, with an average lesion length of 48 ± 64 mm (range 10–300 mm), a reasonable technical success was achieved with less than 30% residual stenosis in 75% of lesions (8). The authors reported technical problems requiring aspiration of emboli and debris in five patients. At six months, restenosis occurred in 27% for primary lesions, 41% for restenotic lesions, and 36% for in-stent restenosis. Reintervention rates were 20%, 37%, and 29%, respectively. A primary assisted clinical success rate exceeding 80% was reported (8).

LASER

The use of laser angioplasty was limited by thermal injury induced by the laser beam. Although the initial success rate was high, aneurysm formation, perforation, or restenosis was frequently identified in the follow-up period. The excimer laser utilizes ultraviolet light in short energy bursts, with a penetration depth of only 50 μm. The mechanism of action is photochemical rather then thermal, and causes only a limited rise in temperature of 5°C (9).

In a series of 318 consecutive long (mean 19 cm) SFA occlusions treated with excimer laser, the initial technical success rate was 90%. Complications included acute reocclusion (1%), perforation (2%), and distal thrombosis/embolization (4%). At one year, primary patency was only 20%, but primary assisted patency and secondary patency were 65% and 75%, respectively (10). In the Peripheral Excimer Laser Angioplasty trial, excimer laser was directly compared with percutaneous transluminal angioplasty (PTA) in patients with long (mean 20 cm) SFA occlusions. The initial technical success rate was 84% for excimer laser and 89% for PTA. In the laser group, fewer stent placements were required than in the PTA group (42% vs. 59%). The one-year patency rates for laser and PTA were similar (79% and 87%, respectively) (11). More recently the Laser Angioplasty for Critical Limb Ischemia trial was directed at patients with critical limb ischemia considered poor candidates for conventional surgery. Here, the excimer laser was used as an adjunct to PTA and optional stenting. Lesions treated comprised occlusions in 92% of cases with a median length of 11 cm. Stents were placed in 45%, and procedural success was 86%. At six-month follow-up, limb salvage was achieved in 92% of surviving patients (12).

The excimer laser is still under development. With the devices presently available, technical problems are posed by the rigidity of the catheters and the small caliber of the intravascular laser tips (2.5 mm).

SEMI-CLOSED ENDARTERECTOMY

In 1946, the Portuguese surgeon Dos Santos described an effective technique to surgically remove the diseased intima from atherosclerotic blood vessels (13)—endarterectomy. Over time, several instruments were specifically designed to facilitate blind dissection of the intima core, and perform this procedure in a minimally invasive fashion. In 1954, DeBakey introduced the ring stripper, consisting of a sharp metal ring placed at a 90° angle on a metal shaft. In 1967, Vollmar modified the ring stripper to the shape that is most frequently used today. The sharp ring was changed into a blunt oval shape and placed on its shaft at a 135° angle (14). When the ring stripper is progressed via a groin incision, the occluded vessel segment can be successfully passed in over 90% of the cases. In single-center series, five-year patency rates for successful procedures reach 71% (15), comparable to above-knee bypass surgery.

REMOTE ENDARTERECTOMY

With the introduction of fluoroscopy in the operating theatre and the development of the ring strip cutter (MollRing Cutter®, Vascular Architects San Jose, California, U.S.A.), the semi-closed technique has evolved into the remote endarterectomy procedure. The ring strip cutter is a device that consists of two rings with sharpened inner edges that mimic a pair of scissors when the two shafts telescope into each other (Fig. 1). This device enables distal endoluminal termination of the intima core through the initial femoral arteriotomy (16). The distal intima is then fixed to the vessel wall with an endovascular stent, thus obviating the need for an additional above-knee incision. This minimizes initial surgical trauma and leaves the possibility for subsequent above-knee bypass surgery.

Clinical results after remote endarterectomy are described in several single (17) and multicenter series (18,19). The initial technical success rate varied from 80% to 90%. The main potential complications are SFA perforation (2%) and distal embolization (<1%) (17). Small perforations can often be left untreated. Larger perforations or inability to pass the occlusion might require a second incision or conversion to bypass surgery (5%). Distal embolization can usually be managed by thrombosuction or balloon thrombectomy.

Reported primary patency rates after remote endarterectomy are 67%, 61%, and 38% after one, three, and five years, respectively (17). Cumulative secondary patency rates approach 49%

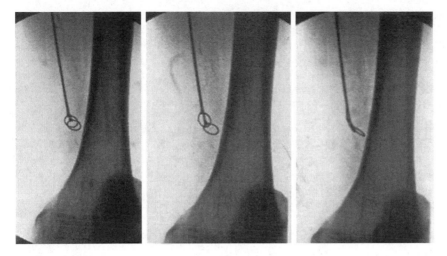

FIGURE 1 Ring cutters.

after five years. During the first year, restenosis occurs in up to 36% of cases and warrants prophylactic balloon angioplasty. When left untreated, 50% of these early restenoses will progress to an occlusion (20). Late restenosis (>1 year post-procedure) is seldom progressive and usually benign. Restenosis is not confined to the stented transition zone but occurs throughout the endarterectomized region. To overcome the problem of restenosis, attempts to completely cover the endarterectomized surface with a balloon-expandable endovascular stent (Endolining, W. L. Gore & Associates, Flagstaff Arizona, U.S.A.) proved unfruitful (21). This was partly due to restenosis at the proximal and distal end of the covered surface. More importantly, endolining entails the sacrifice of all collaterals from the deep femoral artery. We currently prefer the use of a semi-covered spiral stent (aSpire®, Vascular Architects San Jose, California, U.S.A.), which is kink resistant and spares important collaterals at the distal transition zone.

Reocclusion after remote endarterectomy often shows a mild clinical course. This is partly due to patent collaterals and preserved supragenicular pickup. Indeed, the clinical outcome after reocclusion of a remote endarterectomy compares favorably with that after failure of an above-knee bypass. In a large series of primary successful remote endarterectomy procedures, late occlusion led to clinical deterioration in only 18% of cases, of which 6% required an emergency procedure. In a population mix with 27% critically ischemic patients, this resulted in a cumulative amputation rate of only 0.85% (22). This compares favorably with the 7% amputation rate observed after failed above-knee bypass surgery in a similar patient mix (23).

Supporters of this technique propose remote endarterectomy as a first-line treatment for long SFA occlusions when there is a patent popliteal artery, with at least one crural runoff vessel. The goals and results of treatment will be dictated by the presenting symptoms. Measures to improve patency rates include aggressive medical therapy with antiplatelet agents and close duplex surveillance, with angioplasty for restenotic (>70%) lesions. A clinical trial comparing remote endarterectomy to above-knee bypass surgery is currently underway.

CONCLUSION

Over recent decades, the treatment of long SFA occlusions has evolved from surgery to minimally invasive percutaneous therapy. Patients who benefit most from these developments are those with critical limb ischemia and extensive comorbidity, and those with lifestyle-limiting claudication that does not warrant surgical intervention. With improved patency rates for percutaneous techniques, these therapies should also be considered primarily in patients who are otherwise good surgical candidates. When a choice for surgical intervention has been made, a minimally invasive technique such as remote endarterectomy forms an attractive alternative. Patients are subjected to less surgical trauma, and in the case of late failure, the option for conventional bypass surgery still remains open. Future developments in the direction of percutaneous debulking with novel devices or excimer laser show much promise.

REFERENCES

1. Criqui MH, Fronek A, Barrett-Connor E, Klauber MR, Gabriel S, Goodman D. The prevalence of peripheral arterial disease in a defined population. Circulation 1985; 71:510–5.
2. Criqui MH, Langer RD, Fronek A, et al. Mortality over a period of 10 years in patients with peripheral arterial disease. N Engl J Med 1992; 326:381–6.
3. Verhoeven B, Hellings WE, Moll FL, et al. Carotid atherosclerotic plaques in patients with transient ischemic attacks and stroke have unstable characteristics compared with plaques in asymptomatic and amaurosis fugax patients. J Vasc Surg 2005; 42:1075–81.
4. Kher N, Marsh JD. Pathobiology of atherosclerosis—a brief review. Semin Thromb Hemost 2004; 30:665–72.
5. Caro CG, Fitz-Gerald JM, Schroter RC. Arterial wall shear and distribution of early atheroma in man. Nature 1969; 223:1159–60.
6. Lindbom A. Arteriosclerosis and arterial thrombosis in the lower limb: a roentgenological study. Acta Radiol Suppl 1950; 80:1–80.
7. Dormandy JA, Rutherford RB. Management of peripheral arterial disease (PAD). TASC Working Group. TransAtlantic Inter-Society Concensus (TASC). J Vasc Surg 2000; 31:S1–296.
8. Zeller T, Rastan A, Schwarzwalder U, et al. Percutaneous peripheral atherectomy of femoropopliteal stenoses using a new-generation device: six-month results from a single-center experience. J Endovasc Ther 2004; 11:676–85.
9. Wollenek G, Laufer G. Comparative study of different laser systems with special regard to angioplasty. Thorac Cardiovasc Surg 1988; 36(Suppl. 2):126–32.
10. Scheinert D, Laird JR, Jr., Schroder M, Steinkamp H, Balzer JO, Biamino G. Excimer laser-assisted recanalization of long, chronic superficial femoral artery occlusions. J Endovasc Ther 2001; 8:156–66.
11. Laird JR, Jr. PELA Trial: Peripheral Excimer Laser Angioplasty, 2002. (http://www.medscape.com/viewarticle/442691)
12. Laird JR, Zeller T, Gray BH, et al. Limb salvage following laser-assisted angioplasty for critical limb ischemia: results of the LACI multicenter trial. J Endovasc Ther 2006; 13:1–11.
13. Dos Santos JC. Sur la desubstruction des tromboses arterielles anciennes. Mem Acad Chir 1946; 73:409–11.
14. Vollmar J, Laubach K, Trede M. The surgical treatment of chronic arterial occlusions in the femoro-popliteal segment. Report on 546 operations. Langenbecks Arch Chir 1967; 318:102–25.
15. van der Heijden FH, Eikelboom BC, van Reedt Dortland RW, et al. Long-term results of semiclosed endarterectomy of the superficial femoral artery and the outcome of failed reconstructions. J Vasc Surg 1993; 18:271–9.
16. Ho GH, Moll FL, Joosten PP, Van de Pavoordt ED, Overtoom TT. The mollring cutter remote endarterectomy: preliminary experience with a new endovascular technique for treatment of occlusive superficial femoral artery disease. J Endovasc Surg 1995; 2:278–87.
17. Smeets L, Ho GH, Hagenaars T, van den Berg JC, Teijink JA, Moll FL. Remote endarterectomy: first choice in surgical treatment of long segmental SFA occlusive disease? Eur J Vasc Endovasc Surg 2003; 25:583–9.
18. Knight JS, Smeets L, Morris GE, Moll FL. Multi centre study to assess the feasibility of a new covered stent and delivery system in combination with remote superficial femoral artery endarterectomy (RSFAE). Eur J Vasc Endovasc Surg 2005; 29:287–94.
19. Rosenthal D, Schubart PJ, Kinney EV, et al. Remote superficial femoral artery endarterectomy: multicenter medium-term results. J Vasc Surg 2001; 34:428–32.
20. Ho GH, van Buren PA, Moll FL, van der Bom JG, Eikelboom BC. Incidence, time-of-onset, and anatomical distribution of recurrent stenoses after remote endarterectomy in superficial femoral artery occlusive disease. J Vasc Surg 1999; 30:106–13.
21. Ho GH, Moll FL, Tutein Nolthenius RP, van den Berg JC, Overtoom TT. Endovascular femoropopliteal bypass combined with remote endarterectomy in SFA occlusive disease: initial experience. Eur J Vasc Endovasc Surg 2000; 19:27–34.

22. Smeets L, Huijbregts RJT, Ho G, de Vries JP, Moll FL. Clinical outcome after re-occlusion of initially successful remote endarterectomy of the superficial femoral artery. Thesis/dissertation, 2005.
23. Klinkert P, Schepers A, Burger DH, van Bockel JH, Breslau PJ. Vein versus polytetrafluoroethylene in above-knee femoropopliteal bypass grafting: five-year results of a randomized controlled trial. J Vasc Surg 2003; 37:149–55.

6 | Treatment of Restenosis Following Lower Limb Intervention

Manfred Cejna
Zentrales Radiologie Institut, LKH Feldkirch, Feldkirch, Austria

INTRODUCTION

Despite major progress in endovascular therapy over the last two decades, restenosis is still a major limitation in the treatment of lower limb arterial occlusive disease. The extent of restenosis after angioplasty is mainly determined by two mechanisms: negative remodeling and development of neointimal hyperplasia. The literature relating to coronary interventions has demonstrated that stent implantation provides a mechanical scaffold that eliminates recoil and prevents negative remodelling. Stenting may also eliminate arterial dissection or residual stenosis due to calcified plaques. However, enhanced neointimal hyperplasia increases the rates of late failure after stenting.

Despite the magnitude of the clinical problem, the issue of restenosis was not addressed specifically in the TransAtlantic Inter-Society Consensus (TASC) 2000 paper (1). This may be partly explained by the paucity of literature relating to the clinical problem in lower limb disease. In the TASC 2007 update (2), restenosis was also not addressed specifically but recognized as a relevant problem. For TASC classification of femoral popliteal lesions repeat restenotic obstruction (recurrent stenoses or occlusions that need treatment after two endovascular interventions) in femoropopliteal arteries were categorized as TASC C lesions (Recommendation 37. Treatment of femoral popliteal lesions: In TASC C lesions, surgical treatment can be preferred over endovascular treatment in young otherwise healthy patients and upon patient's preferences). The approaches for post-angioplasty and in-stent restenosis are different and will be discussed separately.

RESTENOSIS—EXPERIMENTAL AND CLINICAL DATA

Restenosis is encountered more frequently after treatment of femoropopliteal disease than iliac lesions. This can lead to a significant number of reinterventions (1). Muradin et al. (3) performed a meta-analysis of 19 studies relating to femoropopliteal percutaneous transluminal angioplasty (PTA) and stent implantation between 1999 and 2000, adjusting for lesion type (stenosis vs. occlusion) and indication for treatment (claudication vs. critical limb ischemia). The combined three-year patency rates for PTA alone were 61% and 48% for stenoses and occlusions, respectively. The rates for critical ischemia were 43% for stenoses and 30% for occlusions. The three-year patency rates after stent implantation ranged from 63% to 66%, regardless of the clinical indication or lesion type (3,4).

Despite major recent improvements, including the introduction of nitinol and drug-eluting stents (DES) for the lower extremity, the problem of in-stent restenosis remains significant. A large retrospective study of 104 nitinol stents and 123 stainless steel stents for the treatment of femoropopliteal occlusions demonstrated one- and two-year patency rates of 75% and 69%, respectively, for nitinol stents. At least 25% of patients developed restenoses after treatment of long lesions (5,6). In all these publications, no data were provided for target vessel revascularization (necessary treatment due to reoccurrence of clinical symptoms and retenosis in the previously treated segment). Additionally the number of patients who had to be referred to surgical treatment is of major interest, because these patients ultimately failed endovascular therapy. Recent studies—the FAST trial (7) and the ABSOLUT trial (8)—better addressed the clinical scope of the problem, reporting patency rates and TLR for short and medium femoropopliteal lesions. For the FAST trial (244 patients with a mean femoropliteal lesion length was 45 mm), target lesion revascularization was necessary in 21 patients after angioplasty with selective stenting and in 17 patients after primary stenting. In the ABSOLUT trial (98 patients with a mean femoropliteal lesion length of 101 mm), target lesion revascularization was necessary in 28 patients after angioplasty with selective stenting and in 17 patients after primary stenting. Yet in the latter group, in 3 patients surgical bypass creation was necessary, besides 12 angioplasty only and 2 restenting treatments. For selective stenting, the proportion of stent implantation versus angioplasty only for reintervention was a little but not significantly higher (20 angioplasty only and 8 stent implantation treatments).

Economic impact

Economic issues are most important for the treatment of claudicants. Here uninterrupted (clinical) patency is of utmost importance. Although the definite roles of surgical (vein or prosthetic) bypasss or endovascular treatment or exercise training are not clearly defined due to the lack of appropriate studies, restenosis is the main limitation in this group of patients. For claudicants we are looking for the most cost-effective means to achieve long-term uninterrupted patency.

Since immediate revascularization is the treatment goal for critical ischemia, to promote healing after a deficit in perfusion, in a very often previously balanced state of hypoperfusion. Here angioplasty after subintimal recanalization has been demonstrated as a good tool in a randomized trial, treatment of restenosis is not the main concern in this—often severely ill—cohort of patients with multiple comorbidities.

Post-Angioplasty Restenosis

The restenotic process has been characterized using intravascular ultrasound (IVUS) and magnetic resonance imaging (9,10). It is now clear that restenosis is the net result of vessel recoil, intimal thickening, and vessel remodelling. An IVUS/atherectomy correlation demonstrated that intimal hyperplasia was mostly homogenous and hypoechogenic on IVUS, composed of hypocellular, partly thrombotic material (9). Histological specimens contained more replicating cells than coronary artery specimens, though the overall number was very low, suggesting that replication was not a major factor in the pathophysiology of restenosis (11).

Söder et al. (12) analyzed the angiographic recurrence pattern after femoropopliteal angioplasty. From 263 consecutive patients, follow-up angiography was available in 52 patients with suspected recurrent symptomatic disease during follow-up. In 48 patients 75 lesions were analyzed. Interestingly recurrent stenosis was found more often after treatment of stenotic rather than occlusive disease (92% and 59%, respectively). Reexpansion of the lesion is the key to treatment of post-angioplasty restenosis.

In-Stent Restenosis

Experimental data are not easily transferable to the in vivo situation. Nor are the data regarding coronary restenosis applicable to lower limb interventions. There is still controversy regarding the correct approach to treat in-stent restenosis. To understand peripheral in-stent restenosis we have to rely on data obtained from atherectomy specimens and surgical explants. In-stent restenotic tissue retrieved from atherectomy specimens contain extensive hypercellular foci composed predominantly of smooth muscle cells with ongoing proliferation. Apoptotic cells are detected, along with macrophages and leukocytes. Interestingly organized thrombus was observed in the majority of specimens (13).

Surgically removed Palmaz® (Johnson & Johnson, Miami, Florida, U.S.A.) stent explants demonstrate two distinct pathogenic processes in different zones that contribute to in-stent restenosis. One process is an increase in cell number in the inner intima due to prolonged cellular proliferation. This is in contrast to post-angioplasty restenosis where replication does not contribute to the restenotic process. Secondly, there is an accumulation of matrix around the stent struts. There may also be an association with a reduction in circulating endothelial progenitor cell subset levels. Defective endothelialization with thrombus formation could partially account for the tendency to generate restenotic lesions (14).

In-stent restenosis is more difficult to treat than post-angioplasty restenotic lesions. Atherectomy is an interesting option but long-term follow-up data are not convincing. Cutting balloon angioplasty is also appealing. Data for cryoplasty and DES are, however, lacking.

Restenosis After Stent Grafts

The situation regarding occlusion of stent grafts is different from the usual restenotic process. For the expanded polytetrafluoroethylene stent grafts—the Hemobahn™/Viabahn® (W.L. Gore and Assoc., Flagstaff, Arizona, U.S.A.) devices—thrombotic reocclusions are most often found without preceding restenosis in the stent. Thrombolysis of occluded stent grafts has revealed an absence of in-stent stenosis, yet extension of the stent graft was warranted in some cases because of anastomotic stenoses. In the few cases where in-stent stenoses were detected, angioplasty was sufficient for treatment (15,16).

Some polyethylene-terephtalate (Dacron™) stent grafts seem to have a predisposition to stenose at the proximal and distal ends of the stent in the femoral artery, though not in the iliac system. Additionally incomplete stent expansion has been identified in as many as 42% of cases (17). In the majority of patients, restenosis treated with repeat PTA seems initially sufficient, but secondary patency rates are poor (60% at one year) (18).

Restenosis Due to Incomplete Stent Expansion–Stent Compression and Stent Deformation

Another factor that potentially contributes to in-stent restenosis is incomplete stent expansion, identified in up to 40% of the cases (19). Complete stent expension as documented by IVUS was able to increase patency rates (20). For balloon-expandable stents, external compression has been shown to predispose to restenosis, e.g., pressure within the adductor canal. Redilatation can be of temporary benefit though recompression will occur (21). Self-expandable stents are preferable for target lesions in arteries exposed to external compression, whether by muscle or other external forces. Native artery trauma caused by the motion of the superficial femoral artery (SFA) and popliteal arteries against the ends of nitinol stents appears to contribute to some cases of acute occlusion, as well as to late restenosis. Some stent designs minimize this effect by allowing longitudinal compression which may allow a more favorable response to movement of the limb. Longer stents may increase the likelihood of traumatic arterial wall and stent interaction. Performing leg flexion to 90° before stent placement may allow better planning and prevent stent placement across areas of excessive motion (22). More flexible coil stents might address this problem, though these may have an increased incidence of stent fracture. Coil stents on the other hand are also prone to restenosis. In the Intracoil® (Sulzer, St. Paul, Minnesota, U.S.A.) RCT (a randomized comparison of PTA vs. the Intrastent® Coilstent, the data were not published but available at the FDA homepage www.fda.gov/cdrh/pdf/p000033b.pdf; that was cancelled after 266 patients, 500 patients should have been included) interim results demonstrated compareable 9 month target vessel revascularization rates for both treatment groups (14.3% for the Intrastent® vs. 16.1% for angioplasty) in the treatment of relative short (<4 cm) lesions.

Restenosis Due to Stent Fracture

Stent fracture is increasingly recognized, especially after stenting long SFA lesions. The major cause appears to be twisting. This may expose unpolished bare metal and contribute to increased restenosis.

In a report by Scheinert et al. (23), stent fractures were detected in 45 of 121 treated legs (37.2%) with a mean stented segment of 15.7 cm. In a stent-based analysis, 64 of 261 stents (24.5%) demonstrated fractures, classified as minor (single strut fracture) in 31 cases (48.4%), moderate (fracture of >1 strut) in 17 cases (26.6%), and severe (complete separation of stent segments) in 16 cases (25.0%). Fracture rates were 13.2% for a stented length of 8 cm or less, 42.4% for length 8 to 16 cm, and 52.0% for a stented length greater than 16 cm. In 21 cases (32.8%) there was a restenosis of more than 50% diameter reduction at the site of stent fracture. In 22 cases (34.4%) with stent fracture there was a total stent reocclusion.

Stent fracture is therefore a major contributing factor to restenosis. Treatment of stent fracture–induced restenosis depends on the severity of the stent fracture and of the nature of the stent (18).

In a retrospective analysis by Schlager et al. (24) there was no significant association between fractures and restenosis with Wallstents™ (Boston Scientific, Watertown, Massachusetts, U.S.A.) ($p = 0.57$ by log-rank), but an association was demonstrated with SMART® stents (Johnson & Johnson, Cordis Division, Miami, Florida, U.S.A.) ($p = 0.008$ by log-rank). The length of the stented segment was significantly associated with fractures ($p = 0.046$). No other complications were associated with stent fractures including strut embolization, pseudoaneurysm, or bleeding. All cases were retreated by endovascular therapy or bypass surgery (24). On the contrary the ABSOLUT trial (8) produced a reasonably low stent fracture rate, only 2% with a number of 1.8 stents per patients (with a range of 1–5 stents per patient).

Severe stent fractures are therefore often associated with stent restenosis or reocclusion. If angioplasty alone does not achieve good secondary patency rates, surgical bypass is an alternative. The results of repeat stent-grafting in this situation are unclear.

TREATMENT OF POST-ANGIOPLASTY RESTENOSIS

Angioplasty (±Brachytherapy)

The traditional approach to restenosis is angioplasty. Stent implantation is generally reserved for cases with vascular recoil, dissection or post-angioplasty residual stenosis. It should be recognized that the culprit lesion is histologically and macroscopically different from the de novo lesion and angioplasty in isolation may not be sufficient. In a study of post-angioplasty restenosis (12 of 85 treated limbs), adjunctive stent placement was required in 9 of 12 cases (25).

Brachytherapy has been proposed as an adjunct to the treatment of restenosis (26), which is discussed in detail in Chapter 7.

Angioplasty vs. Stent Implantation

Schillinger et al. presented data regarding 533 consecutive patients with femoropopliteal interventions (27). A retrospective comparison was performed on data from balloon angioplasty and stent implantation in recurrent lesions. The one-year patency of stenting was significantly better than angioplasty (33% and 52%, respectively). For de novo lesions, angioplasty performed better, producing equivalence with stenting (61% compared to 58% one-year patency).

Recurrent stenosis should be treated with stent implantation rather than angioplasty in isolation. Stent implantation for restenosis has comparable patency rates as for treatment of de novo lesions.

TREATMENT OF IN-STENT RESTENOSIS

Background

Most data regarding the treatment of in-stent restenosis are from large-scale coronary studies. Until recently, angioplasty with brachytherapy was thought to be the most effective approach, but DES seem to have superior results (28–30). This is difficult to extrapolate to the situation in the lower limb.

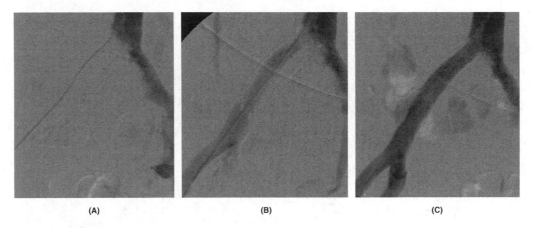

(A)   (B)   (C)

FIGURE 1 Reocclusion of a Palmaz stent in the common iliac artery (**A**) implanted 2 years ago. Repeat angioplasty is not sufficient to achieve a good result (**B**). Another balloon-expandable stent has to be implanted to achieve a good result (**C**).

Iliac Stent Restenosis

Meta-analyses have demonstrated that stent implantation increases patency following iliac intervention (31–33). The Dutch Iliac Stent trial (34–36) compared routine stenting with angioplasty and selective stenting, using the balloon-expandable Palmaz stent. In the stenting group, 33 of 187 (18%) iliac procedures required reintervention over two years.

Self-expanding stents demonstrate superior results. In a retrospective analysis by Vorwerk et al. 26 of 212 patients developed restenosis or reocclusion after iliac Wallstent placement (37). When analyzing stent restenosis ($n=10$), angioplasty was sufficient in nine patients, one requiring a further stent. In cases of occlusion ($n=16$), additional stent placement was necessary in 10 patients. Angioplasty therefore seems sufficient for the treatment of in-stent restenosis but stent occlusion often requires restenting or surgery. Figure 1 demonstrates the failure of angioplasty alone to treat an iliac stent reocclusion 24 months after initial stent implantation. A balloon-expandable stent had to be implanted in the right common iliac artery.

Femoropopliteal Stent Restenosis

Balloon-expandable stents have been used in short lesions of the femoropopliteal arteries in randomized studies (38–41). Results are similar to angioplasty and, according to the TASC recommendations, stents should be reserved for failed PTA (38).

The advent of nitinol stents has changed the approach to long infra-inguinal lesions, which may now be treated with either primary or secondary stent implantation. Nitinol stent placement in iliac and femoral arteries was studied by Henry et al. Restenosis and occlusion occurred mainly in the femoral artery. Over a mean follow-up of 16 months, 64 (16%) developed one or more restenoses (total 79 stenoses), 40 in the first six months. These 79 were treated by angioplasty ($n=41$), surgery ($n=25$), or conservative management ($n=13$) (42).

In a prospective study by Schillinger et al. (8) nitinol stents were used for the treatment of long femoropopliteal lesions (mean lesion length 101 mm), predominantly stenoses. Reintervention following nitinol stent placement was required in 14 of 49 cases, 10 by angioplasty alone, 1 with further stent, and 3 with surgery due to length of occlusion.

Restenosis after short- and long-segment stent implantation in the femoropopliteal arteries are again successfully treated by angioplasty alone. This is illustrated in Figure 2 and Figure 3. Angioplasty alone was sufficient to achieve secondary patency without residual stenosis. Stent implantation is necessary only in a minority of patients.

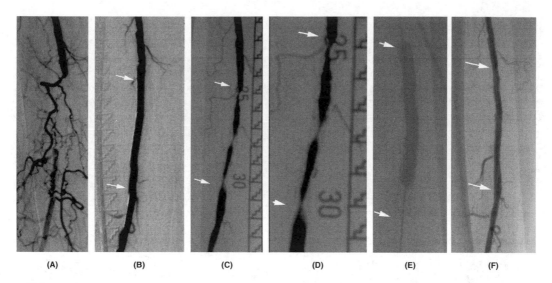

FIGURE 2 Recanalization of a short femoropopliteal occlusion (**A**) with optimal results after implantation of 2 Palmaz stents (**B**). Development of 3 high-grade restenosis (**C**) on the proximal portion, the overlapping portion and the distal portion of the 2 Palmaz stents (**D**, magnification). Angioplasty was able to achieve a good result without residual stenosis (**E,F**). The proximal and distal portion of the Palmaz stents are denoted by arrows.

CUTTING BALLOON

In treating coronary stents, the cutting balloon (Boston Scientific) appears to produce better results than standard angioplasty for in-stent restenosis. Luminal enlargement occurs mainly by in-stent tissue reduction associated with only a moderate degree of stent expansion (43). The latter is probably due to the low pressure of the cutting balloon (recommended balloon pressure <10 atm). Further work has demonstrated plaque compression or shift rather than vessel expansion (44). After cutting balloon angioplasty, there was an increase in mean lumen area and a significant decrease in mean intimal hyperplasia area. This was primarily the result of the neointimal hyperplasia extruding through the stent struts as well as some longitudinal redistribution of the neointimal hyperplasia into the contiguous reference segments (45,46). This mechanism may minimize injury to the intimal membrane and prevent restenosis. Cutting balloon angioplasty therefore seems at least as effective as angioplasty ± brachytherapy, or atherectomy (47) for patients with predominantly diffuse native vessel in-stent restenosis (48).

Additionally cutting balloon angioplasty has been used successfully for the treatment of carotid or renal artery restenosis (49,50). These lesions are often difficult to treat. A short angioplasty balloon tends to move distally or proximally in these smooth lesions, and long balloons are easy to dilate but tend to increase vessel trauma.

There are currently no published data regarding use in lower limb restenosis. M. Schillinger (private communication) had randomized 39 patients to cutting balloon angioplasty and standard balloon angioplasty of long in-stent restenosis. Secondary patency rates were 65% after CBA versus 73% for standard angioplasty at 6 month follow-up. So the cutting balloon does not seem to have a definite advantage in the treatment of long in-stent restenosis. Long-term follow-up data are pending. The cutting balloon may be a useful modality for the treatment of in-stent restenosis (as demonstrated by Figure 4), but published data are required.

CRYOPLASTY

The cryoplasty (Boston Scientific) technique was designed to address the pitfalls of angioplasty, in particular dissection, recoil, and restenosis. This technique utilizes nitrous oxide to produce

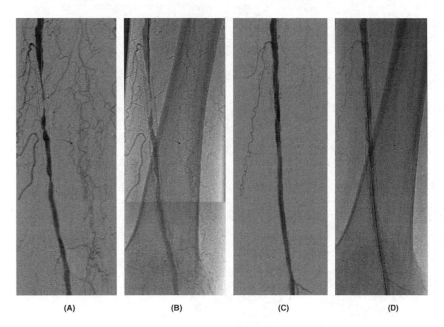

(A)   (B)   (C)   (D)

FIGURE 3 Recanalization of a nitinol stent with high-grade restenosis (**A,B**) one year after recanalization of a 7 cm occlusion. Repeat angioplasty is able to achieve a good result (**C**) but unsubtracted images (**D**) demonstrate presence of neointima, although there is no relevant residual stenosis.

low temperatures, in combination with the dilation force of balloon angioplasty (see chap. 7) (51,52).

In a registry, 11 patients from a series of 70 cases developed restenosis, and all were treated by angioplasty (53). Interestingly the overall rate of bailout stent implantation was only 8.8% and none of the stent-treated patients experienced restenosis at nine months. It could be suggested that cryoplasty creates a favorable basis for stent implantation. The data obtained from this registry provide only short-to-midterm results, and a long-term follow-up is required to assess the enduring impact of cryoplasty (54). In a recent publication by Karthik et al. (55), the role of cryoplasty for the treatment of iliofemoral restenosis was examined. In 12 lesions (which had one to four episodes of restenosis after initial endovascular treatment), technical success was achieved in all lesions, unfortunately the restenosis rate was 100% after 6 month follow-up. This is definitely not a large patient cohort but one can estimate the potential of cryoplasty for the treatment of restenosis. The potential role of cryoplasty for in-stent restenosis has so far not been examined systematically.

DRUG-ELUTING STENTS

No data are currently available regarding the treatment of recurrent stenosis with DES in the peripheral arteries. DES performed only slightly better than standard nitinol stents in randomized trials for primary disease (56), and treatment of restenosis might be an interesting area for further evaluation.

ATHERECTOMY

Plaque or neointima removal is the most appealing idea for the treatment of restenosis. Instead of compressing or crushing the material into wall removal would have its benefits. Yet after treatment, the healing process is started and this process has the side-effect of creating a stimulatory effect on cells which remained in the vessel wall. One of the earliest systems available was the Simpson Atherocath® (DVI, Redwood City, California, U.S.A.). Data are available for the directional Simpson atherectomy catheter™. In a retrospective evaluation of

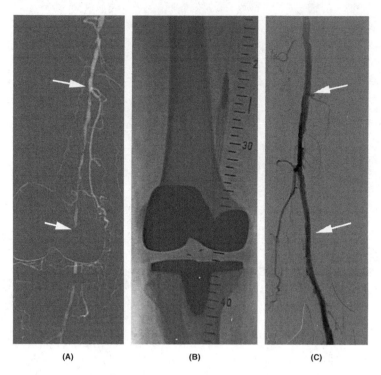

(A)   (B)   (C)

FIGURE 4   Restenosis (**A**) 9 months after recanalization of an occlusion. One pass with a 1 cm long cutting balloon (**B**) is able to achieve a good result (**C**).

directional atherectomy, post-angioplasty restenosis has been successfully treated. The atherectomy specimen obtained during treatment showed a mixture of cell-rich intima (50%), acellular matrix (30%), thrombotic material and elastic fibers (44%) (Fig. 4) (57).

Follow-up data for the treatment of post-angioplasty restenoses are also available for the Redha-Cut® (Sherine Med, Utzendorf, Switzerland) directional atherectomy system. One-year patency rates were poor for restenoses (41% compared to 66% for de novo lesions) (6). Neither of these devices are now available. The Auth Rotablator® (Boston Scientific, Watertown, Massachusetts, U.S.A.) rotational atherectomy system is still available but has rarely been used in peripheral arteries.

The Food and Drug Administration–approved FoxHollow SilverHawk® (FoxHollow, Redwood, California, U.S.A.) device is available, with two series published by the same group (58,60). In their initial report six in-stent restenosis were treated with technical success. In a six-month follow-up study of 27 native vessel restenosis and 14 in-stent restenosis (mean length 40 and 77 mm, respectively), additional angioplasty was performed in 60% of cases. Prior to angioplasty or stent, atherectomy reduced stenosis diameter from 80% to 22% (after 7 passes) and 87% to 31% (after 10 passes), corresponding to mean lumen diameters of 3.8 and 3.3 mm, respectively. The mean lumen diameter increased from 0.8 mm (for both restenosis and in-stent restenosis) to 4.4 or 4.2 mm, respectively. At six-month follow-up, restenosis rates were 41% ($n=11$) and 36% ($n=5$), respectively. Mid-term follow-up of either de novo stenosis (group 1 = 31 limbs), post-angioplasty restenosis (group 2 = 38 limbs) or in-stent restenosis (group 3 = 31 limbs) demonstrated significantly different primary patency rates after 12 and 18 months, 84% and 73% for group 1, 54% and 42% for group 2, and 54% and 49% for group 3, respectively. TLR after 18 months were 22%, 56%, and 49% for groups 1, 2, and 3 respectively. Bypass rates were not significantly different and varied from 9.7%, 15.8% and 12.9% for groups 1, 2, and 3, respectively. On the basis of these studies, randomized trials seem warranted to assess the potential of this atherectomy device.

SUMMARY

Prevention of restenosis is still a significant problem in peripheral arterial disease. Though there are a number of options for treatment, there is little in the literature to support one technique over another. In most centers, angioplasty is available, with reasonable results. Brachytherapy is probably a worthwhile alternative in selected cases but is not available in most centers. The value of debulking atherectomy with various devices is still to be demonstrated, particularly with long-term data. Treatment of femoropopliteal in-stent restenosis as well as post-angioplasty restenosis seldom produces satisfactory secondary patency rates. Treatment of in-stent restenosis is a widely unsolved issue, though for iliac restenosis, reangioplasty produces good results, with stenting for poor technical/hemodynamic results.

REFERENCES

1. Dormandy JA, Rutherford RB, TASC Working Group. Management of peripheral arterial disease (PAD). J Vasc Surg 2000; 31:S1–296.
2. Norgren L, Hiatt WR, Dormandy JA, Nehler MR, Harris KA, Fowkes FG, Nehler MR, TASC II Working Group, Bell K, Caporusso J, et al. Inter-Society Consensus for the Management of Peripheral Arterial Disease (TASC II). Eur J Vasc Endovasc Surg 2007; 33(Suppl 1):S1–75. Epub 2006 Nov 29.
3. Muradin GS, Bosch JL, Stijnen T, Hunink MG. Balloon dilation and stent implantation for treatment of femoropopliteal arterial disease: meta-analysis. Radiology 2001; 221:137–45.
4. Dorrucci V. Treatment of superficial femoral artery occlusive disease. J Cardiovasc Surg (Torino) 2004; 45:193–201.
5. Sabeti S, Schillinger M, Amighi J, et al. Primary patency of femoropopliteal arteries treated with nitinol versus stainless steel self-expanding stents: propensity score-adjusted analysis. Radiology 2004; 232:516–21.
6. Sabeti S, Mlekusch W, Amighi J, Minar E, Schillinger M. Primary patency of long-segment self-expanding nitinol stents in the femoropopliteal arteries. J Endovasc Ther 2005; 12:6–12.
7. Krankenberg H, Schlüter M, Steinkamp HJ, et al. Nitinol stent implantation versus percutaneous transluminal angioplasty in superficial femoral artery lesions up to 10 cm in length: the femoral artery stenting trial (FAST). Circulation 2007; 116(3):285–92. Epub 2007 Jun 25.
8. Schillinger M, Sabeti S, Dick P, et al. Sustained benefit at 2 years of primary femoropopliteal stenting compared with balloon angioplasty with optional stenting. Circulation 2007; 115(21):2745–9. Epub 2007 May 14.
9. Baumgartner I, Redha F, Baumgartner RW, Do DD, Mahler F. Ultrasonic-pathologic comparison of postangioplasty myointimal hyperplasia and primary atheroma of the superficial femoral artery. Ultrasound Med Biol 1996; 22:815–21.
10. Coulden RA, Moss H, Graves MJ, Lomas DJ, Appleton DS, Weissberg PL. High resolution magnetic resonance imaging of atherosclerosis and the response to balloon angioplasty. Heart 2000; 83:188–91.
11. O'Brien ER, Urieli-Shoval S, Garvin MR, et al. Replication in restenotic atherectomy tissue. Atherosclerosis 2000; 152:117–26.
12. Soder HK, Manninen HI, Matsi PJ. Angiographic characteristics of symptomatic recurrent disease after infrainguinal percutaneous transluminal angioplasty. Cardiovasc Intervent Radiol 1999; 22:219–23.
13. Kearney M, Pieczek A, Haley L, et al. Histopathology of in-stent restenosis in patients with peripheral artery disease. Circulation 1997; 95:1998–2002.
14. George J, Goldstein E, Abashidze S, et al. Circulating endothelial progenitor cells in patients with unstable angina: association with systemic inflammation. Eur Heart J 2004; 25:1003–8.
15. Bray PJ, Robson WJ, Bray AE. Percutaneous treatment of long superficial femoral artery occlusive disease: efficacy of the Hemobahn stent-graft. J Endovasc Ther 2003; 10:619–28.
16. Fischer M, Langhoff R, Schulte KL. Hemobahn-endoprosthesis: long-term experience (< or =4 years follow-up) with percutaneous application in stenoses and occlusions of the superficial femoral artery. Zentralbl Chir 2003; 128:740–5.
17. Muller-Hulsbeck S, Schwarzenberg H, Hutzelmann A, Steffens JC, Heller M. Intravascular ultrasound evaluation of peripheral arterial stent-grafts. Invest Radiol 2000; 35:97–104.
18. Ahmadi R, Schillinger M, Maca T, Minar E. Femoropopliteal arteries: immediate and long-term results with a Dacron-covered stent-graft. Radiology 2002; 223:345–50.
19. Schwarzenberg H, Muller-Hulsbeck S, Gluer CC, Wesner F, Heller M. Restenosis of peripheral stents and stent grafts as revealed by intravascular sonography: in vivo comparison with angiography. AJR Am J Roentgenol 1998; 170:1181–5.
20. Buckley CJ, Arko FR, Lee S, et al. Intravascular ultrasound scanning improves long-term patency of iliac lesions treated with balloon angioplasty and primary stenting. J Vasc Surg 2002; 35(2):316–23.

21. Rosenfield K, Schainfeld R, Pieczek A, Haley L, Isner JM. Restenosis of endovascular stents from stent compression. J Am Coll Cardiol 1997; 29(2):328–38.
22. Arena FJ. Arterial kink and damage in normal segments of the superficial femoral and popliteal arteries abutting nitinol stents—a common cause of late occlusion and restenosis? A single-center experience. J Invasive Cardiol 2005; 17:482–6.
23. Scheinert D, Scheinert S, Sax J, et al. Prevalence and clinical impact of stent fractures after femoropopliteal stenting. J Am Coll Cardiol 2005; 45:312–5.
24. Schlager O, Dick P, Sabeti S, et al. Long-segment SFA stenting—the dark sides: in-stent restenosis, clinical deterioration, and stent fractures. J Endovasc Ther 2005; 12:676–84.
25. Karch LA, Mattos MA, Henretta JP, McLafferty RB, Ramsey DE, Hodgson KJ. Clinical failure after percutaneous transluminal angioplasty of the superficial femoral and popliteal arteries. J Vasc Surg 2000; 31:880–7.
26. Zehnder T, von Briel C, Baumgartner I, et al. Endovascular brachytherapy after percutaneous transluminal angioplasty of recurrent femoropopliteal obstructions. J Endovasc Ther 2003; 10:304–11.
27. Schillinger M, Mlekusch W, Haumer M, Sabeti S, Ahmadi R, Minar E. Angioplasty and elective stenting of de novo versus recurrent femoropopliteal lesions: 1-year follow-up. J Endovasc Ther 2003; 10:288–97.
28. Holmes DR, Jr., Teirstein P, Satler L, et al. Sirolimus-eluting stents vs vascular brachytherapy for in-stent restenosis within bare-metal stents: the SISR randomized trial. JAMA 2006; 295:1264–73.
29. Feres F, Munoz JS, Abizaid A, et al. Comparison between sirolimus-eluting stents and intracoronary catheter-based beta radiation for the treatment of in-stent restenosis. Am J Cardiol 2005; 96:1656–62.
30. Iofina E, Radke PW, Skurzewski P, et al. Superiority of sirolimus eluting stent compared with intracoronary beta radiation for treatment of in-stent restenosis: a matched comparison. Heart 2005; 91:1584–9.
31. Bosch JL, Haaring C, Meyerovitz MF, Cullen KA, Hunink MG. Cost-effectiveness of percutaneous treatment of iliac artery occlusive disease in the United States. AJR Am J Roentgenol 2000; 175:517–21.
32. Bosch JL, Hunink MG. Meta-analysis of the results of percutaneous transluminal angioplasty and stent placement for aortoiliac occlusive disease. Radiology 1997; 204:87–96.
33. Bosch JL, Tetteroo E, Mali WP, Hunink MG, Dutch Iliac Stent Trial Study Group. Iliac arterial occlusive disease: cost-effectiveness analysis of stent placement versus percutaneous transluminal angioplasty. Radiology 1998; 208:641–8.
34. Tetteroo E, van der Graaf Y, Bosch JL, et al. Randomised comparison of primary stent placement versus primary angioplasty followed by selective stent placement in patients with iliac-artery occlusive disease. Lancet 1998; 351:1153–9.
35. Klein WM, van der Graaf Y, Seegers J, et al. Dutch iliac stent trial: long-term results in patients randomized for primary or selective stent placement. Radiology 2006; 238:734–44.
36. Klein WM, van der Graaf Y, Seegers J, Moll FL, Mali WP. Long-term cardiovascular morbidity, mortality, and reintervention after endovascular treatment in patients with iliac artery disease: The Dutch Iliac Stent Trial Study. Radiology 2004; 232:491–8.
37. Vorwerk D, Guenther RW, Schurmann K, Wendt G. Late reobstruction in iliac arterial stents: percutaneous treatment. Radiology 1995; 197:479–83.
38. Cejna M, Thurnher S, Illiasch H, et al. PTA versus Palmaz stent placement in femoropopliteal artery obstructions: a multicenter prospective randomized study. J Vasc Interv Radiol 2001; 12:23–31.
39. Grenacher L, Saam T, Geier A. PTA versus Palmaz stent placement in femoropopliteal artery stenoses: results of a multicenter prospective randomized study (REFSA). Rofo 2004; 176:1302–10.
40. Grimm J, Muller-Hulsbeck S, Jahnke T, Hilbert C, Brossmann J, Heller M. Randomized study to compare PTA alone versus PTA with Palmaz stent placement for femoropopliteal lesions. J Vasc Interv Radiol 2001; 12:935–42.
41. Vroegindeweij D, Vos LD, Tielbeek AV, Buth J, vd Bosch HC. Balloon angioplasty combined with primary stenting versus balloon angioplasty alone in femoropopliteal obstructions: a comparative randomized study. Cardiovasc Intervent Radiol 1997; 20:420–5.
42. Henry M, Henry I, Klonaris C, Hugel M. Clinical experience with the OptiMed sinus stent in the peripheral arteries. J Endovasc Ther 2003; 10:772–9.
43. Montorsi P, Galli S, Fabbiocchi F, et al. Mechanism of cutting balloon angioplasty for in-stent restenosis: an intravascular ultrasound study. Catheter Cardiovasc Interv 2002; 56:166–73.
44. Hara H, Nakamura M, Asahara T, Nishida T, Yamaguchi T. Intravascular ultrasonic comparisons of mechanisms of vasodilatation of cutting balloon angioplasty versus conventional balloon angioplasty. Am J Cardiol 2002; 89:1253–6.
45. Ahmed JM, Mintz GS, Castagna M, et al. Intravascular ultrasound assessment of the mechanism of lumen enlargement during cutting balloon angioplasty treatment of in-stent restenosis. Am J Cardiol 2001; 88:1032–4.
46. Muramatsu T, Tsukahara R, Ho M, et al. Efficacy of cutting balloon angioplasty for in-stent restenosis: an intravascular ultrasound evaluation. J Invasive Cardiol 2001; 13:439–44.

47. Adamian M, Colombo A, Briguori C, et al. Cutting balloon angioplasty for the treatment of in-stent restenosis: a matched comparison with rotational atherectomy, additional stent implantation and balloon angioplasty. J Am Coll Cardiol 2001; 38:672–9.
48. Schluter M, Tubler T, Lansky AJ, et al. Angiographic and clinical outcomes at 8 months of cutting balloon angioplasty and beta-brachytherapy for native vessel in-stent restenosis (BETACUT): results from a stopped randomized controlled trial. Catheter Cardiovasc Interv 2005; 66:320–6.
49. Setacci C, de Donato G, Setacci F, et al. In-stent restenosis after carotid angioplasty and stenting: a challenge for the vascular surgeon. Eur J Vasc Endovasc Surg 2005; 29:601–7.
50. Munneke GJ, Engelke C, Morgan RA, Belli AM. Cutting balloon angioplasty for resistant renal artery in-stent restenosis. J Vasc Interv Radiol 2002; 13:327–31.
51. Gage AA, Fazekas G, Riley EE, Jr. Freezing injury to large blood vessels in dogs. With comments on the effect of experimental freezing of bile ducts. Surgery 1967; 61:748–54.
52. Tatsutani KN, Joye JD, Virmani R, Taylor MJ. In vitro evaluation of vascular endothelial and smooth muscle cell survival and apoptosis in response to hypothermia and freezing. Cryo Letters 2005; 26:55–64.
53. Laird JR, Biamino G, McNamara T, et al. Cryoplasty for the treatment of femoropopliteal arterial disease: extended follow-up results. J Endovasc Ther 2006; 13(Suppl. 2):II52–59.
54. Laird J, Jaff MR, Biamino G, et al. Cryoplasty for the treatment of femoropopliteal arterial disease: results of a prospective, multicenter registry. J Vasc Interv Radiol 2005; 16:1067–73.
55. Karthik S, Tuite DJ, Nicholson AA, et al. Cryoplasty for arterial restenosis. Eur J Vasc Endovasc Surg. 2007; 33(1):40–3. Epub 2006 Aug 23.
56. Duda SH, Bosiers M, Lammer J, et al. Sirolimus-eluting versus bare nitinol stent for obstructive superficial femoral artery disease: the SIROCCO II trial. J Vasc Interv Radiol 2005; 16:331–8.
57. Gonschior P, Hofling B, Mack B, et al. Results of directional peripheral atherectomy with reference to histology, histochemistry, and ultrastructure. Angiology 1993; 44:454–63.
58. Zeller T, Rastan A, Schwarzwalder U, et al. Percutaneous peripheral atherectomy of femoropopliteal stenoses using a new-generation device: six-month results from a single-center experience. J Endovasc Ther 2004; 11:676–85.
59. Zeller T, Rastan A, Schwarzwalder U, et al. Midterm results after atherectomy-assisted angioplasty of below-knee arteries with use of the Silverhawk device. J Vasc Interv Radiol 2004; 15:1391–7.
60. Zeller T, Rastan A, Sixt S, et al. Long-term results after directional atherectomy of femoro-popliteal lesions. J Am Coll Cardiol. 2006; 48(8):1573–8. Epub 2006 Sep 26.

7 | Emerging Therapies to Counter Restenosis

Thomas Jahnke
Department of Radiology, University Clinics Schleswig-Holstein (UKSH), Campus Kiel, Kiel, Germany

INTRODUCTION

Percutaneous transluminal angioplasty (PTA) represents the mainstay of treatment for the majority of femoropopliteal lesions in patients with chronic limb ischemia. A disadvantage of the procedure is the high rate of recurrent stenosis, which usually develops 6 to 12 months after treatment (1). Initial failure in the form of elastic recoil and dissection, as well as late negative remodeling, can be addressed by the implantation of stents. During long-term follow-up, however, stent implantation has largely failed to provide superior patency rates when compared to angioplasty alone. In a recent meta-analysis of 19 studies ($\sim$1400 PTA or stent procedures) femoropopliteal PTA resulted in three-year primary patency of 30%, 48%, and 61% for occlusions with critical ischemia, occlusions with claudication, and stenoses with claudication, respectively. The use of femoropopliteal stents resulted in three-year primary patency of 63% to 66%, independent of lesion types and indication (2).

The cellular and molecular mechanisms that occur in the vessel wall after angioplasty and/or stenting lead to smooth muscle cell proliferation, migration and phenotypic change with excessive extracellular matrix synthesis (neointimal hyperplasia and restenosis). These mechanisms are more important in smaller arteries with relatively low shear stress, including the superficial femoral artery (SFA). Stent placement is often associated with a more pronounced intimal hyperplasia than PTA alone, which is in part due to radial force exerted on the artery (3–5). For the infrainguinal territory, additional factors come into play. The femoropopliteal arteries are prone to various stress forces, including torsion, compression, flexion and extension, which can lead to stent fracture (6,7). In addition, the small luminal diameter of the SFA contributes to a less favorable outcome.

Recent studies have indicated that the newer generations of self-expanding coil and mesh stents, with one- and three-year primary patencies of 85% and 70%, respectively (8,9), offer better results than anticipated from earlier trials (10–12). In a retrospective analysis comparing stainless steel balloon-expandable stents ($n = 123$) to nitinol (nickel–titanium) self-expanding stents ($n = 104$), primary patencies at six months, one year, and two years were 85%, 75%, 69% for nitinol stents, and 78%, 54%, 34% for stainless steel stents, respectively. Propensity-adjusted multivariable analysis showed that nitinol stents reduced restenosis with a hazard ratio of 0.44 ($p = 0.014$) compared with stainless steel stents (13). Despite recent advances in stent technology providing multidimensional flexibility, neointimal hyperplasia remains a concern. The purpose of this review is to provide an overview on new techniques for restenosis prevention which may revolutionize the treatment of peripheral arterial disease. Emerging treatment modalities include systemic drug treatment, administration of ionizing radiation, modern stent- and catheter-based technologies.

SYSTEMIC THERAPY

Systemic therapy has largely been investigated for coronary restenosis, but, given the similarities in pathophysiology and revascularization procedures, the results may be extrapolated to restenosis in chronic limb ischemia. The systemic treatment regimens evaluated in clinical studies have targeted the multiple factors involved in the development of restenosis. These included antiplatelet drugs, anticoagulants, statins, calcium channel blockers, angiotensin-converting enzyme (ACE) inhibitors, vitamins, and antiproliferative drugs. Though there is evidence that an adequate antiplatelet and anticoagulation protocol can enhance early results of PTA and stenting in the coronary and peripheral vasculature, the potential to prevent neointimal hyperplasia is limited, with early clinical studies demonstrating disappointing results (14,15). Systemic therapy with statins, ACE inhibitors or vitamins has generated controversial reports, ranging from beneficial outcomes to worsening of restenosis (16–20).

Tranilast is a substance with antiproliferative properties that was evaluated more extensively. In Prevention of REStenosis with Tranilast and its Outcomes (PRESTO) trial, the effect of this oral anti-inflammatory agent on major adverse cardiovascular events and angiographic end points was tested in a double-blind, placebo-controlled study in patients after percutaneous coronary intervention. The primary end point was the first occurrence of major adverse cardiovascular events within nine months, defined as death, myocardial infarction, and/or ischemia-driven target lesion revascularization (TLR). There were no differences in outcomes between the treatment and placebo groups (21).

Recently reports of pharmacotherapy after placement of coronary stents have been more optimistic. In the randomized, double-blind, placebo-controlled "Cilostazol for Restenosis Trial," patients were treated with cilostazol—a phosphodiesterase 3-inhibitor with antithrombotic and antiproliferative properties—for six months, starting immediately after implantation of stents in coronary de novo lesions. Minimal lumen diameter, determined by angiography at six months, was larger among patients treated with cilostazol than placebo (22). A further randomized study investigated the effect of a six-month treatment with the thiazolidinedione "pioglitazone," an oral antidiabetic drug with anti-restenotic properties, following bare-metal stent implantation for de novo coronary lesions. Neointima formation was significantly lower in patients treated with pioglitazone than placebo (23).

A drug repeatedly shown to counter restenosis in preclinical studies is the immunosuppressive macrolid antibiotic "rapamycin." Rapamycin is currently used to inhibit neointimal proliferation by local application using a stent-based platform. Quite recently the systemic application of rapamycin has entered into clinical studies as an adjunct to percutanous procedures. In a retrospective study analyzing a small cohort of patients with recalcitrant restenosis, systemic oral administration of rapamycin provided no benefit (24), though further randomized studies contradict this. The Oral Sirolimus to Inhibit Recurrent In-stent Stenosis (OSIRIS) and Oral Rapamycin to Prevent Restenosis in Patients Undergoing Coronary Stent Therapy showed beneficial effects in restenotic and de novo lesions, respectively (25,26). The OSIRIS study was a randomized, double-blind, placebo-controlled trial for the evaluation of adjunctive sirolimus treatment with an intensified loading dose before coronary intervention. This trial demonstrated a significant improvement in angiographic restenosis in the treatment group. This trial supports a concept of pretreatment, higher loading doses, and shorter treatment times for patients with in-stent restenosis (25). The Oral Rapamune to Inhibit Restenosis trial evaluated safety and feasibility of oral rapamycin in achieving low rates of repeat TLR in de novo coronary lesions. Lower rates of, and delayed, restenosis were observed in two dosing strategies without a dose–response dependency (27). As dose levels and duration of treatment did not affect restenosis, the early loading dose was considered as pivotal, supporting results from previous experimental work (28,29). Regardless of the promising results achieved with systemic application of antiproliferative agents, many questions need to be addressed to define the future value of this approach. Apart from the choice of agent, other factors which may affect restenosis include timing of initiation of therapy, dosage, and duration of treatment.

RADIATION THERAPY

Brachytherapy

Vascular brachytherapy refers to the local application of ionizing radiation directly to the vessel wall by temporary placement of a sealed radioactive source, a beta- (P-32, Y-90 and Sr-90) or gamma-emitter (Ir-192), through a delivery catheter. The major advantage of brachytherapy over external beam therapy is a rapid reduction or "fall-off" in radiation dose beyond the target volume, minimizing toxicity to adjacent tissues. The cellular and molecular mechanisms by which radiation inhibits restenosis are still under investigation. In vitro and animal studies point to several processes, including target cell killing and inactivation, decreased extracellular matrix synthesis, impairment of cellular migration, and inhibition of unfavorable vascular remodeling (30). Catheter-based endovascular delivery of beta- and gamma-radiation has been shown to reduce neointimal formation in animal models (31–34) and in patients with coronary artery disease (35,36). Although most research has concentrated on coronary restenosis, vascular brachytherapy may be beneficial in peripheral vascular disease. Iridium-192 is preferable and has been studied most widely for peripheral intervention, because gamma particles have a greater penetrating capability and can pass through larger vessels with adequate levels of radioactivity. A series of clinical studies—the "Vienna trials"—showed that peripheral brachytherapy reduced restenosis rates after femoropopliteal angioplasty of recurrent, but not de novo lesions (37). In a prospective randomized-controlled trial with centered endovascular gamma irradiation of de novo femoropopliteal lesions, the degree of restenosis was significantly reduced at 6, 12, and 24 months (38). The pilot phase of the Peripheral Artery Radiation Investigational study yielded promising results (39), but clinical and angiographic end points were not assessed (40). The latest of the "Vienna trial" series (Vienna-5 study) evaluated the effectiveness of endovascular gamma irradiation after femoropopliteal stent implantation in high-risk patients. This demonstrated a high incidence of early and late thrombotic occlusions, suggesting a limited role for brachytherapy after stent implantation (41).

Despite clinical studies suggesting that brachytherapy prevents restenosis after femoropopliteal angioplasty (42–44), this technique has not been adopted in routine clinical practice. In addition to the risks of edge effect, catch-up late restenosis, and late aneurysm formation are major drawbacks. Large delivery systems are required (8–9-F), and patients have to be transported to a secondary location with the catheter in position, risking thrombosis at the treatment site. Recent reports indicate that there might be a place for external beam radiation, which is easier to administer. In a randomized study, patients were assigned to placebo or different doses of external beam radiation in a single session 24 hours after femoropopliteal PTA. External beam radiation of 14 Gy of the femoropopliteal angioplasty site significantly reduced restenosis at one year (45).

Radioactive Stents

Beta- and gamma-emitting stents are conventional metal stents made radioactive by direct coating with radioisotope, activation by nuclear bombardment, or ion implantation. Studies in rabbit iliac arteries and porcine coronary arteries demonstrate that implantation of beta-particle-emitting stents inhibits intrastent neointimal cell proliferation (46,47). The safety and feasibility of ^{32}P radioactive beta-emitting stents has been assessed in patients with symptomatic de novo or restenotic coronary lesions. The Insulin Resistance Intervention after Stroke trials, using low-to-intermediate activity stents, showed that the devices can be implanted safely with a high short-term success rate. However, coronary angiography at six-months revealed restenosis within and at the edges of the stent of up to 40% (48). Subsequently, the Milan Dose–Response study, evaluated the safety and efficacy of higher dose ^{32}P radioactive beta-emitting stents. At six months, intrastent neointimal hyperplasia was reduced in a dose-related manner, but there was a high rate of restenosis at the stent edges in all groups. This was explained by low radiation activity at the edges of the stent, referred to as "edge effect" or "candy wrapper" (49). The notion that a further increase of activity in combination with reduced balloon injury outside the stent would reduce edge restenosis has not been confirmed (50). More recently, quite promising physical properties of Re-188-labeled stents were reported in an animal study, suggesting that the problem of edge effect might be addressed by identifying the optimal radioisotope (51).

STENT-BASED TECHNOLOGY

Biodegradable Stents

Stents provide a mechanical scaffolding which eliminates vessel recoil after angioplasty, but the associated long-term radial force is disadvantageous, leading to exaggerated tissue proliferation and in-stent stenosis. Stents composed of a bioabsorbable/biodegradable material could be an alternative, providing short-term vessel scaffolding, but avoiding potential long-term complications (52,53). Absorbable stents made from polymers have been used clinically in the coronary circulation (54). An important drawback is that biodegradable stents do not exert as much radial force as metal stents, limiting the prevention of recoil and negative remodeling. Degradable stents made of a magnesium alloy with a slow degradation rate represent a recent alternative. These devices provide a radial force comparable to conventional metal stents (55). In a clinical study, 20 patients with critical limb ischemia of Rutherford class 4 and 5 and below-knee lesions were treated with magnesium stents. Primary patency at three months was 89.5% with limb salvage of 100%. Although the long-term outcome remains unclear, this initial clinical experience is promising (56).

Passive Stent Coatings

Garasic and co-workers have postulated that stent design significantly affects the restenosis rate (57). Recognized variables include the number and/or thickness of struts and differences in the angular burden of the stent in cross section (58,59). However, given that sufficient scaffolding is crucial to prevent recoil and negative remodeling, variations of design are somewhat limited. More recent work has focussed on surface characteristics of stents which might influence biocompatibility and restenosis (60).

Inert coatings, like chromium, titanium, platinum and gold were thought to prevent corrosion, enhance biocompatibility and improve long-term outcome (61). Gold, however, yielded poor clinical results for reasons that are not entirely clear (62,63). Other passive stent coatings thought to enhance patency included ceramics and polymers (64), but polymer coatings seem to induce a proliferative inflammatory response, which would limit long-term patency (65,66). Modern polymers are more thromboresistant, produce less inflammation and reduce late in-stent stenosis in animal models (67). Carbon coating of coronary stents has proved to generate a low restenosis rate (11%) in clinical studies (68). In a recent pilot trial, the primary success and short-term patency of carbofilm-coated stents were evaluated for high-grade infrapopliteal lesions and seem to be better than PTA alone (69). The future role of carbon coating will be determined by an ongoing international randomized multicenter trial.

Active Stent Coatings

The material and surface patterns of stents play an important role in activating platelets and triggering adherence of inflammatory cells (70). As outlined previously, inert coatings are thought to reduce thrombogenicity and/or minimize the inflammatory reaction. Active stent coatings on the other hand aim to directly prevent smooth muscle cell proliferation and consequent restenosis. Active stent coatings include radioisotopes, antithrombogenic or antiproliferative drugs and/or gene carrying vectors.

Delivery of drugs using a stent-based platform has the advantage of higher local concentrations potentiating the desired action of the agent, without provoking systemic side effects, and has been shown to reduce in-stent neointimal hyperplasia. Randomized clinical safety and feasibility trials with sirolimus (rapamycin)- and paclitaxel-eluting stents have shown promising results, preventing restenosis in de novo coronary lesions and within stents (71,72). Rapamycin is produced by *Streptomyces hygroscopicus*, originally isolated from soil collected from Easter Island (73,74). It acts by binding to the FK-binding protein 12 (FKBP12) and a serine threonine kinase, mammalian target of rapamycin, to inhibit cytokine signals relevant to induction of proliferation of fibroblasts and smooth muscle cells (75). In a randomized study comparing paclitaxel and rapamycin-eluting stents in small coronary vessels, rapamycin-eluting stents were more effective and associated with a lower late of luminal loss (76). The only published study in the peripheral vasculature is the SIROlimus-coated Cordis Self-expandable Stent (SIROCCO) trial. The first part of this mutlicenter study (SIROCCO I) evaluated rapamycin-eluting nitinol shape memory alloy recoverable technology stents in the SFA with quite promising, though nonsignificant, results (0% in-stent and in-segment restenosis versus 18% and 24% in the control group, respectively) (77). Recently, the extended trial results became available (SIROCCO II) and, again, statistical significance was not achieved for any of the preselected end points (78). In addition to theoretical limitations of drug-eluting stents including aneurysm development, edge effect, thrombosis, and stent malapposition, it has been suggested that healing responses in humans might be merely delayed (79,80). Work has clearly shown that the drug-carrying polymer is capable of inducing a proliferative inflammatory response once the active metabolite is lost (81,82). However, the most serious concern is cost particularly for diffuse infrainguinal disease which may require multiple stents.

CATHETER-BASED TECHNOLOGY

Sonotherapy

Cell culture studies in a swine stent-injury model have shown that low-frequency, noncavitational ultrasound may have an impact on smooth muscle cell migration, adhesion and proliferation (83). Seven days after stent implantation, cellular proliferation was significantly reduced when compared to a control group (84). The mechanism of the effect of ultrasound on the vessel wall, the optimal power and duration of administration are unclear. Regar and colleagues have evaluated the effect of sonotherapy on coronary vessels six months after treatment. Sonotherapy was applied in de novo lesion, restenosis or in-stent restenosis in 37 patients using a 5 Fr catheter with three serial ultrasound transducers operating at 1 MHz (85). There was high acute procedural success without major adverse events but late lumen loss and neointimal growth were similar to conventional coronary angioplasty. This prompted a randomized clinical study, the "EUROpean Sonotherapy Prevention of Arterial Hyperplasia" (EURO-SPAH). EURO-SPAH was a multicenter, double-blind, randomized study investigating the efficacy of sonotherapy to reduce in-stent late lumen loss. Four hundred and three patients with multiple first-time stented lesions were randomized to receive sonotherapy or sham. Though the prevention of late stent loss was not achieved, the study emphasized the feasibility and safety of sonotherapy (86). There are currently no clinical data for the effect in the peripheral vasculature.

Photodynamic Therapy

Photodynamic therapy involves the interaction of a photosensitizing drug, light, and tissue oxygen (87). Photosensitizing agents, such as porphyrins, can be administered locally or systemically. At therapeutic concentrations, most photosensitizers have no side effects. Activity requires the local application of light at a wavelength matching the absorption characteristics of the sensitizer, usually from a laser at a power with no significant thermal effects. The timing of light delivery is crucial for achieving the desired response, and varies with the pharmacokinetics of the specific sensitizer. When activated, the agent generates a highly reactive form of oxygen (singlet oxygen) that initiates apoptosis in vascular smooth muscle cells (88). Photodynamic therapy has been demonstrated to inhibit restenosis in several preclinical models (89,90). In a small clinical study, photodynamic therapy was assessed in patients who developed restenosis within six months of angioplasty for SFA disease. Patients were injected with a photosensitizing agent, 5-aminolaevulinic acid, and angioplasty was performed four to six hours later. Immediately following angioplasty, a special fiberoptic catheter was inserted and light was applied to the treated site. There were no immediate complications, and after a mean follow-up of 48 months, only one of the eight lesions developed symptomatic restenosis (91). More recently, photodynamic therapy was assessed in the prevention of restenosis after coronary-stent placement. By 18 months there were no adverse events nor in-stent restenoses and the authors concluded that photodynamic therapy was safe and potentially valuable in preventing in-stent restenosis (92). To date, larger randomized trials are lacking, and there are insufficient data to determine the potential of this technique or compare it with current endovascular procedures.

Cryoplasty

Cryoplasty refers to the combination of conventional balloon dilatation with simultaneous cooling of the target lesion. Cold thermal energy is applied to the vessel by inflating a balloon with nitrous oxide. The liquid nitrous oxide converts to gas on entering the balloon; dilates the vessel and causes an endothermal reaction with a heat sink of $-10°C$. The mechanical principle differs little from conventional angioplasty, but freezing the artery is thought to change the biologic response, resulting in a more benign healing process (93). Cryoplasty produces three effects:

1. A uniform, controlled stretching of the vessel due to the change of plaque microstructure.
2. Freeze-induced alteration of the morphology of collagen and elastin fibers, with short-term loss of vessel elasticity.
3. Apoptosis of vascular smooth muscle cells and reduction of neointima formation (93–95).

Following encouraging results in early clinical reports, a recently published prospective, nonrandomized multicenter registry (94) evaluated the efficacy of cryoplasty for the treatment of femoropopliteal occlusive disease. Primary end points were technical success and freedom from TLR at nine months (clinical patency). Secondary end points were adverse events and nine-month primary patency. In a cohort of 102 patients, no device-related adverse events were recorded. The initial technical success was high (85.3%) with a low rate of balloon-mediated dissection (6.9%). The overall procedural success including "bailout" stenting was 94.1%. For all lesion types, the nine-month clinical and primary patency rates based on ultrasound were 82.2%, and 70.1%, respectively, comparable to previous smaller studies (96). Overall, cryoplasty appears safe and the alteration of the biologic response to angioplasty might enhance long-term outcomes. However, more work is needed to determine the future role of cryoplasty in comparison with current techniques.

Balloon Coating

While drug-eluting stents have shown promising results in clinical trials, non-stent-based local delivery of antiproliferative drugs may offer additional flexibility and reach areas beyond immediate stent coverage. In a study of balloon angioplasty in rabbit carotid arteries the local delivery of paclitaxel using a porous balloon catheter prevented neointimal thickening (97), though in clinical practice these devices did not prove beneficial and concerns were raised about the infusion pressure inducing vessel trauma. This, and the fact that low concentrations of intramural drug were achieved, were defined as factors diminishing the clinical potential of the procedure (98,99).

Recently the concept of local balloon-based drug delivery was revisited in a study by Scheller et al. who compared conventional uncoated and paclitaxel-coated angioplasty balloons in a porcine model of coronary stenting (100). The paclitaxel coating facilitated a dose-dependent reduction of in-stent restenosis. Despite a marked reduction in neointimal proliferation, endothelialization of stent struts was present in all samples and there was no evidence of a significant inflammatory response in the proximity of the stent struts (100). These promising data have recently been confirmed by a randomized, double-blinded German multicenter trial to test the efficacy and tolerance of paclitaxel-eluting balloon catheters in coronary in-stent restenosis (101). From another multicenter study the first results on the use of paclitaxel-coated angioplasty balloons in the peripheral arteries were reported. Early data showed that after six months the drug-coated balloons were significantly more effective than the non-coated balloons at preventing restenosis. There were no serious adverse events ascribed to the drug coating (102). As was emphasized by the investigator, the rationale for coating a balloon with an antiproliferative drug is that the technique allows more of the active substance to come into contact with the vessel wall, since in coated stents the drug is restricted to the area of the stent struts. As a consequence, tissue that is near the struts receives more of the drug than the surrounding tissue. Although paclitaxel-coated balloons are thought to deliver the drug to the vessel wall immediately, and in one dose, early animal research suggests that the effect persists in spite of rapidly decreasing drug concentration.

The currently emerging data on local drug delivery with balloon coating portray a promising new concept, which might have the potential to change the cellular response to balloon angioplasty, and result in a reduction of neointimal hyperplasia and restenosis. Further clinical studies are warranted to show if the success of this procedures can be extended to the long term.

REFERENCES

1. Jeans WD, Amstrong S, Cole SEA. Fate of patients undergoing transluminal angioplasty for lower-limb ischemia. Radiology 1990; 177:559–64.
2. Muradin GS, Bosch JL, Stijnen T, Hunink MG. Balloon dilation and stent implantation for treatment of femoropopliteal arterial disease: meta-analysis. Radiology 2001; 221:137–45.
3. Kearney M, Pieczek A, Haley L. Histopathology of in-stent restenosis in patients with peripheral artery disease. Circulation 1997; 95:1998–2002.
4. Barth KH, Virmani R, Froelich J. Paired comparison of vascular wall reactions to Palmaz stents, Strecker tantalum stents, and Wallstents in canine iliac and femoral arteries. Circulation 1996; 93:2161–9.
5. Cejna M, Thurnher S, Illiasch H, et al. PTA versus Palmaz stent placement in femoropopliteal artery obstructions: a multicenter prospective randomized study. J Vasc Interv Radiol 2001; 12:23–31.
6. Rosenfield K, Schainfeld R, Pieczek A, Haley L, Isner JM. Restenosis of endovascular stents from stent compression. J Am Coll Cardiol 1997; 29:328–38.
7. Allie D, Hebert C, Walker C. Nitinol stent fractures in the SFA. Endovasc Today 2004; 3:1–8.
8. Jahnke T, Voshage G, Muller-Hulsbeck S, Grimm J, Heller M, Brossmann J. Endovascular placement of self-expanding nitinol coil stents for the treatment of femoropopliteal obstructive disease. J Vasc Interv Radiol 2002; 13:257–66.
9. Vogel TR, Shindelman LE, Nackman GB, Graham AM. Efficacious use of nitinol stents in the femoral and popliteal arteries. J Vasc Surg 2003; 38:1178–84.
10. Lugmayr HF, Holzer H, Kastner M, Riedelsberger H, Auterith A. Treatment of complex arteriosclerotic lesions with nitinol stents in the superficial femoral and popliteal arteries: a midterm follow-up. Radiology 2002; 222:37–43.
11. Henry M, Henry I, Klonaris C, Hugel M. Clinical experience with the OptiMed sinus stent in the peripheral arteries. J Endovasc Ther 2003; 10:772–9.
12. Mewissen MW. Self-expanding nitinol stents in the femoropopliteal segment: technique and midterm results. Tech Vasc Interv Radiol 2004; 7:2–5.
13. Sabeti S, Schillinger M, Amighi J, et al. Primary patency of femoropopliteal arteries treated with nitinol versus stainless steel self-expanding stents: propensity score-adjusted analysis. Radiology 2004; 232:516–21.
14. Faxon DP. Effect of high dose angiotensin-converting enzyme inhibition on restenosis: final results of the MARCATOR Study, a multicenter, double-blind, placebo-controlled trial of cilazapril. The Multicenter American Research Trial With Cilazapril After Angioplasty to Prevent Transluminal Coronary Obstruction and Restenosis (MARCATOR) Study Group. J Am Coll Cardiol 1995; 25(2):362–9.
15. Kastrati A, Schuhlen H, Hausleiter J, et al. Restenosis after coronary stent placement and randomization to a 4-week combined antiplatelet or anticoagulant therapy: six-month angiographic follow-up of the Intracoronary Stenting and Antithrombotic Regimen (ISAR) Trial. Circulation 1997; 96(2):462–7.
16. Serruys PW, Foley DP, Hofling B, Puel J, Glogar HD, Seabra-Gomes R, Goicolea J, Coste P, Rutsch W, Katus H, et al. Carvedilol for prevention of restenosis after directional coronary atherectomy: final results of the European carvedilol atherectomy restenosis (EUROCARE) trial. Circulation 2000; 101(13):1512–8.
17. Bertrand ME, McFadden EP, Fruchart JC, et al. Effect of pravastatin on angiographic restenosis after coronary balloon angioplasty. The PREDICT Trial Investigators. Prevention of Restenosis by Elisor after Transluminal Coronary Angioplasty. J Am Coll Cardiol 1997; 30(4):863–9.
18. Boccuzzi SJ, Weintraub WS, Kosinski AS, Roehm JB, Klein JL. Aggressive lipid lowering in postcoronary angioplasty patients with elevated cholesterol (the lovastatin restenosis trial). Am J Cardiol 1998; 81(5):632–6.

19. Kondo J, Sone T, Tsuboi H, et al. Effect of quinapril on intimal hyperplasia after coronary stenting as assessed by intravascular ultrasound. Am J Cardiol 2001; 87:443–5.

20. Ribichini F, Wijns W, Ferrero V, et al. Effect of angiotensin-converting enzyme inhibition on restenosis after coronary stenting. Am J Cardiol 2003; 91(2):154–8.

21. Holmes DR, Jr., Savage M, LaBlanche JM, Grip L, Serruys PW, Fitzgerald P, Fischman D, Goldberg S, Brinker JA, Zeiher AM, et al. Results of Prevention of REStenosis with Tranilast and its Outcomes (PRESTO) trial. Circulation 2002; 106(10):1243–50.

22. Douglas JS, Jr., Holmes DR, Jr., Kereiakes DJ, et al. Coronary stent restenosis in patients treated with cilostazol. Circulation 2005; 112(18):2826–32.

23. Marx N, Wohrle J, Nusser T, et al. Pioglitazone reduces neointima volume after coronary stent implantation: a randomized, placebo-controlled, double-blind trial in nondiabetic patients. Circulation 2005; 112(18):2792–8.

24. Brara PS, Moussavian M, Grise MA, et al. Pilot trial of oral rapamycin for recalcitrant restenosis. Circulation 2003; 107(13):1722–4 (Erratum in: Circulation 2003; 108(17):2170).

25. Hausleiter J, Kastrati A, Mehilli J, et al. Randomized, double-blind, placebo-controlled trial of oral sirolimus for restenosis prevention in patients with in-stent restenosis. The Oral Sirolimus to Inhibit Recurrent In-stent Stenosis (OSIRIS) trial. Circulation 2004; 110:790–5.

26. Rodriguez AE, Alemparte MR, Vigo CF, et al. Pilot study of oral rapamycin to prevent restenosis in patients undergoing coronary stent therapy: Argentina Single-Center Study (ORAR Trial). J Invasive Cardiol 2003; 15(10):581–4.

27. Waksman R, Ajani AE, Pichard AD, et al. Oral rapamycin to inhibit restenosis after stenting of de novo coronary lesions: the Oral Rapamune to Inhibit Restenosis (ORBIT) study. J Am Coll Cardiol 2004; 44(7):1386–92.

28. Uchimura N, Perera GB, Fujitani RM, et al. Dose-dependent inhibition of myointimal hyperplasia by orally administered rapamycin. Ann Vasc Surg 2004; 18(2):172–7.

29. Jahnke T, Schäfer F, Bolte H, et al. Short-term sirolimus for inhibition of neotintima formation after ballon-mediated vessel injury in rats: is there a window of opportunity for systemic prophylaxis of restenosis? J Endovasc Ther 2005; 12(3):332–42.

30. Diamond DA, Vesely TM. The role of radiation therapy in the management of vascular restenosis. Part I. Biologic basis. J Vasc Interv Radiol 1998; 9(2):199–208.

31. Wiedermann JG, Marboe C, Amols H, Schwartz A, Weinberger J. Intracoronary irradiation markedly reduces restenosis after balloon angioplasty in a porcine model. J Am Coll Cardiol 1994; 23:1491–8.

32. Waksman R, Robinson KA, Crocker IR, Gravanis MB, Cipolla GD, King SB. Endovascular low-dose irradiation inhibits neointima formation after coronary artery balloon injury in swine: a possible role for radiation therapy in restenosis prevention. Circulation 1995; 91:1533–9.

33. Weinberger J, Amols H, Ennis RD, Schwartz A, Wiedermann JG, Marboe C. Intracoronary irradiation: dose response for the prevention of restenosis in swine. Int J Radiat Oncol Biol Phys 1996; 36:767–75.

34. Mazur W, Ali MN, Khan MM, et al. High dose rate intracoronary radiation for inhibition of neointimal formation in the stented and balloon-injured porcine models of restenosis: angiographic, morphometric, and histopathologic analyses. Int J Radiat Oncol Biol Phys 1996; 36:777–88.

35. Teirstein PS, Massullo V, Jani S, et al. Catheter-based radiotherapy to inhibit restenosis after coronary stenting. N Engl J Med 1997; 336:1697–703.

36. King SB, III, Williams DO, Chougule P, et al. Endovascular beta-radiation to reduce restenosis after coronary balloon angioplasty: results of the beta energy restenosis trial (BERT). Circulation 1998; 97:2025–30.

37. Wolfram RM, Budinsky AC, Pokrajac B, Potter R, Minar E. Endovascular brachytherapy: restenosis in de novo versus recurrent lesions of femoropopliteal artery—the Vienna experience. Radiology 2005; 236(1):338–42.

38. Krueger K, Zaehringer M, Bendel M, et al. De novo femoropopliteal stenoses: endovascular gamma irradiation following angioplasty–angiographic and clinical follow-up in a prospective randomized controlled trial. Radiology 2004; 231:546–54.

39. Waksman R, Laird JR, Jurkovitz CT, et al. Intravascular radiation therapy after balloon angioplasty of narrowed femoropopliteal arteries to prevent restenosis: results of the PARIS feasibility clinical trial. J Vasc Interv Radiol 2001; 12:915–21.

40. Waksman R. Results of the PARIS trial. In: 2003 Annual Transcatheter Cardiovascular Therapeutics Meeting, Washington, DC, September 2003.

41. Wolfram RM, Budinsky AC, Pokrajac B, Potter R, Minar E. Vascular brachytherapy with 192Ir after femoropopliteal stent implantation in high-risk patients: twelve-month follow-up results from the Vienna-5 trial. Radiology 2005; 236(1):343–51.

42. Gallino A, Do DD, Alerci M, Baumgartner I, Cozzi L, Segatto JM, Bernier J, Tutta P, Kellner F, Triller J, et al. The effect of probucol (P) and brachytherapy (EBVT) on restenosis after angioplasty of the femoro-popliteal arteries: a randomised multicenter trial. Circulation 2004; 108(Suppl. IV):605 (Abstract).

43. Zehnder T, von Briel C, Baumgartner I, et al. Endovascular brachytherapy after percutaneous afterpercutaneous transluminal angioplasty of recurrent femoropopliteal obstructions. J Endovasc Ther 2003; 10:304–11.

44. Pokrajac B, Potter R, Wolfram RM, et al. Endovascular brachytherapy for restenosis prevention after femoro-popliteal angioplasty: the Vienna-3 multicenter trial. Radiother Oncol 2004; 71(Suppl. 1):104.

45. Therasse E, Donath D, Lesperance J, et al. External beam radiation to prevent restenosis after superficial femoral artery balloon angioplasty. Circulation 2005; 111(24):3310–5.

46. Hehrlein C, Stintz M, Kinscherf R, et al. Pure β-particle-emitting stents inhibit neointima formation in rabbits. Circulation 1996; 93:641–5.

47. Carter AJ, Laird JR, Bailey LR, et al. Effects of endovascular radiation from a β-particle-emitting stent in a porcine coronary restenosis model: a dose–response study. Circulation 1996; 94:2364–8.

48. Fischell TA, Carter A, Foster M, Fischell RE, Fischell DR. Lessons from the feasibility radioactive (IRIS) stent trials. In: Waksman R, ed. Vascular Brachytherapy. 2nd ed. Armonk, NY: Futura Publishing Co., 1999:475–81.

49. Albiero R, Adamian M, Kobayashi N, et al. Short- and intermediate-term results of (32)P radioactive beta-emitting stent implantation in patients with coronary artery disease: The Milan Dose–Response Study. Circulation 2000; 101(1):18–26.

50. Albiero R, Colombo A. European high-activity (32)P radioactive stent experience. J Invasive Cardiol 2000; 12(8):416–21.

51. Tepe G, Dietrich T, Grafen F, et al. Reduction of intimal hyperplasia with Re-188-labeled stents in a rabbit model at 7 and 26 weeks: an experimental study. Cardiovasc Intervent Radiol 2005; 28(5):632–7.

52. Zidar J, Lincoff A, Stack R. Biodegradable stents. In: Topol EJ, ed. Textbook of Interventional Cardiology. 2nd ed. Philadelphia, PA: WB Saunders Co., 1994:787–802.

53. Colombo A, Karvouni E. Biodegradable stents: "fulfilling the mission and stepping away.". Circulation 2000; 102:371–3.

54. Tamai H, Igaki K, Kyo E, et al. Initial and 6-month results of biodegradable poly-L-lactic acid coronary stents in humans. Circulation 2000; 102(4):399–404.

55. Erne P, Schier M, Resink TJ. The road to bioabsorbable stents: reaching clinical reality? Cardiovascular Intervent Radiol 2006; 29:11–6.

56. Peeters P, Bosiers M, Verbist J, Deloose K, Heublein B. Preliminary results after application of absorbable metal stents in patients with critical limb ischemia. J Endovasc Ther 2005; 12(1):1–5.

57. Garasic J, Edelman E, Squire JC, Seifert P, Williams M, Rogers C. Stent and artery geometry determine intimal thickening independent of arterial injury. Circulation 2000; 101:812–8.

58. Kastrati A, Mehilli J, Dirschinger J, et al. Intracoronary stenting and angiographic results: strut thickness effect on restenosis outcome (ISAR-STEREO) trial. Circulation 2001; 103(23):2816–21.

59. Schulz C, Herrmann RA, Beilharz C, Pasquantonio J, Alt E. Coronary stent symmetry and vascular injury determine experimental restenosis. Heart 2000; 83(4):462–7.

60. Sprague EA, Palmaz JC. A model system to assess key vascular responses to biomaterials. J Endovasc Ther 2005; 12(5):594–604.

61. Duda S, Poerner TC, Wiesinger B, et al. Drug-eluting stents: potential applications for peripheral arterial occlusive disease. J Vasc Interv Radiol 2003; 14:291–301.

62. vom Dahl J, Haager PK, Grube E. Effects of gold coating of coronary stents on neointimal proliferation following stent implantation. Am J Cardiol 2002; 89(7):801–5.

63. Kastrati A, Schomig A, Dirschinger J, et al. Increased risk of restenosis after placement of gold-coated stents: results of a randomized trial comparing gold-coated with uncoated steel stents in patients with coronary artery disease. Circulation 2000; 101(21):2478–83.

64. Galloni M, Prunotto M, Santarelli A, Laborde F, Dibie A. Carbon-coated stents implanted in porcine iliac and renal arteries: histologic and histomorphometric study. J Vasc Interv Radiol 2003; 14:1053–61.

65. Murphy JG, Schwartz RS, Edwards WD, Camrud AR, Vlietstra RE, Holmes DR, Jr. Percutaneous polymeric stents in porcine coronary arteries: initial experience with polyethylene terephthalate stents. Circulation 1992; 86:1596–604.

66. Goodwin SC, Yoon HC, Chen G, et al. Intense inflammatory reaction to heparin polymer-coated intravascular Palmaz stents in porcine arteries compared to uncoated Palmaz stents. Cardiovasc Intervent Radiol 2003; 26:158–67.

67. Richter GM, Stampfl U, Stampfl S, et al. A new polymer concept for coating of vascular stents using PTFEP poly(bis(trifluoroethoxy)phosphazene) to reduce thrombogenicity and late in-stent stenosis. Invest Radiol 2005; 40(4):210–8.

68. Antoniucci D, Bartorelli A, Valenti R, et al. Clinical and angiographic outcome after coronary arterial stenting with the carbostent. Am J Cardiol 2000; 85:821–5.

69. Rand T, Basile A, Cejna M, et al. PTA versus carbofilm-coated stents in infrapopliteal arteries: pilot study. Cardiovasc Intervent Radiol 2006; 29(1):29–38.

70. Tepe G, Schmehl J, Wendel HP, et al. Reduced thrombogenicity of nitinol stents—in vitro evaluation of different surface modifications and coatings. Biomaterials 2006; 27(4):643–50.
71. Liistro F, Stankovic G, Di Mario C, et al. First clinical experience with a paclitaxel derivate-eluting polymer stent system implantation for in-stent restenosis: immediate and long-term clinical and angiographic outcome. Circulation 2002; 105(16):1883–6.
72. Moses JW, Leon MB, Popma JJ, et al. Sirolimus-eluting stents versus standard stents in patients with stenosis in a native coronary artery. N Engl J Med 2003; 349(14):1315–23.
73. Vezina C, Kudelski A, Sehgal SN. Rapamycin (AY-22,989), a new antifungal antibiotic. I. Taxonomy of the producing streptomycete and isolation of the active principle. J Antibiot (Tokyo) 1975; 28(10):721–6.
74. Sehgal SN, Baker H, Vezina C. Rapamycin (AY-22,989), a new antifungal antibiotic. II. Fermentation, isolation and characterization. J Antibiot (Tokyo) 1975; 28(10):727–32.
75. Sehgal SN. Rapamune (RAPA, rapamycin, sirolimus): mechanism of action immunosuppressive effect results from blockade of signal transduction and inhibition of cell cycle progression. Clin Biochem 1998; 31(5):335–40.
76. Mehilli J, Dibra A, Kastrati A, et al. Randomized trial of paclitaxel- and sirolimus-eluting stents in small coronary vessels. Eur Heart J 2006; 27(3):260–6.
77. Duda SH, Pusich B, Richter G, et al. Sirolimus eluting stents for the treatment of obstructive superficial femoral artery disease: six-month results. Circulation 2002; 106:1505–9.
78. Duda SH, Bosiers M, Lammer J, et al. Sirolimus-eluting versus bare nitinol stent for obstructive superficial femoral artery disease: the SIROCCO II trial. J Vasc Interv Radiol 2005; 16:331–8.
79. Virmani R, Liistro F, Stankovic G, et al. Mechanism of late in-stent restenosis after implantation of a paclitaxel derivate-eluting polymer stent system in humans. Circulation 2002; 106(21):2649–51.
80. Tanabe K, Serruys PW, Degertekin M, Grube E, Guagliumi G, Urbaszek W, Bonnier J, Lablanche JM, Siminiak T, Nordrehaug J, et al. Incomplete stent apposition after implantation of paclitaxel-eluting stents or bare metal stents: insights from the randomized TAXUS II trial. Circulation 2005; 111(7):900–5.
81. Virmani R, Guagliumi G, Farb A, et al. Localized hypersensitivity and late coronary thrombosis secondary to a sirolimus-eluting stent: should we be cautious? Circulation 2004; 109(6):701–5.
82. Faxon DP. Systemic drug therapy for restenosis, "Déjà Vu All Over Again". Circulation 2002; 106:2296–8.
83. Lawrie A, Brisken AF, Francis SE, et al. Ultrasound enhances reporter gene expression after transfection of vascular cells in vitro. Circulation 1999; 99(20):2617–20.
84. Fitzgerald PJ, Takagi A, Moore MP, et al. Intravascular sonotherapy decreases neointimal hyperplasia after stent implantation in swine. Circulation 2001; 103(14):1828–31.
85. Regar E, Thury A, van der Giessen WJ, et al. Sonotherapy, antirestenotic therapeutic ultrasound in coronary arteries: the first clinical experience. Catheter Cardiovasc Interv 2003; 60(1):9–17.
86. Serruys PW, Hoye A, Grollier G, Colombo A, Symons J, Mudra H. A European multi-center trial investigating the anti-restenotic effect of intravascular sonotherapy after stenting of de novo lesions (EUROSPAH: EUROpean Sonotherapy Prevention of Arterial Hyperplasia). Int J Cardiovasc Intervent 2004; 6(2):53–60.
87. Dougherty TJ, Gomer CJ, Henderson BW, et al. Photodynamic therapy. J Natl Cancer Inst 1998; 90(12):889–905.
88. Mansfield R, Bown S, McEwan J. Photodynamic therapy: shedding light on restenosis. Heart 2001; 86(6):612–8.
89. Wakamatsu T, Saito T, Hayashi J, Takeichi T, Kitamoto K, Aizawa K. Long-term inhibition of intimal hyperplasia using vascular photodynamic therapy in balloon-injured carotid arteries. Med Mol Morphol 2005; 38(4):225–32.
90. Waksman R, Leitch I, Roessler J, et al. Intracoronary photodynamic therapy reduces neointimal growth without suppressing re-endothelialization in a porcine model. Heart (Epub ahead of print).
91. Mansfield RJ, Jenkins MP, Pai ML, Bishop CC, Bown SG, McEwan JR. Long-term safety and efficacy of superficial femoral artery angioplasty with adjuvant photodynamic therapy to prevent restenosis. Br J Surg 2002; 89(12):1538–9.
92. Usui M, Miyagi M, Fukasawa S, et al. A first trial in the clinical application of photodynamic therapy for the prevention of restenosis after coronary-stent placement. Lasers Surg Med 2004; 34(3):235–41.
93. Gage A, Fazekas G, Riley E. Freezing injury to large blood vessels in dogs. Surgery 1967; 61:748–54.
94. Laird J, Jaff MR, Biamino G, et al. Cryoplasty for the treatment of femoropopliteal arterial disease: results of a prospective, multicenter registry. J Vasc Interv Radiol 2005; 16(8):1067–73.
95. Tatsutani KN, Joye JD, Virmani R, Taylor MJ. In vitro evaluation of vascular endothelial and smooth muscle cell survival and apoptosis in response to hypothermia and freezing. Cryo Letters 2005; 26:55–64.
96. Fava M, Loyola S, Polydorou A, et al. Cryoplasty for femoropopliteal arterial disease: late angiographic results of initial human experience. J Vasc Interv Radiol 2004; 15(11):1239–43.

97. Oberhoff M, Kunert W, Herdeg C, et al. Inhibition of smooth muscle cell proliferation after local drug delivery of the antimitotic drug paclitaxel using a porous balloon catheter. Basic Res Cardiol 2001; 96(3):275–82.
98. Kalinowski M, Tepe G, Schieber A, et al. Local administration of ramiprilat is less effective than oral ramipril in preventing restenosis after balloon angioplasty in an animal model. J Vasc Interv Radiol 1999; 10(10):1397–404.
99. Westedt U, Barbu-Tudoran L, Schaper AK, Kalinowski M, Alfke H, Kissel T. Effects of different application parameters on penetration characteristics and arterial vessel wall integrity after local nanoparticle delivery using a porous balloon catheter. Eur J Pharm Biopharm 2004; 58(1):161–8.
100. Scheller B, Speck U, Abramjuk C, Bernhardt U, Bohm M, Nickenig G. Paclitaxel balloon coating, a novel method for prevention and therapy of restenosis. Circulation 2004; 110(7):810–4.
101. Scheller B, Hehrlein C, Bocksch W, et al. Randomised trial for the treatment of in-stent restenosis by a paclitaxel coated balloon catheter—PACCOCATH ISR. In: Congress of the European Society of Cardiology, Stockholm, Sweden, September 2005.
102. Tepe G. Drug-coated balloons for prevention of restenosis in the SFA and popliteal arteries. In: 18th Annual International Symposium on Endovascular Therapy, Miami Beach, Florida, U.S.A., January 2006.

8 Emerging Therapies for Chronic Lower Limb Ischemia (Novel Strategies Using Growth Factors, Gene Transfer, and Cellular Techniques to Promote Angiogenesis)

Richard Donnelly
School of Medical and Surgical Sciences, University of Nottingham, Nottingham and Derby City General Hospital, Derby, U.K.

Timothy Rowlands
Derby Hospitals NHS Foundation Trust, Derby, U.K.

INTRODUCTION

Chronic lower limb ischemia is common, especially in the elderly, and often associated with troublesome symptoms of intermittent claudication. There is also an increased risk of ischemic ulceration leading to infection and amputation. The focus of medical treatment includes disease-modifying agents such as angiotensin-converting enzyme inhibitors and statins to encourage stabilization and regression of atherosclerotic plaques, and to reduce the risk of acute limb or life-threatening cardiovascular events. Revascularization is effective, but only in a highly selected subset of patients with refractory symptoms due to discrete, proximal stenoses that are amenable to an endovascular or bypass procedure. For the majority of patients with chronic lower limb ischemia there are few, if any, effective treatments to achieve sustained improvements in distal blood flow in order to provide relief from symptoms and preservation of tissue viability.

There is good clinical evidence that collateral vessel formation has a favorable effect on the clinical presentation and outcome from atherosclerotic disease involving major vessels in the heart and lower limbs. For example, the presence of collateral vessels at the time of a myocardial infarction reduces infarct size and mortality (1). In chronic lower limb arterial disease, collateralization, and vascular remodeling can create new networks of blood vessels which maintain muscle and skin blood flow despite significant occlusive disease in major conduit vessels (2).

Experimental studies 15 years ago began to explore the regulation of new vessel formation and the feasibility of enhancing collateralization in animal models of lower limb ischemia (3). Since then, considerable progress has been made in developing molecular, genetic, and cellular-based interventions for human use. This chapter will summarize some of the major clinical studies that have evaluated different forms of therapeutic angiogenesis in patients with severe atherosclerotic disease (myocardial ischemia and lower limb ischemia).

REGULATION OF NEW BLOOD VESSEL FORMATION

The development of new blood vessels is a complex physiologic process which occurs as part of normal growth and development, and as a crucial step in tissue maintenance and repair (4). In the context of chronic lower limb ischemia, the duration and severity of ischemia are important determinants of any compensatory angiogenic response, but sheer stress, endothelial function, inflammation, and metabolic factors (e.g., diabetes) can have important effects on the rate of formation, structure, and effectiveness of collateral networks which circumvent significant stenoses in native lower limb arteries (4).

Biologic Processes and Terminology

Angiogenesis

Angiogenesis is the sprouting of new capillaries from existing vascular structures, and involves activation, migration, and proliferation of endothelial cells followed by tubule formation and expansion of the surrounding connective tissue and smooth muscle components. Sprouting of new vessels includes branching points, and angiogenesis creates a network of fragile new vessels with a lumen and endothelial lining.

Vasculogenesis

Vasculogenesis is the formation of new blood vessels from circulating bone marrow-derived endothelial progenitor cells (EPCs) which differentiate into endothelial cells and fuse into luminal structures. Vasculogenesis was previously considered exclusively an embryologic process but there is increasing evidence that neovascularization in adult tissues involves a combination of vasculogenesis and angiogenesis (5). The number of circulating EPCs increases in response to ischemia, but vasculogenesis is impaired in patients with diabetes (6).

Arteriogenesis

This term refers to an increase in the diameter of pre-existing arteriolar collateral vessels by recruitment of perivascular cells and expansion and remodeling of the surrounding cellular matrix (7). Arteriogenesis seems to promote wall thickness of collateral vessels, and is stimulated mainly by sheer stress rather than hypoxia (8). This essentially converts thin-walled capillary structures into more robust arterioles capable of withstanding arterial pressure. Thus, a major element of arteriogenesis includes migration, differentiation, and proliferation of smooth muscle cells, matrix components and tissue macrophages. This maturation of collateral vessels is associated with up to a 20-fold increase in lumen diameter, and with the formation of a smooth muscle layer within the vessel wall (9).

Thus, establishing a network of new collateral vessels in the lower limb involves a combination of angiogenesis, vasculogenesis, and arteriogenesis. The regulation and interaction of these processes involve complex pathways linking cellular, biochemical, and endocrine signals.

Angiogenic Growth Factors

Angiogenesis requires activation of endothelial cells, e.g., by ischemia, hemodynamic or circulating factors, which then triggers individual cells to begin a process of migration and proliferation leading to capillary budding and local release of matrix metalloproteinases. The migrating endothelial cells form bands which then develop into loops and eventually canalize to create a luminal structure. The major steps in angiogenesis, i.e., endothelial cell activation, migration, proliferation, and reorganization, are tightly regulated in a complex balance between pro- and anti-angiogenic mechanisms. Over the last 30 years a number of growth factors and cytokines have been identified which either stimulate or inhibit angiogenesis (10).

Three groups of angiogenic growth factors have been exploited in experimental studies of therapeutic angiogenesis: (*i*) the vascular endothelial growth factor (VEGF) family; (*ii*) the fibroblast growth factor (FGF) family; and (*iii*) granulocyte–monocyte-colony stimulating factor (GM-CSF).

Vascular Endothelial Growth Factor

This family of growth factors includes VEGF-A, VEGF-B, VEGF-C, and VEGF-D (11). VEGF-A is subject to post-transcriptional modification which results in three different isoenzymes: $VEGF_{121}$, $VEGF_{165}$ and $VEGF_{189}$ (12,13). The binding of VEGF to endothelial cells triggers an increase in endothelial permeability and proliferation of endothelial cells which triggers angiogenesis. VEGF is markedly upregulated by hypoxia (14), and platelets are a major source of circulating VEGF.

Fibroblast Growth Factor

FGF, in contrast to VEGF, are non-secreted growth factors that are released only during cell death or ischemic cell injury. The FGF family of cytokines is not endothelial cell specific, and there are at least 20 different members of this family of growth factors (15). The major FGFs of interest in studies of therapeutic angiogenesis include FGF-2 (also known as basic FGF) and FGF-4 (16–18).

Granulocyte–Monocyte Colony Stimulating Factor

GM-CSF activates circulating monocytes and stimulates release of bone marrow-derived EPCs (18). In two studies, injection of GM-CSF was shown to mobilize EPCs from bone marrow and promote collateral vessel growth in patients with coronary artery disease (19,20).

NOVEL THERAPEUTIC STRATEGIES

Local Administration of Recombinant Human Proteins

Local intramuscular or intra-arterial administration of recombinant cytokines and growth factors into the coronary or femoral arteries, or intramuscular injection into the ischemic lower limb, has been evaluated as a simple and practical approach to therapeutic angiogenesis. Three specific proteins have been evaluated in this way in placebo-controlled clinical trials: $VEGF_{165}$, FGF-2 and GM-CSF (Table 1) (15,16,20,21). These trials have been conducted mainly in patients with myocardial ischemia, but one trial, the therapeutic angiogenesis with recombinant FGF-2 for intermittent claudication (TRAFFIC) study (16), evaluated FGF-2 in patients with stable lower limb arterial disease (Fontaine stage II).

The TRAFFIC study was a randomized, double-blind placebo-controlled trial of single or repeat-dose intra-arterial recombinant FGF-2 30 mg/kg (16). FGF-2 was formulated as a 146-amino acid, 16.5-kDa protein produced genetically from yeast. Patients with intermittent claudication and reproducible exercise tolerance on a treadmill received half the dose of FGF-2 down each femoral artery via a single arterial puncture and a crossover catheter. Inclusion criteria included evidence of >70% stenosis of the femoral, popliteal or tibial arteries on angiography and a resting ankle-brachial pressure index (ABPI) <0.8 on the most affected limb. A total of 190 patients were randomized to placebo, single-dose FGF-2 or two sequential doses of FGF-2 (second dose administered 30 days later). The primary endpoint for the study was maximum walking distance at 90 days after FGF-2 administration.

The trial reported a statistically significant improvement in peak walking time, but there was no difference between single and repeated doses of FGF-2 (Fig. 1). Compared with baseline, patients in the placebo group increased their peak walking time by 0.6 min (14%), while patients in the single-dose group increased walking time by 1.77 min (34%) and those patients in the double-dose group increased walking distance by 1.54 min (20%) (Fig. 1) (16). The results on an "intention-to-treat" analysis ($n=190$) showed a significant difference between the three groups ($p=0.034$) (Fig. 1) (16). Active therapy also produced a small but significant increase in ABPI ($p<0.04$).

Three pre-specified subgroups were evaluated in terms of their response to FGF-2: patients with diabetes, those aged >68 years and non-current smokers. All three of these groups showed a smaller improvement in peak walking time in response to FGF-2 treatment. Surprisingly,

TABLE 1 Randomized, Placebo-Controlled Trials of Single-Dose, Local Administration of Recombinant Human Proteins to Stimulate Angiogenesis in Patients with Coronary Artery Disease or Peripheral Arterial Disease

Trial (Ref.)	Protein	Route of administration	No. of patients	Disease	Primary end point	Result
TRAFFIC (16)	FGF-2	Intrafemoral	172	PAD	Peak walking distance	Positive
FIRST (15)	FGF-2	Intracoronary	337	CAD	Exercise tolerance	Negative
VIVA (21)	$VEGF_{165}$	Intramyocardial	178	CAD	Exercise tolerance	Negative
Seiler et al. (20)	GM-CSF	Intracoronary	21	CAD	Coronary flow index	Positive

Abbreviations: CAD, coronary artery disease; PAD, peripheral arterial disease.

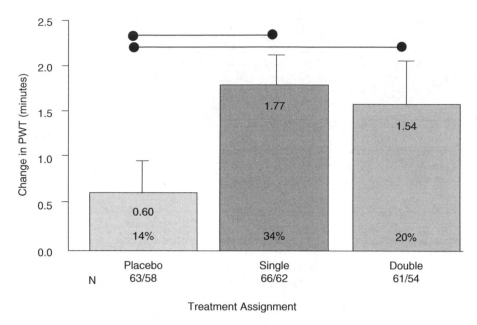

FIGURE 1   The TRAFFIC study. Effects of single- or double-dose administration of bFGF (FGF-2) on peak walking time (PWT). *Source*: From Ref. 16.

current smokers showed a greater increase in peak walking time than the group as a whole: 1.25, 2.10, and 2.26 min for placebo, single-dose, and double-dose FGF-2, respectively (16).

   Over 700 patients with lower limb or myocardial ischemia were randomized in the four major trials summarized in Table 1 (15,16,20,21). The results were mixed with only modest and inconsistent evidence of efficacy. Current evidence suggests that single-dose administration of individual proteins may be insufficient to initiate a sustained therapeutic angiogenic response (22,23). In addition, recent experimental studies in animal models of lower limb ischemia have shown that longer periods of exposure to angiogenic proteins are required for a therapeutic effect (24–26).

Gene Therapy

As proteins have a short half-life and single-dose administration of recombinant protein has been largely ineffective in clinical trials (Table 1), interest has turned to gene transfer strategies in an effort to initiate sustained expression of the transgene with chronic increases in local growth factor protein synthesis (27). A gene can be transferred using either a plasmid (naked DNA) vector or a viral vector (adenoviral or retroviral vectors are used). Viral-based vectors are incapable of replicating within the cell. Plasmids have a low rate of gene transfer both in vitro and in vivo but are perceived to be safer; only a fraction of plasmid DNA enters the cell nucleus. Plasmid-based gene transfer leads to increased local expression of the transgene for up to one month (28).

   Using viral-based vectors to facilitate transfer of the gene of interest into a target tissue results in a higher rate of gene transfer compared with plasmids (29). Adenoviral-based vectors, for example, enter proliferating and non-proliferating cells and, like plasmid vectors, give rise to a relatively short period of transgene expression (30). The advantage of adenoviral-based vectors is that gene transfer efficiency is much higher, but these vectors can trigger immunologic and inflammatory reactions which renders them less well tolerated and raises concerns about longer term safety (29).

   Retroviral-based vectors transfer RNA into the target cells. DNA is formed by reverse transcription, and incorporated into the host cell genome which, theoretically, should lead to

TABLE 2 Clinical Gene Therapy Trials to Stimulate Angiogenesis in Patients with Coronary Artery Disease or Peripheral Arterial Disease

Trial (Ref.)	Vector	Route of administration	No. of patients	Disease	Follow-up (wks)	Primary end point	Result
RAVE (31)	$VEGF_{121}$ (adenoviral)	Intramuscular	105	PAD	12 and 26	Exercise tolerance	Negative
REVASC (32)	$VEGF_{121}$ (adenoviral)	Intramyocardial	67	CAD	12 and 26	Not defined	Positive[a]
KAT (33)	$VEGF_{165}$ (adenoviral vs. plasmid)	Intracoronary	103	CAD	24	Not defined	Positive[b]
AGENT II (17)	FGF-4 (adenoviral)	Intracoronary	79	CAD	12	—	Negative
AGENT II (30)	FGF-4 (adenoviral)	Intracoronary	415	CAD	12 and 25	Exercise duration	Negative

[a] Time to ST depression positive at 26 weeks.
[b] Myocardial perfusion positive in adenoviral group only.
Abbreviations: CAD, coronary artery disease; PAD, peripheral arterial disease.

indefinite overexpression of the transgene (10). This strategy offers the possibility of permanent increases in local growth factor production following a single gene transfer procedure. Indeed several genes might be administered in order to create a cocktail of local growth factors that is conducive to new vessel formation.

There have been several gene transfer studies in patients with coronary or peripheral arterial disease (Table 2) (17,30–33). The Regional Angiogenesis with VEGF trial used an adenoviral vector to transfer the gene for $VEGF_{121}$ ($AdVEGF_{121}$) in patients with critical lower limb ischemia and reproducible unilateral claudication (31). Patients were randomized to one of two doses of $AdVEGF_{121}$, or placebo, and follow-up measurements of exercise tolerance were performed at 12 and 26 weeks after gene transfer. A single intramuscular injection of $AdVEGF_{121}$ was ineffective in this study (31), and similarly FGF-4 gene transfer using an adenoviral vector has been disappointing in patients with coronary disease (17,30).

Over 900 patients have been treated in gene therapy trials (Table 2). Although plasmid and adenoviral vectors were well tolerated, neither approach, for single gene transfer, has been effective. This may be due to low gene transfer efficiency, non-sustained and/or insufficient local expression of the angiogenic growth factor ($VEGF_{121}$ or FGF-4), or because multiple genes need to be transferred to produce an angiogenic response.

Bone Marrow-Derived Endothelial Progenitor Cells

EPCs in the CD34 stem-cell fraction of peripheral blood are involved in new vessel formation (mainly vasculogenesis) (34), and experimental studies have shown that peripheral blood mononuclear cells increase capillary density in models of hindlimb ischemia (35). Bone marrow stromal cells secrete many angiogenic cytokines, and in animal models of lower limb ischemia there is evidence that implantation of bone marrow mononuclear cells promotes collateral vessel formation with incorporation of EPCs into new networks of capillaries (36).

On this basis, there have been some clinical studies of bone marrow transplantation into ischemic limbs and myocardium. The Therapeutic Angiogenesis Using Cell Transplantation study was a randomized controlled trial of autologous bone marrow-derived mononuclear cells, including EPCs, which were implanted into critically ischemic limbs (37). The primary endpoints for the study were safety and feasibility of treatment, and improvements in ABPI, transcutaneous oxygen pressure and rest pain.

The bone marrow mononuclear cells contained $CD34^+$ and $CD34^-$ cells, and fluorescence activated cell sorting analysis in each patient showed that 18% of $CD34^+$ cells had the characteristics of EPCs (37). The authors postulated that these cells might release angiogenic factors as well as providing a local supply of EPCs for vasculogenesis. The placebo group in this trial were given peripheral blood mononuclear cells with 500-fold fewer EPCs.

Clinical improvements (decreased rest pain) were recorded in 39 out of 45 patients, and there was a significant increase in mean ABPI from 0.35 at baseline to 0.47 after four weeks ($p < 0.001$) (37). The improvements were sustained after 24 weeks, and there were no significant adverse effects.

CONCLUSIONS

New vessel formation to create a network of collateral vessels is a physiologic compensatory response to ischemia which occurs gradually in patients with atherosclerotic disease. Strategies to augment this response involve stimulation of angiogenesis, vasculogenesis, and arteriogenesis by manipulating the local concentrations of, and responses to, angiogenic growth factors, especially VEGF and FGF. These novel therapeutic strategies have been evaluated in animal models of lower limb ischemia and in randomized controlled trials in patients with stage II and III peripheral arterial disease.

It has become clear that single-dose administration of a single growth factor protein is insufficient to produce a sustained angiogenic response. Even single gene transfer, which may trigger local growth factor production for up to four weeks, is inadequate for developing a network of collateral vessels. New gene therapy approaches are seeking to increase the efficiency of gene transfer and the duration of increased gene expression.

For newly formed vessels to function properly, remodeling, thickening, and smooth muscle deposition are essential. This complex sequence of events requires several growth factors, working in concert, to develop new vessels capable of withstanding arterial pressure. It is likely, therefore, that therapeutic angiogenesis will involve a multi-modality approach if it is to achieve a sustained and effective clinical response.

REFERENCES

1. Charney R, Cohen M. The role of the coronary collateral circulation in limiting myocardial ischaemia and infarct size. Am Heart J 1993; 126:937–45.
2. Lehoux S, Levy BI. Collateral artery growth: making the most of what you have. Circ Res 2006; 99:567–9.
3. Baffour R, Berman J, Garb J, Rhee S, Kaufman J, Friedmann P. Enhanced angiogenesis and growth of collaterals by in vivo administration of recombinant bFGF in a rat model of acute lower limb ischaemia: dose–response effect of bFGF. J Vasc Surg 1992; 2:181–91.
4. Risau W. Mechanisms of angiogenesis. Nature 1997; 386:671–4.
5. Isner JM, Asahara T. Angiogenesis and vasculogenesis as therapeutic strategies for postnatal neovascularization. J Clin Invest 1999; 103:1231–6.
6. Tepper OM, Galiano RD, Capla JM, et al. Human endothelial progenitor cells from type II diabetics exhibit impaired proliferation, adhesion and incorporation into vascular structures. Circulation 2002; 106:2781–6.
7. Ito WD, Arras M, Scholz D, Winkler B, Htun P, Schaper W. Angiogenesis but not collateral growth is associated with ischaemia after femoral artery occlusion. Am J Physiol 1997; 273:H1255–65.
8. Schaper W, Ito WD. Molecular mechanisms of coronary collateral vessel growth. Circ Res 1996; 79:911–9.
9. Buschmann I, Heil M, Jost M, Schaper W. Influence of inflammatory cytokines on arteriogenesis. Microcirculation 2003; 10:371–9.
10. Staudacher DL, Preis M, Lewis BS, Grossman PM, Flugelman MY. Cellular and molecular therapeutic modalities for arterial obstructive syndromes. Pharm Ther 2006; 109:263–73.
11. Tammela T, Enholm B, Alitalo K, Paavonen K. The biology of vascular endothelial growth factors. Cardiovasc Res 2005; 65:550–63.
12. Robinson CJ, Stringer SE. The splice variants of vascular endothelial growth factor (VEGF) and their receptors. J Cell Sci 2001; 114:853–65.
13. Shweiki D, Itin A, Soffer D, Keshet E. Vascular endothelial growth factor induced by hypoxia may mediate hypoxia-initiated angiogenesis. Nature 1992; 359:843–5.
14. Gerwins P, Skoldenberg E, Claesson-Welsh L. Function of fibroblast growth factors and vascular endothelial growth factors and their receptors in angiogenesis. Crit Rev Oncol Hematol 2000; 34:185–94.
15. Simons M, Annex B, Laham R, Kleiman N, Henry T, Dauerman H. Pharmacological treatment of coronary artery disease with recombinant FGF-2: FIRST study. Circulation 2002; 105:788–93.

16. Lederman RJ, Mendelsohn FO, Anderson RD, Saucedo JF, Hermiller JB. Therapeutic angiogenesis with recombinant fibroblast growth factor-2 for intermittent claudication (TRAFFIC study). Lancet 2002; 359:2053–8.
17. Grines CL, Watkins MW, Mahmarian JJ, et al. A randomised, double-blind placebo-controlled trial of Ad5FGF-4 gene therapy and its effect on myocardial perfusion in patients with stable angina. J Am Coll Cardiol 2003; 42:1339–47.
18. Carmeliet P. Mechanisms of angiogenesis and arteriogenesis. Nat Med 2000; 6:389–95.
19. Takahashi T, Kalka C, Masuda H, et al. Ischaemia and cytokine-induced mobilization of bone marrow-derived endothelial cells for neovascularization. Nat Med 1999; 5:434–8.
20. Seiler C, Pohl T, Wustmann K, et al. Promotion of collateral growth by granulocyte–macrophage colony-stimulating factor in patients with coronary artery disease: a randomised, double-blind, placebo-controlled study. Circulation 2001; 104:2012–7.
21. Henry TD, Annex BH, Mckendall GR, et al. The VIVA trial: vascular endothelial growth factor in ischaemia for vascular angiogenesis. Circulation 2003; 107:1359–65.
22. Collinson DJ, Donnelly R. Therapeutic angiogenesis in peripheral arterial disease: can biotechnology produce an effective collateral circulation? Eur J Vasc Endovasc Surg 2004; 28:9–23.
23. Freedman SB, Isner JM. Therapeutic angiogenesis for coronary artery disease. Ann Intern Med 2002; 136:54–71.
24. Sun Q, Chen RR, Shen Y, Mooney DJ, Rajagopalan S, Grossman PM. Sustained vascular endothelial growth factor delivery enhances angiogenesis and perfusion in ischaemic hind limb. Pharm Res 2005; 22:1110–6.
25. von Degenfeld G, Banfi A, Springer ML, et al. Microenvironmental VEGA distribution is critical for stable and functional vessel growth in ischaemia. FASEB J 2006; 20:2657–9.
26. Greve JM, Chico TJ, Goldman H, et al. Magnetic resonance angiography reveals therapeutic enlargement of collateral vessels induced by VEGF in a murine model of peripheral arterial disease. J Magn Reson Imaging 2006; 24:1124–32.
27. Yla-Herttuala S, Martin JF. Cardiovascular gene therapy. Lancet 2000; 355:213–22.
28. Laham RJ, Simons M, Selke F. Gene transfer for angiogenesis in coronary artery disease. Annu Rev Med 2001; 52:485–502.
29. Brody SL, Crystal RG. Adenovirus-mediated in vivo gene transfer. Ann N Y Acad Sci 1994; 716:90–101.
30. Penny WF, Hammond HK. Clinical use of intracoronary gene transfer of fibroblast growth factor for coronary artery disease. Curr Gene Ther 2004; 4:225–31.
31. Rajagopalan S, Mohler ER, Lederman RJ, et al. Regional angiogenesis with vascular endothelial growth factor in peripheral arterial disease: a phase II randomised, double-blind, controlled study of adenoviral delivery of $VEGF_{121}$ in patients with disabling intermittent claudication. Circulation 2003; 108:1933–8.
32. Stewart DJ. Late-breaking clinical trial abstracts: a phase II, randomised, multicentre, 26-week study to assess the efficacy and safety of BIOBYPASS (AdVEGF$_{121}$) delivered through minimally invasive surgery versus maximum medical treatment in patients with severe angina, advanced coronary artery disease and no options for revascularization. Circulation 2002; 106:2986a.
33. Hedman M, Hartikainen J, Syvanne M, et al. Safety and feasibility of catheter-based local intracoronary VEGF gene transfer in the prevention of postangioplasty in-stent restenosis and in the treatment of chronic myocardial ischaemia: phase II results of the Kupio Angiogenesis Trial (KAT). Circulation 2003; 107:2677–83.
34. Asahara T, Murohara T, Sullivan A, et al. Isolation of putative progenitor endothelial cells for angiogenesis. Science 1997; 275:964–7.
35. Murohara T, Ikeda H, Duan J, et al. Transplanted cord blood-derived endothelial precursor cells augment postnatal neovascularisation. J Clin Invest 2000; 105:1527–36.
36. Shintani S, Murohara T, Ikeda H, et al. Augmentation of postnatal neovascularisation with autologous bone marrow transplantation. Circulation 2001; 103:895–7.
37. Tateishi-Yuyama E, Matsubara H, Murohara T, et al. Therapeutic angiogenesis for patients with critical limb ischaemia using autologous bone marrow cell transplantation. Lancet 2002; 360:427–35.

9 | Recent Trials for Chronic Lower Limb Ischemia

Donald J. Adam and Andrew W. Bradbury
University Department of Vascular Surgery, Heart of England NHS Foundation Trust, Solihull, Birmingham, U.K.

INTRODUCTION

The treatment of patients with chronic lower limb ischemia should be tailored to the individual's clinical presentation, general health and pattern of disease. Many patients with intermittent claudication (IC) will be best served by conservative management, instituting best medical therapy and enrolling them in an exercise program. For a large proportion of patients with critical lower limb ischemia (CLI) and a salvageable limb, or those with severe lifestyle limiting IC unresponsive to conservative management, some form of revascularization procedure will be required. Increasingly more complex atherosclerotic lesions are now being successfully managed using endovascular techniques where previously only surgical revascularization would have been offered. The present chapter reviews the results of randomized trials of the management of patients with chronic lower limb ischemia with particular emphasis on (*i*) stenting versus angioplasty, (*ii*) surgery versus angioplasty and (*iii*) exercise therapy versus angioplasty.

Given the vast number of patients with lower limb ischemia who present to vascular interventionalists every year, the randomized evidence supporting differing treatments is sparse.

TRIALS COMPARING STENTING AND ANGIOPLASTY

Iliac Occlusive Disease

A meta-analysis of 1300 patients in six iliac percutaneous transluminal angioplasty (PTA) studies and 816 patients in eight iliac stenting studies demonstrated no significant difference in rates of immediate technical success, complications and mortality but improved long-term patency with iliac stenting (1). For PTA, the four-year primary patency rates in patients with IC were 65% for stenoses and 54% for occlusions and in patients with CLI were 53% for stenoses and 44% for occlusions. For stenting, the four-year primary patency rates in patients with IC were 77% for stenoses and 61% for occlusions and in patients with CLI were 67% for stenoses and 53% for occlusions.

The subsequent publication of the results of the Dutch Iliac Stent trial, however, failed to support the findings of the meta-analysis. In this prospective multicenter trial, 279 patients with IC due to >50% iliac artery stenotic disease or short (≤ 5 cm) occlusions were randomized to primary iliac stenting (*n* = 143) or primary PTA (*n* = 136) with selective stenting performed for a poor PTA result (residual mean pressure gradient >10 mm Hg) in 43% of patients. At a mean follow-up of 9.3 months (range 3–24 months), initial hemodynamic success rates were 81% after primary stenting and 82% after primary PTA. At 24 months, clinical success rates were 78% after primary stenting and 77% after primary PTA, and cumulative patency rates were 71% and 70%, respectively (2). Health-related quality of life improved equally after primary stenting and primary PTA with selective stenting (3). At mean follow-up of 5.6 years (4), there were no significant differences in iliac reintervention (primary stenting, 18% vs. primary PTA, 20%), risk of cardiovascular events (myocardial infarction, stroke, extracranial bleeding; primary stenting, 13% vs. primary PTA, 11%) or risk of death (primary stenting, 15% vs. primary PTA, 16%). At five to eight years after treatment (5), PTA and selective stenting was associated with significantly better symptomatic outcome but there was no difference in iliac patency, ankle-brachial pressure index (ABPI) or quality of life between the groups.

These data support a policy of primary iliac PTA with selective stenting for patients with IC. This is less expensive than primary stenting and associated with equivalent clinical outcomes.

Infra-inguinal Occlusive Disease

There have been a total of seven published randomized trials of stenting versus angioplasty for infra-inguinal arterial occlusive disease and all but the two most recently published reports have failed to demonstrate a significant benefit for stenting over PTA alone.

Vroegindeweij et al. (6) randomized 51 patients with symptomatic femoropopliteal disease to PTA and stenting ($n=24$) or PTA alone ($n=27$). At 12 months, there was no significant difference in clinical and hemodynamic success rates (stenting, 74% vs. PTA, 85%) and primary patency rates (stenting, 62% vs. PTA, 74%). Zdanowski et al. (7) subsequently reported on 32 patients with femoropopliteal occlusions and disabling IC or CLI who were randomized to PTA and stenting ($n=15$) or PTA alone ($n=17$). At 12 months, there was no significant difference in the rate of clinical improvement or reocclusion rate on angiography (stent, 33% vs. PTA alone, 75%) while the restenosis rate was significantly higher after stenting (50% vs. PTA alone, 25%; $p=0.033$). In another trial (8), 53 patients with femoropopliteal disease were randomized to PTA and Palmaz® (Cordis Corporation, Miami Lakes, Florida, U.S.A.) stenting ($n=30$) or PTA alone ($n=23$). At midterm follow-up, there was no significant difference in primary or secondary patency rates between the groups: the primary and secondary patency rates after PTA and Palmaz stenting were 62% and 90%, respectively, at a median follow-up of 29 months; at a median follow-up of 34 months, the primary and secondary patency rates after PTA alone were 68.4% and 89.5%, respectively.

In a 2001 meta-analysis of 19 English language studies (9), the three-year patency rates after 923 femoropopliteal PTAs were 48% to 61% for IC and 30% to 43% for CLI with lower patency rates for occlusions compared with stenotic disease. The three-year patency rates after 473 femoropopliteal stent implantations were 63% to 66% and were not related to clinical indication. Based upon these data, the authors concluded that PTA and stenting were equally effective in the long term for the management of IC and stenotic disease but stenting was more effective for more advanced disease (occlusions and CLI). A subsequent Cochrane Review published in 2003 (10) included only two randomized trials of femoropopliteal PTA alone versus PTA and (Palmaz) stenting in a total of 104 patients with IC. There was no significant difference in patency rates between the treatment strategies and the authors recommended that large multicenter trials be performed to address this clinical issue.

A trial reported by Cejna and colleagues (11) was published in 2001 but not included in the Cochrane Review. In this study, a total of 144 limbs in 141 patients with IC or CLI and less than 5 cm of femoropopliteal stenotic or occlusive disease were randomized to PTA and Palmaz stenting ($n=77$) or PTA alone ($n=77$). The technical success rate was significantly higher in the stent group (99% vs. PTA alone, 84%; $p=0.009$). At two years, however, there was no significant difference in the hemodynamic and clinical success rates (PTA alone, 65% vs. stenting, 65%), and primary (53% both groups) and secondary angiographic patency rates (PTA alone, 74% vs. stenting, 73%). Becquemin and colleagues (12) randomized 227 patients with disabling IC or CLI and less than 7 cm of stenosed or occluded superficial femoral artery (SFA) to selective ($n=112$) or systematic Palmaz stenting ($n=115$). A total of 15% of patients required selective stenting due to a suboptimal angioplasty result. At 12-month follow-up, there was no significant difference in the treatment failure rate or 50% restenosis rate on angiography (selective stenting, 32.3% vs. systematic stenting, 34.7%). There was no significant difference between the groups in terms of patient survival or survival free from new vascular events in the treated limb up to four years follow-up. The authors concluded that Palmaz stenting should be reserved for suboptimal angioplasty result and not used routinely.

Unlike previous studies that used the Palmaz stent, the most recent prospective randomized study to report (13) compared primary stenting using the self-expanding Guidant Absolute™ (Guidant Corporation, Indianapolis, Indiana, U.S.A.) nitinol stent ($n=51$) and PTA alone ($n=53$) in 104 patients with severe IC or CLI secondary to stenotic or occlusive disease of the SFA. Secondary stenting was required in 32% of patients randomized to PTA alone. At 12 months, primary stenting was associated with a significantly lower duplex-detected restenosis rate (stent, 37% vs. PTA alone, 63%; $p=0.01$) and a significantly better treadmill claudication distance. To date, there is only one published trial comparing stenting and angioplasty in the infrapopliteal arterial segment (14). In this study, a total of 95 infrapopliteal lesions in 51 patients with CLI were prospectively randomized to PTA alone (53 lesions in 27 patients) or stenting using carbofilm-coated stents (42 lesions in 24 patients). A total of 57 lesions in 37 patients were available for review at six months. The six-month cumulative primary patency at the 50% and 70% restenosis rates were significantly higher in the stented group (83.7% and 79.7% vs. PTA alone, 61.1% and 45.6%; $p<0.05$). In the hands of experienced interventionalists, the short-term outcome associated with infrapopliteal stenting for CLI appears superior to PTA alone.

The results of Phase II of the RESILIENT trial have been reported but not yet published. In this prospective multicenter trial of femoropopliteal stenting using the nitinol Edwards Lifesciences LifeStent NT™ (Edwards Lifesciences, Irvine, California, U.S.A.) compared with PTA alone in patients with severe IC, the six-month clinical success rate was 86.1% for stenting and 72.2% for PTA with primary patency rates of 84% and 53.8%, respectively. The early results from these three most recent trials are encouraging and seem to demonstrate the significant advances in stent technology, which have been made over the traditional Palmaz stent. Medium-to-long-term durability data from these trials will be eagerly awaited as will the results of the ongoing trials comparing femoropopliteal stenting and PTA alone, which include the FAST trial using the Bard LUMINEXX™ (Bard Inc., Murray Hill, New Jersey, U.S.A.) stent and the SUPER trial using the Cordis SMART® (Cordis Corporation, Miami Lakes, Florida, U.S.A.) stent.

TRIALS COMPARING DIFFERENT TYPES OF STENTS

Iliac Occlusive Disease

The Cordis Randomized Iliac Stent Project-U.S. (15) was a prospective, multicenter trial that randomized 203 patients to implantation of the SMART nitinol self-expanding stent ($n=102$) or the Boston Wallstent® (Boston Scientific, Natick, Massachusetts, U.S.A.) ($n=101$) after suboptimal iliac PTA. Although the technical success rate was significantly better with the SMART stent (98.2% vs. Wallstent, 87.5%; $p=0.002$), there was no significant difference in primary patency (SMART stent, 94.7% vs. Wallstent, 91.1%) or functional and hemodynamic improvement at 12 months.

Infra-inguinal Occlusive Disease

The SIROCCO trials were designed to assess the efficacy of drug-eluting stents (DES) in reducing neointimal hyperplasia in the femoropopliteal segment (16–18). In the prospective randomized multicenter double-blind SIROCCO II trial (17), 57 patients with IC or CLI due to SFA stenotic or occlusive disease were randomized to receive the sirolimus-eluting SMART nitinol self-expanding stent ($n=29$) or a bare SMART nitinol stent ($n=28$). At six months, there was no significant difference in patency rates or in-stent mean lumen diameter, target lesion diameter, percent stenosis or binary restenosis rates with 50% cutoff (DES, 0% vs. bare stent, 7.7%). The 18-month patency rate in both groups was high at 80%. Long-term outcome (18) was subsequently reported for all 93 patients with TransAtlantic Inter-Society Consensus type C SFA disease who were randomized within the two phases of the SIROCCO trial. A total of 47 patients received the sirolimus-eluting SMART stent and 46 received the bare SMART stent. At a mean follow-up of 24 months, there was no significant difference in the improvement in ABPI, claudication symptoms and restenosis rates (DES, 22.9% vs. bare stent, 21.1%). The target lesion revascularization rate for the DES group was 6% and for the bare stent group was 13%. The target vessel revascularisation rate for the DES group was 13% and for the bare stent group was 22%. The authors concluded that sirolimus-eluting and bare SMART stents were effective, safe, and free from restenosis in the majority of patients for up to 24 months and there was no significant difference in restenosis rates between the two types of stent. In an ongoing study of

SFA stenting, the SUPER-SL trial, the bare SMART stent is being compared directly with the Bard Luminexx stent.

TRIALS COMPARING STENT-GRAFTING AND ANGIOPLASTY

There are few data comparing stent-grafting with PTA alone in patients with chronic limb ischemia. Two non-randomized studies reporting the use of self-expanding nitinol supported expanded polytetrafluoroethylene (ePTFE) stent grafts (Hemobahn®, W.L. Gore & Associates, Flagstaff, Arizona, U.S.A.) in patients with chronic lower limb ischemia deserve attention. In an international study, Lammer et al. (19) implanted ePTFE stent grafts in 127 patients with symptomatic iliac (61 limbs) and SFA disease (80 limbs) with 100% technical success. The 12-month primary and secondary patency rates for iliac stent grafts were 91% and 93%, respectively, and for the SFA stent grafts were 79% and 93%, respectively. In another study (20), Hemobahn stent grafts were implanted in 52 patients with femoropopliteal artery occlusions (present in 82.7%) or stenoses with a minimum lesion length of 3 cm. Technical success was 100% and at 12 and 24 months, the primary patency rates were 78.4% and 74.1%, respectively, and secondary patency rates were 88.3% and 83.2%, respectively. These encouraging patency rates were supported by the results of a single-center experience (21) reported as part of a U.S. multicenter prospective randomized trial of the Hemobahn stent graft versus PTA alone for femoropopliteal stenoses or occlusions. In this study, 28 patients with IC or CLI were randomized to PTA alone ($n=13$) or PTA and implantation of a Hemobahn stent graft ($n=15$). The technical success rate was 100% in the stent-graft group and 92% in the PTA group. The 24-month primary patency rates were significantly better in the stent-graft group (87% vs. PTA alone, 25%; $p=0.002$) as was clinical outcome. While these results and those from the non-randomized studies are encouraging, the results from the full U.S. trial of femoropopliteal stent-grafting have not yet been reported so the single-center data must be interpreted with caution. The VIBRANT multicenter randomized trial is an ingoing study comparing the Viabahn® (W.L. Gore & Associates) stent graft and bare nitinol stents in patients with symptomatic SFA disease.

TRIALS COMPARING ENDOVASCULAR AND SURGICAL REVASCULARIZATION

There are a total of four published trials comparing PTA and surgery (22–25) and one published trial comparing stent-grafting and bypass surgery for SFA disease (26). There are no published trials comparing (iliac or infra-inguinal) stenting and surgery or stent-grafting with surgery for the management of iliac disease.

In the first reported study (22), which was performed in the late 1980s, a total of 102 patients with disabling IC or CLI were randomized to PTA or surgical revascularization. The study failed to demonstrate a significant difference in the immediate and one-year clinical outcomes in the two groups but PTA required a significantly shorter hospital stay. In a subsequent study from the U.S.A. published in the early 1990s (23), 263 men with IC or CLI due to iliac and/or femoropopliteal atherosclerotic disease were randomized to bypass surgery ($n=126$) or PTA ($n=129$) with eight patients receiving no treatment. As for the previous study, no significant difference in primary technical success, patient survival or limb salvage was demonstrated between the two groups at a median follow-up of four years.

There have been two more recent European trials comparing surgery and PTA. In one multicenter trial (24), 56 patients with IC or CLI due to long (5–15 cm) SFA disease were randomized to PTA ($n=31$) or above-knee femoropopliteal bypass grafting ($n=25$)]. The cumulative one-year patency after PTA and bypass grafting were 43% and 82%, respectively, and the authors concluded that above-knee femoropopliteal bypass was better than PTA for symptomatic patients with long SFA disease. In the BASIL trial (25), a U.K. prospective multicenter randomized controlled trial, 452 patients with CLI due to infra-inguinal disease were randomized to a bypass surgery first ($n=228$) or PTA first ($n=224$) treatment strategy. Overall, there was no significant difference in amputation-free survival or quality of life between the groups during follow-up. Bypass surgery was more expensive than PTA in the short term but, after two years follow-up, it appeared to be associated with a significantly reduced risk of amputation and/or death compared with PTA. The authors concluded that PTA was probably the best treatment for patients with limited life expectancy and significant comorbidity, whereas surgery may be the better option in patients expected to live for more than two years and who have usable vein for bypass.

To date, there has been one published randomized trial comparing stent-grafting and surgery (26). In this study, 100 limbs in 86 patients with IC or CLI due to femoropopliteal arterial occlusive disease were randomized to PTA and implantation of Viabahn ePTFE stent grafts (50 limbs) or above-knee prosthetic femoropopliteal bypass (50 limbs). At a median follow-up of 18 months, ABPI and duplex ultrasound demonstrated no significant difference in primary or secondary patency rates between the groups. The 12-month primary and secondary patency rates after stent graft were 73.5% and 83.9%, respectively, and after bypass were 74.2% and 83.7%, respectively, for the surgery group. Further follow-up is necessary to support these encouraging early results.

TRIALS COMPARING PTA ALONE AND EXERCISE TRAINING FOR CLAUDICATION

There is little doubt that exercise in patients with IC is associated with improved pain-free and maximum walking distance (27). In a Cochrane Review (28), only two randomized trials were identified comparing PTA alone versus nonsurgical management in a total of 98 patients with IC.

In the Edinburgh study (29), a total of 62 patients with mild or moderate IC due to SFA or iliac occlusive disease were randomized to PTA and best medical therapy (aspirin, advice on smoking and exercise) ($n=30$) or best medical therapy alone ($n=32$). At six-month follow-up, PTA was associated with a significantly greater improvement in pain-free walking distance, ABPI and quality of life and significantly less disease progression compared with the best medical therapy alone. At two-year follow-up (30), there was no significant difference in claudication symptoms, treadmill maximum walking distance, ABPI or quality of life between the groups. Those treated by PTA, however, continued to demonstrate significantly less disease progression. In the Oxford study (31), a total of 56 patients with stable unilateral IC were randomized to PTA or supervised exercise training. Exercise training was associated with the most significant changes in claudication and maximum walking distance from six months onward, with the greatest functional improvement observed in patients with SFA disease treated by exercise training. At approximately six years follow-up, there was no significant difference between the groups.

These data comparing PTA and nonsurgical management in IC appear to compare rather poorly with the results of surgery. In a prospective randomized trial (32), 75 patients with IC were randomized to surgery, surgery with physical training and physical training alone. At 13 months, symptom-free and maximal walking distance improved in all three groups. Surgery alone or in combination with subsequent training was superior to physical training alone.

SUMMARY

Randomized trials published to date demonstrate the following:

1. In patients with IC due to iliac disease, primary PTA with selective stenting is equivalent to primary stenting and is less expensive.
2. There is no robust evidence to support a policy of primary stenting of femoropopliteal disease compared with primary PTA and selective stenting. Early results from recent trials are encouraging, but long-term follow-up is required and the results of ongoing trials are awaited.
3. There is no evidence to support the use of drug-eluting nitinol stents in the femoropopliteal segment.
4. The early results of implanting self-expanding nitinol supported ePTFE stent grafts in the femoropopliteal segment appear better than PTA alone and equivalent to prosthetic above-knee femoropopliteal bypass.

5. In patients with chronic lower limb ischemia who can be managed with either surgery or PTA, both treatment strategies are associated with broadly similar outcomes.
6. There is no evidence that PTA is associated with a better long-term outcome compared with medical management alone in patients with IC.

REFERENCES

1. Bosch JL, Hunink MG. Meta-analysis of the results of percutaneous transluminal angioplasty and stent placement for aortoiliac occlusive disease. Radiology 1997; 204:87–96.
2. Tetteroo E, van der Graaf Y, Bosch JL, et al. Randomised comparison of primary stent placement versus primary angioplasty followed by selective stent placement in patients with iliac artery occlusive disease. Dutch Iliac Stent Trial Study Group. Lancet 1998; 351:1153–9.
3. Bosch JL, van der Graaf Y, Hunink MG. Health-related quality of life after angioplasty and stent placement in patients with iliac artery occlusive disease: results of a randomized controlled clinical trial. The Dutch Iliac Stent Trial Study Group. Circulation 1999; 99:3155–60.
4. Klein WM, van der Graaf Y, Seegers J, Moll FL, Mali WP. Long-term cardiovascular morbidity, mortality, and reintervention after endovascular treatment in patients with iliac artery disease: The Dutch Iliac Stent Trial Study. Radiology 2004; 232:491–8.
5. Klein WM, van der Graaf Y, Seegers J, et al. Dutch iliac stent trial: long-term results in patients randomized for primary or selective stent placement. Radiology 2006; 238:734–44.
6. Vroegindeweij D, Vos LD, Tielbeek AV, Buth J, vd Bosch HC. Balloon angioplasty combined with primary stenting versus balloon angioplasty alone in femoro-popliteal obstructions: a comparative randomized study. Cardiovasc Intervent Radiol 1997; 20:420–5.
7. Zdanowski Z, Albrechtsson U, Lundin A, et al. Percutaneous transluminal angioplasty with or without stenting for femoro-popliteal occlusions? A randomized controlled study. Int Angiol 1999; 18:251–5.
8. Grimm J, Muller-Hulsbeck S, Jahnke T, et al. Randomized study to compare PTA alone versus PTA with Palmaz stent placement for femoro-popliteal lesions. J Vasc Interv Radiol 2001; 12:935–42.
9. Muradin GS, Bosch JL, Stijnen T, Hunink MG. Balloon dilation and stent implantation for treatment of femoropopliteal arterial disease: meta-analysis. Radiology 2001; 221:137–45.
10. Bachoo P, Thorpe P. Endovascular stents for intermittent claudication. Cochrane Database Syst Rev 2003; 1:CD003228.
11. Cejna M, Thurnher S, Illiasch H, et al. PTA versus Palmaz stent placement in femoro-popliteal artery obstructions: a multicentre prospective randomized study. J Vasc Interv Radiol 2001; 12:23–31.
12. Becquemin JP, Favre JP, Marzelle J, et al. Systematic versus selective stent placement after superficial femoral artery balloon angioplasty: a multicentre prospective randomised study. J Vasc Surg 2003; 37:487–94.
13. Schillinger M, Sabeti S, Loewe C, et al. Balloon angioplasty versus implantation of nitinol stents in the superficial femoral artery. N Eng J Med 2006; 354:1879–88.
14. Rand T, Basile A, Cejna M, et al. PTA versus carbofilm-coated stents in infrapopliteal arteries: pilot study. Cardiovasc Intervent Radiol 2006; 29:29–38.
15. Ponec D, Jaff MR, Swischuk J, et al. The Nitinol SMART stent vs Wallstent for suboptimal iliac artery angioplasty: CRISP-US trial results. J Vasc Interv Radiol 2004; 15:911–8.
16. Duda SH, Pusich B, Richter G, et al. Sirolimus-eluting stents for the treatment of obstructive superficial femoral artery disease: six-month results. Circulation 2002; 106:1505–9.
17. Duda SH, Bosiers M, Lammers J, et al. Sirolimus-eluting versus bare nitinol stent for obstructive superficial femoral artery disease: the SIROCCO II trial. J Vasc Interv Radiol 2005; 16:331–8.
18. Duda SH, Bosiers M, Lammers J, et al. Drug-eluting and bare nitinol stents for the treatment of atherosclerotic lesions in the superficial femoral artery: long-term results from the SIROCCO trial. J Endovasc Ther 2006; 13:701–10.
19. Lammer J, Dake MD, Bleyn J, et al. Peripheral arterial obstruction: prospective study of trearment with a transluminally placed self-expanding stent-graft. International Trial Study Group. Radiology 2000; 217:95–104.
20. Jahnke T, Andresen R, Muller-Hulsbeck S, et al. Haemobahn stent-grafts for treatment of femoropopliteal arterial obstructions: midterm results of a prospective trial. J Vasc Interv Radiol 2003; 14:41–51.
21. Saxon RR, Coffman JM, Gooding JM, et al. Long-term results of ePTFE stent-graft versus angioplasty in the femoro-popliteal artery: single center experience from a prospective randomised trial. J Vasc Interv Radiol 2003; 14:303–11.
22. Holm J, Arfvidsson B, Jivegard L, et al. Chronic lower limb ischaemia. A prospective randomised controlled study comparing the 1-year results of vascular surgery and percutaneous transluminal angioplasty (PTA). Eur J Vasc Surg 1991; 5:517–22.

23. Wolf GL, Wilson SE, Cross AP, Deupree RH, Stason WB. Surgery or balloon angioplasty for peripheral vascular disease: a randomised clinical trial. Principal investigators and their Associates of Veterans Administration Cooperative Study Number 199. J Vasc Interv Radiol 1993; 4:639–48.
24. Van der Zaag ES, Legemate DA, Prins MA, et al. Angioplasty or bypass for superficial femoral artery disease? A randomized controlled trial. Eur J Vasc Endovasc Surg 2004; 28:132–7.
25. Adam DJ, Beard JD, Cleveland T, et al. BASIL trial participants. Bypass versus angioplasty in severe ischaemia of the leg (BASIL): multicentre, randomised controlled trial. Lancet 2005; 366:1925–34.
26. Kedora J, Hohmann S, Garrett W, Munschaur C, Theune B, Gable D. Randomised comparison of percutaneous Viabahn stent grafts vs prosthetic femoral-popliteal bypass in the treatment of superficial femoral arterial occlusive disease. J Vasc Surg 2007; 45:10–6.
27. Leng GC, Fowler B, Ernst E. Exercise for intermittent claudication. Cochrane Database Syst Rev 2000; 2:CD000990.
28. Fowkes FG, Gillespie IN. Angioplasty (versus non surgical management) for intermittent claudication. Cochrane Database Syst Rev 2000; 2:CD000017.
29. Whyman MR, Fowkes FG, Kerracher EM, et al. Randomised controlled trial of percutaneous transluminal angioplasty for intermittent claudication. Eur J Vasc Endovasc Surg 1996; 12:167–72.
30. Whyman MR, Fowkes FG, Kerracher EM, et al. Is intermittent claudication improved by percutaneous transluminal angioplasty? A randomised controlled trial. J Vasc Surg 1997; 26:551–7.
31. Perkins JM, Collin J, Creasy TS, Fletcher EW, Morris PJ. Exercise training versus angioplasty for stable claudication. Long and medium term results of a prospective, randomised trial. Eur J Vasc Endovasc Surg 1996; 11:409–13.
32. Lundgren F, Dahllof AG, Lundholm K, et al. Intermittent claudication, surgical reconstruction or physical training? A prospective randomized trial of treatment efficiency. Ann Surg 1989; 209:346–55.

10 Endovascular Management of Endovascular Complications (Troubleshooting Guide for Retrieval of Emboli, Misplaced Stents, Vascular Perforation, Dissection)

David O. Kessel
Department of Radiology, Leeds Teaching Hospitals, St. James's University Hospital, Leeds, U.K.

INTRODUCTION

Endovascular procedures are performed using a variety of catheters, guidewires and other tools which are manipulated within the vessel lumen. Like laparoscopic and endoscopic procedures the devices are inserted at a remote site. The advantage of all these minimally invasive techniques is reduction in trauma to the patient allowing a more rapid recovery following intervention. The most important disadvantage of a remote approach is lack of immediate access in case of a complication. For this reason operators need to be able to recognize and repair problems before they become irreversible. It is essential to be familiar with the devices and manoeuvers that can be used to rescue endovascular complications. Similarly it is indefensible to perform procedures without immediate access to the equipment to manage the most common complications which are likely to lead to open surgery. The basic principles underpinning this chapter are to minimize harm by adopting the maxim "prevention is better than cure" and recognition of when it is either safer to do nothing or use an open surgical option.

The most frequently encountered problems are complications resulting from angioplasty / stenting and the management of iatrogenic intravascular foreign bodies (Fig. 1). Clearly there is some overlap between these general areas, as distal atheroembolism and stent migration are amongst the commonest complications of endovascular management of arterial occlusive disease.

COMPLICATIONS OF ANGIOPLASTY AND STENTING

Complications of angioplasty and stenting are reported to occur in 1% to 4% of procedures and range from trivial events to potentially life-threatening disasters. Operators must recognize that when dealing with sensitive end-organs a complication that would be trivial in the peripheral circulation may result in devastating consequences such as stroke or renal failure. This is the key reason for regarding these territories as "advanced angioplasty." Broadly speaking the complications of angioplasty and stenting relate to arterial trauma either at the puncture site or the treatment itself (Table 1).

Puncture Site

Puncture site complications will not be discussed in detail other than these can be considered as "the 3 Bs"—bruising, bleeding, and blockage. The latter two may require emergency care, which may include the use of a balloon to tamponade the hole in the artery. This may be life saving especially in the presence of large hematoma in a hypotensive patient.

It is important to consider the implications of puncture site complications when planning procedural approach. For example if using the brachial artery the left arm is often the best

TABLE 1 Complications of Angioplasty and Stenting

Puncture site
  Bruising
  Bleeding
  Blockage
Related to angioplasty/stenting
  Spasm
  Vascular perforation
  Dissection
  Rupture
  Distal embolization
  Stent malposition
  Stent migration

choice as the catheter will pass fewest cerebral arteries and it is usually also the nondominant arm in case of puncture-related spasm or occlusion.

Spasm

Certain arteries are more prone to spasm than others. These include the crural circulation, the brachial, internal carotid, renal (Fig. 2) and the visceral arteries. These vessels should be treated particularly gently; low profile balloon and wire systems are less traumatic than larger and stiffer catheters and wires. Prophylactic or therapeutic antispasmodic agents such as glyceryl trinitrate (GTN) and papaverine should be considered in the arm, calf, and visceral vessels.

Arterial Perforation

Guidewire perforation is often self-limiting but if continued may result in formation of a large hematoma or compartment syndrome. Perforation occurs typically during extraluminal recanalization (Fig. 3). In this case although the degree of extravasation can be alarming it is usually self-limiting as flow has not been established. Unfortunately, this may preclude recanalization of the target vessel as the guidewire tends to pass repeatedly down the same tract. Perforation also occurs when a wire is inadvertently passed down a small branch artery mimicking the desired course of the wire. It is for this reason that it is essential to confirm true lumen entry after traversing an occlusion, as balloon angioplasty of a branch vessel is likely to result in rupture. Simple perforation of a branch vessel is more troublesome than perforation in the context of extraluminal recanalization, as this is the equivalent of arterial trauma in a

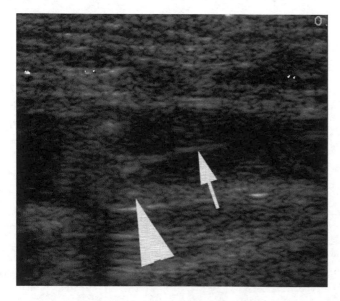

FIGURE 1 Angioseal device (*arrowhead*) occluding the common femoral artery; the thread (*arrow*) remains attached. The device was removed through an arteriotomy.

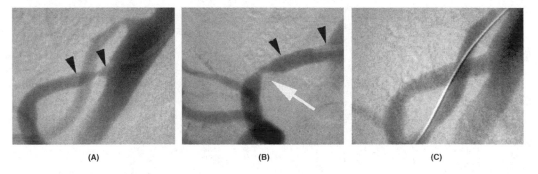

FIGURE 2　(**A**) Recurrent stenosis in a caudal renal transplant artery (*arrowheads*). (**B**) The stenosis has been stented (*black arrowheads*) but there is flow-limiting spasm (*white arrow*) beyond it. (**C**) Following glyceryl trinitrate (GTN) the spasm has resolved.

heparinized patient. In this instance it is usually best to inflate an angioplasty balloon across the origin of the branch to occlude it for 5 to 10 minutes. If the bleeding does not stop after this then consider whether the vessel can be removed, if yes then coil embolization will usually quickly and permanently occlude the vessel and stop further bleeding.

Arterial Dissection

Arterial dissection is an inevitable component of angioplasty and is the correlate of plaque rupture. Fortunately dissection is not typically flow limiting and in most cases is safely ignored. If the dissection obstructs flow then further intervention is necessary. The first step is to perform prolonged low pressure balloon inflation at the dissection site. If this does not improve the

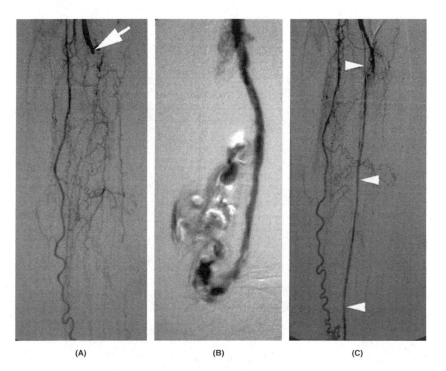

FIGURE 3　(**A**) Occlusion of all three crural arteries (*arrow*) in a patient with critical limb ischemia. (**B**) Guidewire perforation of the anterior tibial artery close to the ankle during attempted recanalization. (**C**) Completion angiogram following recanalization of the peroneal artery (*arrowheads*). As there is no flow in the anterior tibial artery, the extravasation was self-limiting.

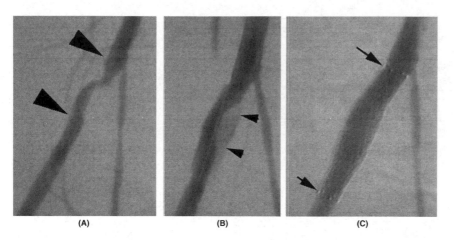

(A)   (B)   (C)

FIGURE 4 (**A**) External iliac artery stenosis (*arrowheads*). (**B**) Flow-limiting dissection persisted following prolonged balloon inflation (*arrowheads*). (**C**) Final appearance following stent deployment (*arrows*).

clinical situation, the options are to leave alone, stent (Fig. 4) or perform surgery. There are many anecdotal experiences where an apparently appalling outcome to angioplasty has "remodeled" to yield an excellent clinical and angiographic result. Equally there are many occasions when the angioplasty site thromboses. There is no scientifically proven answer to this issue, hence a strategy can be adopted based around the do no harm principle as given in the algorithm below:

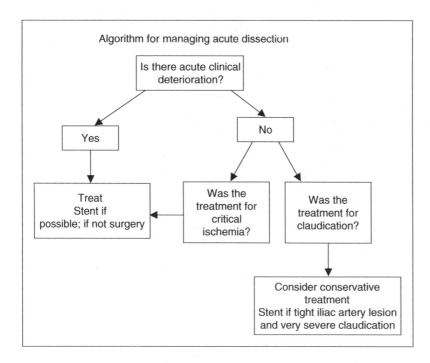

Vascular Rupture

This is one of the most serious complications of angioplasty and stenting. Although rare it is important to be able to recognize the situations in which it is likely to occur, the symptoms and angiographic signs and be able promptly to manage the situation. The most common cause of rupture is over zealous angioplasty of a small calcified external iliac artery usually in a female patient. This clinical scenario should invite caution from the outset! The clinical clues heralding

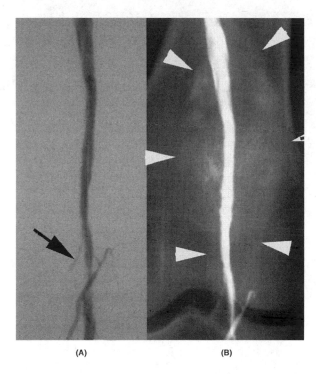

(A)   (B)

FIGURE 5 (**A**) Following extraluminal recanalization of a popliteal artery occlusion there is an apparent small branch vessel (*black arrow*). (**B**) Review of the unsubtracted image shows that this represents a tear with a large hematoma (*white arrowheads*). The leak resolved following five minutes balloon inflation with no clinical sequelae.

hypotensive collapse are usually yawning and restlessness or agitation. If this occurs check the pulse and blood pressure immediately and prepare to resuscitate the patient. The angiographic signs of rupture range from a subtle blush adjacent to the angioplasty site (Fig. 5) to frank extravasation of contrast.

When rupture is diagnosed it is time to act swiftly before the patient becomes shocked. The first step in management is to control bleeding. This is normally readily achieved by inflating the angioplasty balloon proximal to or across the leak.

Arresting Hemorrhage

There are limited options for arresting hemorrhage, the simplest being prolonged balloon inflation. This may suffice with small leaks but is unlikely to work with more major injury. In this case whilst it is possible that a simple stent might repair a small rent in the artery wall, a covered stent is a better option. Consider the best approach for deploying the stent graft, if possible use a separate access point as this will allow the balloon tamponade to be maintained until the stent graft is almost in position to be deployed. This minimizes the time during which bleeding will occur. This principle also applies when removing a line that has been placed intra-arterially.

Distal Atheroembolism

Detection of distal emboli is the reason for performing completion angiography of the runoff circulation. Distal embolization can be considered in terms of the size of the embolic material. Plaque rupture with distal cholesterol embolization is a feared complication of angiography and intervention. Cholesterol emboli occlude capillaries irreversibly. The commonest manifestation of this is livedo reticularis but more severe problems result if the embolic shower occludes a vital vascular bed such as the kidney, intestine or brain. Unfortunately there is little that can be done to treat these microemboli and prevention by gentle catheter and wire manipulation is the key. Larger emboli occlude larger vessels and their manifestation depends on the vessel affected. Embolic occlusion of a vital vessel will produce acute ischemia in its territory and require immediate management. Fortunately most emboli will affect small branch vessels, which may be treated conservatively. Management of clinically significant emboli

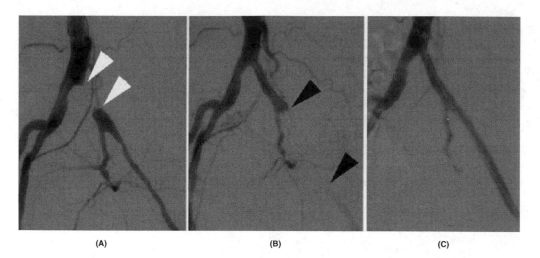

(A)   (B)   (C)

FIGURE 6   (**A**) Common iliac occlusion (*white arrowheads*). (**B**) Following stenting the external iliac artery has been occluded by plaque embolus (*black arrowheads*). (**C**) After deployment of a second stent over the embolus, flow has been restored.

depends on the size and site of the occlusion. Small emboli can be aspirated through large lumen guide catheters with removable hubs. If this fails some may respond to thrombolysis but larger or refractory emboli may require surgery or stenting in selected cases (Fig. 6). Stenting is possible in the iliac arteries and also the superficial femoral artery but should be avoided at points of flexion such as the hip and knee joints where repeated flexion and compression will inevitably lead to stent failure.

Stent Migration and Misplacement

Balloon-mounted stents may dislodge from the angioplasty balloon during passage to the deployment site or during balloon inflation. Fortunately, this is uncommon with premounted stents unless attempting to pass the stent around challenging anatomy. If this problem is recognized early it is simple to manage as the stent will not have been expanded, this allows some chance of capturing it and either deploying it at the target site or at least in a position where it is unlikely to cause harm. The most favorable scenario is when the stent has stayed in the correct position but the balloon has displaced due to asymmetric expansion (Fig. 7). In this case it may be possible to anchor the stent in place by fully deflating the balloon (this is most readily achieved with a 50-mL syringe) and attempting to reposition it within the stent then

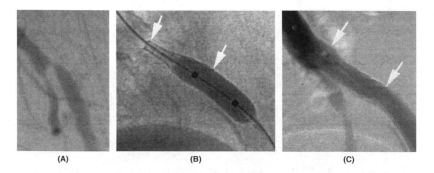

(A)   (B)   (C)

FIGURE 7   (**A**) External iliac artery stenosis. (**B**) The partially expanded balloon expandable stent (*arrows*) has remained in position but the angioplasty balloon has moved caudally during inflation. (**C**) Completion angiogram; the stent is in excellent position (*arrows*) and has been fully expanded by repositioning the balloon.

starting again. Unfortunately a deflated angioplasty balloon seldom regains its initial low profile and is more likely to snag on the stent and displace it. If this happens the stent can be brought back to a safe place such as the iliac artery and deployed. When the stent comes right off the balloon the situation becomes more complicated. If it is still on the guidewire it can usually be brought back into a large arterial sheath. This usually requires exchange of the sheath before attempts to recover the stent. Recovery is accomplished either by passing a low-profile balloon through the stent to capture it or by snaring the stent on the wire. The former may require exchanging the guidewire for a 0.018-in. wire. If the stent has come off the guidewire it will probably only be retrievable with a snare. The snare and stent combination tend not to align perfectly. If this is the case consider seriously whether it would be safer to leave the stent where it is.

Problems can also occur when balloon mounted and self-expanding stents are deployed in a suboptimal position. Recovering and repositioning a fully expanded stent risks causing significant vascular trauma and whenever possible they should be left where they are.

RETRIEVAL OF INTRAVASCULAR FOREIGN BODIES

Snares

A key tool in recovering and repositioning intravascular devices is a snare. This is simply a form of lasso which can be used to grab the free end of a catheter, wire or stent. Snares come in different forms and sizes to suit different vessels. The principle behind their use is the same; the snare is introduced through a shaped steerable catheter. It opens when pushed out of the guide catheter and closes when retracted into the catheter. The snare is manoeuvered into position and opened, then either advanced over the target object or alternatively if capturing a guidewire the snare is kept still and then the wire advanced through it. In either case the snare is tightened by keeping it still and advancing the guide catheter (Fig. 8). Most snares incorporate a pin vice on the snare wire which can be positioned against the catheter hub and

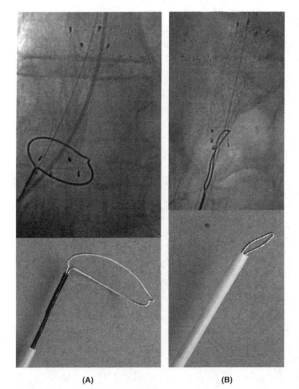

(A) (B)

FIGURE 8   A self-expanding stent being captured by a gooseneck snare. (**A**) The open snare is maneuvered around the stent. (**B**) The snare is closed and the stent pulled back into a safe position in the common iliac vein.

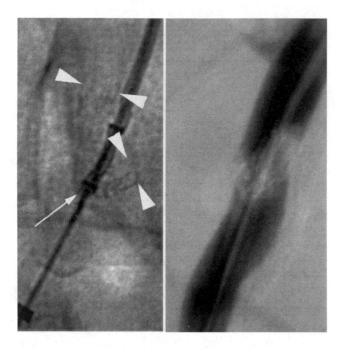

FIGURE 9 A thrombosed balloon expandable stent (*arrowheads*) has been removed from a renal artery and brought down to the external iliac artery. The stent is kinked (*arrow*) and fills the artery lumen and hence is too big to bring into a sheath. The patient was heparinized and the stent removed through a surgical cutdown.

tightened locking the snare closed. Once the object has been grasped it can then be repositioned or retrieved. When removing something from the circulation ensure that a large enough sheath is used to accommodate the snare and the object together. With very large objects this is not possible, in this case bring the object to a safe place and perform a surgical cutdown and arteriotomy or venotomy (Fig. 9).

SUMMARY

It is almost inevitable that anyone performing endovascular procedures will occasionally need to be able to manage complications. The Learning Points stress a safety first ethos which is in the best interests of both clinicians and patients.

Learning points:
- Prevention is always better than cure.
- Be honest about your ability and ask for help when working in unfamiliar scenarios.
- Learn to recognize actions that lead to complications.
- Think ahead try to anticipate potential difficulties and how they might be prevented or managed.
- Be familiar with the tools that will get you out of trouble and ensure that your "repair kit" is available.
- Always leave the wire in place when doing the first angiographic control.

When a problem has occurred:
- Try to recognize it before the situation becomes critical.
- *Stay calm*: This not always easy but maximizes the chances of saving the day.
- *Stabilize the patient*: Stop the bleeding quickly, resuscitate the patient, and call for appropriate help.
- Consider whether fixing the problem is necessary; sometimes the repair will cause more harm than good.
- Plan your approach and ensure that the necessary equipment is ready.

BIBLIOGRAPHY

There is no comprehensive list of references for management of complications of angiography and intervention. The reader might find some of the following helpful.

Beek FJ, Kaatee R, Beutler JJ, et al. Complications during renal artery stent placement for atherosclerotic ostial stenosis. Cardiovasc Intervent Radiol 1997; 20:184–90.

Belli A-M, Cumberland DC, Knox AM, et al. The complication rate of percutaneous peripheral balloon angioplasty. Clin Radiol 1990; 41:380–3.

Egglin TPK, Dickey KW, Rosenblatt M, et al. Retrieval of intravascular foreign bodies: experience in 32 cases. AJR 1995; 164:1259–64.

Gabelmann A, Kramer S, Gorich J. Percutaneous retrieval of lost or misplaced intravascular objects. AJR 2001; 176:1509–13.

Hartnell GG, Gates J, Soujanen JN, et al. Transfemoral repositioning of malpositioned central venous catheters. Cardiovasc Intervent Radiol 1996; 19:329–31.

Hartnell GG. Techniques for intact removal of vascular foreign bodies. Intervent Radiol 1996; 11:29–37.

Kessel D, Robertson I. Interventional Radiolgy: A Survival Guide. 2nd ed. New York: Chuchill Livingstone, 2005 (ISBN 0443062897).

Matsi PJ, Manninen HI. Complications of lower limb percutaneous transluminal angioplasty: a prospective analysis of 410 procedures on 295 consecutive patients. Cardiovasc Intervent Radiol 1998; 21:361–6.

Slonim SM, Dake MD, Razavi MK, et al. Management of misplaced or migrated endovascular stents. J Vasc Interv Radiol 1999; 10:851–9.

Spies JB, Berlin L. Complications of femoral artery puncture. AJR 1998; 170:9–11.

Standards of Practice Committee, Society of Cardiovascular and Interventional Radiology. Standard for diagnostic arteriography in adults. J Vasc Interv Radiol 1993; 4:385–95.

Trerotola SO. Management of hemorrhagic complications. J Vasc Interv Radiol 1996; 7:92–4.

Wagner HJ, Starck EE. Acute embolic occlusions of the infrainguinal arteries: percutaneous aspiration embolectomy in 102 patients. Radiology 1992; 182:403–7.

11 Brachiocephalic and Subclavian Artery Occlusive Disease

Jowad Raja and Anna-Maria Belli
Department of Radiology, St. George's Hospital, London, U.K.

INTRODUCTION

Occlusive disease of the brachiocephalic artery and subclavian arteries is often asymptomatic because of the extensive collateral network of the upper limb arteries. However it is an important cause of extracranial cerebrovascular disease and upper limb ischemia due to occlusion or distal embolization (1). The commonest cause of occlusive disease is atherosclerosis, followed by Takayasu's disease. Other causes of occlusive disease are shown in Table 1. The pattern of disease and the age at presentation reflects the underlying etiology. Endovascular methods of treatment are the same as those used in the lower limb arteries, but anatomical differences direct the choices made during treatment and the risks related to the procedure.

ETIOLOGY

In the Western world the commonest cause is atherosclerosis (2). Atherosclerotic disease can occur at any site along the subclavian or brachiocephalic arteries but is most likely to cause symptoms when located at the ostium as this is most likely to compromise formation of effective collaterals. Ostial lesions are usually the result of aortic plaque impinging on the origin of the vessel. Disease at the origin of the right subclavian artery may also affect the right common carotid artery origin. The left subclavian artery is the most common aortic arch branch vessel affected by atherosclerosis (Fig. 1) and causes subclavian steal syndrome three times more commonly than the right. Subclavian steal syndrome occurs when the subclavian artery is occluded or stenosed proximal to the origin of the vertebral artery. When the arm is exercised, blood flows retrogradely down the vertebral artery and the patient may develop neurological symptoms such as dizziness and syncope, due to vertebro-basilar ischemia (3). In a study of extracranial arterial occlusive disease, subclavian or brachiocephalic artery stenosis was reported in 17% of cases. Flow reversal within the vertebral artery occurred in 2.5% of these cases, and of those with angiographic steal only 5.3% (9 patients of 168) had neurological symptoms (1). If blood flow to the arm is inadequate, the patient may present with arm claudication.

The subclavian artery may become narrowed or occluded as a result of chronic extrinsic compression in thoracic outlet syndrome as the artery passes medial to the scalene triangle in the costoclavicular space or within the scalene triangle itself. The relatively small size of these spaces means that muscular hypertrophy, congenital abnormalities (e.g., cervical rib) or pathological masses (e.g., clavicular fractures with callus formation) may cause compression of vascular structures. Compression is exacerbated in certain positions and imaging investigations should be performed in the neutral and hyperabducted positions. Repeated compression leads to intimal injury with fibrosis and luminal narrowing with post-stenotic dilatation and aneurysm formation. Formation of mural thrombus either at the lesion or in the area of post-stenotic dilatation may lead to embolization, resulting in digital ischemia or symptoms mimicking Raynaud's phenomenon. Thoracic outlet syndrome is more common in women and age at presentation ranges from 10 to 50 years.

TABLE 1   Causes of Occlusive Disease of Subclavian
and Brachiocephalic Arteries

Atherosclerosis
Thoracic outlet syndrome
Takayasu's arteritis
Giant cell arteritis
Radiation-induced arteritis
Trauma
Fibromuscular dysplasia
Aortic dissection
Cardiogenic emboli

Takayasu's disease and giant cell arteritis are important causes of occlusive disease affecting the upper extremity large vessels although their incidence is low. The incidence of Takayasu's disease varies geographically, but in Europe one to three new cases per million per year are observed (2). Takayasu's disease is a chronic arteritis affecting large vessels, predominantly the aorta and its main branches (5,6). Its incidence is higher in females and the median onset of age is 25 years (7). In giant cell arteritis, giant cells (i.e., macrophages, lymphocytes, and mononuclear cells), infiltrate all layers of the arterial wall causing segmental inflammation, which leads to wall thickening and fibrosis mainly involving arteries originating from the aortic arch. Typical angiographic features include stenoses (Fig. 2) and microaneurysm formation. Symptoms are usually related to involvement of the external carotid artery (headache, scalp tenderness and blindness). Giant cell arteritis affects patients older than 50 years, again with prevalence for female patients. Treatment of the arterial occlusive disease by angioplasty and stenting must be accompanied by medical treatment of the underlying arteritis.

INDICATIONS FOR TREATMENT

The commonest indications for treatment are symptoms of vertebro-basilar insufficiency, upper limb ischemia and blue digits due to embolization from a proximal lesion. An important

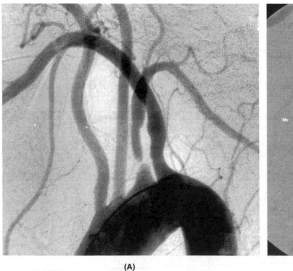
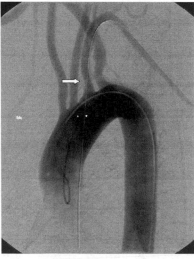

(A)   (B)

FIGURE 1   (**A**) An arch aortogram showing a stenosis in the proximal left subclavian artery. The projection is left anterior oblique. Note the aberrant right subclavian artery. (**B**) A post percutaneous transluminal angioplasty angiogram showing a good result (*white arrow*). In this case an 8 mm balloon was used. Access was obtained from the ipsilateral brachial artery and right common femoral artery.

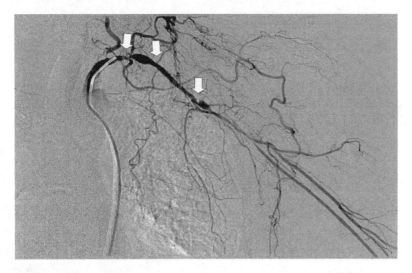

FIGURE 2 A selective left subclavian arteriogram in a patient with giant cell arteritis. This shows multiple stenoses with post stenotic dilatation along the subclavian artery (*highlighted by white arrows*). The axillary artery is also affected and shows a long stenosis.

indication for treatment is as an adjunct to surgery to relieve any inflow obstruction prior to placing a by-pass graft, or to treat a lesion which develops after such surgery, e.g., internal mammary artery to coronary artery and axillo-femoral by pass grafts. Other indications include transient ischemic attacks and stroke. In all cases of neurological symptoms careful assessment of other possible causes should be investigated.

IMAGING TECHNIQUES

Ultrasound

Ultrasound (US) is a useful noninvasive modality although it is operator dependent. Duplex US can detect stenosis greater than 50% with a moderate high sensitivity (80%) and has an excellent negative predictive value, greater than 95% (8). Duplex US can demonstrate reversal of flow in the vertebral artery if subclavian steal syndrome is suspected. It will also demonstrate if the vertebral artery is occluded.

The brachiocephalic artery is difficult to examine and the ostium of the left subclavian artery cannot be directly visualized but useful information can be obtained from the subclavian artery where it is visible. A normal Doppler waveform is triphasic. If there is loss of the sharp systolic peak associated with loss of triphasic waveform and presence of turbulence, this would infer a significant proximal stenosis. US is easy to perform with the patient in various positions during assessment of thoracic outlet syndrome.

Multi-Slice Computed Tomography Angiography

This is a noninvasive modality which is excellent for evaluating the subclavian and brachiocephalic arteries. It has the advantages of not being operator dependent and is able to assess the origins of the supra-aortic vessels, but has the disadvantages of using ionizing radiation and requiring iodinated contrast medium. Thin collimation (1–3 mm) with contrast enhancement can produce images comparable to digital subtraction angiography (DSA). However, the images are degraded in the presence of metal artifacts such as stents.

Magnetic Resonance Angiography

Magnetic resonance angiography (MRA) is another noninvasive modality for imaging the subclavian and brachiocephalic arteries with the advantages of no ionizing radiation or iodinated contrast medium. Gadolinium enhanced 3D acquisitions provide excellent detail of the aortic arch and vessel origins. Phase contrast MRA encode the direction of flow and can show subclavian stenosis and reversal of flow in the vertebral artery.

Digital Subtraction Angiography

DSA is an invasive method for evaluating disease of the subclavian and brachiocephalic arteries. However it provides high temporal and spatial resolution, hence the images give clear visualization of the arteries and any stenoses or occlusions. DSA shows direction of flow within the vertebral arteries but carries the same risks of all arteriographic techniques, with the added risk of stroke and so is reserved for those patients where there is ambiguity on other imaging modalities. It is important to examine the patient with the arm in neutral and hyperabducted when investigating thoracic outlet syndrome (Fig. 3A,B). Angiography is an essential prerequisite for endovascular treatment.

ENDOVASCULAR METHODS OF TREATMENT

Percutaneous transluminal angioplasty (PTA) is a simple, safe, and effective treatment for stenotic disease of the subclavian and brachiocephalic arteries whatever the underlying etiology and site of the lesion (9–11). In the presence of a complete occlusion, primary stenting is the treatment of choice, to avoid potential complications of displacing a large volume of occlusive material and to improve patency rates. Complex stenoses may also be treated by primary stenting to reduce the risk of embolization (12,13). Some operators advocate primary stenting for all lesions (14) but others reserve stenting for failed PTA when there is a residual significant stenosis or occluding dissection flap (12,15). Stent grafts may be used in treating acute iatrogenic or traumatic ruptures and aneurysms but are not the subject of this chapter.

Before a stent is placed, consideration of the anatomic site is essential. If the site to be treated is secondary to extrinsic compression, e.g., by a rib anomaly, a stent may fracture by repeated compression leading to restenosis or reocclusion (Fig. 4). Either a stent should not be placed or the underlying cause addressed, e.g., rib resection should be performed first.

Radiation induced stenoses and those secondary to arteritides may be very fibrotic and resistant to balloon dilatation. In such cases cutting balloon angioplasty (CBA) may have a place (16). (See the section entitled Troubleshooting.)

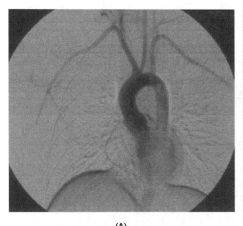 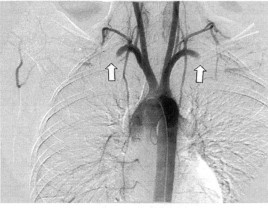

(A)   (B)

FIGURE 3 Arch aortogram in a patient with thoracic outlet obstruction. The image in (**A**) was taken with arms down; (**B**) was taken with arms up. Note compression of the subclavian arteries (*white arrows*) is only seen with arms raised.

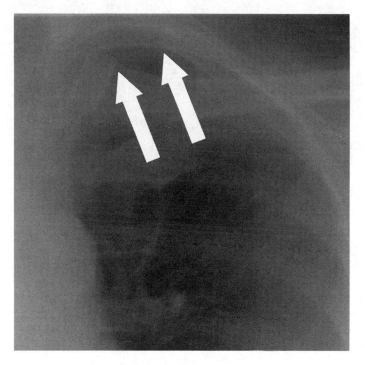

FIGURE 4   This chest x-ray shows a fractured stent (*white arrows*). The stent was placed in the left subclavian artery one year previously for stenotic disease. The patient was asymptomatic at the time of control.

ENDOVASCULAR TECHNIQUE

The procedure is performed under local anaesthetic. Arterial access in most cases will be obtained via the brachial and/or common femoral arteries. Other potential arterial access sites are the radial and axillary arteries. The approach depends on the site of the lesion and experience of the operator.

Ostial lesions, particularly complete occlusions, can be difficult to recanalize from the aortic arch. In these situations a pigtail catheter is passed into the aortic arch from a femoral approach and this allows diagnostic images to be obtained as a "roadmap" to guide recanalization attempts which are made from the ipsilateral arm via a brachial, radial or axillary approach. The access site selected depends on local expertise, diameter of vessels and size of sheath required. A 6 or 7 F sheath or guiding catheter is adequate for most cases. An arm approach facilitates recanalization by providing a shorter route with more guidewire and catheter control and avoids the difficulties of maneuvering in large, tortuous vessels. However, should this fail, a guiding catheter may be lodged into the proximal part of the artery being treated to provide support and angiographic guidance for recanalization.

Heparin is given intra-arterially as a bolus (5000 IU) and antispasmodic agents are given to prevent spasm and occlusion in a brachial or more distal artery. The lesion is crossed using the operator's standard technique for crossing stenoses and occlusions. Although this varies with different operators, a hydrophilic wire such as the 0.035 in. Terumo (Radiofocus® Guidewire M) with a curved catheter providing directional control and support, is commonly used. The diameter of the target artery is estimated on angiographic images and the appropriate size of stent or balloon selected accordingly. Very accurate measurement is rarely required in this territory but if more accurate measurement is required, the operator may use their preferred method, i.e., calibration with a catheter. The subclavian and brachiocephalic arteries are generally of large diameter ranging from 7 to 12 mm.

The method of determining whether PTA has been successful is by measuring the pressure gradient across the lesion ($<$10% of the systemic systolic gradient is usually

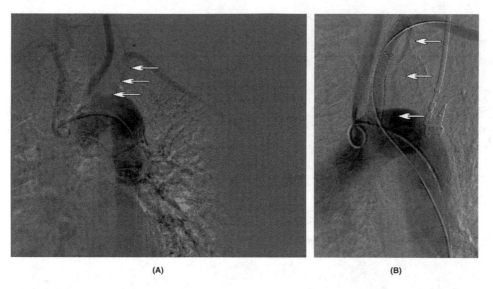

(A)   (B)

FIGURE 5 Arch aortogram showing a long occlusion of the left subclavian artery (*white arrows*). In (**A**) The left vertebral artery is seen filling retrogradely. Primary stenting with self expanding stents produced a successful result. (**B**) Note the origins of the left vertebral and internal thoracic arteries are not covered.

deemed acceptable) (13). Alternatively on angiography, less than 30% residual stenosis is deemed a successful result. Stenting is considered if the PTA result is unsatisfactory. Primary stenting is undertaken for complete occlusions (Fig. 5A,B) and is analogous to primary stenting of complete occlusions of the iliac arteries. Some operators would consider primary stenting in all subclavian lesions (13).

Balloon expandable stents (Fig. 6) are preferred at the ostium of the artery as they can be placed highly accurately with only a few millimeters projecting into the aorta (analogous to renal artery stenting at the ostium) and they provide higher radial force than self-expanding stents. They are ideal for short occlusions where the artery is not curved. For longer occlusions or occlusions distal to the origin of the vertebral artery, self-expanding stents are preferred to allow for curvature and mobility.

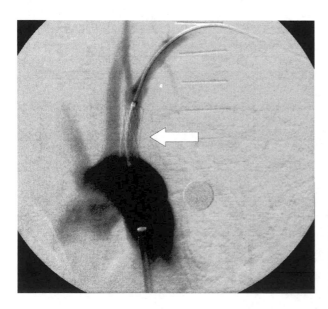

FIGURE 6 A ballooned expandable stent is deployed across the ostium of the left subclavian artery (*white arrow*). This patient had a short ostial stenosis. Note only a few millimeters of the stent projects into the aorta. Balloon expandable stents allow greater accuracy in deployment.

Protection of vulnerable adjacent arteries is controversial. Protection of a patent vertebral artery by using an inflated balloon or cerebral protection device prior to PTA of the subclavian artery has been advocated (15) but flow is usually reversed in these patients and this is thought to act as inherent protection, preventing microemboli reaching the posterior cerebral circulation. Protection of the common carotid artery during brachiocephalic intervention or when treating disease at the origin of the right subclavian artery may have a role and has been reported in small numbers of patients with good results (17,18).

TROUBLESHOOTING

This section deals with specific problems encountered during endovascular treatment of brachiocephalic and subclavian arterial lesions.

How to Puncture Small, Pulseless Arteries

The initial problem is to secure arterial access in an artery of small caliber, prone to spasm or is pulseless. US guidance is essential to do this without trauma to the vessel. A 7 to 12 MHz linear probe will show the artery longitudinally and in cross section. Color flow and Doppler are helpful though not essential. The artery is usually punctured with the probe showing it in cross section. The puncture is less traumatic if a micropuncture set is used (4 Fr) and once access is secured a bolus of antispasmodic agent, e.g., 150 µg of glyceryl trinitrate is given immediately.

What to Do if Recanalization from the Ipsilateral Arm Fails

For the reasons specified in the previous section an ipsilateral arm approach is preferred, but should this fail or not be feasible, recanalization from the aortic arch is required. Although endovascular intervention of supra-aortic vessels via a contralateral arm approach is undoubtedly feasible and has been described, in most situations a femoral approach is used. Here there are several options.

Bilateral femoral punctures allow a pigtail catheter to be inserted from one side to provide angiographic guidance, whilst a pre-shaped catheter such as a Mani, Sidewinder or Cobra from the other side is manipulated to catheterize the artery to be treated. If the diseased segment is several centimeters beyond the origin, it should be possible to pass a guidewire far enough into the vessel to allow the catheter to advance to a stable position from which an attempt to recanalize the occluded segment can be made (Fig. 7A,B). If the disease extends to the aortic arch, this is more difficult. In such cases attempts should be made to lodge the tip of a guiding catheter in the origin and tentatively try to advance guidewires of various types and diameter without dislodging the guiding catheter. Hydrophilic 0.035-in. guidewires are particularly useful, but smaller 0.014- or 0.018-in. wires with long or short floppy tips can also be successful.

What to Do if the Catheter Will Not Track over the Wire

Having recanalized the lesion, it is occasionally difficult to pass a catheter across the lesion. This may be because of extreme tortuosity of the arteries causing the wire to buckle in the arch, or because of the fibrotic and calcified nature of the underlying disease process. A Van Andel® catheter (Cook Medical Bloomington Indiana, U.S.A.) has a graduated tip and may pass over the wire. Hydrophilic catheters may also pass where others fail due to their slippery coating.

If any of these catheters do pass, it is then possible to replace the wire through them with a stiffer wire such as an Amplatz Super Stiff™ (Boston Scientific Natick, Massachusetts, U.S.A.) or Lunderquist (Cook) so that a balloon catheter or stent can be passed over them more easily. Pre-dilatation with a balloon catheter of small diameter, i.e., 4 mm, may allow easier passage of the definitive balloon catheter or stent.

If it proves impossible to pass any catheter over the recanalizing wire or the very stiff support wire cannot be advanced through the tortuous vessels without losing position, it may

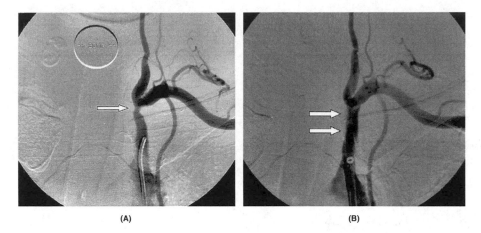

FIGURE 7 (A) Left subclavian arteriogram showing a left subclavian artery stenosis several centimeters from the origin (*white arrow*). (B) In this case a guiding catheter can be introduced from the right common femoral artery allowing percutaneous transluminal angioplasty and check angiography through the guiding catheter while maintaining the guidewire across the lesion in case stenting is required.

be necessary to snare the wire (either in the arm or aorta) and pull it though the second arterial access site. This will only be possible with a femoral and arm approach and with an exchange length wire (260 cm). This will then allow the operators to put tension on the wire from both ends to facilitate passage of a catheter.

What to Do if Thrombus Is Present

If the presence of fresh thrombus is suspected catheter-guided thrombolysis may be performed. Alternatively if the lesion is in the brachiocephalic artery then a combined surgical and radiological approach is useful. The right common carotid artery is surgically exposed and the lesion treated retrogradely via the common carotid artery, with cross clamping of the common carotid artery during stent deployment to prevent cerebral embolization (12).

What to Do If the Lesion Involves Vertebral Artery Origin

Subclavian disease may involve the origin of the vertebral artery. Although placement of stents across vertebral artery origins should be avoided, such cases have been reported with no significant complications. In one study no significant neurological complications occurred on follow up even when the vertebral artery became occluded (12).

What to Do if the Artery Resists Dilatation

Stenoses due to radiation-induced arteritis, in stent restenosis and arteritides such as giant cell, may be very resistant to balloon dilatation. Balloon dilatation should be attempted first as many of these lesions will respond favorably. In one study (19) repeat PTA was successful in 50% of restenoses. However, if the balloon cannot be inflated to its full diameter within the lesion, CBA may be helpful (20,21). The cutting balloon should be undersized in relation to the vessel being treated to avoid rupture of the artery. If this is successful, it can be followed by balloon dilatation or stenting with a device of the required diameter. There are several case reports in the literature describing the role of CBA in arteritides (22).

REVIEW OF LITERATURE

There are no randomized controlled trials comparing surgery with endovascular repair and no systematic reviews in the English literature. There is one recent comparative non-matched study (23) of bypass surgery using an extra-anatomic approach versus angioplasty for atherosclerotic disease of the supra-aortic vessels. A prospective database was used to collect information on 76 patients, 35 treated by surgery and 41 by angioplasty/stenting. No information was supplied about the selection process but the angioplasty cohort did not include any carotid or brachiocephalic arteries (only subclavian and axillary arteries) and the surgical group included five patients who required a carotid to carotid bypass graft prior to thoracic stent-graft insertion. In the surgical group there were five complications, but no peri-operative strokes, deaths or limb amputations and a secondary patency of 97% at mean five year follow-up. In the endovascular group there were four complications including one major peri-procedural stroke but no deaths or limb amputations. There were eight technical failures. The primary patency rate for technically successful angioplasties was 82% at four years.

Symptomatic atherosclerotic disease of the supra-aortic vessels was traditionally treated by bypass from the aortic arch to the carotid or subclavian vessels. The patency of these grafts was excellent and reported as 94% and 88% at five and ten years, respectively (24), but with a stroke and death rate of 16%. This led to the introduction of extra-anatomic bypass procedures, which have equivalent graft patency rates but a reduced mortality of between 0% and 3% (24–26) and a complication rate of 13% (27). Endovascular methods of treatment should be compared with this surgical approach.

The majority of evidence on endovascular treatment is based on case series. Some of the largest and most recent case series from the English literature, reporting key outcomes are reported in Table 2.

The technical success rate ranges from 84% to 97%, but is much higher for stenoses than occlusions. The number of occlusions reported in each series is very small, but the success rate in occlusions is of the order of 50%. The patency rates range from 72% to 89% at five years. Most reports are for treatment of atherosclerotic disease but the results in Takayasu's disease are similar with secondary patency rates of 82% at 82 months (22).

Complication rates range widely from 4.5% to 19% with minor complications reported. Thirty day mortality and stroke rates range from 1% to 9%. The major complications of this technique are stroke, transient ischemic attack, arm embolization and ischemia. Less frequently occurring, but reported complications include stent infection, cerebral hyperperfusion and arterial rupture (31). Recurrent disease is successfully managed by a repeat endovascular procedure in half the cases. There is still insufficient evidence to show whether the results of primary stenting are better than for PTA, although in one series (14) it was noted that there were no cerebrovascular complications and the restenosis rate was lower but this was based on only 21 patients.

CONCLUSION

Endovascular treatment of subclavian and brachio-cephalic arterial disease avoids some of the complications associated with open surgery. The recovery rate is quicker than with surgery and hospital stay shorter.

Endovascular treatment does not require a general anaesthetic and so is clearly indicated in those patients who are a poor anaesthetic risk. The high technical success and patency rates in focal stenoses also make it the procedure of choice in such disease. Total occlusions may be technically unsuccessful, but as in other vascular territories it is worthwhile attempting an endovascular approach first, as the results are good if technically successful and if unsuccessful, surgery is still possible.

The immediate complication rates are similar and although the durability and long-term results are not as good as with surgery, they are reasonable out to five years. It is also likely that results with systematic stenting will improve long term patency. The overall patient survival in this group of patients is 76% at five years (28) as they tend to be elderly and have multiple co-morbidities and in these patients many authors would advocate PTA/stenting as first line treatment (9,12,13,19,27). If the patient is young and relatively fit, then surgery may be the preferred option.

TABLE 2 Results of Case Series of Endovascular Treatment of Subclavian and Brachiocephalic Arterial Disease

Reference	No. of patients	Site	Stenosis vs. occlusion	PTA (%) /stent (%)	Technical success (%)	Primary patency	Follow-up (months)	Combined 30 day major stroke and death rate (%)	Total comp. rate (%)	Comments
De Vries et al. 2004 (19)	110	Subclavian	90 vs. 20	42/58	93	89% at 5 yr	Mean 34 Max 120	3.6	4.5	Higher technical failure in occlusions Numbers too small to detect difference between PTA and stenting Restenosis occurred within 2 yr
Amor et al. 2004 (14)	86	Subclavian	76 vs. 13	0/100	93.3	88% at 3 yr	Mean 38 Max 50	2.3	10.1	54% technical success in occlusions Primary stenting vs. stenting post dilatation showed lower re-stenosis and no major complications
Brountzos et al. 2004 (12)	48	Subclavian (49) and brachiocephalic (10)	42 vs. 7	0/100	96	77% at 2 yr	Mean 16.7 Max 68	4.2	8.3	Two patients with thrombus in brachiocephalic lesions were treated by a combined surgical and radiological approach with surgical cut down on the ipsilateral CCA Two patients died within 30 days from unrelated causes
Bates et al. 2004 (28)	91	Subclavian	NR	0/100	97	72% at 5 yr	Mean 36 Max 109	1	14	Death within 30 days unrelated to procedure

Study	N	Vessel				Follow-up (mo)			Comments
Huttl et al. 2002 (17)	89	Brachiocephalic	84 vs. 5	99/1	96.4	93% at 16–117 mo	Mean 33 Max 117	2	7.9	Only one patient stented Experience over 19 yrs reported
Korner et al. 1999 (29)	37	Subclavian (38) and brachiocephalic (4)	NR	NR	84	72% at 100 mo	Mean 15 Max 100	9	19	Double balloon technique used in three high risk cases to reduce cerebrovascular complications
Henry et al. 1999 (30)	113	Subclavian	94 vs. 19	55/45	91	75% at 8 yr	Mean 38 Max 50	0.9	5.3	Possible crossover with some cases reported by Amor et al. (2004) Majority of recurrences were in unstented arteries
Sullivan et al. 1998 (13)	83	Subclavian (66), brachiocephalic (7) and common carotid (14)	73 vs. 10	0/100	94.3	84% at 35 mo	Mean 14 Max 49	4.8	17.8	Two strokes occurred in 14 CCAs treated
Motarjeme 1996 (11)	112	Subclavian (80), brachiocephalic (13), common carotid (8), vertebral (39)	127 vs. 13	98/2	93	95.5% at 5 yr	Max 60	0.9	2.7	Retrospective review article

Abbreviations: CCA, common carotid artery; NR, not reported; PTA, percutaneous transluminal angioplasty.

REFERENCES

1. Fields WS, Lemark NA. Joint study of extracranial arterial occlusion. Subclavian steal: a review of 168 cases. JAMA 1972; 222:1139–43.
2. Shadman R, Criqui MH, Bundens WP, et al. Subclavian artery stenosis: prevalence, risk factors, and association with cardiovascular diseases. J Am Coll Cardiol 2004; 44(3):618–23.
3. Kaufman J. Upper-extremity arteries. In: Kaufman J, Lee MJ, eds. Vascular and Interventional Radiology. The Requisites. Philadelphia, PA: Elsevier, 2004:149–53.
4. Arend WP, Michel BA, Bloch DA, et al. The American College of Rheumatology 1990 criteria for the classification of Takayasu arteritis. Arthritis Rheum 1990; 33(8):1129–34.
5. Lupi-Herrera E, Sanchez-Torres G, Marcushamer J, et al. Takayasu's arteritis. Clinical study of 107 cases. Am Heart J 1977; 93:94–103.
6. Purkayastha S, Jayadevan ER, Kapilamoorthy TR, et al. Suction thrombectomy of thrombotic occlusion of the subclavian artery in a case of Takayasu's arteritis. Cardiovasc Intervent Radiol 2006; 29(2):289–93.
7. Subramanyan R, Joy J, Balakrishnan KG. Natural history of aortoarteritis (Takayasu's disease). Circulation 1989; 80(3):429–37.
8. Kalaria VG, Jacob S, Irwin W, et al. Duplex ultrasonography of vertebral and subclavian arteries. J Am Soc Echocardiogr 2005; 18(10):1107–11.
9. Bogey WM, Demasi RJ, Tripp MD, et al. Percutaneous transluminal angioplasty for subclavian artery stenosis. Am J Surg 1994; 60:103–6.
10. Farina C, Mingoli A, Schultz RD, et al. Percutaneous transluminal angioplasty versus surgery for subclavian artery occlusive disease. Am J Surg 1989; 158(6):511–4.
11. Motarjeme A. Percutaneous transluminal angioplasty of supra-aortic vessels. J Endovasc Surg 1996; 3(2):171–81.
12. Brountzos EN, Peterson B, Binkert C, et al. Primary stenting of subclavian and innominate artery occlusive disease: a single center's experience. Cardiovasc Intervent Radiol 2004; 27(6):616–23.
13. Sullivan TM, Gray BH, Bacharach JM, et al. Angioplasty and primary stenting of the subclavian, innominate, and common carotid arteries in 83 patients. J Vasc Surg 1998; 28(6):1059–65.
14. Amor M, Eid-Lidt G, Chati Z. Endovascular treatment of the subclavian artery: stent implantation with or without predilatation. Catheter Cardiovasc Interv 2004; 63(3):364–70.
15. Sadato A, Satow T, Ishii A, et al. Endovascular recanalization of subclavian artery occlusions. Neurol Med Chir (Tokyo) 2004; 44:447–55.
16. Henry M, Rath PC, Lakshmi G, et al. Percutaneous transluminal angioplasty using a new peripheral cutting balloon for stenosis of arch vessels in aorto arteritis. Int Angiol 2004; 23(4):403–9.
17. Huttl K, Nemes B, Simonffy A, et al. Angioplasty of the innominate artery in 89 patients: experience over 19 years. Cardiovasc Intervent Radiol 2002; 25(2):109–14 (Epub 2002 Jan 17).
18. Ohki T, Marin M, Lyon R. Ex vivo human carotid artery bifurcation stenting: correlation of lesion characteristics with embolic potential. J Vasc Surg 1998; 27(3):463–71.
19. De Vries JP, Jager LC, Van den Berg JC, et al. Durability of percutaneous transluminal angioplasty for obstructive lesions of proximal subclavian artery: long term results. J Vasc Surg 2005; 41(1): 19–23.
20. Engelke C, Sandu C, Morgan RA, et al. Using 6-mm cutting balloon angioplasty in patients with resistant peripheral artery stenosis: preliminary results. AJR Am J Roentgenol 2002; 179(3): 619–23.
21. Munneke GJ, Engelke C, Morgan RA, et al. Cutting balloon angioplasty for resistant renal artery in-stent restenosis. J Vasc Interv Radiol 2002; 13(3):327–31.
22. Joseph S, Mandalam KR, Rao VR, et al. Percutaneous transluminal angioplasty of the subclavian artery in nonspecific aortoarteritis: results of long-term follow-up. J Vasc Interv Radiol 1994; 5(4):573–80.
23. Modarai B, Ali T, Dourado R, et al. Comparison of extra-anatomic bypass grafting with angioplasty for atherosclerotic disease of the supra-aortic trunks. Br J Surg 2004; 91:1453–7.
24. Berguer R, Morasch MD, Kline RA. Transthoracic repair of innominate and common carotid artery disease: immediate and long-term outcome for 100 consecutive surgical reconstructions. J Vasc Surg 1998; 27:34–41.
25. AbuRahma AF, Robinson PA, Jennings TG. Carotid-subclavian bypass grafting with polytetrafluoroethylene grafts for symptomatic subclavian artery stenosis or occlusion: a 20-year experience. J Vasc Surg 2000; 32:411–8.
26. Raithel D. Our experience of surgery for innominate and subclavian lesions. J Cardiovasc Surg (Torino) 1980; 21:423–30.
27. Hadjipetrou P, Cox S, Piemonte T, et al. Percutaneous revascularization of atherosclerotic obstruction of aortic arch vessels. J Am Coll Cardiol 1999; 33(5):1238–45.
28. Bates MC, Broce M, Lavigne PS. Subclavian artery stenting: factors influencing long-term outcome. Catheter Cardiovasc Interv 2004; 61(1):5–11.

29. Korner M, Baumgartner I, Mahler F, et al. PTA of the subclavian and innominate arteries: long-term results. Vasa 1999; 28(2):117–22 (Review).
30. Henry M, Amor M, Henry I, et al. Percutaneous transluminal angioplasty of the subclavian arteries. J Endovasc Surg 1999; 6:33–41.
31. Broadbent LP, Moran CJ, Cross DT, et al. Management of ruptures complicating angioplasty and stenting of supraaortic arteries: report of two cases and a review of the literature. AJNR Am J Neuroradiol 2003; 24(10):2057–61 (Review).

12 | Current Status of Peripheral Arterial Thrombolysis

Robert J. Hinchliffe
Endovascular Department, University Hospital, Malmo, Sweden
Bruce D. Braithwaite
Department of Vascular and Endovascular Surgery, University Hospital, Nottingham, U.K.

INTRODUCTION

Thrombolysis was first used clinically in 1955 by Tillett and the intra-arterial technique was pioneered by Dotter in the 1970s. However, it was not until the 1980s that thrombolysis became widely available.

Current thrombolytic agents, mode of action is to activate fibrin-bound plasminogen in thrombus. A high local concentration of the active enzyme plasmin is generated which breaks down fibrin, reestablishing blood flow in an occluded vessel.

Thrombolysis has distinct theoretical advantages over conventional thromboembolectomy. It is less invasive, reduces patient discomfort, diminishes the risks associated with anesthesia and allows better definition of underlying atherosclerotic lesions. Furthermore, it does not directly damage the vascular endothelium and has the capacity to clear small vessels of thrombus.

The overall clinical success of thrombolytic therapy is limited by delays in achieving arterial reperfusion and the development of bleeding complications. In addition there are logistic and cost issues. Some patients may require open surgery following thrombolysis.

THE EVIDENCE FOR THROMBOLYSIS

Despite the widespread use of thrombolysis in lower limb ischemia the evidence for its use is limited. A recent systematic review of published data found 10 reports of randomized controlled trials (1). Only five of these trials compared lysis directly with surgery. The majority concern thrombolysis of native arterial occlusions. A subgroup of patients identified from the Surgery versus Thrombolysis for the Ischemic Lower Extremity (STILE) trial, specifically reported the results of surgery or thrombolysis in patients with occluded bypass grafts of less than six-month duration (2). Although the randomized studies provide the most reliable data currently available, each one has its limitations.

In addition to the randomized studies, a large national database of thrombolysis, the National Audit of Thrombolysis in Acute Leg Ischemia (NATALI) was maintained in the U.K. The evidence base evaluating thrombolysis will now be described.

Rochester Trial

The first randomized trial was from Rochester, New York. In a single center over a three-year period, 114 patients with severe upper or lower extremity ischemia were recruited (3). All patients had symptoms of seven days duration or less (mean two days). Patients were randomized to thrombolysis (intra-arterial urokinase) or primary surgery. Only patients with limb-threatening ischemia were included. The primary end points were patient survival and limb salvage during follow-up.

STILE Trial

The STILE trial was a multi-center trial. Patients were eligible for the trial if they had lower extremity ischemic symptoms of less than six-month duration (4). Only 30% of patients had ischemia of less than 14-day duration. Consequently, a heterogeneous group of patients were randomized. All occlusions were native arterial and non-embolic (based on clinical and angiographic assessment). Randomization took place in to one of three treatment groups. These comprised thrombolysis with recombinant tissue plasminogen activator (rt-PA), thrombolysis with urokinase or surgery. The primary outcome was composite (adverse outcome index), consisting of ischemia, amputation, major morbidity and mortality. A total of 393 patients were randomized. Randomization was performed on an intention-to-treat basis. Successful catheter placement for thrombolysis was not possible in 28% of patients (no significant difference between centers). Conclusions were based on an intention to treat and per-protocol analysis.

The trial was terminated at the first interim analysis due to inferior outcome (primary end point) in the thrombolysis arm. This may have limited the trials' power. Subsequently an arbitrary cutoff of 14-day duration of ischemia was made for analysis and the two thrombolytic groups were combined because they were found to have similar outcomes.

There were two publications arising from the STILE trial. These were 12-month reports of subgroup analysis of native artery occlusion and bypass graft occlusion (5,2).

Any conclusions drawn from these studies must be interpreted with caution due to the smaller number and inherent weaknesses associated with subgroup analysis.

TOPAS Study

The Thrombolysis or Peripheral Arterial Surgery trial (TOPAS) comprised two multicenter studies (TOPAS I and TOPAS II) (6,7). The trial recruited from 113 centers across North America and Europe. Patients were enrolled with lower limb arterial occlusion of less than 14-day duration. The first study (TOPAS I) was a dose ranging study (213 patients) and the second (544 patients) a comparison of urokinase with open surgery. The primary end point of the dose-ranging study was the extent of lysis on an angiogram taken at four hours following the start of lysis. The results of the first study determined the dosage regimen used in the second. The second part of the study (TOPAS II) was powered to detect a difference in amputation-free survival at six months between surgery and thrombolysis.

The primary end point of amputation-free survival at six months may have introduced bias by evaluating the risks of the therapies rather than the benefits. Not all patients presenting with critical limb ischemia will require amputation. At six months, many of these patients will have died of other pre-morbid conditions rather than the treatment (8).

The TOPAS study recruited from a large number of centers. The limited number of patients (less than five) per center may indicate selection bias. A significant variation in practice between centers was another possible confounding factor.

Nilsson

A small randomized trial of 20 patients to either surgery ($n=9$) or thrombolysis ($n=11$) from Lund, Sweden (9). No difference was found between the groups in rates of successful revascularization, mortality or major hemorrhage. The trial was underpowered to detect any difference between the two groups and will not be discussed further.

NATALI Registry

The Thrombolysis Study Group was formed in 1990 by a group of surgeons and radiologists from 14 district and teaching hospitals in the U.K. who wished to conduct research into peripheral thrombolysis (10). Indications and outcomes of thrombolysis were standardized and data were submitted, mainly contemporaneously, to a computer database. Over 1000 episodes of thrombolysis were recorded on the database, which was completed in 2000. Thrombolytic techniques and dosages were not standardized. The primary outcomes, which were standardized, were measured at 30 days as amputation-free survival, major amputation and death.

Recruitment to the database tailed off in the late 1990s and only 11/14 centers fulfilled the criteria for final analysis. NATALI resulted in five publications; thrombolysis in acute onset claudication, the effect of aspirin on outcome, the effect of different thrombolytic regimes on outcome and a paper on thrombolysis complications (11). The final results were published in 2004 (12).

SYSTEMATIC REVIEWS

Two comprehensive reviews of the literature have been undertaken (1,13). The first was a systematic review of the literature with meta-analysis and the second a Cochrane review of randomized studies comparing thrombolysis with surgery in the management of acute limb ischemia.

Palfreyman's systematic review found a total of 10 randomized controlled trials published 1980–2000. The objective of his review was to determine the relative effectiveness of intra-arterial thrombolysis compared with surgery for the treatment of lower limb ischemia.

In the Cochrane review, a total of five randomized trials were found from the published literature and conference proceedings. These trials included a total of 1283 patients and formed the basis of the analysis.

INDICATIONS/PATIENT SELECTION

The majority of studies of intra-arterial thrombolysis have investigated its use in acute limb ischemia. There are isolated reports of successful thrombolysis in chronic occlusions (14). However, the STILE trial demonstrated that success of thrombolysis was related to duration of symptoms (age of thrombus). In a post hoc subgroup analysis, patients with symptoms less than 14 days had a lower amputation rate when treated with thrombolysis compared with surgery. Chronic ischemia was better treated with surgery. Although most patients describe a deterioration of symptoms it is possible to refine patient selection. Fresh thrombus may be identified using both magnetic resonance imaging techniques and intravascular ultrasound (15,16). However, neither of these techniques has found its way in to routine clinical practice.

Surgery has generally not been recommended for claudication because of the associated morbidity and mortality. In the NATALI database, 108 patients who presented with acute onset claudication because of native arterial or bypass graft occlusion were analyzed (17). After 30 days four patients (8%) had a major amputation, seven (13%) had died, 32 (62%) were symptom free and nine (17%) had persistent claudication. Three patients (6%) suffered a major hemorrhage. The outcome of this group of patients was similar to those treated for critical ischemia. The recommendation from the U.K. Thrombolysis Study Group was therefore to reserve thrombolysis for those patients who progressed to critical limb ischemia.

Many patients who present with acute limb ischemia are simply too old and frail to undergo major surgery. Although thrombolysis is "minimally invasive," retrospective studies and registry data suggest it is associated with significant morbidity and mortality in the elderly. A report of acute leg ischemia in elderly (>75 years) patients found an overall mortality at 30 days of 42% (38% of those receiving active intervention) (18). Initial successful revascularization was more likely following surgery (29 of 33 vs. 25 of 43 events with thrombolysis, $p < 0.01$), but the 30-day outcome was similar in the actively treated groups owing to subsequent morbidity and mortality. Lambert analyzed 102 patients who underwent thrombolysis for acute limb ischemia and stratified outcome related to age (19). Complications occurred in 40% of those patients greater than 80 years of age.

An analysis of the TOPAS II trial suggested that longer vessel occlusions (>30 cm) treated with thrombolysis first resulted in an improved amputation-free survival compared with surgery (20). The improved outcome may be related to the ability of thrombolysis to reveal a target vessel for subsequent bypass surgery. Other studies confirmed that the absolute volume of thrombus does not appear to be predictive of successful lysis. However, greater loads of thrombus correlate with increased reperfusion and infusion time (21).

TECHNIQUE

Delivery

The technique of thrombolysis itself can have a significant effect on outcome.

Systemic administration of thrombolytic agents has been abandoned in peripheral arterial (both native and bypass) occlusions due to the high number of bleeding complications and the more favorable results achieved by direct intra-thrombus delivery (22).

Although end hole lysis may be performed with lower doses and result in less distal emboli it takes longer to perform than direct intra-thrombus delivery (23).

Failure to commence thrombolysis due to access difficulties is a significant problem, especially in patients with bypass grafts, where the occlusion is flush with the native vessel. In the STILE trial, failure to catheterize occurred in 41% bypass grafts and 22% native arteries. Failure to cross an occluded segment with a guidewire prior to starting thrombolysis suggests the thrombus is chronic and harder to lyse (24). An inability to embed a catheter in the proximal thrombus may also be predictive of failure (21).

Access to the thrombus or embolus was possible in 95% (224/256) patients in the TOPAS I study and 96% (55/57) in the Rochester trial. The higher failure rate in the STILE trial reflects a higher proportion of graft occlusions, chronic occlusions (up to six months) and less experience (multiple centers).

In patients with occluded bypass grafts, an alternative technique is to perform direct graft puncture. This technique is particularly useful in patients with extra-anatomic prosthetic bypass grafts (25). Prophylactic antibiotics are required where direct puncture is undertaken.

Once the vessel is catheterized, successful revascularization of the occluded artery is not guaranteed. In the Rochester trial, complete lysis was only achieved in 30%.

Graft occlusions may take longer to successfully lyse than their native arterial counter-parts, even when using pulsed spray techniques (93 vs. 65 minutes in one study) (26). The TOPAS II study also confirmed that graft occlusions require higher doses of lytic agent.

Types of Thrombolytic Agent

Thrombolytic agents may be divided in to four groups, the streptokinase compounds, the urokinase compounds, the tissue plasminogen activators (t-PAs) and an additional miscellaneous group consisting of novel agents (27).

t-PA has theoretical advantages over other commonly used and studied thrombolytic agents. Both streptokinase and urokinase have little affinity for fibrin and therefore do not discriminate between circulating plasminogen and fibrin-bound plasminogen. (t-PA), on the other hand has a high affinity for plasminogen in the presence of fibrin. This should make for an increased lytic effect with a reduction of systemic complications compared with the non-fibrin selective agents. The increased lytic effects of t-PA over streptokinase were confirmed in coronary trials Global Utilization of Streptokinase and Tissue Plasminogen Activator for Occluded Coronary Arteries (GUSTO-1).

Unfortunately, patient heterogeneity, differing dosage regimes, delivery techniques and study criteria have made it difficult to compare the efficacy and complications related to various thrombolytic agents in peripheral vascular disease.

A recent multicenter randomized study of rt-PA versus urokinase for the treatment of femoropopliteal occlusions concluded that rt-PA had a more pronounced lytic effect than urokinase (22). However, lysis was combined (as necessary) with additional catheter interventions to restore patency. Any benefit of rt-PA over urokinase gained from improved lysis was negated by secondary interventions performed. There were no differences in local or systemic complication rates between the two agents in that study.

Initial trials, which suggested high-dose urokinase regimes were better than standard low-dose streptokinase, were confirmed by later studies (28).

In a trial by Lonsdale where patients treated with rt-PA were closely matched with those receiving streptokinase, rt-PA resulted in more rapid thrombolysis (29). No difference in haemorrhagic complications was detected between the groups. Other centers have been unable to detect any improvement with t-PA thrombolysis in terms of lytic action or side effect profile (30). Similarly, the STILE trial was unable to demonstrate any difference between urokinase and rt-PA in safety and efficacy terms, although, in the native artery subgroup, thrombolysis was achieved more rapidly with rt-PA (8 vs. 24 hours $p < 0.05$).

The development of antibodies is a major disadvantage of streptokinase. Antibodies may have an adverse effect on future thrombolysis and retain the potential for serious adverse allergic reactions for several years.

Newer highly fibrin-specific lytic agents have emerged such as tenecteplase, a bio-engineered alteration of rt-PA and recombinant staphylokinase (31,32). All of these agents have been specifically designed to improve lysis and reduce complications. They are safe, but whether they improve outcome or reduce complications compared to more established agents remains unproven.

In 1998 the Food and Drug Administration withdrew urokinase from the U.S. market due to concerns over possible viral disease transmission. A subsequent review of thrombolytic agents by Valji concluded that more evidence was required to find the safest and most effective thrombolytic agent (33).

At the time of writing, a new thrombolytic agent, Alfimerprase, was being studied. Dose-ranging studies had been completed and the drug, with more specificity for fibrin, appeared to produce fewer hemorrhagic side effects than other agents.

Thrombolytic Dose Regimens

A variety of different dosing regimes exist for thrombolysis. Many studies of thrombolysis use a graded dose regime. The thrombus is first laced with a high dose of lytic agent after which a continuous infusion is started (34,35).

Dose-ranging studies of individual thrombolytic agents usually demonstrate a dose-related safety and efficacy profile. Increasing dosages/administration rates usually increase the rate of thrombolysis at the expense of slightly increased frequency of bleeding complications (36). Unfortunately the TOPAS I study was too small to identify any difference among the three urokinase dosages.

In a report of native arterial thrombolysis there was no difference with respect to limb salvage or complications following low- or high-dose therapy. The data may have been skewed by the greater number of secondary procedures performed in those patients receiving the high dose regime (37). Others have confirmed no difference in limb salvage between high- and low-dose regimes (38).

The issue of infusion techniques for peripheral arterial thrombolysis has been the subject of a Cochrane review (39). Six randomized trials were analyzed. The authors concluded that high-dose regimes achieved vessel patency in less time than low-dose infusions but at the expense of more bleeding complications and no increase in patency rates or improvement in limb salvage at 30 days.

Adjunctive Pharmacological Treatment

Heparin

The use of heparin in acute limb ischemia is meant to prevent further ischemic deterioration by the prevention of thrombus propagation. A consensus document supports its use, although there is little evidence (40). When heparin is administered down the sheath during thrombolysis it helps prevent peri-catheter thrombus formation (0.8% in NATALI). Whether the presence of heparin increases the bleeding complications or improves the lytic action of thrombolytic agents remains controversial. Results from the TOPAS II study suggested that heparin does significantly increase the incidence of bleeding complications (19% vs. 9%).

In contrast, in a single study of thrombolysis that omitted heparin, the incidence of major haemorrhage remained high at 11% (3).

Aspirin

Many patients with risk factors for or established peripheral vascular disease are already on antiplatelet therapy. Evidence from the NATALI database over 10 years ago suggested the use of aspirin prior to thrombolysis resulted in approximately a 10% greater limb salvage rate (41). Aspirin did not appear to confer any protection against reocclusion, amputation or death and there was no increase in major haemorrhage.

More potent antiplatelet agents have been studied but have concentrated on safety and side effect profiles rather than efficacy. These trials examining efficacy have significant limitations.

The multicenter RELAX (ReoPro and REtapbase Lysis of Arterial Occlusions in the Lower Extremities) trial was designed specifically to establish the safety of combining a thrombolytic agent with a glycoprotein IIb/IIIa inhibitor (42). Patients also received aspirin and low-dose heparin. The authors concluded that the addition of a glycoprotein platelet inhibitor did not increase bleeding risk. Although not powered to detect any difference in efficacy, the patients receiving ReoPro had reduced risk of embolization during lysis.

The Platelet Receptor AntibOdies to Manage Peripheral Artery Thrombosis randomly assigned patients to abciximab or no lysis adjunct (43). There appeared to be an increased limb salvage rate at 90 days in the abciximab group with no difference in bleeding complications. There was significant heterogeneity between groups. Some 40% of patients in the abciximab group and 15% in the control group did not have critical limb ischemia.

A randomized trial of aspirin versus abciximab found that abciximab reduced the time required to successful thrombolysis (75 vs. 110 minutes) (44). The results of this trial must be interpreted with some caution because of the high proportion of patients treated for noncritical ischemia.

Intraoperative/Perioperative Thrombolysis

Intraoperative lysis has been suggested as a useful adjunct to open surgery in an attempt to clear thrombus from distal vessels, particularly in acute limb ischemia.

A prospective, randomized, blinded, and placebo-controlled study using three doses of urokinase for routine revascularization for chronic ischemia suggested there was no significant fibrinogen depletion or increased operative blood loss or wound hematoma formation (45).

Intraoperative slow bolus injection of thrombolytic agents was used in a study of 38 patients with acute ischemia over a six-year period (46). All patients had acute occlusion of the runoff vessels due to incomplete operative thromboembolectomy. Limb salvage was possible in 28 patients. There was one systemic hemorrhagic complication.

A group of patients who may benefit from intraoperative thrombolysis are those presenting acutely with popliteal aneurysm thrombosis. Evidence from a U.K. multicenter study suggested that patients treated with thrombolysis first line for acute thrombosis of popliteal aneurysm may be more likely to suffer acute limb deterioration compared with native arterial occlusions (13% vs. 1.5%) (47). A recent review therefore suggested that thrombolysis should be reserved as an intraoperative adjunct for the clearance of thrombus from distal vessels rather than first-line management (48).

The loss of distal tissue perfusion sufficient for limb salvage following restoration of inflow to an acutely ischemic extremity has been referred to as the "no-reflow" phenomenon. The group from University of California, Los Angeles (UCLA) hypothesized that this group of patients may benefit from a prolonged postoperative intra-arterial infusion of the thrombolytic agent urokinase (49). Using this technique they were able to salvage 6 out of 12 limbs at a median follow-up of 24.9 months. Seven patients required transfusion for local bleeding complications during a mean of 47 hours of thrombolysis. There were no systemic bleeding complications.

Mechanical Clot Dissolution

Prolonged thrombolysis is likely to be associated with higher doses of lytic agent, more bleeding complications and is more costly (see chap. 14). There are methods for reducing the duration of thrombolysis using mechanical techniques.

The pulse spray technique achieves thrombolysis through the delivery of lytic agent under pressure via a multi-side hole catheter. The pressure created contributes to the mechanical lysis of thrombus. The technique has been shown in randomized clinical trials to significantly shorten the time to achieve local thrombolysis compared to standard infusion techniques (195 vs. 1390 minutes) (50). In another study using pulse spray exclusively for bypass graft occlusion only 27% of patients required an infusion of thrombolytic agent outside the radiology suite (51). Lysis using pulse spray alone took 118 minutes, whereas requirement for an infusion increased the time to 13.5 hours. The disadvantage of pulse spray is the more expensive catheter and infusion systems. Consequently, the technique was only used in 13% of patients in the NATALI database (52).

There are other techniques to reduce thrombus volume prior to or during lysis including aspiration thromboembolectomy (using end-hole catheters), rheolytic thrombectomy and ultrasound. Rheolytic thrombectomy requires devices such as rotational thrombectomy catheters (53). Ultrasound applied externally with low frequencies and high intensities can enhance thrombolytic drug-induced clot dissolution in vitro and in animal studies (54). Others have demonstrated in controlled experiments in animals that it is possible to achieve successful thrombolysis with the a microbubble agent (intravenous administration of perfluorocarbon-exposed sonicated dextrose albumin) and transcutaneous delivery of ultrasound without the need for other thrombolytic agents (55).

LOGISTICS AND COST

Thrombolysis is a labor-intensive technique. Patients usually require multiple visits to the endovascular suite. In a study by Browse, on average, four angiograms were required in every patient (56). Few hospitals can currently provide this service. Additionally, monitoring in a critical care environment is required.

In the Rochester trial despite equivalent hospital stay between thrombolysis and surgery, the costs were higher with thrombolysis ($15,672 vs. $12,703) (3). In 1997, Rickard calculated that an additional $2440 (Australian) were spent during the thrombolytic procedure alone, above and beyond the cost of simple angiography (57). However, work from the Cleveland Clinic, U.S.A. demonstrated little cost difference between bypass surgery and thrombolysis in native arterial occlusion. Using data from the TOPAS II trial, Patel and colleagues constructed a Markov model to determine the cost effectiveness of thrombolysis relative to surgery for a hypothetical cohort of patients with acute lower extremity arterial occlusion (58). The lifetime costs were $57,429 for surgery versus $76,326 for thrombolysis. They concluded that initial surgery provides the most efficient and economical utilization of resources for acute lower extremity arterial occlusion.

Two separate surveys in the early 1990s of over 100 U.K. vascular surgeons attempted to clarify the issues regarding the apparently poor uptake of intra-arterial thrombolysis (59,60). In both studies approximately half of surgeons contacted used thrombolysis. In the latter study, 38% of surgeons never used thrombolysis. Where stated, the main reasons for this limited use were the doubts about efficacy (45%) and lack of radiological support (47%).

Galland performed a follow-up questionnaire some 10 years later (61). In the interim the number of publications on thrombolysis had significantly increased, the U.K. NATALI database had been completed and data had become available from randomized trials. This time, the questionnaire was sent to members of the Thrombolysis Study Group (24 centers), all of whom had significant thrombolysis experience and submitted data to NATALI. Eighty-six percent reported a decline in the use of thrombolysis. Most centers still used thrombolysis selectively, although the indications were variable. Only three centers had not experienced a decline in use. Interestingly the reasons for this decline were similar to those stated in the early 1990s, namely questions about efficacy (particularly long term), and logistics (staffing issues, critical care and interventional radiology availability).

COMPLICATIONS OF THROMBOLYSIS

The accepted overall mortality from thrombolysis in the peri-procedural period is in the region of 3% to 5%. The majority will perish from stroke, myocardial infarction or hemorrhagic complications.

The results of complications reported in retrospective and nonrandomized studies should be interpreted with caution. Nonobjective personnel without clear criteria often measure outcomes and these studies are prone to bias. In the TOPAS II and Rochester studies significant bleeding occurred in more patients (12.5% and 11%, respectively) than is often quoted from less-rigorous studies. A study from Nottingham reported a figure of 5% for major hemorrhage, 15% minor hemorrhage and 1% suffered a stroke (62).

The risk factors for haemorrhage during thrombolysis continue to be debated. In a systematic review, Semba found the major haemorrhage rate was 5% from rt-PA in his review of the literature and appeared to be related to the overall dose and duration of infusion (63). Patients with bleeding complications in the STILE trial tended to be older (71 vs. 67 years) but did not reach statistical significance.

There are theoretical reasons why some thrombolytic agents may cause less bleeding. For example, staphylokinase is known to reduce the depletion of fibrinogen. Whether these theoretical advantages demonstrate clinical benefit required further investigation. A recent review of publications comparing the complications of low-molecular-weight urokinase with rt-PA suggested urokinase had a lower incidence of any haemorrhagic complications and a reduced transfusion requirement (64). However, a major confounding factor of the review was the significantly higher mean age in the rt-PA patients studied. Furthermore, patients undergoing rt-PA lysis were more likely to have chronic occlusions.

It is prudent to avoid arterial puncture in anatomical areas where vessels cannot be compressed, especially the axilla and advisable to keep the duration of thrombolysis and lytic agent as low as possible.

Evidence from the NATALI database suggests that patients undergoing graft thrombolysis have more bleeding complications. Prosthetic grafts in particular seem to have more local complications, which may be related to the increased doses required for successful lysis. However, Dacron graft occlusions should not undergo thrombolysis for at least four weeks after implantation because of the ongoing risk of hemorrhage.

In Rickard's experience, more complications were experienced with prosthetic graft lysis (53%) compared with vein graft (41%) and native artery (29%), although these figures did not reach statistical significance (57). Furthermore, acute worsening of ischemia due to embolization appeared to be almost twice as common in graft thrombolysis (2.7% vs. 1.5%) (47). In that study of 19 patients, 11 required amputation and two died despite further lysis or surgery. Paradoxically, lower rates of hemorrhagic complications occurred in patients with bypass graft occlusions in the TOPAS trial and no difference could be demonstrated with regard to major morbidity at one year in the STILE trial.

Because many of the factors that increase the risk of bleeding remain uncertain it is probably better to direct efforts to the early detection and appropriate management of hemorrhage. Patients who develop low levels of fibrinogen during thrombolysis are more prone to bleeding. A protocol for the treatment of thrombolysis complications may reduce their severity and simplify patient management.

RESULTS OF THROMBOLYSIS

No study declared the overall admission rate of patients with leg ischemia during the recruitment period. This would have been important demographic data to exclude significant selection bias. It is therefore not possible to determine the applicability of thrombolysis in patients presenting with acute leg ischemia. Many patients may have been unsuitable for thrombolysis because of immediately threatened viability, contraindications to thrombolysis or logistic issues. Other patients may have received primary amputation or have been too unfit for any intervention.

The outcome of both thrombolysis and surgery may be affected by the nature of arterial occlusion. In the Rochester trial, outcome was improved for patients treated (surgery and thrombolysis) for embolic rather than thrombotic occlusion. In contrast there was no difference in perioperative amputation or death in embolic compared with thrombotic patients in TOPAS II. Emboli were excluded on the basis of clinical assessment and angiography in the STILE trial.

In the STILE trial, patency was restored in 81% of bypass grafts and 69% of native arteries ($p = $NS) once thrombolysis was successfully started. Those randomized to thrombolysis permitted a lesser invasive procedure to be performed subsequent to lysis in 56% of cases. Patients who have failed thrombolysis retain a surgical option. In the STILE trial, the amputation rate of patients with acute ischemia who had failed primary surgery was 67%, whereas in the thrombolysis group the amputation rate was 30%.

Thrombolysis may allow early reperfusion and then treatment of an underlying lesion later at elective angioplasty or surgery. In the Rochester trial, thrombolysis uncovered anatomic lesions in 21 (37%) of patients who subsequently underwent angioplasty ($n = 2$) or surgery ($n = 19$). The underlying cause of thrombotic bypass occlusion is likely to affect outcome (65). Early occlusions are usually the result of technical failure or the wrong operation and are unlikely to benefit from thrombolysis. Occlusions in the mid- to long-term may have an underlying cause (intimal hyperplasia, vein graft stenosis) amenable to correction. Sullivan confirmed the outcome of thrombolysis was improved if an underlying lesion could be unmasked and treated by either angioplasty or open surgery (66). Two-year patency rates were 79% in those with an underlying lesion versus 9.8% without.

In another study, the major factor associated with poor long-term patency was an inability to detect and treat underlying lesions (67). In those patients receiving thrombolysis in the Rochester trial, 64% of patients required surgery at 12-month follow-up.

Over the past 15 years since trial recruitment, there have been significant advances in endovascular technology. One may speculate that an increasing proportion of these patients would now have been amenable to endovascular therapy rather than open surgery. The high rate of secondary open procedures (even if directed) may have accounted for the length of hospital stay which was similar (mean 11 days) in both the thrombolytic arm and the open surgical arm of the trial.

Open surgery is usually thought to be a more durable option than endovascular treatment, requiring less secondary interventions. However, in the TOPAS II study, a total of 551 surgical patients required further surgery. Open surgical interventions were required in 315 of the patients who received thrombolysis six months after randomization. In the same time period, percutaneous procedures were required on 55 and 128 occasions, respectively.

The chronic symptoms of patients (70% of patients had ischemia of more than one month duration) entered into the STILE trial had an impact on early outcome compared with the other randomized studies. The low rates of major morbidity and mortality also suggest that some of these patients did not have limb threatening ischemia (estimated to be 31%) (68). At one month following treatment in the STILE trial, the mortality in each group was 5%, with major amputations in 6% of surgical and 5% of lysis patients. In comparison, mortality at 30 days in the Rochester trial was 18% following surgery and 12% following lysis. Amputation rates were 14% and 9%, respectively.

The native artery subgroup of STILE demonstrated increased rates of amputation in the thrombolysis group (10% vs. 0%). In contrast, amputation was lower in patients receiving thrombolysis for acute (<14 days) graft occlusion.

In the two meta-analyses, there was no significant difference in limb salvage or death at 30 days, 6 months or 1 year between initial surgery and initial thrombolysis. The findings of the systematic reviews underscore the importance of patient selection. Patients need to be identified who might do well or poorly with either thrombolysis or surgery. In the U.K. there is evidence to suggest that more appropriate patient selection for thrombolysis is now taking place with improved outcomes. In NATALI, the 30-day amputation-free survival following thrombolysis was 65% in 1990 compared with 80% in 1999.

In the final analysis of NATALI, the 30-day mortality following thrombolysis was 12.4%. The commonest causes of death were myocardial infarction and stroke. 12.4% of patients required a major amputation (amputation-free survival at 30 days was 75.2%). In the TOPAS II study, amputation-free survival was not statistically different at discharge from hospital (84% thrombolysis vs. 89% surgery).

There was a significantly lower mortality in the thrombolytic group at one year (58% vs. 84%) in the Rochester trial. This difference in mortality was attributed to the greater number of cardiopulmonary complications which developed perioperatively in the surgical group (41% vs. 16%). Over 50% of patients developing cardiovascular complications were dead at 12 months. However, mortality rates were low (8% and 14%, respectively) without these complications. The surgical arm of the Rochester trial was associated with significantly higher perioperative cardiopulmonary morbidity compared to TOPAS II patients. One explanation may be that patients chosen for the TOPAS II study were a healthier group than in the Rochester trial as perioperative mortality was only 6%. In the Rochester trial, 63% of patients had major (graft replacement) or moderate (graft revision) surgical procedures. Only 37% of patients underwent the lesser procedure of thromboembolectomy. In contrast, 66% of patients in TOPAS II underwent thromboembolectomy. The complex nature of vascular reconstructions in the Rochester trial may have accounted for the high number of cardio-pulmonary complications. The reduced mortality in the TOPAS II trial compared to the Rochester trial persisted at 12 months. After one year in the TOPAS II trial, the mortality in the surgical group was 17% and 20% in the thrombolysis group.

There is further evidence to suggest that aggressive surgical management of bypass graft occlusion is associated with significant morbidity and mortality. In a study of bypass graft occlusion by the Portland group, where all patients underwent graft replacement, only 12% of patients were alive at five years (69). Many patients are simply too frail to undergo further major arterial bypass surgery. However, the long-term survival following lysis of occluded bypass grafts is encouraging. In Nackman's paper 89% of patients were still alive at two years and 84% of patients in another study were alive at 42 months (70,71).

In the TOPAS study, one year amputation-free survival was 65% in the thrombolysis group and 70% in the surgical group. In the native artery subgroup of the STILE trial, at one year there was a significant reduction in amputation (10% vs. 0%) and recurrent ischemia (64% vs. 35%) in those who had surgery. There was no difference in mortality.

Outcomes following thrombolysis for graft occlusions were related to the duration of ischemia, this was not the case with native artery occlusions. In the graft group, early ischemia resulted in a major amputation rate of 48% in the surgery group compared with 20% in the lysis group ($p=0.03$). In contrast there was no difference in limb salvage at one year in ischemia of greater than two-week duration, although there was a greater proportion of ongoing/recurrent ischemia in the lysis group. In the Rochester trial, the primary end point was amputation-free survival. No difference in major amputation (18% at 12 months in each group) was detected but there was a statistically significant lower amputation-free survival (75% vs. 52%) in the thrombolysis group.

A review of the available results published in the literature prior to 1992 by Browse and colleagues demonstrated an improved outcome in patients undergoing thrombolysis for suprainguinal bypass occlusion compared with those obtained from infrainguinal lysis (56). Galland's analysis of the NATALI database was unable to support this finding. There was no difference in patency between the two sites (72). Comerota's analysis of bypass graft outcome was unable to detect any difference between supra- and infrainguinal position. In the native artery subgroup of STILE, patients with femoropopliteal occlusions had a significantly inferior outcome to those with iliofemoral occlusions. Other factors associated with poor outcome were the presence of diabetes and critical ischemia. These results from the STILE trial subgroups should be interpreted with caution owing to the small number of patients on which analysis was performed.

In their series of 43 infrainguinal grafts, vein grafts had significantly better patency in the longer term (69.3% vs. 28.6% at 30 months) compared with prosthetic grafts after successful thrombolysis (66). These results and those of other studies suggest that concerns over the effects of vein wall ischemia during graft occlusion are probably exaggerated. Probably more important than arguments over vein versus prosthetic graft outcome following thrombolysis are the duration of occlusion and the presence of a correctable underlying lesion. In a study by Conrad, patients with vein-graft occlusion who underwent successful lysis followed by angioplasty or surgical revision of a lesion had a limb salvage rate of 95% at five years (73). However, of the 48 occluded vein grafts studied (successfully lysis in 43), only 22 underlying lesions were identified. As a consequence the five-year cumulative patency rate was a more modest 65%. In contrast, in Galland's study of 75 bypass graft occlusions, only 27 adjunctive procedures were performed. The one-year patency rate was 20%.

CONCLUSIONS

The exact role of thrombolysis in patients with lower limb ischemia remains elusive. Previous studies have defined patient groups and indications that are more or less likely to benefit. Thrombolysis should be used with caution in the elderly, those presenting with sudden onset claudication, patients with limb ischemia more than two-week duration and popliteal aneurysm thrombotic occlusion.

rt-PA and urokinase may produce more rapid thrombolysis than streptokinase.

There is probably little difference in terms of the side effect profiles of various thrombolytic agents.

High-dose thrombolysis regimes and pulse spray reduce the time to perform thrombolysis but may not necessarily reduce the dose of lytic agent required and do not affect overall outcome. High-dose regimes may achieve rapid thrombolysis at the expense of slightly more complications. The role of mechanical thrombectomy devices as an adjunct to thrombolysis has not been investigated.

Meta-analysis of randomized trials suggests there is no significant difference in limb salvage or death at 30 days, 6 months or 1 year between initial surgery and initial thrombolysis for acute limb ischemia. Major hemorrhage and stroke are more common following thrombolysis.

Improved early results in the U.K. with thrombolysis suggest more appropriate patient selection. However, the number of patients receiving intra-arterial thrombolysis for acute limb ischemia is declining. Vascular surgeons surveyed in the U.K. believe the long-term outcomes are not improved over surgery and the technique is more labor intensive. Thrombolysis is also more expensive.

The randomized trials have their limitations but represent the best data currently available. They were all performed over a decade ago. Since then endovascular technology has progressed significantly whilst surgical techniques remain broadly similar. It is now unlikely that careful patient selection and current technology would give the high-treatment crossovers seen in the STILE trial. It is doubtful that trials performed today would produce similar results.

REFERENCES

1. Palfreyman SJ, Booth A, Michaels JA. A systematic review of intra-arterial thrombolytic therapy for lower limb ischaemia. Eur J Vasc Endovasc Surg 2000; 19:143–57.
2. Comerota AJ, Weaver FA, Hosking JD, et al. Results of a prospective, randomised trial of surgery versus thrombolysis for occluded lower extremity bypass grafts. Am J Surg 1996; 172:105–12.
3. Ouriel K, Shortell CK, DeWeese JA, et al. A comparison of thrombolytic therapy with operative revascularization in the initial treatment of acute peripheral arterial ischemia. J Vasc Surg 1994; 19:1021–30.
4. The STILE Investigators. Results of a prospective randomized trial evaluating surgery versus thrombolysis for ischemia of the lower extremity. The STILE trial. Ann Surg 1994; 220:251–66.
5. Weaver FA, Comerota AJ, Youngblood M, et al. Surgical revascularization versus thrombolysis for nonembolic lower extremity native artery occlusions: results of a prospective randomized trial. The STILE Investigators. Surgery versus Thrombolysis for Ischemia of the Lower Extremity. J Vasc Surg 1996; 24:513–21.
6. Ouriel K, Veith FJ, Sasahara AA. Thrombolysis or peripheral arterial surgery: phase I results. TOPAS Investigators. J Vasc Surg 1996; 23:64–73.
7. Ouriel K, Veith FJ, Sasahara AA. A comparison of recombinant urokinase with vascular surgery as initial treatment for acute arterial occlusion of the legs. Thrombolysis or Peripheral Arterial Surgery (TOPAS) Investigators. N Engl J Med 1998; 338:1105–11.

8. Porter JM. Thrombolysis for acute arterial occlusion of the legs. N Engl J Med 1998; 338:1148–50.
9. Nilsson L, Albrechtsson U, Jonung T, et al. Surgical treatment versus thrombolysis in acute arterial occlusion: a randomised controlled study. Eur J Vasc Surg 1992; 6:189–93.
10. Braithwaite BD, Ritchie AW, Earnshaw JJ. NATALI—a model for National Computer Databases in the investigation of new therapeutic techniques. J R Soc Med 1995; 88:511–5.
11. Thomas SM, Gaines PA. Vascular surgical society of great britain and ireland: avoiding the complications of thrombolysis. Br J Surg 1999; 86:710.
12. Earnshaw JJ, Whitman B, Foy C. National Audit of Thrombolysis for Acute Leg Ischemia (NATALI): clinical factors associated with early outcome. J Vasc Surg 2004; 39:1018–25.
13. Berridge DC, Kessel D, Robertson I. Surgery versus thrombolysis for acute limb ischaemia: initial management. Cochrane Database Syst Rev 2002; (3):CD002784.
14. Lammer J, Pilger E, Justich E, et al. Fibrinolysis in chronic arteriosclerotic occlusions: intrathrombotic injections of streptokinase. Work in progress. Radiology 1985; 157:45–50.
15. Berridge DC, Perkins AC, Frier M, et al. Detection and characterization of arterial thromboses using a platelet-specific monoclonal antibody (P256 Fab′). Br J Surg 1991; 78:1130–3.
16. Kwan D, Dries A, Burton T, et al. Thrombus characterization with intravascular ultrasound: potential to predict successful thrombolysis. J Endovasc Ther 2003; 10:90–8.
17. Braithwaite BD, Tomlinson MA, Walker SR, et al. Peripheral thrombolysis for acute-onset claudication. Thrombolysis Study Group. Br J Surg 1999; 86:800–4.
18. Braithwaite BD, Davies B, Birch PA, et al. Management of acute leg ischaemia in the elderly. Br J Surg 1998; 85:217–20.
19. Lambert AW, Trkulja D, Fox AD, et al. Age-related outcome for peripheral thrombolysis. Eur J Vasc Endovasc Surg 1999; 17:144–8.
20. Ouriel K, Veith FJ. Acute lower limb ischemia: determinants of outcome. Surgery 1998; 124:336–41.
21. Ouriel K, Shortell CK, Azodo MV, et al. Acute peripheral arterial occlusion: predictors of success in catheter-directed thrombolytic therapy. Radiology 1994; 193:561–6.
22. Berridge DC, Gregson RH, Hopkinson BR, Makin GS. Randomized trial of intra-arterial recombinant tissue plasminogen activator, intravenous recombinant tissue plasminogen activator and intra-arterial streptokinase in peripheral arterial thrombolysis. Br J Surg 1991; 78:988–95.
23. Mahler F, Schneider E, Hess H. Steering Committe, Study on Local Thrombolysis. Recombinant tissue plasminogen activator versus urokinase for local thrombolysis of femoropopliteal occlusions: a prospective, randomized multicenter trial. J Endovasc Ther 2001; 8:638–47.
24. Meyerovitz MF, Goldhaber SZ, Reagan K, et al. Recombinant tissue-type plasminogen activator versus urokinase in peripheral arterial and graft occlusions: a randomized trial. Radiology 1990; 175:75–8.
25. Guest P, Buckenham T. Thrombolysis of the occluded prosthetic graft with tissue-type plasminogen activator–technique, results and problems in 23 patients. Clin Radiol 1992; 46:381–6.
26. Valji K, Roberts AC, Davis GB, Bookstein JJ. Pulsed-spray thrombolysis of arterial and bypass graft occlusions. Am J Roentgenol 1991; 156:617–21.
27. Ouriel K. Current status of thrombolysis for peripheral arterial occlusive disease. Ann Vasc Surg 2002; 16:797–804.
28. McNamara TO, Fischer JR. Thrombolysis of peripheral arterial and graft occlusions: improved results using high-dose urokinase. Am J Roentgenol 1985; 144:769–75.
29. Lonsdale RJ, Berridge DC, Earnshaw JJ, et al. Recombinant tissue-type plasminogen activator is superior to streptokinase for local intra-arterial thrombolysis. Br J Surg 1992; 79:272–5.
30. Earnshaw JJ, Scott DJ, Horrocks M, Baird RN. Choice of agent for peripheral thrombolysis. Br J Surg 1993; 80:25–7.
31. Allie DE, Hebert CJ, Lirtzman MD, et al. Continuous tenecteplase infusion combined with peri/postprocedural platelet glycoprotein IIb/IIIa inhibition in peripheral arterial thrombolysis: initial safety and feasibility experience. J Endovasc Ther 2004; 11:427–35.
32. Heymans S, Vanderschueren S, Verhaeghe R, et al. Outcome and one year follow-up of intra-arterial staphylokinase in 191 patients with peripheral arterial occlusion. Thromb Haemost 2000; 83:666–71.
33. Valji K. Evolving strategies for thrombolytic therapy of peripheral vascular occlusion. J Vasc Interv Radiol 2000; 11:411–20.
34. Traughber PD, Cook PS, Micklos TJ, Miller FJ. Intraarterial fibrinolytic therapy for popliteal and tibial artery obstruction: comparison of streptokinase and urokinase. Am J Roentgenol 1987; 149:453–6.
35. Sullivan KL, Gardiner GA, Jr., Shapiro MJ, et al. Acceleration of thrombolysis with a high-dose transthrombus bolus technique. Radiology 1989; 173:805–8.
36. Ouriel K, Kandarpa K, Schuerr DM, et al. Prourokinase versus urokinase for recanalization of peripheral occlusions, safety and efficacy: the PURPOSE trial. J Vasc Interv Radiol 1999; 10:1083–91.
37. Braithwaite BD, Buckenham TM, Galland RB, et al. Prospective randomised trial of high-dose bolus versus low-dose tissue plasminogen activator infusion in the management of acute limb ischaemia. Br J Surg 1997; 84:646–50.

38. Cragg AH, Smith TP, Corson JD, et al. Two urokinase dose regimens in native arterial and graft occlusions: initial results of a prospective, randomized clinical trial. Radiology 1991; 178:681–6.
39. Kessel DO, Berridge DC, Robertson I. Infusion techniques for peripheral arterial thrombolysis. Cochrane Database Syst Rev 2004; (1):CD000985.
40. Thrombolysis in the management of lower limb peripheral arterial occlusion—a consensus document. Working Party on Thrombolysis in the Management of Limb Ischemia. Am J Cardiol 1998; 81:207–18.
41. Braithwaite BD, Jones L, Yusuf SW, et al. Aspirin improves the outcome of intra-arterial thrombolysis with tissue plasminogen activator. Thrombolysis Study Group. Br J Surg 1995; 82:1357–8.
42. Ouriel K, Castaneda F, McNamara T, et al. Reteplase monotherapy and reteplase/abciximab combination therapy in peripheral arterial occlusive disease: results from the RELAX trial. J Vasc Interv Radiol 2004; 15:229–38.
43. Duda SH, Tepe G, Luz O, et al. Peripheral artery occlusion: treatment with abciximab plus urokinase versus with urokinase alone—a randomized pilot trial (the PROMPT Study). Platelet Receptor Antibodies in Order to Manage Peripheral Artery Thrombosis. Radiology 2001; 221:689–96.
44. Schweizer J, Kirch W, Koch R, et al. Short- and long-term results of abciximab versus aspirin in conjunction with thrombolysis for patients with peripheral occlusive arterial disease and arterial thrombosis. Angiology 2000; 51:913–23.
45. Comerota AJ, Rao AK, Throm RC, et al. A prospective, randomized, blinded, and placebo-controlled trial of intraoperative intra-arterial urokinase infusion during lower extremity revascularization. Regional and systemic effects. Ann Surg 1993; 218:534–41.
46. Comerota AJ, White JV, Grosh JD. Intraoperative intra-arterial thrombolytic therapy for salvage of limbs in patients with distal arterial thrombosis. Surg Gynecol Obstet 1989; 169:283–9.
47. Galland RB, Earnshaw JJ, Baird RN, et al. Acute limb deterioration during intra-arterial thrombolysis. Br J Surg 1993; 80:1118–20.
48. Galland RB. Popliteal aneurysms: controversies in their management. Am J Surg 2005; 190:314–8.
49. Law MM, Gelabert HA, Colburn MD, et al. Continuous postoperative intra-arterial urokinase infusion in the treatment of no reflow following revascularization of the acutely ischemic limb. Ann Vasc Surg 1994; 8:66–73.
50. Yusuf SW, Whitaker SC, Gregson RH, et al. Prospective randomised comparative study of pulse spray and conventional local thrombolysis. Eur J Vasc Endovasc Surg 1995; 10:136–41.
51. Hye RJ, Turner C, Valji K, et al. Is thrombolysis of occluded popliteal and tibial bypass grafts worthwhile? J Vasc Surg 1994; 20:588–96.
52. Gaines PA, Braithwaite BD, Earnshaw JJ. Thrombolytic treatment. Pulse spray infusion works faster but is more expensive. Br Med J 1995; 311:1505–6.
53. Schmitt HE, Jager KA, Jacob AL, et al. A new rotational thrombectomy catheter: system design and first clinical experiences. Cardiovasc Intervent Radiol 1999; 22:504–9.
54. Siegel RJ, Atar S, Fishbein MC, et al. Noninvasive transcutaneous low frequency ultrasound enhances thrombolysis in peripheral and coronary arteries. Echocardiography 2001; 18:247–57.
55. Birnbaum Y, Luo H, Nagai T, et al. Noninvasive in vivo clot dissolution without a thrombolytic drug: recanalization of thrombosed iliofemoral arteries by transcutaneous ultrasound combined with intravenous infusion of microbubbles. Circulation 1998; 97:130–4.
56. Browse DJ, Torrie EPH, Galland RB. Low-dose intra-arterial thrombolysis in the treatment of occluded vascular grafts. Br J Surg 1992; 79:86–8.
57. Rickard MJ, Fisher CM, Soong CV, et al. Limitations of intra-arterial thrombolysis. Cardiovasc Surg 1997; 5:634–40.
58. Patel ST, Haser PB, Bush HL, Jr., Kent KC. Is thrombolysis of lower extremity acute arterial occlusion cost-effective? J Surg Res 1999; 83:106–12.
59. Earnshaw JJ, Shaw JF. Survey of the use of thrombolysis for acute limb ischaemia in the U.K. and Ireland. Br J Surg 1990; 77:1041–2.
60. Browse DJ, Barr H, Torrie EP, Galland RB. Limitations to the widespread usage of low-dose intra-arterial thrombolysis. Eur J Vasc Surg 1991; 5:445–9.
61. Richards T, Pittathankal AA, Magee TR, Galland RB. The current role of intra-arterial thrombolysis. Eur J Vasc Endovasc Surg 2003; 26:166–9.
62. Berridge DC, Makin GS, Hopkinson BR. Local low dose intra-arterial thrombolytic therapy: the risk of stroke or major haemorrhage. Br J Surg 1989; 76:1230–3.
63. Semba CP, Murphy TP, Bakal CW, et al. Thrombolytic therapy with use of alteplase (rt-PA) in peripheral arterial occlusive disease: review of the clinical literature. The Advisory Panel. J Vasc Interv Radiol 2000; 11(2 Pt 1):149–61.
64. Ouriel K, Kandarpa K. Safety of thrombolytic therapy with urokinase or recombinant tissue plasminogen activator for peripheral arterial occlusion: a comprehensive compilation of published work. J Endovasc Ther 2004; 11:436–46.
65. Graor RA, Risius B, Young JR, et al. Thrombolysis of peripheral arterial bypass grafts: surgical thrombectomy compared with thrombolysis. A preliminary report. J Vasc Surg 1988; 7:347–55.

66. Sullivan KL, Gardiner GA, Jr., Kandarpa K, et al. Efficacy of thrombolysis in infrainguinal bypass grafts. Circulation 1991; 83(Suppl. 2):I99–105.
67. McNamara TO, Bomberger RA. Factors affecting initial and 6-month patency rates after intraarterial thrombolysis with high dose urokinase. Am J Surg 1986; 152:709–12.
68. The STILE Investigators. Results of a prospective randomized trial evaluating surgery versus thrombolysis for ischemia of the lower extremity. The STILE trial (discussion). Ann Surg 1994; 220:266–8.
69. Edward JE, Taylor LM, Porter JM. Treatment of failed lower extremity bypass grafts with new autogenous vein bypass grafting. J Vasc Surg 1990; 11:136–45.
70. Nackman GB, Walsh DB, Fillinger MF, et al. Thrombolysis of occluded infrainguinal vein grafts: predictors of outcome. J Vasc Surg 1997; 6:1023–31.
71. Hye RJ, Turner C, Valji K, et al. Is thrombolysis of occluded popliteal bypass grafts worthwhile? J Vasc Surg 1994; 4:588–96.
72. Galland RB, Magee TR, Whitman B, et al. Patency following successful thrombolysis of occluded vascular grafts. Eur J Vasc Endovasc Surg 2001; 22:157–60.
73. Conrad MF, Shepard AD, Rubinfeld IS, et al. Long-term results of catheter-directed thrombolysis to treat infrainguinal bypass graft occlusion: the urokinase era. J Vasc Surg 2003; 37:1009–16.

13 | Peripheral Arterial Thrombolysis for Acute Limb Ischemia

Tim Buckenham
Radiology Services, Christchurch Hospital, Christchurch, New Zealand

INTRODUCTION

Peripheral arterial thrombolysis (PAT) is an important technique in the management of acute limb ischemia. Like many techniques, the interest in PAT was strong in the 10 years after its introduction and a large amount of literature was generated during the 1990s. Since 2000, the focus of the literature on thrombolysis has been concentrated on the investigation of new lytic agents and alternative applications of PAT. There has been a general decline in the use of PAT in the management of acute limb ischemia, resulting from evidence-based practice limiting it to limb-threatening ischemia in younger patients. Its present role is primarily in the management of acute limb-threatening ischemia where temporal constraints allow, usually Rutherford 2A and selected 2B ischemia, often as a prelude to subsequent angioplasty or surgery (Table 1).

ACUTE LIMB-THREATENING ISCHEMIA

PAT has an established role in the management of acute limb-threatening ischemia, irrespective of etiology, by facilitating limb reperfusion by dissolution of the occluding thrombus or embolus (1).

The causes of limb-threatening ischemia that may be treated with PAT include acute thrombosis of an arterial segment secondary to atherosclerotic disease, embolic occlusion, popliteal aneurysm disease, or thrombosis associated with extrinsic arterial compression, e.g., popliteal entrapment or cystic adventitial disease. It is important to determine the cause of ischemia once lysis is completed, as management of the underlying cause by surgery, angioplasty or anticoagulation is often required.

The severity of ischemia needs to be defined, as it is an important determinant of outcome. Patients with Rutherford 1 (non-limb-threatening ischemia, e.g., those with acute onset claudication) should not be treated with intra-arterial thrombolysis, as their PAT-treated outcomes differ little from those with acute limb-threatening ischemia (2) and should only be considered for lysis if their ischemia progresses to Rutherford 2A or 2B (Table 1) (3). For those patients with severe ischemia where rapid reperfusion is essential (Rutherford 2B and 3), thrombolysis may also be contraindicated. Patients with Rutherford 2A or 2B ischemia without major contraindications can be considered for treatment with a thrombolysis-first strategy if time allows.

PRETREATMENT IMAGING

Prior to the commencement of PAT, good quality noninvasive imaging has an important role in determining occluded segments and facilitating optimal catheter access. Where conventional catheter-directed diagnostic angiography has been performed, this may limit the operator to the retrograde common femoral puncture that has been used for the diagnostic procedure and may be suboptimal for thrombolysis. Removal of the diagnostic arterial catheter and repuncturing at another site exposes the patient to the risk of bleeding from the original

TABLE 1 Severity of Acute Leg Ischemia

	Category	Description	Capillary return	Muscle paralysis	Sensory loss	Doppler signals Arterial	Doppler signals Venous
I	Viable	Not immediately threatened	Intact	None	None	Audible	Audible
IIa	Threatened	Salvageable if treated	Intact/slow	None	Partial	Inaudible	Audible
IIb	Threatened	Salvageable if treated as emergency	Slow/absent	Partial	Partial	Inaudible	Audible
III	Irreversible	Primary amputation frequently required	Absent	Complete	Complete	Inaudible	Inaudible

Source: Modified from Refs. 1, 3.

puncture site. Color Doppler ultrasound, multidetector computerized tomography, or magnetic resonance angiography are all preferable methods of defining distribution of disease and facilitating planning of thrombolysis.

Occlusive disease may be approached from a contralateral access with the catheter placed over the bifurcation and down the affected limb, but this approach may limit subsequent endovascular intervention. Therefore, an ipsilateral antegrade approach is preferable as it does not require significant catheter manipulation and facilitates complementary techniques such as aspiration thromboembolectomy (4) and percutaneous balloon dilatation, but may be limited by obesity or occlusions lying close to the access site.

TECHNIQUES

Intravenous administration of a thrombolytic agent for management of acute limb-threatening ischemia of arterial etiology has largely been abandoned, and all current techniques are a variation on the intrathrombic instillation of lytic agent (5). These techniques can be divided into low-dose infusions or high-dose pulsed techniques. There are a small number of randomized trials that have compared the low-dose infusion techniques with the higher dose pulsed techniques. These are difficult to compare due to a heterogeneity of indications, lytic agents and techniques.

The infusional technique relies on an angiographic catheter being placed in the occluded segment via percutaneous access of a patent artery. Techniques vary as to the optimal catheter site, but most operators use the guidewire traversal test to assess the thrombus then place the catheter in the proximal occlusion. This may be from a contralateral approach, ipsilateral antegrade or retrograde approach, or less commonly, from upper limb access. Progress is monitored by periodic angiography and catheter position adjusted as appropriate.

High-dose pulsing techniques require either the lacing of the thrombosed segment with a percutaneous single end hole catheter, or the positioning of a multiple side hole catheter placed in the occluded segment and multiple pulses of the lytic agent delivered (Fig. 1).

High-dose bolusing of recombinant tissue plasminogen activator [rt-PA (5 mg×3 followed by infusion of 0.5 mg/hr)] was prospectively compared with a low-dose infusional technique by Braithwaite (6). Amputation-free survival in both groups was the same, as were bleeding complications. The only significant difference between the two groups was duration of lysis, the high-dose technique achieving more rapid reperfusion. Kandarpa (7) compared pulse spray with continuous infusion of urokinase and, similar to the Braithwaite study, there was no significant difference in amputation-free survival. Yusuf (8) compared a conventional infusion with pulse spray using rt-PA and again outcomes were similar in both groups. These studies enable a conclusion that high-dose pulsed regimes reduce the duration of thrombolysis though amputation-free survival is similar, but the cost of reducing the time of lysis may be increased bleeding complications (9) and increased radiological procedure time. Infusion techniques, which take longer to achieve lysis, may be less suitable for patients with more severe limb-threatening ischemia, e.g., Rutherford 2B. Infusion techniques have the advantage of requiring less operator time and are less labor-intensive.

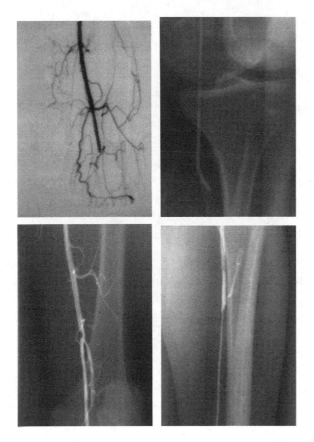

FIGURE 1 Patient presenting with an occluded femoropopliteal bypass. Thrombolysis was instituted, which resulted in complete lysis and graft salvage.

OUTCOMES

The most significant Level 1 evidence for outcomes arises from the Surgery Versus Thrombolysis for Ischemia of the Lower extremity trial (10), which was a prospective randomized trial comparing surgery and thrombolysis. Amputation-free survival, on an intention to treat basis, did not differ between the two groups. However, subgroup analysis demonstrated that patients with acute ischemia <14 days treated with thrombolysis had improved amputation-free survival rates at six months and a reduction in the magnitude of surgery. The Rochester study (11) of acute limb ischemia compared surgical intervention alone with thrombolytic therapy prior to surgical revascularization. The one-year cumulative limb salvage rate was similar. Further Level 1 evidence from the thrombolysis or peripheral artery surgery study (12) showed no difference in mortality or amputation rate, or reduction in the magnitude of surgery.

It is difficult to determine from the literature the influence of the etiology of occlusion in determining outcome. Most studies do not report the cause of occlusion. There is some evidence from a single center study that suggested both restoration of patency of the affected segment and clinical outcome were superior in those with embolic occlusions. It is difficult to explain the reason for the superiority of thrombolysis for embolic occlusions over in situ thrombotic occlusions, as many emboli are organized thrombus arising from the heart. In many clinical practices thrombolysis for embolic occlusion has been supplanted by aspiration thromboembolectomy, particularly because patients with embolic occlusions may have less of an atheromatous burden in the affected arterial segment, facilitating the aspiration of emboli. (See also chap. 12.)

OTHER INDICATIONS

Upper Limb Ischemia

Acute upper limb-threatening ischemia is considerably rarer than lower limb-threatening ischemia, and more likely to be of an embolic etiology. It is more difficult to manage with thrombolysis. The principles of thrombolytic treatment are the same, but if the occlusion is proximal, the catheter may have to be placed from the femoral artery with the catheter lying across the carotid and vertebral if on the right side or the vertebral artery if on the left side. High-dose pulsed techniques risk the displacement of thrombus into the vertebral or carotid artery. If the occlusion lies more distally in the upper limb, such as the brachial artery or radial and ulnar arteries, using femoral access requires very long catheters to reach the occlusion. If the occlusion is distal to the brachial artery, an antegrade brachial artery puncture using micropuncture equipment is an alternative, but conservative therapy is best in most cases unless limb-threatening ischemia persists.

Phlegmasia Syndromes

Phlegmasia cerulea dolens is a limb- and life-threatening condition which is characterized by patency of the arterial inflow but venous occlusive disease, resulting in venous gangrene of the affected limb. Multiple small series have been reported in the literature using thrombolytic agents to treat this condition. A thrombolytic agent may be introduced via an ipsilateral arterial approach (13). Alternatively, it may be introduced via an intravenous route by accessing the deep venous system via the short saphenous vein (14,15). Other investigators have used a combination of thrombectomy and isolated limb perfusion.

Insufficient evidence is available to make recommendations as to the use of thrombolytic agents in phlegmasia syndromes, but catheter-directed thrombolysis from either the intra-arterial or intravenous route may have a role in managing this condition.

Popliteal Aneurysms

Complicated popliteal aneurysms represent a difficult condition to treat (16). Patients usually present with acute or chronic limb ischemia secondary to aneurysm, thrombosis and/or distal embolization. Forty percent of the symptomatic popliteal aneurysms present with acute limb ischemia. Catheter-directed PAT has a role in the management of severe acute limb ischemia secondary to popliteal aneurysms in restoring crural circulation to facilitate bypass grafting (17). Technically these patients may be challenging, and it is important to place the catheter tip in the crural circulation beyond the aneurysm rather than in the thrombosed popliteal aneurysm sac. Lysis of the popliteal aneurysm itself may cause further embolization of thrombus and exacerbate ischemia. Many popliteal aneurysms are tortuous and may extend up into the subsartorial canal and significant catheter manipulation may have to be performed in order to enter the crural circulation. Microcatheters may have to be used. Peroperative thrombolysis may be used to reestablish crural patency at the time of bypass if the limb ischemia will not stand a trial of lysis.

Inadvertent Intra-arterial Drug Injection

Thrombolytic agents have been used in the management of inadvertent intra-arterial drug injections, predominantly in the upper limb. Investigators have used thrombolytic agents alone or in combination with prostanoids (18). The evidence is not sufficient to make recommendations, but intra-arterial thrombolysis may have a role in reperfusing an ischemic limb secondary to intra-arterial drug injection, probably by dissolving the associated thrombus.

CONTRAINDICATIONS TO THROMBOLYSIS

Absolute Contraindications

These have been proposed and published in the consensus document on PAT, and republished by the Society of Interventional Radiology (Table 2). These are common sense contraindications based on clinical experience and should be used as guidelines.

Relative Contraindications

These are listed in Table 2 and, similarly to the absolute contraindications, are proposed on the basis of clinical experience and their importance should be considered on a case-by-case basis.

Other Contraindications

Age

Hemorrhagic complications of PAT are age-related. The curve-relating risk to age is parabolic, with the risk of complications relating to lysis greatly increasing after age 80. Amputation-free survival is worse in patients over 70 who are treated with a PAT-first strategy, but also have poor outcome in a similar cohort treated primarily with surgery. On balance, amputation-free survival favors a surgery-first strategy in the elderly. This is probably related to the significant hemorrhagic complications in the PAT group.

Therefore, a cautious approach must be taken before embarking on primary thrombolysis in elderly patients. If the occlusion is clinically embolic, the use of a Fogarty embolectomy catheter or fluoroscopically guided aspiration may offer a better outcome (19). In thrombotic occlusion, consideration should be given to a surgery-first strategy (20).

THROMBOLYTIC AGENTS

Presently there are a number of different thrombolytic agents that have been described in the literature for clinical use. They are all plasminogenic activators and do not degrade fibrinogen. Thrombolytic agents may be divided into two groups according to their origin:

TABLE 2   Contraindications

Absolute
1. Established cerebrovascular event (including TIAs within last 2 months)
2. Active bleeding diathesis
3. Recent gastrointestinal bleeding (<10 days)
4. Neurosurgery (intracranial and spinal) within last 3 months
5. Intracranial trauma within last 3 months

Relative major
1. Cardiopulmonary resuscitation within last 10 days
2. Major nonvascular surgery or trauma within last 10 days
3. Uncontrolled, hypertension: >180 mmHg systolic or >110 mmHg diastolic
4. Puncture of noncompressible vessel
5. Intracranial tumor
6. Recent eye surgery

Minor
1. Hepatic failure, particularly those with coagulopathy
2. Bacterial endocarditis
3. Pregnancy
4. Diabetic hemorrhagic retinopathy

Abbreviation: TIA, transient ischemia attack.
Source: Modified from Ref. 1.

1. Recombinant
2. Those produced by bacteria

For practical terms, the thrombolytic agents fall into the following groups:

1. *Streptokinase.* This was the first thrombolytic agent used, and although limited by the presence of antibodies in many patients, this may be dose-dependent resistant. More serious limitations include allergy. The use of streptokinase has largely been replaced.
2. *Urokinase.* This is available in either a tissue culture origin or as a recombinant form. The clinical efficacy of the two versions is similar.
3. *Prourokinase.* Is a precursor of urokinase, but little clinical information is available on its safety and efficacy, though the PURPOSE trial did suggest that it was a useful clinical thrombolytic trial (21).
4. *Recombinant Tissue Plasminogen Activators.* This is produced by endothelial cells and occurs naturally. This has been extensively studied as a lytic agent in PAT and has a well-defined safety and efficacy record.
5. *Reteplase.* This has an advantage over rt-PA in that it has a longer half-life. This has been studied in two small peripheral arterial trials and its safety and efficacy appears to be similar to that of rt-PA (22,23).

Prospective randomized studies that compare different agents directly are few and it is difficult to determine the optimal thrombolytic agent. It is also difficult to compare clot dissolving activity in the various dosages between the lytic agents. The recent review by Ouriel and Kandarpa suggested that urokinase may be associated with a lower incidence of complications than rt-PA in the treatment of peripheral arterial occlusions, quoting an incidence of major hemorrhage in the urokinase group of 6.2% and the rt-PA group of 8.4% ($p=0.07$). They also conclude the overall incidence of intracerebral hemorrhage was significantly lower for urokinase -0.4% vs 1.1% for rt-PA ($p=0.02$), with amputation-free survival being equal (24,25).

ADJUVANT DRUG THERAPY

Aspirin

There is evidence that patients on concomitant aspirin treatment undergoing PAT have improved outcomes (26).

Heparin

There is no scientific data that specifically addresses the potential advantages or disadvantages of heparin during PAT (1).

Abciximab

This drug is a glycoprotein IIb/IIIa antagonist and has been used in combination with the newer lytic agents such as reteplase. A number of small studies using this combination of agents suggest that there may be an improvement in amputation-free survival with no increase in complication rates, but further investigation is required to facilitate case selection to optimize the use of this combination therapy (27–29).

OTHER APPLICATIONS

Peroperative Thrombolysis

This technique enables the dissolution of residual thrombus after mechanical removal techniques such as balloon embolectomy, or to improve the crural circulation in patients treated surgically. Most of the published series suggest there is no increase in bleeding complications. The use of peroperative thrombolysis to dissolve thrombi in small or distal vessels, such as the reestablishment of crural circulation or in popliteal aneurysm disease, has been described and in one randomized trial patients receiving peroperative urokinase for elective infrainguinal reconstruction had a lower mortality than placebo controls (30). Many techniques have been described in the administration of peroperative thrombolytic agents, including direct instillation into the exposed artery or as isolated limb perfusion. Continuation of the thrombolytic therapy postoperatively is associated with a higher complication rate.

Isolated Limb Perfusion

Modified PAT techniques have been used for the severely ischemic limb. A catheter is placed in the inflow artery, brachial or femoral, and an outflow catheter placed in the popliteal or brachial vein with the application of a proximal tourniquet. A high-dose thrombolytic agent is infused into the isolated limb via the arterial catheter and drained out the venous catheter. A small series have reported good limb salvage results in those patients facing amputation with no surgical revascularization option (31).

COMPETING TECHNIQUES

Due to the systemic complications associated with PAT, investigators have been working on options to obviate the need for thrombolysis in the management of acute limb-threatening ischemia. The traditional surgical technique for the retrieval of intra-arterial clot involving an embolectomy balloon has a diminishing role in modern vascular practice, due to the reduction in cases presenting with acute embolic occlusion. In non-atherosclerotic arteries, an embolectomy catheter remains a very effective tool for revascularization in this clinical situation, but current disease patterns are predominantly in situ thrombosis of diseased segments.

This has led investigators to develop many thromboembolectomy devices which use a variety of physical methods to remove or macerate thrombus, including impellers, and devices which utilize the Venturi effect (32,33). None of these techniques has succeeded in replacing peripheral thrombolysis, due to their expense, technical difficulty, and the problem of peripheral embolization. Other investigators have attempted to recanalize acutely thrombosed iliac arteries by stent placement in the iliac arteries via a patent common femoral artery, under intravenous heparin protection. This is a reasonable alternative to thrombolysis for patients who cannot tolerate the time delay to achieve lysis or who have contraindication to lysis, but the evidence for this approach is limited (34). (See also chap. 14.)

CONCLUSION

Although its utilization has diminished over the last decade, PAT is still a useful treatment option for patients presenting with acute lower limb ischemia. It is difficult to determine its exact role or when it should be used in the initial treatment of acute limb-threatening ischemia, but risks preclude its use in non-limb-threatening ischemia.

A thrombolysis-first strategy in the management of acute limb-threatening ischemia is probably associated with a higher incidence of complications, including stroke, major hemorrhage and distal embolization. In terms of amputation-free survival, there is little difference between a thrombolysis-first and a surgery-first strategy.

Ultimately, a combined approach between endovascular practitioners and vascular surgeons is advised to identify patients who are at low risk of complications (which are primarily age-related) and have the appropriate time to undergo thrombolysis, in this group catheter-directed intra-arterial thrombolysis is an acceptable initial strategy. Most nonembolic cases will require correction of an underlying lesion with angioplasty or surgery.

REFERENCES

1. Working Party on Thrombolysis in the Management of Limb Ischemia. Thrombolysis in the management of lower limb peripheral arterial occlusion—a consensus document. J Vasc Interv Radiol 2003; 14(9 Pt 2):S337–49 (Review).
2. Braithwaite BD, Tomlinson MA, Walker SR, Davies B, Buckenham TM, Earnshaw JJ. Peripheral thrombolysis for acute-onset claudication. Thrombolysis Study Group. Br J Surg 1999; 86(6):800–4.
3. Rutherford RB, Flanigan DP, Gupta SK, et al. Suggested standards for reports dealing with lower extremity ischemia. J Vasc Surg 1986; 4:80–94.
4. Cleveland TJ, Cumberland DC, Gaines PA. Percutaneous aspiration thromboembolectomy to manage the embolic complications of angioplasty and as an adjunct to thrombolysis. Clin Radiol 1994; 49(8):549–52.
5. Kessel DO, Berridge DC, Robertson I. Infusion techniques for peripheral arterial thrombolysis. Cochrane Database Syst Rev 2004;(1):CD000985 (DOI: 10.1002/14651858.CD000985.pub2).
6. Braithwaite BD, Buckenham TM, Galland RB, Heather BP, Earnshaw JJ. Prospective randomized trial of high-dose bolus versus low-dose tissue plasminogen activator infusion in the management of acute limb ischaemia. Thrombolysis Study Group. Br J Surg 1997; 84(5):646–50.
7. Kandarpa K, Chopra PS, Áruny JE, et al. Intraarterial thrombolysis of lower extremity occlusions: prospective, randomized comparison of forced periodic infusion and conventional slow continuous infusion. Radiology 1993; 188(3):861–7.
8. Yusuf SW, Whitaker SC, Gregson RH, Wenham PW, Hopkinson BR, Makin GS. Prospective randomised comparative study of pulse spray and conventional local thrombolysis. Eur J Vasc Endovasc Surg 1995; 10(2):136–41.
9. Braithwaite BD, Birch PA, Poskitt KR, Heather BP, Earnshaw JJ. Accelerated thrombolysis with high dose bolus t-PA extends the role of peripheral thrombolysis but may increase the risks. Clin Radiol 1995; 50(11):747–50.
10. The STILE Investigators. Results of a prospective randomised trial evaluating surgery versus thrombolysis for ischaemia of the lower extremity. The STILE trial. Ann Surg 1994; 220(3):251–66 (discussion 266–8).
11. Ouriel K, Veith FJ, Sasahara AA. A comparison of recombinant urokinase with vascular surgery as initial treatment for acute arterial occlusion of the legs. Thrombolysis or Peripheral Arterial Surgery (TOPAS) Investigators. N Engl J Med 1998; 338(16):1105–11.
12. Ouriel K, Veith FJ, Sasahara AA. Thrombolysis or peripheral arterial surgery: phase I results. TOPAS Investigators. J Vasc Surg 1996; 23(1):64–73 (discussion 74–5).
13. Wlodarczyk ZK, Gibson M, Dick R, Hamilton G. Low-dose intra-arterial thrombolysis in the treatment of phlegmasia caerulea dolens. Br J Surg 1994; 81(3):370–2.
14. Tardy B, Moulin N, Mismetti P, Decousus H, Laporte S. Intravenous thrombolytic therapy in patients with phlegmasia caerulea dolens. Haematologica 2006; 91(2):281–2.
15. Patel NH, Plorde JJ, Meissner M. Catheter-directed thrombolysis in the treatment of phlegmasia cerulea dolens. Ann Vasc Surg 1998; 12(5):471–5.
16. Galland RB. Popliteal aneurysms: controversies in their management. Am J Surg 2005; 190(2):314–8 (Review).
17. Dorigo W, Pulli R, Turini F, et al. Acute leg ischaemia from thrombosed popliteal artery aneurysms: role of preoperative thrombolysis. Eur J Vasc Endovasc Surg 2002; 23(3):251–4.
18. Hering J, Angelkort B. Acute ischemia of the hand after intra-arterial injection of flunitrazepam. Local combined fibrinolysis therapy in three cases. Dtsch Med Wochenschr 2006; 131(24):1377–80 (German).
19. Jivegard L, Holm J, Schersten T. The outcome in arterial thrombosis misdiagnosed as arterial embolism. Acta Chir Scand 1986; 152:251–6.
20. Braithwaite BD, Davies B, Birch PA, Heather BP, Earnshaw JJ. Management of acute leg ischaemia in the elderly. Br J Surg 1998; 85(2):217–20.
21. Ouriel K, Kandarpa K, Schuerr DM, Hultquist M, Hodkinson G, Wallin B. Prourokinase versus urokinase for recanalization of peripheral occlusions, safety and efficacy: the PURPOSE trial. J Vasc Interv Radiol 1999; 10(8):1083–91.
22. Ouriel K, Katzen B, Mewissen M, et al. Reteplase in the treatment of peripheral arterial and venous occlusions: a pilot study. J Vasc Interv Radiol 2000; 11(7):849–54.
23. Valji K. Evolving strategies for thrombolytic therapy of peripheral vascular occlusion. J Vasc Interv Radiol 2000; 11(4):411–20 (Review).
24. Ouriel K, Kandarpa K. Safety of thrombolytic therapy with urokinase or recombinant tissue plasminogen activator for peripheral arterial occlusion: a comprehensive compilation of published work. J Endovasc Ther 2004; 11(4):436–46 (Review).
25. Ouriel K. Current status of thrombolysis for peripheral arterial occlusive disease. Ann Vasc Surg 2002; 16(6):797–804 (Review).
26. Braithwaite BD, Jones L, Yusuf SW, et al. Aspirin improves the outcome of intra-arterial thrombolysis with tissue plasminogen activator. Thrombolysis Study Group. Br J Surg 1995; 82(10):1357–8.

27. Tepe G, Hopfenzitz C, Dietz K, et al. Peripheral arteries: treatment with antibodies of platelet receptors and reteplase for thrombolysis–APART trial. Radiology 2006; 239(3):892–900.
28. Ouriel K, Castaneda F, McNamara T, et al. Reteplase monotherapy and reteplase/abciximab combination therapy in peripheral arterial occlusive disease: results from the RELAX trial. J Vasc Interv Radiol 2004; 15(3):229–38.
29. Drescher P, McGuckin J, Rilling WS, Crain MR. Catheter-directed thrombolytic therapy in peripheral artery occlusions: combining reteplase and abciximab. AJR Am J Roentgenol 2003; 180(5):1385–91.
30. Comerota AJ, Rao AK, Throm RC, et al. A prospective, randomized, blinded, and placebo-controlled trial of intraoperative intra-arterial urokinase infusion during lower extremity revascularization. Regional and systemic effects. Ann Surg 1993; 218(4):534–41 (discussion 541–3).
31. Ali AT, Kalapatapu VR, Bledsoe S, Moursi MM, Eidt JF. Percutaneous isolated limb perfusion with thrombolytics for severe limb ischemia. Vasc Endovascular Surg 2005; 39(6):491–7.
32. Reekers JA, Kromhout JG, van der Waal K. Catheter for percutaneous thrombectomy: first clinical experience. Radiology 1993; 188(3):871–4.
33. Self SB, Coe DA, Normann S, Seeger JM. Rotational atherectomy for treatment of occluded prosthetic grafts. J Surg Res 1994; 56(2):134–40.
34. Berczi V, Thomas SM, Turner DR, Bottomley JR, Cleveland TJ, Gaines PA. Stent implantation for acute iliac artery occlusions: initial experience. J Vasc Interv Radiol 2006; 17(4):645–9.

14 Mechanical Thrombectomy in Acute Leg Ischemia

Dierk Vorwerk
Department of Diagnostic and Interventional Radiology, Klinikum Ingolstadt, Krumenauerstrasse, Ingolstadt, Germany

CURRENT CONCEPTS

According to the TransAtlantic Inter-Society Consensus document (1), treatment of acute ischemia depends on the clinical stage. In stages I (viable) and IIa (threatened: marginal), surgical treatment with open embolectomy or thrombectomy as well as thrombolysis are accepted concepts. In stage IIb (threatened: immediate), fogarty embolectomy is the treatment of choice, while thrombolysis is not recommended due to potential complications that may result from bleeding into revascularized tissue resulting in compartment syndrome. In early stage III (irreversible), surgical thrombectomy may be utilized, but in advanced stage III cases, only amputation remains the principal option.

To achieve a successful and enduring result, at least one lower limb artery or a major collateral has to be reopened down to the foot in order to establish a sufficient outflow and to avoid early rethrombosis. Thrombolysis has some drawbacks that prevent widespread use in acute limb ischemia. It may be time-consuming and rapid revascularization is rare. In particular, in advanced stages, treatment duration of up to 24 hours may worsen the clinical situation with an unpredictable outcome. Local bleeding may occur at the entry site that complicates an adjunctive surgical approach, if required. Coagulopathy after thrombolysis may also interfere with surgery. Furthermore, the subset of patients with acute ischemia is frequently of older age and their comorbidities often contraindicate the use of thrombolytic agents (2).

Fogarty embolectomy via a femoral or popliteal approach is effective in cases of circumscribed thrombi but may become difficult in concomitant atherosclerotic stenoses or extensive thromboses affecting the lower limb arteries. In older thrombi, wall adhesion of the occluding clots can complicate removal.

INSTRUMENTS FOR MECHANICAL THROMBECTOMY

Many of the difficulties with surgical thromboembolectomy and thrombolysis might be solved by a reliable method of percutaneous clot retrieval. Mechanical removal of thrombo-embolic material may utilize the following techniques:

- Manual aspiration
- Hydrodynamic thrombectomy
- Rotational thrombectomy
- Atherectomy
- Stent placement

In addition, there are a number of other devices or treatment options which are under development and evaluation.

Manual Clot Aspiration

Manual aspiration is the key technique of mechanical thrombectomy (Fig. 1). It is simple to perform and easy to learn, is inexpensive and rapid. It is therefore surprising that its use is frequently underestimated in clinical practice. This technique was first described by Starck et al. (3) as well as Sniderman et al. (4) and is applicable to emboli as well as thrombosis of iatrogenic or intrinsic origin.

There are some techniques that facilitate success:

1. A sheath with a removable hub is mandatory at the access site to allow safe removal of the aspirated clot, together with the aspiration catheter, without removing the sheath from the artery.
2. End-hole catheters of appropriate diameter must be chosen according to the size of the artery. As a guideline, for the superficial femoral and popliteal artery 8- to 9-F catheters, for

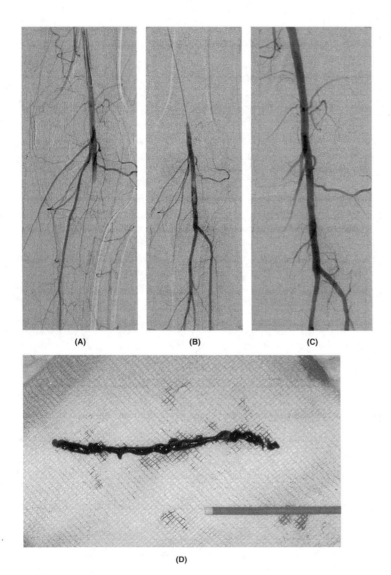

(A)   (B)   (C)

(D)

FIGURE 1 (**A**) Acute occlusion of the popliteal artery. (**B**) Popliteal artery after partial success with aspiration thrombectomy. (**C**) Complete aspiration of clot. (**D**) Aspiration catheter and retrieved clot.

the proximal lower limb arteries 6-F catheters and for the tibial arteries 4-F catheters are required. By use of a hydrophilic guidewire, the catheters may be directed into the tibial and peroneal arteries down to the foot. For tibial arteries diagnostic end-hole catheters of 4-F in a vertebral configuration are useful.

3. When aspirating the clot, the end of the catheter is brought into contact with the proximal end of the clot and suction is applied by use of a 20- or 50-cm^3 syringe which is continued while the catheter is pulled back into the sheath. Suction is discontinued once easy aspiration of blood occurs during suction. This indicates loss of the thrombus or successful aspiration of smaller particles into the syringe.

4. After each suction maneuver the syringe, sheath and the catheter have to be carefully checked for retained clot material and should be flushed and cleaned.

In very difficult cases, ballooning of the clot may help to disintegrate the clot into smaller fragments which may be aspirated. This technique is only recommended if the outflow is still blocked by additional clots as there is a risk of peripheral embolization.

The results for percutaneous aspiration embolectomy (PAE) have been reported as favorable. Wagner et al. (5) reported on 85 patients that underwent 90 PAEs for embolic occlusions below the inguinal ligament between October 1987 and September 1992 in a prospective study with a 96% follow-up. The first PAE was clinically successful in 77 limbs (86%). In eight cases, major amputation was necessary. Eleven out of thirteen failures were observed in limbs with severe ischemia, but the success rate was independent of the time interval from embolism to the procedure. The 30-day mortality rate was 3.5%. The cumulative primary patency rate at one and four years was 68% and 58%, respectively. The limb salvage rate was 88% after one year and 86% after four years (5).

Canova et al. (6) reported on 88 procedures in patients with acute embolic occlusions. Forty-three patients had limb threatening ischemia while 45 patients suffered from severe claudication. Technical success was 96.6%; major and minor complications occurred in two patients each. Follow-up was an average of 3.7 years and patency after two years was 81.7%. It is important to note that failure during follow-up was due to recurrent embolization in 10 out of 16 instances.

Hydrodynamic Thrombectomy

There are three devices of this type that have been used for treating arterial occlusions. All of them utilize the Venturi principle for thrombus removal. Saline solution is injected through a small bore channel that ends into a large exhaust lumen at the tip of the catheter. At this point a flow vortex is created that removes surrounding clot material while the fluid leaves the body through the exhaust lumen. Under ideal circumstances, the procedure is isovolumetric avoiding fluid overload in the patient. The systems work well in nonorganized clots and fresh thrombus, but have some limitations in older material as well as in large diameter vessels, as the efficacy is limited once the diameter exceeds 8 mm.

Two of the systems, the Cordis hydrolyzer and the Boston Scientific Oasis system of 6- and 7-F, both use a conventional injection pump usually used for contrast media application. Relatively few data exist on the use of these two systems in the arterial circulation. Henry et al. (7) presented a single-center experience with the hydrolyzer in native arteries, veins, and bypass grafts. The device was used in 41 patients with recent thromboses (aged 1–30 days, mean 8.7±8.5), measuring from 4 to 35 cm. The occlusions were located in native lower limb arteries ($n=28$), bypass grafts ($n=8$), superior vena cava ($n=2$), axillary vein ($n=1$), and pulmonary arteries ($n=2$). Immediate technical success (residual clot <50% of lumen diameter) was achieved in 34 patients (83%): 22 out of 28 native arteries (78%), 7 out of 8 bypass grafts (87%), and all pulmonary arteries, superior vena cava, and the axillary vein. The seven failed patients were treated surgically adjunctive procedures were used to maximize luminal diameter: angioplasty ($n=29$, with 13 immediate stent implantations), thromboaspiration ($n=17$), and thrombolysis ($n=10$). One case of distal embolism was the only complication (treated by thromboaspiration). At 30 days, 30 (73%) vessels remained patent.

Hoepfner et al. (8) reported on 64 patients, 12 with viable and 52 with threatened limbs. All limbs were successfully treated. Residual thrombi, underlying atherosclerotic vessel disease and occluded arteries with a small diameter made adjunctive interventions (balloon angioplasty, percutaneous aspiration thrombectomy, lysis) were necessary. Primary patency was 72%, 70%, 67%, and 65%; the limb salvage rates were 81%, 78%, 75%, and 73% for 1, 3, 12, and 24 months respectively.

Kasirajan (9) reported the use of the Angiojet system. A total of 86 (acute, $n=65$; subacute, $n=21$) patients were available for retrospective analysis. Angiographic success was evaluated in 83 out of 86 patients (guidewire unable to traverse lesion in three patients). The procedure failed in 13 out of 83 (15.6%) patients, partial success was seen in 19 out of 83 patients (22.9%), and successful recanalization was noted in 51 out of 83 patients (61.4%). Adjunctive thrombolysis was used in 50 out of 86 patients (58%). However, thrombolysis resulted in angiographic improvement in only 7 out of 50 of these patients (14%). Adjunctive thrombolysis was uniformly unsuccessful in patients in whom initial hydrodynamic thrombectomy failed. Success was more likely in the setting of in situ thrombosis, with 61 out of 68 (90%) procedures successful, compared to embolic occlusions, with 9 out of 15 (60%) procedures successful. Angiographic outcome was not dependent on the duration of occlusion or the type of vessel. Follow-up data were available in 56 patients for patency assessment at a median of 3.9 months. Patency at six months was 79%. Systemic complications occurred in 16.3% of patients, local complications were noted in 18.6%, and one-month amputation and mortality rates were 11.6% and 9.3%, respectively. At present, few cases of hemodynamics thrombectmy are performed worldwide.

Rotational Thrombectomy

The group of rotational thrombectomy devices contains a number of different instruments that all fragment the thrombus into small pieces which are small enough to pass the capillary bed. This, of course, is not always effective since embolization of larger pieces may cause complications.

The oldest device of this group is the Amplatz clot buster. This comprises a 7- or 8-F catheter that carries housing at its distal end. An impeller is mounted within the housing which can rotate up to 1,000,000 rpm and create a vortex around the catheter tip that sucks in clot material which is pulverized and destructed. Due to repeat exposure to the impeller, under ideal circumstances, the clot is macerated into very small pieces that allow passage through the capillary bed. The catheter cannot be guided over a guidewire and has a blunt tip making passage through curved vessels difficult. The principle only works if no or low flow is present as the vortex will be destroyed by the arterial flow. It therefore becomes difficult to remove remaining wall-adherent clot material once flow has been reestablished.

Görich et al. (10) reported their experience with the Amplatz thrombectomy device for recanalization of acute occlusions of both the superficial and the deep femoral arteries. Eighteen patients with acute occlusions of the femoral arteries (8 males, 10 females; 10–87 years old) were treated using the Amplatz thrombectomy clot macerator. The duration of occlusion was 16 ± 8 hours. Eighteen patients underwent treatment of the deep femoral artery, and 16 patients had additional involvement of the superficial femoral artery. After primary recanalization of the deep femoral artery, the superficial femoral artery was also recanalized using the Amplatz thrombectomy device. Nine patients required additional aspiration thrombectomy of the tibial arteries, five patients required additional aspiration thrombectomy of side branches of the deep femoral artery, and 12 patients required additional local thrombolysis with urokinase. In 14 (78%) out of 18 patients, recanalization of the deep femoral artery was complete without demonstrable residual thrombi. Arterial spasm was observed in five patients (28%). The rate of limb salvage was 94% at a mean follow-up interval of 8.9 ± 4.1 months. No severe complications were reported.

An alternative device is the Rotarex catheter (Straub Medical, Inc.) that combines thrombus destruction with suction. A double catheter head consisting of a stator and a rotator crushes and macerates surrounding thrombus material while the pieces are sucked into the catheter and transported backwards by a rotating Archimedes spiral, driven by a motor unit. The device is guided over an 0.018 in. guidewire and requires an 8-F sheath.

This device is effective in removing both organized and fresh thrombus from arteries the size of the femoral and popliteal. To be effective and safe the artery needs to be somewhat larger in diameter than the catheter. If the catheter acts in a wedged position, there is a high risk of vessel wall damage. This is also the case if the device is used in arterial spasm that may be encountered in young patients. It is not recommended that the device is used in arteries less than 4–5 mm since there is a risk of damaging the arterial wall especially once the catheter hits an atherosclerotic plaque.

Zeller et al. (11) evaluated the acute and long-term results after recanalization of thrombotic occlusions of infra-aortic native arteries, stented arteries and bypass-grafts using the Rotarex device. In 98 patients with a mean duration of occlusion of 31 ± 33 (range 0–140) days, and a mean occlusion length 21 ± 11 cm, 100 procedures were performed. The primary success rate was 96% (ipsilateral interventions 99%, crossover 40%). The restenosis rate after a mean follow-up of 13 ± 4 months was 33% for native arteries, 74% for instent-recanalizations and 86% for bypass-graft occlusions. In 3%, severe complications occurred.

Stents

In some instances, stents may be used to treat soft thrombotic occlusions. This is done more frequently than usually reported as many femoropopliteal occlusions contain underlying thrombus. After percutaneous transluminal angioplasty (PTA), these lesions tend to remain a problem and frequently undergo stenting to overcome the remaining stenosis. It is difficult to decide angiographically whether the residual disease process is atherosclerotic or thrombotic. The mechanical properties of the lesion are more helpful under those circumstances. Once a guidewire passes the occlusion smoothly without any resistance it is very likely that at least parts of the lesion contain thrombus material, particularly if accompanied by recent onset of symptoms.

If an occlusion appears to contain fresh material, the author prefers to perform a mechanical thrombectomy before PTA.

Stents are able to displace clot material to the periphery of the vessel wall and can be utilized as a last resort if mechanical clot removal fails. Stenting should be used with care since the long-term results of stents in the femoropopliteal region are poor at the present time.

Other Devices

High-frequency ultrasound may be used in two different ways for thrombus removal. Intra-arterial thrombolysis may be enhanced by additional application of ultrasound, designed to break fibrin bonds in order to accelerate completion of thrombolysis. Early clinical experiences were moderately successful using the Acolysis system but trials were prematurely halted. New data will hopefully become available soon.

Ultrasound energy as a tool for thrombus destruction was used by the Angiosonic system (Omnisonics, New York, NY), but there are little clinical data at present.

DIFFERENTIAL APPLICATION OF TECHNIQUES

There are many concepts available for mechanical thrombectomy and little evidence exists to suggest which approach is the best. It is important that each institution builds an individual strategy using treatment modalities that are available. It is mandatory to perform these interventions via an antegrade ipsilateral femoral approach.

Popliteal and Lower-Limb Arteries

The author's basic technique relies on aspiration embolectomy which is the principle technique for the popliteal artery and runoff vessels. If simple aspiration fails in the popliteal artery, the author continues with a mechanical device using clot maceration (Amplatz-clot buster, Rotarex) in order to reduce the clot burden. We do not reopen the trifurcation and distal popliteal arteries with these devices in order to retain a distal clot in place that prevents uncontrolled downward embolization of occlusive material into the pedal arteries.

The most distal clot is then aspirated by the usual technique.

If the tibial arteries are also occluded, the strategy is to establish flow down one artery into the foot. If possible, as many arteries are recanalized as possible, but under difficult circumstances, one open artery is used as an endpoint.

In cases where the distal popliteal artery and the trifurcation are open, a cuff is positioned around the calf and inflated to the individual systolic pressure whilst the thrombectomy process is ongoing with mechanical rotational instruments. This technique is utilized to prevent downward embolization of the very distal portion of the clot. Aspiration thrombectomy is then used to remove the last clot before the cuff is deflated.

If it is not possible to reopen at a single lower limb artery with sufficient outflow to the foot, local thrombolysis is attempted by injecting 5–10 mg of recombinant tissue plasminogen activator directly into the occluded artery. This is followed by prolonged heparinization and IV application of prostaglandins.

Superficial Femoral Artery

In long segment thrombosis of the superficial femoral artery, a mechanical rotational instrument using the Amplatz clot buster or the Rotarex thrombectomy device is used as first line therapy. If adherent thrombus remains, the patient is anti-coagulated for a three-day period and another angiogram is performed. In cases of residual thrombus, a stent is used. If fresh thrombosis occurs within a stent, the Rotarex catheter is used as a primary instrument followed by balloon angioplasty.

CONCLUSION

Mechanical thrombectomy is a feasible concept for acute thrombosis in arteries below the femoral bifurcation. In most instances it allows removal of the clot material, rapid revascularization and avoids lengthy procedures with repeat angiography. Mechanical thrombectomy requires knowledge of a variety of different devices—from low-cost aspiration catheters to expensive mechanical systems—but is a concept that may replace thrombolysis in selected patients. Single-center and single-arm studies report high-technical success and encouraging follow-up results. Randomized data comparing these techniques to surgery or thrombolyis are lacking.

REFERENCES

1. TASC working group TASC. Management of peripheral arterial disease. Transatlantic intersociety consensus. Int Angiol 2000; 152(Suppl. 1):161–3.
2. Ouriel K, Veith FJ, Sasahara AA. A comparison of recombinant urokinase with vascular surgery as initial treatment for acute arterial occlusion of the legs. Thrombolysis or Peripheral Arterial Surgery (TOPAS) Investigators. N Engl J Med 1998; 338(16):1105–11.
3. Starck EE, McDermott JC, Crummy AB, Turnipseed WD, Acher CW, Burgess JH. Percutaneous aspiration thromboembolectomy. Radiology 1985; 156(1):61–6.
4. Sniderman KW, Bodner L, Saddekni S, Srur M, Sos TA. Percutaneous embolectomy by transcatheter aspiration. Work in progress. Radiology 1984; 150(2):357–61.
5. Wagner HJ, Starck EE, Reuter P. Long-term results of percutaneous aspiration embolectomy. Cardiovasc Intervent Radiol 1994; 17(5):241–6.
6. Canova CR, Schneider E, Fischer L, Leu AJ, Hoffmann U. Long-term results of percutaneous thrombo-embolectomy in patients with infrainguinal embolic occlusions. Int Angiol 2001; 20(1):66–73.
7. Henry M, Amor M, Henry I, Tricoche O, Allaoui M. The Hydrolyser thrombectomy catheter: a single-center experience. Endovasc Surg 1998; 5(1):24–31.
8. Hopfner W, Bohndorf K, Vicol C, Loeprecht H. Percutaneous hydromechanical thrombectomy in acute and subacute lower limb ischemia. Rofo 2001; 173(3):229–35 (German).
9. Kasirajan K, Gray B, Beavers FP, et al. Rheolytic thrombectomy in the management of acute and subacute limb-threatening ischemia. J Vasc Interv Radiol 2001; 12(4):413–21.

10. Görich J, Rilinger N, Sokiranski R, et al. Mechanical thrombolysis of acute occlusion of both the superficial and the deep femoral arteries using a thrombectomy device. AJR Am J Roentgenol 1998; 170(5):1177–80.
11. Zeller T, Frank U, Burgelin K, et al. Long-term results after recanalization of acute and subacute thrombotic occlusions of the infra-aortic arteries and bypass-grafts using a rotational thrombectomy device. Rofo Fortschr Geb Rontgenstr Neuen Bildgeb Verfahr 2002; 174(12):1559–65.

15 | Combined Endovascular/Surgical Approach to Acute Lower Limb Ischemia

Ian M. Loftus
St. George's Vascular Institute, St. George's Hospital, London, U.K.

INTRODUCTION

Over recent years the applications and indications for endovascular therapy have expanded. Endovascular techniques have become more sophisticated in parallel with developments in equipment and devices. Learning and adapting endovascular skills is essential for modern vascular practice, and surgical and radiological interventions should no longer be considered in isolation. Rather, they should be seen in combination, complementing one another, expanding the range of options available for treating common vascular problems. Acute lower limb ischemia, a problem previously seen as predominantly surgical rather than radiological, is one area where a combined approach can be very successful. An in-depth knowledge of surgical and radiological techniques combine to offer increased flexibility in the management of acute ischemia.

Acute lower limb ischemia may be embolic in origin, or secondary to thrombus formation over preexisting atheroma. The advent of endovascular aneurysm repair (EVAR) and iliac stents has seen a further spectrum of ischemic complications associated with device failure or maldeployment, stent kinking and narrowing (1). In the acute situation, where thrombus is likely to represent a significant contributor to arterial obstruction, angioplasty is unadvisable due to the risk of embolization. Historically, acute limb ischemia has been treated either surgically, or by thrombolysis. While the latter gained popularity for a while, historical review of data suggests that a shift away from thrombolysis in recent years has improved clinical outcomes (2). However, data also suggest that thrombectomy alone is often not sufficient, and adjunctive techniques are often required to achieve a good clinical outcome (3).

Interventionists now have a variety of mechanical thrombectomy devices and endovascular adjuncts to the treatment of acute occlusion (see chap. 14) (4,5), and there is some evidence to suggest that a minimally invasive approach is better than surgery alone (6). However, much of the evidence for this is anecdotal and published in the form of case reports and individual center series. The variable nature of presentation and extent of disease make randomized trials in this area difficult; each case must be treated on an individual basis, depending upon the presentation and the cause of acute ischemia.

THE "OVER-THE-WIRE" FOGARTY CATHETER

One of the most useful adjuncts to the surgical treatment of acute leg ischemia is the over-the-wire Fogarty® catheter (Edwards™ Lifesciences Inc., Irvine, California, U.S.A.) (Fig. 1). Designed for the retrieval of soft embolus and thrombus, these through-lumen catheters have the advantage of being guidewire compatible allowing radiological guidance through occluded, tortuous or stenotic arteries. They have stainless steel brushings under both proximal and distal balloon windings to assure accurate visualization during fluoroscopy. There are a variety of available sizes: the 3-F catheter is compatible with a 0.018 guidewire, 4-F with a 0.025 guidewire and 5.5, 6, and 7-F catheters with a 0.035 guidewire. There are two lengths available, 40 and 80 cm. Through a femoral exposure and they can be passed proximally through tortuous or diseased iliac vessels. Despite being radiopaque, contrast

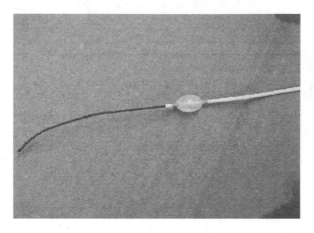

FIGURE 1   The "over-the-wire" Fogarty® catheter.

injection should be performed regularly to assess position of the catheter and ensure that dissection does not occur. Once positioned under fluoroscopy, the technique is the same as for the conventional Fogarty catheter, though the double lumen device can be visualized radiographically as it is retrieved (Fig. 2A,B). The same approach can be used for popliteal and distal vessel thrombus (Fig. 3), with the advantage over conventional Fogarty catheters that the double lumen device can be guided into all three distal vessels by guidewire manipulation. A completion angiogram can be performed through the catheter, and if deemed appropriate, thrombolysis may also be given (Fig. 4).

The over-the-wire Fogarty technique is particularly useful for thombus retrieval for acute limb occlusion following EVAR.

ACUTE LOWER LIMB ISCHEMIA FOLLOWING EVAR

Limb occlusion is a recognized complication of EVAR, especially with difficult iliac anatomy (7). Most series suggest that the rate of limb ischemia is around 1%, though this is likely to be higher if more challenging cases are tackled by endovascular rather than conventional methods. In a series of 311 patients, 21 developed lower limb ischemia (1). Of these, 15 were due to limb occlusion, 3 secondary to embolization and 3 were the result of common femoral

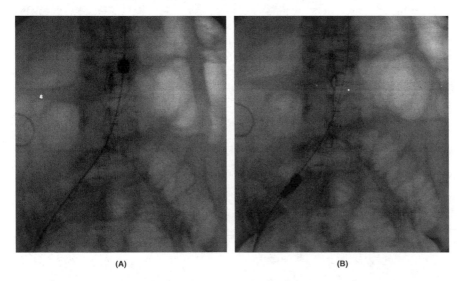

(A)   (B)

FIGURE 2   (**A**) and (**B**) Use of the "over-the-wire" Fogarty® catheter for performing a thrombectomy for acute iliac artery occlusion.

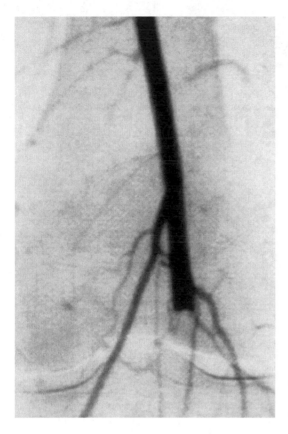

FIGURE 3 Angiogram revealing acute femoral embolus. The "over-the-wire" Fogarty® catheter can be used to perform a thrombectomy, distal vessel embolectomy, angiogram and thrombolysis if required.

artery thrombosis. Limb occlusions were managed with thrombectomy and further stent placement ($n=4$), femorofemoral bypass ($n=7$), explantation due to a persistant endoleak ($n=1$) or expectant management ($n=3$). The other six patients were managed by a combination of endarterectomy, embolectomy and patch angioplasty.

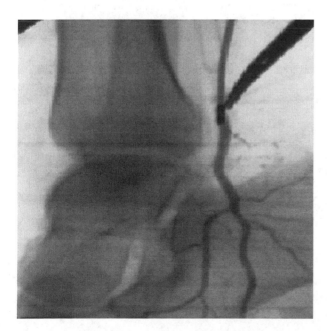

FIGURE 4 Completion angiography following distal vessel embolectomy with an "over-the-wire" Fogarty® catheter. This can be directed in to all three calf vessels by guidewire manipulation.

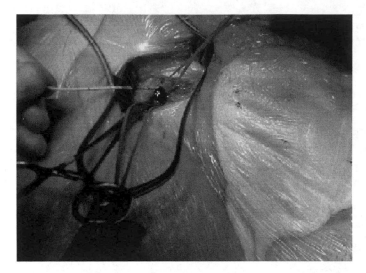

FIGURE 5 Retrievel of fresh thrombus from the thrombosed right limb of an endovascular aneurysm stent graft using the "over-the-wire" Fogarty® catheter.

The preference of the authors is to perform a completion angiogram following EVAR with all wires removed so that any tortuosity or abuttal of the end of the stent graft against the vessel wall is identified and corrected by the deployment of further stents. If angiography is performed with wires in situ, such tortuosity or kinking can be missed. Despite this, limb occlusion still occasionally occurs, and is best treated with the groin reopened, the distal vessel clamped to prevent distal embolization, and an over-the-wire Fogarty passed up the limb under angiographic control (Fig. 5). Once thrombus is cleared from the limb, an angiogram can be performed to detect any underlying problem with the limb of the device, such as narrowing or kinking of the stent graft. If this can be corrected by the placement of further stents or angioplasty, this is the preferred method of limb salvage.

COMBINED ENDARTERECTOMY AND ENDOVASCULAR PROCEDURES

Angiographic retrieval of iliac thrombus may be combined with femoral endarterectomy when there is severe occlusive disease of the common femoral artery and bifurcation. This has also been described in combination with angioplasty stenting of the infrarenal aorta and common iliac arteries. Palmaz stents may be used in the distal aorta above kissing iliac stents and femoral endarterectomies to revascularize the aortoiliofemoral axis (8). This should be considered as a viable alternative to laparotomy in selected patients with total infrarenal aortic occlusion.

In cases of acute limb ischemia secondary to thrombosis in preexisting severe athero-sclerotic disease, if disease extends more proximally into the common femoral and external iliac artery, there is reluctance to position stents across the inguinal ligament. However, combined thrombus retrieval, femoral endarterectomy extending into the extrenal iliac artery, and iliac angioplasty offers an attractive solution which prevents the need for either femorofemoral cross over or ilio femoral bypass.

In a retrospective analysis of 34 patients who underwent intraoperative external iliac stenting and common femoral endarterectomy/patch angioplasty between 1997 and 2000, the combined endovascular and surgical approach demonstrated excellent results (9). External iliac stent deployment incorporated the stenotic iliac segment and the proximal end point of the endarterectomy in all patients, without crossing the inguinal ligament. Four patients (12%) also needed common iliac angioplasty at the same time, for proximal iliac disease, and 14 patients (41%) needed distal revascularization for associated femoropopliteal or tibial disease. Technical and hemodynamic success were achieved in all patients with a complication rate of 15%. With a mean follow-up period of 13 months (range, 0.5–28 months), one-year primary patency and primary-assisted patency rates were 84% and 97%, respectively. No perioperative mortality was seen.

Iliac stenting as an adjunct to common femoral endarterectomy/patch angioplasty allows for more localized surgery than conventional bypass with excellent technical success and patency rates.

ACUTE LIMB ISCHEMIA ASSOCIATED WITH AORTIC DISSECTION

Acute aortic dissection may present with acute limb ischemia. Such cases can be technically challenging and a combined surgical and endovascular approach should be considered, whenever intervention is deemed appropriate. In 458 patients from an International Registry for Acute Aortic Dissection (IRAD), acute limb ischemia was present in 6% of cases, though this was higher in a single institutional series from the same publication (10).

One option is unilateral aorto-iliac stenting combined with femoro-femoral cross over bypass (11). In a case report of lower limb ischemia, computed tomography (CT) scan revealed occlusion of the right iliac artery due to acute descending aortic dissection with a thrombosed false lumen. Three days after femorofemoral crossover bypass, ischemia of both legs developed and angiography demonstrated occlusion of the infrarenal aorta and left common iliac artery. Two overlapping stents were deployed in these vessel segments. Completion angiography confirmed successful recanalization with adequate distal flow and good patency of the crossover bypass. Peripheral pulses were restored associated with symptomatic relief.

The authors have recently performed a combined open/endovasular procedure in a 71-year-old man who presented with an acutely ischemic right leg and dissection without bypass grafting. A CT scan revealed an acute type B aortic dissection associated with right common iliac occlusion (Fig. 6). Under a general anesthetic bilateral groin cut downs were performed and the common femoral artery controlled on both sides. With some difficulty, a guidewire was directed under radiographic control through the occluded right iliac system into the aortic true lumen. Over this, a pigtail catheter was positioned in the arch of the aorta. A 20 cm 34 mm Valiant™ (Medtronic Ave Inc., Santa Rosa, California, U.S.A.) stent graft was positioned to seal the dissection entry tear, covering the origin of the left subclavian artery, without complication. Angiography revealed complete right iliac occlusion immediately distal to the common iliac bifurcation. A self expanding stent was positioned across the dissection

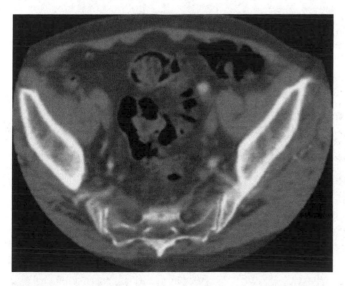

FIGURE 6 Acute aortic dissection extending into both iliac arteries, leading to occlusion of the right external iliac and acute lower limb ischemia.

flap in the right iliac artery, after which an over-the-wire Fogarty catheter was used to retrieve a large amount of fresh thrombus. After thorough flushing, flow was restored with excellent inflow and with repair of the arteriotomy, all leg pulses returned. Completion angiography demonstrated an excellent result (Fig. 7) and the patient made a swift and uneventful recovery.

There have now been a number of other case reports describing the management of acute limb ischemia secondary to aortic dissection using a combination of endovascular stent graft placement and fenestration (12,13).

The outcome for patients with acute type B dissection and acute limb ischemia was studied from the IRAD database from 1996 to 2002, along with data from a single institutional database (University of Michigan, U.S.A.) (10). Univariate and multivariate statistics were used to delineate factors associated with morbidity and mortality outcomes. The overall mortality was 12%. Endovascular intervention was more commonly performed in patients with acute limb ischemia and was associated with increased risk of acute renal failure, acute mesenteric ischemia and death. The single institution analysis revealed acute limb ischemia occurred in 28 of 93 patients. Aortic fenestration or aorto-iliac stenting was the primary therapy in 93% though surgical bypass was required in 7%. Limb salvage was 93% at a mean of 18-month follow-up. Acute limb ischemia secondary to acute aortic dissection is therefore predictive of death and visceral ischemia, and in these high-risk patients, an aggressive combined surgical and endovascular approach confers excellent limb salvage.

Combined treatment with either crossover bypass, iliac stenting or fenestration and endovascular stenting of the aorta should be considered as a preferable alternative to open surgery in cases of complicated acute dissection with limb ischemia (14).

ISCHEMIA ASSOCIATED WITH TRAUMA

Endovascular treatment of thoracic transection is now well described, but a combined endovascular and surgical approach should be considered for other vascular injuries. Endovascular repair of blunt intra-abdominal aorto-iliac injuries is possible and should be particularly considered when fecal contamination, pelvic hematoma, or multiple associated injuries make conventional repair problematic (15). Such an approach has been described in a young patient with a crush injury to the lower abdomen and pelvis. Vascular examination revealed absent femoral pulses, no pedal signals bilaterally, and minimal left leg and no right leg motor function. Arteriograms revealed right common iliac artery and external iliac artery occlusion

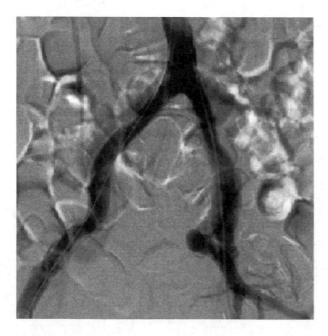

FIGURE 7 Completion angiogram after successful thoracic stent graft and uncovered iliac stent for acute dissection and external iliac occlusion, presenting with acute right limb ischemia.

and a 2-cm near occlusion of the left external iliac artery. Bilateral common femoral artery cut-downs were performed; retrograde arteriograms revealed bilateral common iliac occlusions and extravasation of contrast from the external iliac artery. An angled glidewire was successfully traversed both vascular injuries, which were treated with covered stents. After calf fasciotomy, exploratory laparotomy revealed a severe sigmoid colon injury, requiring resection and colostomy. Postoperatively the patient regained palpable bilateral pedal pulses.

CONCLUSION

A thorough understanding of both the surgical and endovascular options allows a combined approach to acute lower limb ischemia. This is particularly useful in the management of the acutely ischemic limb following EVAR and in the presence of an acute aortic dissection. Such a combined approach may avoid more extensive surgery, minimize the risk to patients and optimize the results of intervention.

REFERENCES

1. Maldonado TS, Rockman CB, Riles E, et al. Ischaemic complications after endovascular abdominal aortic aneurysm repair. J Vasc Surg 2004; 40(4):703–9.
2. Eliason JL, Wainess RM, Proctor MC, et al. A national and single institutional experience in the contemporary treatment of acute lower extremity ischaemia. Ann Surg 2003; 238(3):382–9.
3. Kalinowski M, Wagner HJ. Adjunctive techniques in percutaneous mechanical thrombectomy. Tech Vasc Interv Radiol 2003; 6(1):6–13.
4. Kasirajan K, Haskal ZJ, Ouriel K. The use of mechanical thrombectomy devices in the management of acute peripheral arterial occlusive disease. J Vasc Interv Radiol 2001; 12:405–11.
5. Vordwerk D. Mechanical thrombectomy is an alternative way to go: the European experience commentary on: quality improvement guidelines for percutaneous management of acute limb ischaemia. Cardiovasc Intervent Radiol 2006; 29(1):7–10.
6. Ouriel K. Comparison of surgical and thrombolytic treatment of peripheral arterial disease. Rev Cardiovasc Med 2002; 3(Suppl. 2):S7–16.
7. Gabrielli L, Baudo A, Molinari A, Domanin M. Early complications in endovascular treatment of abdominal aortic aneurysm. Acta Chir Belg 2004; 104(5):519–26.
8. Castelli P, Caronno R, Piffaretti G, et al. Hybrid treatment for juxtarenal aortic occlusion: successful revascularisation using iliofemoral semiclosed endarterectomy and kissing stents technique. J Vasc Surg 2005; 42(3):449–63.
9. Nelson PR, Powell RJ, Schermerhorn ML, et al. Early results of external iliac artery stenting combined with common femoral artery endarterectomy. J Vasc Surg 2002; 35(6):1107–13
10. Henke PK, Williams DM, Upchurch GR, Jr., et al. Acute limb ischaemia associated with type B dissection: clinical relevance and therapy. Surgery 2006; 140(4):532–9.
11. Frahm C, Widmer MK, Brossman J, Do DD. Bilateral leg ischaemia due to descending aortic dissection: combined treatment with femoro-femoral cross over bypass and unilateral stenting. Cardiovasc Intervent Radiol 2002; 25(5):444–6.
12. Yamaguchi M, Sugimoto K, Tsuji Y, et al. Percutaneous balloon fenestration and stent placement for lower limb ischaemia complicated with type B aortic dissection. Radiat Med 2006; 24(3):233–7.
13. Vedantham S, Picus D, Sanchez LA, et al. Percutaneous management of ischaemic complications in patients with type-B aortic dissection. J Vasc Interv Radiol 2003; 14(2 Pt 1):181–94.
14. Kim JS, Choi D, Yoo KJ. Complete revascularization of total obstruction of both subclavian arteries and descending abdominal aorta by combined surgery and percutaneous transluminal angioplasty. J Invasive Cardiol 2004; 16(9):508–10.
15. Sternberg WC, III, Conners MS, III, Ojeda MA, Money SR. Acute bilateral iliac artery occlusion secondary to blunt trauma: successful endovascular treatment. J Vasc Surg 2003; 38(3):589–92.

16 | Current Status of Carotid Artery Stenting

A. Ross Naylor
Department of Vascular Surgery, Leicester Royal Infirmary, Leicester, U.K.

HISTORICAL PERSPECTIVE

Until 1950, it was generally assumed that most ischemic, carotid territory strokes followed in situ intracranial thrombosis, largely because the carotid arteries were used for embalming and never subjected to autopsy examination. The pioneering work of Miller Fisher subsequently showed the internal carotid artery (ICA) to be an important site for atherosclerosis and secondary thromboembolism into the brain (1). In 1954, Eastcott et al. were credited with having performed the first carotid endarterectomy (CEA; although it was actually a resection with primary reanastomosis) in a patient with repeated transient ischemic attacks (TIA) (2). However, the first CEA may have been performed by DeBakey one year earlier in 1953, although this was not reported until 1975 (3). Over the next 50 years, CEA became the most frequently performed vascular procedure in the Western world, but it would be fair to concede that it has remained one of the most controversial and scrutinized procedures of all time.

To understand why carotid surgery (and by implication, carotid angioplasty) has elicited such polarized opinions around the world requires a pragmatic review of the etiology of stroke (Table 1). For every 100 strokes destined to occur in the community, 80% will be ischemic and 20% hemorrhagic. For every 100 ischemic strokes, approximately 80% will involve the carotid territory and 20% will be vertebrobasilar. Thus, overall, approximately 60% of all strokes destined to occur will be "ischemic carotid territory." Within this subgroup, 50% will be secondary to "nonextracranial" pathology such as intracranial small vessel disease, cardio-embolism, hematological and "miscellaneous" causes (Table 1). This leaves a subgroup of 30 patients with thromboembolism from the extracranial ICA as the cause of stroke (i.e., approximately 30% of all strokes are secondary to thromboembolic, extracranial ICA disease). However, two-thirds will not be found to have significant ICA disease. Thus from the outset, practitioners of both CEA and carotid angioplasty and stenting (CAS) must accept that even if they could identify and treat every symptomatic and asymptomatic patient in their community (without any risk), they could only ever prevent about 10% of all strokes from occurring. This is clearly an impossible task and the true figure is probably 5%, i.e., 19 of 20 strokes will still occur despite the best efforts of surgeons and interventionists.

By the mid-1970s, the role of CEA had moved from treating symptomatic patients to recommending intervention in asymptomatic patients on the basis that they were a cohort of patients who were (otherwise) being denied prophylactic intervention. By the 1980s, concerns amongst neurologists and stroke physicians regarding the overall appropriateness of CEA became the catalyst for several multicenter randomized trials (4–8), most notably the European Carotid Surgery trial (ECST), the North American Symptomatic Carotid Endarterectomy trial (NASCET), the Asymptomatic Carotid Atherosclerosis study (ACAS) and the Asymptomatic Carotid Surgery Trial (ACST).

The principal results from these trials are summarized in Table 2. All showed significant benefit for CEA over "best medical therapy" (BMT), although the magnitude of benefit varied according to the degree of stenosis and whether the patient was symptomatic or asymptomatic. Most importantly, the two main symptomatic trials (ECST and NASCET) used different

TABLE 1 Etiology of the Next 100 Strokes in Your Community

Subgroup	*n*
Hemorrhage (ICH, SAH)	20
Ischemic vertebrobasilar	20
Ischemic carotid territory	60
Nonextracranial carotid etiology (n=30)	
Small vessel intracranial disease	15
Cardioembolic	9
Hematological	3
Miscellaneous	3
Extracranial carotid thromboembolism (n=30)	
Mild/moderate ICA stenosis	20
Severe ICA stenosis	10
Previous TIA	2
Previously asymptomatic	8

Abbreviations: ICA, internal carotid artery; ICH, intracranial hemorrhage; SAH, subarachnoid hemorrhage; TIA, transient ischemic attack.

methods for measuring stenosis. This explains the apparent discrepancy between the two trials and practitioners of CEA and CAS must be clear about what stenosis measurement method they are using when planning management.

In order to minimize confusion regarding the apparently "discordant" conclusions from NASCET and ECST, the Carotid Endarterectomy Trialists' Collaboration combined all of the data from ECST, NASCET and the Veterans Affairs (VA) study (9). This required a reanalysis of all of the prerandomization angiograms in 5092 patients using the NASCET method. The principal data from this overview are presented in Table 3 and provide the most extensive evidence base upon which outcomes for CAS and "modern" BMT should be compared.

Following publication of the randomized trials, surgeons probably anticipated an unparalleled increase in the numbers of CEAs worldwide. While this was initially true, the emergence of CAS meant that there was now an alternative. Angioplasty is an accepted treatment in the coronary and peripheral arterial circulations, but it has been slow to gain acceptance in the carotid artery, primarily because of the perceived risk of embolic stroke. A number

TABLE 2 Five-Year Risk of Stroke (Including Perioperative Stroke or Death)

Trial stenosis (%)	Surgical risk (%)	Medical risk (%)	ARR (%)	RRR (%)	NNT	Strokes prevented per 1000 CEAs
ECST						
<30	9.8 at 5 yr	3.9 at 5 yr	−5.9	n/b	n/b	n/b
30–49	10.2 at 5 yr	8.2 at 5 yr	−2.0	n/b	n/b	n/b
50–69	15.0 at 5 yr	12.1 at 5 yr	−2.9	n/b	n/b	n/b
70–99	10.5 at 5 yr	19.0 at 5 yr	+8.5	45	12	83 at 5 yr
NASCET						
30–49	14.9 at 5 yr	18.7 at 5 yr	+3.8	20	26	38 at 5 yr
50–69	15.7 at 3 yr	22.2 at 3 yr	+6.5	29	15	67 at 3 yr
70–99	8.9 at 3 yr	28.3 at 3 yr	+19.4	69	5	200 at 3 yr
ACAS						
60–99	5.1 at 5 yr	11.0 at 5 yr	+5.9	53	17	59 at 5 yr
ACST						
60–99	6.4 at 5 yr	11.8 at 5 yr	+5.4	46	19	53 at 5 yr

Abbreviations: ACAS, Asymptomatic Carotid Atherosclerosis Study; ACST, Asymptomatic Carotid Surgery Trial; ARR, absolute risk reduction; CEA, carotid endarterectomy; CVA/1000, number of strokes prevented at five years by performing 1000 CEAs; ECST, European Carotid Surgery Trial; NASCET, North American Symptomatic Carotid Endarterectomy Trial; NNT, number of CEAs to prevent one ipsilateral stroke at specified time interval; n/b, no benefit; RRR, relative risk reduction.

TABLE 3 Five-Year Risk of Stroke/Death: CETC Overview of European Carotid Surgery Trial, North American Symptomatic Carotid Endarterectomy Trial and Veterans Affairs Study

Stenosis	Surgery (%)	Medical (%)	ARR (%)	RRR	NNT	CVA/1000
Any stroke at five years (including operative stroke/death)						
<30%	18.36	15.71	−2.6	1.17	n/b	n/b
30–49%	22.80	25.45	2.6	0.90	38	26
50–69%	20.00	27.77	7.8	0.72	13	78
70–99%	17.13	32.71	15.6	0.52	6	156
Near occlusion	22.40	22.30	−0.1	0.98	n/b	n/b
Ipsilateral stroke at five-years (including operative stroke/death)						
<30%	12.05	9.78	−2.2	1.23	n/b	n/b
30–49%	14.78	18.06	3.2	0.82	31	32
50–69%	13.61	18.18	4.6	0.75	21	46
70–99%	10.36	26.24	15.9	0.39	6	159
Near occlusion	16.82	15.15	−1.7	1.11	n/b	n/b

Note: All angiograms reexamined and measured using the NASCET method.
Abbreviations: ARR, absolute risk reduction; CVA/1000, number of strokes prevented at five years by performing 1000 carotid endarterectomies; NNT, number of carotid endarterectomies to prevent one ipsilateral stroke at specified time interval; RRR, relative risk reduction; n/b, no benefit.
Source: Adapted from Ref. 9.

of small case series were, however, published during the 1980s, but were largely ignored by the surgical community. In 1992, Brown undertook a systematic review of the available data and observed that following 123 carotid angioplasties (utilizing neither stents nor protection devices), there were no deaths, no major strokes and only one minor stroke to give a 30-day death and/or stroke rate of <1% (10).

Despite these extremely good results following angioplasty alone (which, in retrospect, clearly reflected good case selection) the late 1990s saw an increasing trend toward recommending the insertion of a stent. The rationale being that it would reduce procedural thromboembolism, prevent recoil and give a better technical result. Following the introduction of routine stenting, the next major advances were (*i*) improved catheter technology (microcatheter systems, dedicated carotid stents), (*ii*) a recognition that dual antiplatelet therapy (usually aspirin and clopidogrel) was preferable to monotherapy, and (*iii*) the evolution of cerebral protection systems. The rationale underlying cerebral protection was that filter or balloon occlusion of the ICA (during the actual angioplasty) should prevent embolization and so reduce the procedural risk.

Over the last 10 years, there has been a proliferation of interest in CAS which has generated an enormous amount of conflicting literature. In order to inform the reader of its "current status," the results of CAS will be presented as four subgroups: (*i*) the randomized trials of CEA versus CAS (including the Cochrane systematic review), (*ii*) outcomes from worldwide registries and systematic reviews of published case series, (*iii*) results from commercially funded "high-risk" registries, and (*iv*) an overview of the results of CAS for treating recurrent stenosis after CEA.

THE RANDOMIZED TRIALS OF CAS VS. CEA

Background

Carotid angioplasty has been compared with CEA in a number of randomized trials around the world. To date, seven have either published interim results or have been suspended. Five were undertaken in symptomatic patients (11–15), one in an asymptomatic cohort (16), while another contained a mixture of symptomatic and asymptomatic patients (17). Two other trials [Carotid Revascularisation Endarterectomy vs. Stenting Trial (CREST) in North America and International Carotid Stenting Study in U.K./Europe] continue to randomize symptomatic patients (18–20). Of the 10 ongoing (or completed) studies, five were nationally funded multicenter trials (12,15,18–20), three were single center one funded by a national stroke charity (11) and two without external funding (14,16), while two were commercially funded (13,17). As will be seen, while each evolved with improving angioplasty technology and antiplatelet therapy, almost all have courted controversy! Three other studies (TACIT, ACST II and ACT I) are in the planning stage and aim to randomize asymptomatic patients who would otherwise be considered for CEA (21–23).

THE LEICESTER TRIAL

Methodology

The Leicester trial was funded by the U.K. Stroke Association and planned to recruit 300 patients with recent (<6 months) ipsilateral, carotid territory TIA/minor stroke and a severe (70–99%) stenosis (11). Diagnostic angiography was not performed prior to randomization. It was a condition of ethical approval that the independent Data Monitoring Committee (DMC) undertook interim analyses after every 20 patients were treated. In order to minimize the risk that repeated analyses might influence the overall level of significance, the group sequential statistical method was employed whereupon the DMC was instructed to invoke the "stopping rule" should any interim analysis yield a p-value of <0.0086. All patients were seen preoperatively and postoperatively by an independent neurologist.

Endpoints

Endpoints criteria were: (*i*) 30-day death/stroke, (*ii*) cumulative stroke at three years, (*iii*) restenosis, and (*iv*) impairment of cognitive function (dedicated psychologist employed for the trial). In this trial, the definition of procedural stroke included any new neurological deficit persisting for >24 hours.

Techniques

Following randomization, diagnostic angiography was performed immediately prior to CAS. Endarterectomy patients did not undergo angiography unless indicated. All patients received aspirin therapy (75 mg daily) throughout the periprocedural period. CAS was performed with systemic heparinization, predilatation as necessary and routine stenting (Wallstent™; Schneider, Minneapolis, U.S.A.). Cerebral protection devices (CPDs) were not available at that time. CAS was performed by an experienced radiologist who had performed a small series of uncomplicated CAS procedures prior to starting the trial. No proctoring was employed.

CEA was performed under normocarbic, normotensive general anesthesia, using systemic heparinization, routine shunting, routine polyester patching, intraoperative and postoperative transcranial Doppler monitoring and completion angioscopy.

Results

The DMC invoked the stopping rule after 23 patients had been randomized, during which time, 17 had received their allocated treatment. No deaths/strokes occurred in the 10 patients undergoing CEA. In the CAS group, five of seven patients suffered a stroke within 30 days (four during the procedure and one on day 8). Overall, three were disabling. The trial never restarted, largely because it was never possible to achieve equipoise for further randomization.

Comment

This was the first randomized trial to report and was undertaken in an era preceding protection devices and combination antiplatelet therapy. Although much criticized regarding its methodology, power and the experience of the radiologist (although his experience was greater than many in Brown's 1992 overview), it did send a "warning" to the stroke community that symptomatic patients who would otherwise undergo CEA (on the basis of ultrasound alone) required further imaging/evaluation before being selected for CAS.

CAROTID AND VERTEBRAL ARTERY TRANSLUMINAL ANGIOPLASTY STUDY

Methodology

The Carotid and Vertebral Artery Transluminal Angioplasty study (CAVATAS) was a multi-center, international randomized trial funded by the U.K. Medical Research Council with an independent DMC (12,24). Five hundred and four patients were randomized, 251 to CAS and 253 to CEA. All were assessed pre- and postoperatively by an independent neurologist. For inclusion, patients were meant to have symptoms within six months and a 50% to 99% stenosis. Stenosis was measured centrally in the Trial Office using the "common carotid technique," where the numerator was the residual luminal diameter within the stenosis and the denominator was the diameter of disease-free common carotid artery below the bifurcation.

Endpoints

Endpoints were: (*i*) 30-day death, (*ii*) 30-day death/disabling stroke, (*iii*) 30-day death/any stroke, (*iv*) restenosis, and (*v*) late ipsilateral stroke. In this study, the definition of procedural stroke was any new neurological deficit persisting for >7 days and not any new deficit for > 24 hours.

Techniques

Because this was a multicenter study, surgeons were allowed to use whatever operative/anesthetic techniques were standard in their institution. The majority of CAS procedures (78%) involved balloon dilatation alone. Fifty-five CAS procedures involved stenting (four as a rescue intervention after a procedural stroke). Primary stenting was not routinely available when the trial started in 1992. After 1994, stenting was performed at the discretion of the CAS practitioner utilizing the Wallstent, Streker™ stent (MediTech, U.S.A.) or Palmaz® stent (Johnson & Johnson, U.S.A.). All CAS and CEA practitioners were required to submit their experience with CEA and angioplasty prior to trial entry. "Centers with little skill in carotid angioplasty received training and assistance from a radiologist from a more experienced center." All CEA and CAS patients should have been on aspirin (150 mg) or another antiplatelet equivalent.

Results

Ninety percent of CAVATAS patients were symptomatic within six months of randomization, 7% had symptoms >6 months and 3% were later considered to be asymptomatic. Although the trial included some patients with vertebrobasilar symptoms, numbers were very small and they were excluded from analysis. The majority of patients had a >70% stenosis and the median delay from randomization to treatment was 20 days for CAS patients and 27 days for CEA.

Thirty-Day Procedural Risk

The principal, procedural risks are summarized in Table 4. There was no significant difference between CEA and CAS regarding early outcomes. CAS was successful in 224 (89%) patients. Of the 27 undergoing an initially unsuccessful CAS, four (15%) suffered a procedural stroke.

Six major events occurred between randomization and intended treatment and were censored from the 30-day outcomes, but not from long-term survival. One CEA patient died following complications after cardiac pacing. Three patients randomized to CAS died before receiving their treatment allocation [perforated duodenal ulcer (*n*=1), fatal stroke (*n*=2)]. One patient in each treatment limb suffered a nonfatal stroke and never received their allocated treatment.

Late Outcomes

The three-year rate of death/disabling stroke (in any vascular territory) was 14.3% in CAS patients and 14.2% after CEA (*p*=ns). A cohort of 347 patients underwent duplex imaging at one year with assessment of symptom status. The results are summarized in Table 5. The one-year rate of restenosis >70% was 18.5% after CAS and 5.2% following CEA (*p*=0.0001).

TABLE 4 Principal Endpoints in the Carotid and Vertebral Artery Transluminal Angioplasty Study

	CAS (*n*=251) (%)	CEA (*n*=253) (%)
30-day risks[a]		
Death	3	2
Death/disabling stroke	6.4	5.9
Death/any stroke	10.0	9.9[b]
Cranial nerve injury		8.7
"Significant" hematoma (groin/neck)	1.2	6.7
Long-term risks		
1-yr restenosis >70%	19	5
3-yr death/any stroke	14	14

[a] See text for censored events.
[b] This endpoint did not include strokes lasting >1 to <7 days.
Abbreviations: CAS, carotid angioplasty and stenting; CEA, carotid endarterectomy.

However, there was *no* association between recurrent stenosis and ipsilateral stroke. In a subanalysis of the CAS patients found to have a restenosis >70% at one year, it was observed that 38% had evidence of a residual severe stenosis at the one-month scan indicating that a poor anatomical result was present from the outset.

Comments

CAVATAS was criticized because of the high 30-day risk (CEA and CAS). However, as with the Leicester study, CAVATAS was undertaken in an era preceding newer technological advances and dual antiplatelet therapy. However, two issues do require comment. Notwithstanding the explanations of the Investigators regarding case mix, the procedural risk following both CEA and CAS was excessive. It should be noted that the 10% risk only included strokes lasting for >7 days. Inclusion of deficits lasting >24 hours to seven days would clearly increase the procedural risk even further. Evidence suggests that with a procedural risk of 10%, neither CAS nor CEA will confer any long-term benefit in symptomatic patients. Second, CAVATAS was the first randomized trial to demonstrate that (in the long-term) CAS was just as durable as CEA in terms of stroke prevention. The latter observation is probably the most important conclusion from this study.

THE WALLSTENT STUDY

Methodology

Multicenter randomized trial in 21 U.S. centers involving patients with recent (<120 days) carotid territory TIA/minor stroke and a 60% to 99% stenosis (13,25). Although commercially funded (Schneider U.S.A., Inc.), there was an independent DMC and Critical Events Committee who received data every three months from the trial sponsor. Power calculations were based on proving "equivalence" anticipating a 3% reduction in ipsilateral stroke at 12 months following CAS (5% vs. 8% after CEA). Seven hundred patients were to be recruited. All participants had to submit a track record of experience. Practitioners of CAS had to have done >10 cases of

TABLE 5 One-Year Restenosis and Risk of Ipsilateral Stroke (CAVATAS)

	Restenosis (%)	*n*	Ipsilateral stroke	
			Yes	**No**
CAS	<70	141	3 (2%)	138 (98%)
	>70	32	1 (3%)	31 (97%)
CEA	<70	165	5 (3%)	160 (97%)
	>70	9	0 (0%)	9 (100%)

Abbreviations: CAS, carotid angioplasty and stenting; CEA, carotid endarterectomy.
Source: From Ref. 24.

CAS with a 30-day death/stroke rate of <10%. Less experienced interventionists could be proctored. Surgeons had to have performed at least 30 CEAs within 24 months with a 30-day death/stroke rate of <6%.

Endpoints

Endpoints were: (*i*) 30-day death/stroke, (*ii*) 30-day death/ipsilateral stroke, (*iii*) one-year ipsilateral stroke/procedure-related death/vascular death, and (*iv*) restenosis (>60%).

Techniques

CAS was performed with predilatation and stenting (Wallstent). No protection devices were available. Surgeons could perform CEA using the technique standard in their center. All CAS patients received aspirin (325 mg bid and ticlopidine 250 mg bid) starting three days preprocedure and continued for four weeks. Thereafter the ticlopidine was stopped. All surgical patients received 325 mg aspirin bid (starting three days preoperatively) and continued thereafter. Ticlopidine could be added at the surgeon's discretion.

Results

The trial was suspended after 219 patients were enrolled (CAS 107, CEA 112). While this makes it the third largest randomized trial, the results have only been published as an abstract.

Thirty-Day Procedural Risk
The 30-day death/stroke rate was 12.1% following CAS versus 4.5% after CEA ($p=0.049$). No other surgical complications were listed, but severe bradycardia complicated 7% of CAS procedures and groin hematomas occurred in 4% of stent patients.

Late Outcomes
The one-year ipsilateral stroke/procedure-related death/vascular death rates were 12.1% (CAS) and 3.6% after CEA ($p=0.022$).

Comment

In concluding the abstract, it was noted that "this study did not find that CAS was equivalent to CEA in patients with symptomatic carotid artery stenosis. Based on these data and a futility analysis, the study was terminated before the planned maximum of 700 patients was enrolled." Notwithstanding possible commercial pressures and a negative outcome, this is one of the largest studies undertaken. It is extremely disappointing, therefore, that the results have only been published as an abstract. Interestingly, while the original WALLSTENT "study design" paper had eight authors, only one was listed on the results abstract!

LEXINGTON I

Methodology

This was a single-center randomized trial (based in a community hospital) in patients with recent (<3 months) carotid territory TIA/minor stroke and a 70% to 99% stenosis (14). The study was apparently powered to demonstrate equivalence between CAS and CEA, although no details were provided in the paper. All patients were assessed by a neurologist or research nurse. A commercial company provided the endovascular devices. There was no independent DMC and the trial neurologist was responsible for providing "independent oversight."

Endpoints

Endpoints were: (*i*) 30-day death, (*ii*) 30-day death/any stroke, (*iii*) cranial nerve injury, (*iv*) significant hematoma, (*v*) stroke at two years, and (*vi*) restenosis at two years.

Techniques

One hundred and four patients were randomized; 51 to CAS with stenting (Wallstent) and routine predilatation, but using no protection devices and 53 to CEA. All patients (CEA and CAS) received 325 mg aspirin and 75 mg clopidogrel throughout the perioperative period.

Results

Thirty-Day Procedural Risk
All patients were treated within 6 weeks of randomization. In the CAS group, there were no deaths or strokes. In the CEA group, one patient died following a myocardial infarction (MI), but there were no strokes. The 30-day death/stroke rate was 0.0% and 1.9% following CAS and CEA respectively. One CAS patient suffered acute limb ischemia following popliteal artery thrombosis and ultimately required a below-knee amputation, three (5.7%) developed significant groin hematomas and seven (13%) required temporary pacing. One surgical patient developed a significant neck hematoma requiring drainage and four (8%) suffered a cranial nerve injury.

Late Outcomes
At 24 months, no patient in this study had suffered a stroke or developed a significant restenosis in either limb of the trial. Magnetic resonance imaging was performed at 6 and 12 months and no patient was found to have an asymptomatic area of infarction.

Comment

This trial was underpowered from the outset. It is also unique in that (as with Lexington II) no patients suffered any stroke (or restenosis) either in the perioperative period or during the 24-month period of follow-up.

ENDARTERECTOMY VS. ANGIOPLASTY IN PATIENTS WITH SYMPTOMATIC SEVERE CAROTID STENOSIS

Methodology

This was a French national multicenter trial of patients with recent carotid territory TIA or minor stroke and a 70% to 99% carotid stenosis (15). It was supported by "national research organization" funding. To qualify, each CAS interventionist had to submit their track record of either 12 cases of CAS or 5 CAS+30 endovascular treatments of other supra-aortic vessels. Interventionists with less experience were proctored by experts from another center until considered "self-sufficient." All patients were assessed by an independent neurologist and there was an independent DMC.

Endpoints

The endpoints were: (*i*) 30-day risk of stroke/death, (*ii*) 30-day death/disabling stroke, and (*iii*) long-term risk of ipsilateral stroke.

Techniques

At the time of writing, no details regarding surgical techniques had been released. All patients randomized to CAS underwent stenting and received aspirin and either ticlopidine (250 mg bid) or clopidogrel (75 mg daily) for three days prior to treatment and for one month thereafter. The use of CPDs was optional at the start of the trial.

Results

The Endarterectomy versus Angioplasty in Patients with Symptomatic Severe Carotid Stenosis (EVA-3S) investigators issued a clinical alert in January 2003 after 80 patients had been randomized into the angioplasty limb of the study, primarily because of concerns about unprotected CAS. No data regarding surgical outcomes have been released.

Thirty-Day Procedural Risk

The mortality rate following CAS was 1.25% (death described as "sudden"). Overall, the 30-day risk of death/stroke was 15%, while the 30-day risk of death/disabling stroke was 5%. Four of 15 patients undergoing unprotected CAS (27%) either died or suffered a procedural stroke when compared with 6 of 58 (10%) undergoing CAS utilizing a protection device. A subsequent review of practice indicated that the adverse outcomes were scattered across numerous centers with no evidence of clustering. The DMC recommended resuming the trial with a recommendation that all CAS procedures should now be performed using a protection device.

Comment

EVA-3S aroused considerable debate, not least because it was never powered to make this recommendation (protected vs. unprotected CAS). In fact, the actual difference in risk when the trial was suspended was not statistically significant! Accordingly, this was not really a decision that the DMC had to make and did not conform with accepted stopping rules. Notwithstanding how the decision to restart the trial would affect the original power calculation, the release of the CAS outcomes (especially knowledge of the 15% risk) will inevitably have altered equipoise amongt the participating centers. More interesting, however, is the observation that if CPDs are so effective, why were they associated with a 10% stroke risk? EVA-3S did resume recruitment but was suspended (again) in October 2005.

Late Addendum

EVA-3S resumed recruitment after the initial alert was published but it was again suspended in October 2005 after 527 patients had been recruited. Limited information is, as yet, available but the decision to abandon the trial was taken because of the excess procedural stroke risk in CAS patients (9.5% vs. 3.8%). This was despite the obligatory use of protection devices in patients randomized to CAS.

LEXINGTON II

Methodology

Single-center randomized trial (based in a community hospital) of CEA versus CAS in neurologically asymptomatic patients with an 80% to 99% carotid stenosis (16). No data was forthcoming to indicate how a study of 85 patients could ever be reasonably powered. No external funding was received for this trial and all patients were assessed by an independent neurologist.

Endpoints

These were: (*i*) 30-day death, (*ii*) 30-day death/any stroke, (*iii*) cranial nerve injury, (*iv*) significant hematoma, (*v*) stroke at four years, and (*vi*) restenosis at four years.

Techniques

CEA was performed under general anesthesia with continuous electroencephalography monitoring. All patients randomized to CAS were stented following predilatation (Wallstent) but no protection devices were used. All CEA and CAS patients received 325 mg aspirin and 75 mg clopidogrel.

Results

Thirty-Day Procedural Risk

No perioperative strokes occurred in any patient in either limb of this study. Five CAS patients required treatment for profound bradycardia but (unlike Lexington I), none needed pacing.

No groin complications were reported after CAS. Three CEA patients suffered cranial nerve injuries.

Four-Year Outcomes

No patient in either limb of this study suffered a stroke or significant restenosis during four years of follow-up.

Comments

It is hard to understand how a randomized trial of 85 patients was accepted by the Ethics Committee as being appropriately powered. Lexington I and II remain the only randomized studies of CEA and CAS where no patient suffered any stroke or restenosis at any point during the perioperative period or during follow-up.

SPACE

Methodology

Multicenter randomized trial recruiting patients with a recently symptomatic (<180 days) ipsilateral 50% to 99% carotid stenosis from 35 centers in Germany, Austria and Switzerland (26). It was supported by funding from the Federal Ministry of Education and Research, the German Research Foundation, the German Society of Neurology, the German Society of Neuroradiology, the German Radiological Society together with commercial sponsorship from Boston Scientific, Guidant and Sanofi-Aventis. To participate, each surgeon and interventionist had to submit a track record of their preceding 25 cases. One-fourth of centers wishing to participate in the trial were, thereafter, prevented from randomizing patients following a review of their track record.

Unlike all the other randomized trials, SPACE aimed to demonstrate that CAS was "not inferior" to CEA. This is totally different from proving "superiority" or "equivalence." In this type of study, a predetermined margin of noninferiority is determined from the outset whose value will take into account (*i*) the power calculation, (*ii*) the likely magnitude of risk to be encountered, and (*iii*) an allowance for whether a slightly increased procedural risk following CAS might be offset by other important benefits (e.g., no incision, no cranial nerve injury, etc.). In SPACE, the predefined limit for "noninferiority" was that the upper confidence interval (CI) for the actual difference for the primary endpoint should be <2.5%. Power calculations had anticipated recruiting 1900 patients. All patients were reviewed by independent neurologists.

Endpoints

Endpoints were: (*i*) 30-day risk of death/ipsilateral stroke (primary endpoint), (*ii*) 30-day death/disabling stroke, (*iii*) 30-day death/any stroke, and (*iv*) procedural failure.

Techniques

Patients randomized to CAS received combination antiplatelet therapy for three days prior and 30 days after intervention (100 mg aspirin +75 mg clopidogrel). All CAS patients were stented (stents had to be CE marked) but the choice was left to the clinician as was the decision (type) of protection device and the need for predilatation. Patients randomized to surgery received 100 mg aspirin throughout the perioperative period. The choice of anesthesia and policy regarding shunting, patching, etc., were left to individual surgeons.

Results

Thirty-Day Procedural Risk

The mortality rate following CAS was 0.7% and 0.9% after CEA (p=ns). On an intention to treat basis, the primary endpoint was 6.84% following CAS as opposed to 6.34% for CEA (absolute difference 0.51%, 90% CI −1.89 to +2.91%). On a per protocol basis, the absolute difference was 1.32% (90% CI −1.1 to +3.76%). As the upper 90% CI exceeded 2.5%, noninferiority for CAS could not be proven. However, as the lower 90% CIs were below zero, the differences were not statistically significant. The 30-day death/*any* stroke rates were 7.68% following CAS when compared with 6.51% for CEA (p=ns).

SPACE also published three subgroup analyses. First, approximately 25% of CAS interventions involved the use of a protection device in whom the 30-day death/ipsilateral stroke rate was 7.3% when compared with 6.7% in those not using a CPD. Second, the primary endpoint was identical in each limb of the trial for patients aged <75 years. Patients aged >75 years incurred a higher procedural risk following CAS than after CEA (11.01% vs. 7.53%) but the difference was not statistically significant. Third, there was no apparent gender effect on outcomes following either procedure.

Long-Term Outcomes
None published to date.

Comment

SPACE suspended recruitment following its second interim analysis after only 1200 of the 1900 patients were randomized. The paper cites a number of methodological and logistical reasons for not continuing until the planned cohort had been recruited, but a lack of further funding was probably the most important consideration. Because this was a "noninferiority" trial, interpretation of the findings are almost unique for CEA versus CAS trials. As far as surgeons are concerned, SPACE showed that CAS was "not as good as" CEA. As far as the interventionists are concerned, there was no statistically significant difference! Perhaps the most significant observation from SPACE was that (as was also noted in EVA-3S), protection devices were no panacea against procedural stroke during CAS.

CREST

Methodology

This is an ongoing prospective, multicenter randomized trial comparing protected CAS with CEA in recently symptomatic patients (<180 days) with a 50% to 99% carotid stenosis (27–29). The trial is funded by the U.S. National Institute of Neurological Disorders and Stroke with additional funding by a device manufacturer (Guidant). Unlike any other trial comparing CEA with CAS, interventionists were first required to submit a track record of 10 to 30 cases of CAS. Successful applicants *then* entered a credentialing phase. Here the "potential" interventionist had to perform 20 CAS procedures [using the Acculink™ stent and the Accunet™ protection device (both from Guidant)] in patients who were either symptomatic (50–99% stenosis) or asymptomatic (70–99%). To date, only results from the credentialing phase have been published. All patients were assessed by a neurologist and there was an independent DMC.

Endpoints

Endpoints were: (*i*) stroke, MI, or death within 30 days and (*ii*) late ipsilateral stroke.

Techniques

No data on CEA technique have been published. Interventionists performed CAS using pre-dilatation (as necessary), routine stenting (Acculink) and cerebral protection (Accunet). All patients received aspirin (325 mg) and clopidogrel (75 mg) daily starting 48 hours pre-CAS and then for 30-days postprocedure.

Results

CREST has released results from the credentialing phase (i.e., prior to randomizing patients). One hundred thirty-four interventionists (cardiologists 40%, interventional neuroradiologists 23%, vascular Surgeons 16%, interventional radiologists 11%, neurosurgeons 7% and neurologists 3%) performed 862 CAS procedures in the "lead-in" phase. The two interim papers published outcomes on 749 patients with complete data. The 30-day death/stroke rate following CAS, performed by vascular/neurosurgeons was 5.3% when compared with 4.4% for other practitioners ($p=$ns). In view of emerging concerns about increased morbidity and mortality amongst elderly patients, CREST also analyzed outcomes relative to age. Using logistic regression, CREST observed that the worst 30-day death/stroke rates were found in the elderly patient (<60 years 1.7%, 60–69 years 1.3%, 70–79 years 5.3%, >80 years 12.1%, $p=0.00006$).

Comment

The interim CREST data suggest that the discipline of the interventionist does not significantly influence outcome. However, the excessively high procedural risk seen following CAS in patients aged >80 years has led to a recommendation from the CREST investigators that they be excluded from the credentialing phase but not randomization within the trial.

SAPPHIRE

Methodology

Multicenter (commercially funded) randomized trial of symptomatic patients with a 50% to 99% stenosis or an asymptomatic 80% to 99% stenosis and at least one factor that made them "high risk" (Table 6) (17). The study was powered to test the hypothesis that CAS was not inferior to CEA. All participants had to submit a "track record" of their previous surgical/ interventional results. Surgeons had to demonstrate outcomes within American Heart Association guidelines, while practitioners of CAS had to have a procedural death/stroke rate <6% (although no reference was made as to whether this was in symptomatic or asymptomatic patients). Patients randomized to surgery were not required to undergo diagnostic angiography. Cerebral angiography was performed routinely before stenting.

Patients were only randomized if the surgeon, interventionist and neurologist were in agreement that the patient was suitable for CEA and CAS. If the surgeon declined to operate, the patient was treated by CAS and followed up in a registry. The converse applied if the interventionist declined to undertake CAS. By 2002, the rate of recruitment had declined significantly (attributed to the publication of CAS outcomes from "high-risk" registries) and the trial was suspended.

Endpoints

Primary endpoints were: (*i*) 30-day death/stroke/MI and (*ii*) ipsilateral stroke between 31 days and 1 year. Secondary endpoints were (*i*) target vessel revascularization at one year, (*ii*) cranial nerve palsy, and (*iii*) complications at the surgical or vascular access site. Procedural stroke was defined as a new neurological deficit persisting for >24 hours. MI was defined as a creatinine kinase level higher than two times the upper limit of normal with a positive myocardial-bound fraction.

TABLE 6   Criteria for Entering SAPPHIRE

Symptoms	+50–99% carotid stenosis
Asymptomatic	+80–99% carotid stenosis
Plus at least one of the following:	
Clinically significant cardiac disease (congestive cardiac failure, abnormal stress test, open heart surgery required)	
"Severe" pulmonary disease	
Contralateral carotid occlusion	
Contralateral recurrent laryngeal nerve palsy	
Previous radical neck surgery or neck irradiation	
Recurrent stenosis after endarterectomy	
Age >80 yr	

Source: From Ref. 17.

Techniques

All patients received 80 to 325 mg aspirin for three days prior to treatment. CAS patients also received 75 mg clopidogrel 24 hours pre-CAS and then for two to four weeks thereafter. Surgeons were allowed to use whatever operative/anesthetic techniques were standard within their institution. Primary stenting was employed in all CAS patients (Smart/Precise™; Cordis, U.S.A.) and the same CPD was used routinely (Angioguard™/Angioguard XP™; Cordis, U.S.A.). The stents and devices were supplied by the sponsoring company.

Results

Seven hundred forty-seven patients were considered for randomization. Of these, only 334 (44%) were randomized within the trial (CAS 167, CEA 167). The remaining 413 patients were not randomized (preferential CAS 406, preferential surgery 7). Out of the randomized cohort of 334 patients, it is noteworthy that 71% were neurologically asymptomatic and 28% of the overall cohort had a recurrent stenosis after previous CEA.

Thirty-Day Procedural Risk

Mean hospital stay was 1.8 days for CAS and 2.8 days for CEA. There were no differences in surgical/access site bleeding complications and the prevalence of cranial nerve injury after CEA was 4.9%. The principal results have been presented in varying formats and they are summarized in Table 7. Some of the data were derived from presentations to national societies, having not been included in the main publication.

The overall 30-day death/stroke rate was 4.4% following CAS and 7.3% after CEA (p=ns). However, the majority of patients (71%) were asymptomatic in whom the 30-day death/stroke rate was 5.8% (CAS) and 6.1% following CEA (p=ns). One important outcome not referred to in the SAPPHIRE paper was whether any CAS patients were excluded after suffering an angiographic stroke.

In contrast to all other studies, SAPPHIRE developed a new composite endpoint (30-day death/stroke/MI). Overall, the 30-day risk of suffering a "major adverse cardiovascular event" was 4.8% after CAS and 9.8% following CEA (p=ns). Parallel data for symptomatic and asymptomatic subgroups are detailed in Table 7.

One-Year Outcomes

Readers are cautioned to clearly check which parameter is being reported. The cumulative one-year risk of ipsilateral stroke (including the 30-day stroke/death risk) was 5.5% following CAS and 8.4% after CEA (p=ns). However, the cumulative one-year risk of ipsilateral stroke

TABLE 7 Principal Results from SAPPHIRE

		CAS (%)	CEA (%)	*p*
30-day outcomes				
Death/any stroke	All	4.4	7.3[a]	
	Asymp	5.8	6.1[a]	
Death/MI/stroke	All	4.8	9.8	0.09
	Asymp	5.4	10.2	0.20
	Symp	2.1	9.3	0.18
1-yr outcomes				
Ipsilateral stroke/death (including 30-day stroke/death)	All	5.5	8.4	0.36
Ipsilateral stroke/death (including 30-day stroke/death/MI)	All	12.2	20.1	0.05
	Asymp	9.9	21.5	0.02
	Symp	16.8	16.5	0.95
Revascularization of treated artery		0.6	4.3	0.04

[a] Data not provided in principal paper (17) but reported at national and international symposia.
Abbreviations: CAS, carotid angioplasty and stenting; CEA, carotid endarterectomy; MI, myocardial infarction.

(now including the 30-day death/stroke and MI risk) was 12.2% following CAS and 20.1% after CEA ($p = 0.05$). Parallel data for asymptomatic and symptomatic patients are detailed in Table 7. Finally, CAS patients were less likely to undergo repeat revascularization at one year (0.6%) versus 4.3% in surgical patients.

Comment

If there was ever a trial to have evoked the most polarized interpretations and conclusions, SAPPHIRE is surely it! In the discussion section of the paper, the authors comment that "we studied patients for whom the risk posed by surgery was high." Awareness of this sentence is fundamental to interpreting this paper.

SAPPHIRE introduced two new concepts to traditional trial methodology. The first (the inclusion of MI in a composite endpoint) is, actually, not unreasonable despite the protestations of many surgeons. The available data from SAPPHIRE do suggest that perioperative MI is a predictor of a worse cardiovascular outcome in the long term. The second is the concept of only randomizing the "high-risk" patient. Though laudable in its aim, SAPPHIRE's conclusions have probably influenced practice in a manner that cannot be justified by critical examination of the data. Most clinicians now simply remember that CAS is not inferior to CEA and is, therefore, probably the optimal treatment for "high-risk" patients.

Notwithstanding the fact that almost 60% of the patients were not actually randomized in the trial, the key issue remains the definition of "high risk." Is this high risk for stroke or high risk for treatment? The trial investigators clearly meant the latter (see above), but many now assume that it also includes the former. This is, quite simply, untrue.

For example, contralateral occlusion is a proven predictor for a higher risk of stroke in symptomatic patients (medically treated and following CEA), but not in asymptomatic patients (30). In fact, ACAS showed that patients with contralateral occlusion may not benefit from CEA (31). Second, asymptomatic recurrent stenosis after CEA could never be claimed to be a high-risk predictor for late stroke, but it does increase the risk of stroke following redo CEA. Third, CEA confers no benefit in asymptomatic patients aged >75 years (7), but age >80 years was a specific criterion for increased risk. Fourth, asymptomatic patients made up the majority of patients in SAPPHIRE in whom the risk of stroke in ACAS and ACST was approximately 2% per annum (6,7) and not the 5% to 6% quoted in the methodology of the paper. A 5% to 6% annual stroke rate is more consistent with that observed in *symptomatic* patients with 50% to 70% NASCET stenoses (30). Fifth, there is compelling evidence from ACAS and ACST (Fig. 1) that asymptomatic women gain little benefit from prophylactic CEA (32), so how could they ever be considered a "high-risk" subgroup for inclusion in this trial? This is an important point as few clinicians currently consider gender differences when planning management.

Finally, the 30-day risk of death/stroke in asymptomatic patients in SAPPHIRE was 5.8% after CAS and 6.1% following CEA. No natural history study (and certainly neither ACST nor ACAS) has ever shown that *any* intervention with this level of risk will prevent stroke long term. Accordingly, an alternative conclusion from SAPPHIRE might be that where no intervention was necessary in the first place, CAS is probably safer than CEA!

In conclusion, the concept of "high risk" is indeed important, but it must refer (primarily) to the risk for *stroke*. High-risk inclusion criteria should, therefore, always include the word "symptomatic." Sadly, this was a missed opportunity to answer a really important question.

Summary of the Randomized Trials

The Cochrane Group have performed an overview of the published randomized trials. There were no differences in the 30-day rates of death/any stroke, death/disabling stroke or death/stroke/MI between CEA and CAS (33). The absence of significant benefit (relative to CEA or CAS) was also maintained at one year.

Notwithstanding the inevitable references to "historical" trials (i.e., Leicester, CAVATAS I and WALLSTENT), the three most important contemporary trials are EVA-3S, SPACE and SAPPHIRE. The French trial is important for three reasons. First, it reflects outcomes in the era of modern technology and dual antiplatelet therapy. Second, poor overall outcomes were,

Subgroup	Events/Patients Surgical	Medical	OR	95% CI
Males				
ACST	51 /1021	97 /1023	0.50	0.35–0.72
ACAS	18 /544	38 /547	0.46	0.26–0.81
Total	69 /1565	135 /1570	0.49	0.36–0.66
Females				
ACST	31 /539	34 /537	0.90	0.55–1.49
ACAS	15 /281	14 /287	1.10	0.52–1.82
Total	46 /820	48 /824	0.96	0.63–1.45

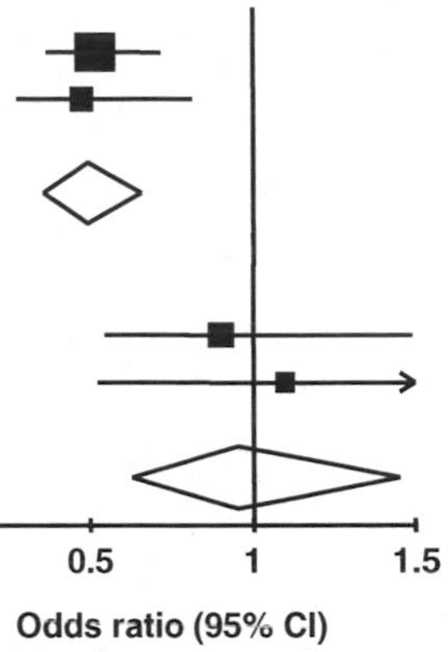

Odds ratio (95% CI) — 0   0.5   1   1.5

FIGURE 1 Reanalysis of data from Asymptomatic Carotid Atherosclerosis Study and Asymptomatic Carotid Surgery Trial (ACST) regarding the benefit of carotid endarterectomy (CEA) in asymptomatic males and females. This analysis now includes the operative risk which was originally not included in the ACST paper. Note that both trials showed that CEA conferred significant benefit in males. Neither trial showed that women (as a whole) gained benefit from prophylactic CEA. *Abbreviations*: CI, confidence interval; OR, odds ratio. *Source*: From Ref. 31.

once again, observed in symptomatic patients undergoing CAS. Third is the inevitable observation that if CPDs are so good, why was there a 10% stroke rate associated with their use in this study? This cannot be simply attributed to inadequacies in the French trial as similar results were observed in the SPACE trial (26).

However, SAPPHIRE is, without doubt, the most "influential" trial to have reported in the last five years. To many clinicians, this trial has shown that CAS is "not inferior" to CEA (although for many that has changed to being superior) and no further debate is required. The concept of seeing whether "high-risk" patients are better treated by CAS is very laudable but, to many, meaningful interpretation of the study was confounded by the inclusion of too many asymptomatic patients.

Finally, it is interesting to observe that in the seven published/abandoned trials, not one CAS patient seemed to have suffered a stroke following diagnostic angiography which was a prerequisite to proceeding to CAS. Did none of the manuscript reviewers question whether some patients underwent angiography, suffered a stroke and were then not randomized?

OVERVIEWS AND INTERNATIONAL REGISTRIES

The modern era of improved communications and electronic publishing has enabled systematic reviews of published case series and international registries to be undertaken with relative ease. Results from these can, therefore, quickly inform contemporary practice, but have the inevitable disadvantage of being "voluntary" with regard to the reporting of adverse events. Accordingly, they are never as reliable as outcome data from randomized trials.

In a recent systematic review of 60 case series involving >22,000 CAS procedures, the mean 30-day risk of stroke/death was 4.5% (34). Unfortunately, other than providing a "ballpark" figure regarding risk, this type of data does not really inform the reader, largely because the constituent studies are (inevitably) very heterogeneous with varying combinations of symptomatic and asymptomatic patients.

The Global Stent Registry has published outcomes from its voluntary (and predominantly retrospective) register since 1997 (Table 8). In the 2003 release (35), data following 12,392 CAS procedures were published and the principal results are summarized in Table 9. Approximately 50% of patients were symptomatic. Overall, CAS was technically successful in 98.9% of

TABLE 8 Summary of Outcomes from the World Stent Registry

	CPD	No CPD	All
30-day stroke plus procedural death [a]			
Overall	2.23% (*n*=4221)	5.29% (*n*=6753)	5.23% (*n*=12,392)
Symptomatic	2.70% (*n*=2111)	6.04% (*n*=4282)	4.94% (*n*=6392)
Asymptomatic	1.75% (*n*=2110)	3.97% (*n*=2471)	2.95% (*n*=4581)

[a] Note this is 30-day stroke plus *procedural* death (not all deaths). Not all the columns will add up as not all respondents filled in all of the CPD data.
Abbreviation: CPD, cerebral protection device.
Source: Adapted from Ref. 35.

cases with an overall 30-day stroke/procedural death of 5.2%. This definition of risk is, however, unusual in that it did not include "all deaths <30 days" as is otherwise conventional. Results from the Global Registry suggest that procedural risk after CAS diminishes with operator experience (50–20 cases 4.04%, 200–500 cases 2.85%, >500 cases 1.56%).

Data from the Global Stent Registry also suggest that for both symptomatic and asymptomatic patients, the procedural risk is less if a protection device is used (Table 9). However, this is by no means a universally accepted recommendation and the results of EVA-3S and SPACE suggest that protection devices are no panacea against procedural stroke.

Late follow-up data from the Global Registry is limited. Cumulative data are not available but the proportional risks of "restenosis >50%" are 2.7% at one year, 2.4% at three years and 5.6% at four years. These figures are considerably less than that noted previously in CAVATAS (24).

"HIGH-RISK" REGISTRIES

One of the reasons why SAPPHIRE closed recruitment was because a number of "high-risk" registries were reporting good results following CAS. Thereafter, these data have been quoted as confirming that CAS is the preferred option for treating "higher-risk" patients, when compared with historical outcomes following CEA.

All of these registries had inclusion criteria similar to SAPPHIRE, they were all commercially funded and none have been published in peer reviewed journals. Table 10 summarizes the principal results from ARCHeR, CHRS, SECURITY, BEACH, CABERNET, MAVERiC and CREATE, the data having been sourced from multiple Internet web pages. Most were designed to test a new stent or protection system provided by the sponsoring company.

As with SAPPHIRE, the reader should be cautious when interpreting these data. As can be seen, the majority were composed of asymptomatic patients and a significant proportion had recurrent stenoses after CEA. Two did not report 30-day death/stroke rates, while four had death/stroke rates >5% (three >6%). Only one documented a procedural risk <4%. All preferred to focus attention on the 30-day death/stroke/MI rates.

The principal conclusion from the "high-risk" registries has been that they support the preferential use of CAS. Unfortunately, closer inspection of the data does not support this. All of the criticisms leveled at SAPPHIRE apply again. Most of the patients may have been at higher risk from redo CEA, but there is little evidence that they faced a significantly higher risk of stroke than if left on "BMT."

CAS FOR TREATING RESTENOSIS AFTER CEA

Seventeen studies (36) have reported outcomes following CAS for the treatment of restenosis after CEA (Table 10). The 30-day risk of death/stroke varied considerably, but was generally lowest in publications which included the highest proportion of asymptomatic patients. Not surprisingly, there were no cranial nerve injuries which are accepted to be a problem with redo CEA. Table 10 also shows that secondary restenosis after CAS is relatively common, although few of the constituent studies undertook redo CAS unless the patients were symptomatic.

TABLE 9 Outcomes in "High-Risk" Carotid Stent Registries

	ARCHeR	CHRS	SECURITY	BEACH	CABERNET	MAVERiC	CREATE
n	437	161	305	480	454	498	419
Sponsor	Guidant	Boston	Abbott	Boston	Boston	Medtronic	ev3
Protection device	Accunet	FilterWire	Emboshield	FilterWire	FilterWire	PercuSurge	SPIDER
Criteria[a]	>80%A, >50%S	>80%A, >70%S	>50%S, >80%A	>50%S, >80%A	>60%A, >50%S		>50%S, >70%A
Restenosis after CEA	32%	41%	21%	41%			23%
Symptoms[b]	48%A, 52%S	75%A, 25%S	79%A, 21%S	76%A, 24%S	76%A, 24%S		83%A, 17%S
30-day death	2.3%	1.2%	1.0%	1.6%	0.5%	1.0%	1.0%
30-day stroke	5.3%	6.2%	6.9%	4.6%	3.4%	3.6%	5.5%
30-day death/stroke	6.6%	6.8%	6.9%	5.3%	3.6%		
30-day death/stroke/MI	7.8%	7.5%	3.5%	5.8%	3.8%	5.9%	6.2%

None of the studies have been reported in peer-reviewed journals. These data have been obtained from numerous Internet publications.
[a] Stenosis thresholds for including symptomatic (S) and asymptomatic (A) patients in the registry.
[b] Proportion of registry cohort who were asymptomatic (A) or symptomatic (S).
Abbreviations: CEA, carotid endarterectomy; MI, myocardial infarction.

TABLE 10 Outcomes for Carotid Angioplasty for Recurrent Stenosis after Carotid Endarterectomy

Study	n	30-day m+m (%)	% Asymp	Rec sten/mo FU
Miotto (38)	20	0.0		15% at 37 mo (>50%)
Alric (39)	17	0.0	76	0.0% at 17 mo (>50%)
Koebbe (40)	23	0.0		4.5% at 36 mo (>50%)
Hobson (41)	19	0.0	53	0.0% at 11 mo (>50%)
Lanzino (42)	25	0.0		16% at 27 mo (>50%)
Leger (43)	8	0.0	75	75% at 12 mo (>50%)
McDonnell (44)	30	0.0	80	10% at 20 mo (>90%)
Cohen (45)	10	0.0		
Hobson (46)	54	1.9	65	0.0% (>50%)
New (47)	342	3.7	61	6% at 14 mo (>50%)
Yadav (48)	25	4.0	23	0% at 8 mo (>50%)
Vitek (49)	110	4.0	40	No data
AbuRahma (50)	22	4.5	23	48% at 60 mo (>50%)
Bowser (51)	52	5.7	40	43% at 26 mo (>50%)
Rockman (52)	16	6.3	69	14% at 14 mo (>50%)
Bergeron (53)	15	13	7	0.0% at 37 mo (>50%)
AbuRahma (54)	25	16	28	56% at 42 mo (>50%)

Abbreviations: 30-day m+m, 30-day death/stroke risk; rec sten/mo FU, prevalence of recurrent stenosis at ψ months follow-up after angioplasty.
Source: From Ref. 36.

As with the preceding sections, interpretation of these data are difficult because of the inclusion of large numbers of patients with asymptomatic restenoses in whom the "natural history" risk of stroke is small. Most appeared to justify treatment on the basis of the ACAS and ACST findings (6,7), although restenoses were specifically excluded from these trials. The American Heart Association guidelines recommend that reintervention (which was redo CEA at the time of publication) was appropriate if the 30-day procedural risk was <10% (37). This threshold has been used to justify the treatment of restenoses worldwide, but it cannot be supported by contemporary natural history data unless the procedural risk is <4% in asymptomatic individuals.

WHAT IS THE CURRENT STATUS OF CAS?

Definite Conclusions

- Dual antiplatelet therapy improves outcomes after CAS.
- Dedicated "carotid" technology has improved outcomes after CAS.
- The 30-day death/stroke risk following CAS in randomized trials of symptomatic patients is generally poor, including two contemporary studies using CPDs.
- No randomized trial or registry has ever reported a diagnostic angiographic stroke in a CAS patient.
- Patients can undergo CEA on the basis of noninvasive imaging, unlike for CAS.
- CAS avoids cranial nerve injury, a condition which can (on occasions) be as debilitating as a stroke.
- Following successful CAS, long-term prevention of stroke is equivalent to CEA, i.e., it is durable.
- Meaningful interpretation of the outcomes following CAS is hampered by the use of "nonstandard" endpoints, e.g., 30-day procedural stroke/death rather than 30-day any stroke/death.
- Many of the randomized trials were beset with methodological problems (underpowered, $n=3$), never published ($n=1$), abandoned ($n=4$), inappropriate stopping rules ($n=1$), possible commercial obstruction to publication ($n=1$).
- CAS is associated with higher rates of restenosis but it does not seem to matter.
- The definition of "high risk" in all of the CAS trials (to date) has been inappropriate.
- The benefits of CEA (and thus by inference CAS) are not equal regarding gender.

■ Practitioners of CEA and CAS are very keen to adopt the positive findings from randomized trials, while disregarding other "unpalatable" data from the same studies (e.g., negative effect of gender, role of procedural risk on overall benefit).

Probable Conclusions

■ CEA wound and CAS access complications are probably comparable and of no long-term relevance.

■ With appropriate training and experience, the "medical discipline" of the interventionist performing CAS probably does not matter.

■ The 30-day risk following CAS is high in symptomatic patients aged >80 years and caution should be exercised.

■ As with the randomized trials of CEA, there is currently no association between recurrent stenosis after CAS and late ipsilateral stroke.

■ CAS is probably safer than redo CEA for treating recurrent stenosis after CEA and abolishes the risk of cranial nerve injury.

Unproven Conclusions

■ Protection devices will make CAS safer in the long term.

■ CAS is safer in "high-risk" patients. To be considered "high risk," patients must (at least) be symptomatic and should preferably (*i*) be male, (*ii*) have recent onset symptoms, (*iii*) have a contralateral occlusion, (*iv*) have plaque irregularity, and (*v*) have a 70% to 99% stenosis.

■ CAS is generalizable. To date, all of the CAS randomized trials and registries have been undertaken in highly specialized centers. In NASCET, only 0.5% of patients undergoing CEA in 1989 were randomized within the study (30). This led to questions about how generalizable the results were for "all surgeons." Community-based studies have confirmed that the results may not be generalizable. The same problem will inevitably apply to CAS practitioners.

■ How do we get round the problem of the "learning curve" when expanding the role of CAS?

■ Restenosis rates following CAS will improve with drug-eluting stents.

■ The modern concept of "BMT" now renders the results of ACAS and ACST obsolete regarding the future role for CEA and CAS in asymptomatic patients?

REFERENCES

1. Fisher M. Occlusion of the internal carotid artery. Arch Neurol Psychiatry 1951; 65:346–77.
2. Eastcott HH, Pickering GW, Robb CG. Reconstruction of internal carotid artery in a patient with intermittent attacks of hemiplegia. Lancet 1954; 267:994–6.
3. DeBakey ME. Successful carotid endarterectomy for cerebrovascular insufficiency: nineteen year follow-up. JAMA 1975; (233):1083–5.
4. European Carotid Surgery Trialists' Collaborative Group. Randomised trial of endarterectomy for recently symptomatic carotid stenosis: final results of the MRC European Carotid Surgery Trial (ECST). Lancet 1998; 351:1379–87.
5. Barnett HJM, Taylor DW, Eliasziw M, et al. Benefit of carotid endarterectomy in patients with symptomatic moderate or severe stenosis. N Engl J Med 1998; 339:1415–25.
6. Executive Committee for the Asymptomatic Carotid Atherosclerosis Study. Endarterectomy for asymptomatic carotid artery stenosis. JAMA 1995; 273:1421–8.
7. Asymptomatic Carotid Surgery Trial Collaborators. The MRC Asymptomatic Carotid Surgery Trial (ACST): carotid endarterectomy prevents disabling and fatal carotid territory strokes. Lancet 2004; 363:1491–502.
8. Mayberg MR, Wilson E, Yatsu F, et al. Carotid endarterectomy and prevention of ischaemia in symptomatic carotid stenosis. JAMA 1991; 266:3289–94.
9. Rothwell PM, Eliasziw M, Gutnikov SA, et al. Analysis of pooled data from the randomised controlled trials of endarterectomy for symptomatic carotid stenosis. Lancet 2003; 361:107–16.
10. Brown MM. Balloon angioplasty for cerebrovascular disease. Neurol Res 1992; 14:159–63.
11. Naylor AR, Bolia A, Abbott RJ, et al. Randomized study of carotid angioplasty and stenting versus carotid endarterectomy: a stopped trial. J Vasc Surg 1998; 28(2):326–34.

12. CAVATAS Investigators. Endovascular versus surgical treatment in patients with carotid stenosis in the Carotid and Vertebral Artery Transluminal Angioplasty Study (CAVITAS): a randomised trial. Lancet 2001; 357:1729–37.
13. Alberts MJ, WALLSTENT. Results of a multicenter prospective randomized trial of carotid artery stenting versus carotid endarterectomy. Stroke 2001; 32:325 (Abstract).
14. Brooks WM, McClure RR, Jones MR, Coleman TC, Breathitt L. Carotid angioplasty and stenting versus carotid endarterectomy: randomized trial in a community hospital. J Am Coll Cardiol 2001; 38:1589–95.
15. EVA-3S Investigators. Carotid angioplasty and stenting with and without cerebral protection: clinical alert from the endarterectomy versus angioplasty in patients with symptomatic severe carotid stenosis. Stroke 2004; 35:e18–20.
16. Brooks WH, McClure RR, Jones MR, Coleman TL, Breathitt L. Carotid angioplasty and stenting versus carotid endarterectomy for treatment of asymptomatic carotid stenosis: a randomised trial in a community hospital. Neurosurgery 2004; 54:318–24.
17. Yadav JS, Wholey MH, Kuntz RE, et al. Protected carotid artery stenting versus endarterectomy in high-risk patients. N Engl J Med 2004; 351:1493–501.
18. Hobson RW, Howard VJ, Roubin GS, et al. Credentialing of surgeons as interventionalists for carotid artery stenting: experience from the lead-in phase of CREST. J Vasc Surg 2004; 40:952–7.
19. Ringleb PA, Kunze A, Allenberg JR, et al. The Stent-Supported Percutaneous Angioplasty of the Carotid Artery vs. Endarterectomy Trial. Cerebrovasc Dis 2004; 18:66–8.
20. Featherstone RL, Brown MM, Coward LJ, for the Investigators. International carotid stenting study: protocol for a randomised clinical trial comparing carotid stenting with endarterectomy in symptomatic carotid artery stenosis. Cerebrovasc Dis 2004; 18:69–74.
21. Gaines PA, Randall MS. Carotid artery stenting for patients with asymptomatic carotid disease (and news on TACIT). Eur J Vasc Endovasc Surg 2005; 30:461–3.
22. http://www.ptca.org/pr_abbott/20050118.html
23. Halliday A, Marro J. Rationale for a randomised trial (surgery versus stenting) in asymptomatic carotid stenosis: ACST II. In: Becquemin J-P, Alimi YS, Watelet J, eds. Controversies and Updates in Vascular Surgery. Torino: Minerva Medica, 2005:277–84.
24. McCabe DJH, Pereira AC, Clifton A, Bland JM, Brown MM, for the CAVATAS Investigators. Restenosis after carotid angioplasty or endarterectomy in the CAVATAS Study. Stroke 2005; 36:281–6.
25. Alberts MJ, McCann R, Smith TP, et al. A randomized trial of carotid stenting vs. endarterectomy in patients with symptomatic carotid stenosis: study design. J Neurovasc Dis 1997; 2:228–34.
26. SPACE Collaborators. Stent protected angioplasty versus carotid endarterectomy in symptomatic patients: 30 days results from the SPACE trial. Lancet 2006; 368:1239–47.
27. Hobson RW, Howard VJ, Brott TG, et al. Organizing the Carotid Revascularization Endarterectomy versus Stenting Trial (CREST): national institutes of health, health care financing administration, and industry funding. Curr Cont Trials Cardiovasc Med 2001; 2:160–4.
28. Hobson RW, Howard VJ, Roubin GS, et al. Credentialing of surgeons as interventionalists for carotid artery stenting: experience from the lead-in phase of CREST. J Vasc Surg 2004; 40:952–7.
29. Hobson RW, Howard VJ, Roubin GS, et al. Carotid artery stenting is associated with increased complications in octogenarians: 30-day stroke and death rates in the CREST lead-in phase. J Vasc Surg 2004; 40:1106–11.
30. Naylor AR, Rothwell PM, Bell PRF. Overview of the principal results and secondary analyses from the European and the North American randomised trials of carotid endarterectomy. Eur J Vasc Endovasc Surg 2003; 26:115–29.
31. Baker WH, Howard VJ, Howard G, Toole JF, for the ACAS Investigators. Effect of contralateral occlusion on long-term efficacy of endarterectomy in the Asymptomatic Carotid Atherosclerosis Study (ACAS). Stroke 2000; 31:2330–4.
32. Rothwell PM. ACST: which subgroups will benefit most from carotid endarterectomy? Lancet 2004; 364:1122–3.
33. Coward LJ, Featherstone RL, Brown MM. Safety and efficacy of endovascular treatment of carotid artery stenosis compared with carotid endarterectomy: a Cochrane Systematic Review of the randomised evidence. Stroke 2005; 36:905–11.
34. Sullivan TM. Current indications, results and technique of carotid angioplasty/stenting. Sem Vasc Surg 2005; 18:87–94.
35. Wholey MH, Al-Mubarek N, Wholey MH. Global experience in cervical carotid artery stent placement. Catheter Cardiovasc Interv 2003; 60:259–66.
36. Naylor AR, Chng S, Awad S. Intervention for recurrent carotid stenosis: the role of carotid angioplasty and stenting. Endovascular Therapies: Current Evidence. Shrewsbury, U.K.: TFM Publishing 2006:123–31.
37. Biller J, Feinberg WM, Castaldo JE, et al. Guidelines for carotid endarterectomy: a statement for healthcare professionals from a special writing group of the Stroke Council. American Heart Association. Stroke 1998; 29:554–62.

38. Miotto D, Picchi G, Rettore C. Endovascular treatment for recurrent carotid stenosis. Radiol Med 2001; 101(5):355–9.
39. Alric P, Branchereau P, Berthet JP, Mary H, Marty-Ane C. Carotid artery stenting for stenosis following revascularization or cervical irradiation. J Endovasc Ther 2002; 9(1):14–9.
40. Koebbe CJ, Liebman K, Veznedaroglu E, Rosenwasser R. The role of carotid angioplasty and stenting in carotid revascularization. Neurol Res 2005; 27(Suppl. 1):S53–8.
41. Hobson RW, Goldstein JE, Jamil Z, et al. Carotid restenosis: operative and endovascular management. J Vasc Surg 1999; 29(2):228–35.
42. Lanzino G, Mericle RA, Lopes DK. Percutaneous transluminal angioplasty and stent placement for recurrent carotid artery stenosis. J Neurosurg 1999; 90(4):688–94.
43. Leger AR, Neale M, Harris JP. Poor durability of carotid angioplasty and stenting for treatment of recurrent artery stenosis after carotid endarterectomy: an institutional experience. J Vasc Surg 2001; 33(5):1008–14.
44. McDonnell CO, Legge D, Twomey E, et al. Carotid artery angioplasty for restenosis following endarterectomy. Eur J Vasc Endovasc Surg 2004; 27(2):163–6.
45. Cohen JE, Gomori JM, Ratz G, Ben Hur T, Umansky F. Protected stent-assisted carotid angioplasty in the management of late post-endarterectomy restenosis. Neurol Res 2005; 27(Suppl. 1):S64–8.
46. Hobson RW, Lal BK, Chakhtoura EY, et al. Carotid artery closure for endarterectomy does not influence results of angioplasty-stenting for restenosis. J Vasc Surg 2002; 35(3):435–8.
47. New G, Roubin GS, Iyer SS. Safety, efficacy, and durability of carotid artery stenting for restenosis following carotid endarterectomy: a multicenter study. J Endovasc Ther 2000; 7(5):345–52.
48. Yadav JS, Roubin GS, King P, Iyer S, Vitek J. Angioplasty and stenting for restenosis after carotid endarterectomy. Initial experience. Stroke 1996; 27(11):2075–9.
49. Vitek JJ, Roubin GS, New G, Al-Mubarek N, Iyer SS. Carotid angioplasty with stenting in post-carotid endarterectomy restenosis. J Invasive Cardiol 2001; 13(2):123–5.
50. AbuRahma AF, Bates MC, Wulu JT, Stone PA. Early postsurgical carotid restenosis: redo surgery versus angioplasty/stenting. J Endovasc Ther 2002; 9(5):566–72.
51. Bowser AN, Bandyk DF, Evans A. Outcome of carotid stent-assisted angioplasty versus open surgical repair of recurrent carotid stenosis. J Vasc Surg 2003; 38(3):432–8.
52. Rockman CB, Bajakian D, Jacobowitz GR, et al. Impact of carotid artery angioplasty and stenting on management of recurrent carotid artery stenosis. Ann Vasc Surg 2004; 18(2):151–7.
53. Bergeron P, Chambran P, Benichou H, Alessandri C. Recurrent carotid disease: will stents be an alternative to surgery? J Endovasc Surg 1996; 3(1):76–9.
54. AbuRahma AF, Bates MC, Stone PA, Wulu JT. Comparative study of operative treatment and percutaneous transluminal angioplasty/stenting for recurrent carotid disease. J Vasc Surg 2001; 34(5):831–8.

17 | Techniques of Carotid Percutaneous Transluminal Angioplasty and Stenting

Trevor J. Cleveland
Sheffield Vascular Institute, Sheffield Teaching Hospitals NHSFT, Northern General Hospital, Sheffield, U.K.

INTRODUCTION

The concept of treating diseases of the carotid bifurcation using endovascular means is not new, but has lagged behind endovascular treatments in other body segments as a result of the fear of cerebral embolization. Considering the nature of atheroma at the carotid bifurcation, and the exquisite sensitivity of the brain to embolic insult, this is perhaps not surprising. However, to the surprise of many clinicians, carotid angioplasty and stenting have been shown to have an acceptable safety profile in many situations (see chap. 17) (1–8). In addition an improved understanding of patient selection and technological advances has made the performance of the procedure more controlled and probably safer for the patient (8–14). This chapter is designed to describe the procedural details and techniques that can be employed to minimize the chances of complications. Chapter 18 addresses the issue of managing these complications, should they occur, and they will do so despite attention to detail. However, the frequency of such problems can be kept to a minimum by technical skill and experience.

HISTORICAL PERSPECTIVES

As noted above, treating carotid bifurcation atheromatous disease by endovascular means has developed some years behind similar treatments in other regions of the body. This was unsurprising for two reasons. Firstly, disease at the carotid bifurcation rarely causes cerebral compromise as a result of blood flow limitation. Treatment is therefore directed toward the effective removal of an embologenic focus at the carotid bifurcation. The prospect of preventing embolic stroke as a result of angioplasty was less apparent than the removal of the embologenic material at endarterectomy. Secondly it is well established that balloon angioplasty may cause pieces of the plaque material to become dislodged, and in the context of carotid disease embolize to the brain and cause a stroke (15,16). In addition, balloon angioplasty alone, may have a suboptimal primary result in terms of reestablishing a satisfactory lumen. This may be due to resistance to angioplasty, or recoil. Similarly dissection flaps that are an inevitable result (to a greater or lesser extent) of percutaneous transluminal angioplasty (PTA) may cause flow limitation and subsequent thrombosis.

Despite such concerns, balloon angioplasty was applied to the carotid bifurcation, usually because the alternative options were limited by comorbidity, and found to have results comparable with carotid endarterectomy (CEA) (1–8). The procedure utilized during the early experiences with PTA was very different to the techniques used in modern day practice, and the data generated at that time should be interpreted with that knowledge (3). In order that the carotid stenosis could be approached, bilateral femoral punctures were performed and a 5-F sheath placed in one groin, and a 7-F sheath in the other. Using the 7-F access, the common carotid artery (CCA) was selectively catheterized, using a shaped catheter of the operators' choice. Controlled catheterization was achieved and the internal carotid stenosis was traversed with a 0.035-in. guidewire (260 cm long) under roadmap control. Once the roadmap was established, this was used for the remainder of the PTA procedure. If the patient moved, considerable difficulties were encountered, ultimately requiring use of the contralateral access site to perform further selective catheterization (with its attendant potential risks) to produce an updated roadmap. With a 0.035-in. wire in place, a 5-F shaft balloon catheter was positioned (the diameter having been determined by prior measurement) and balloon dilatation performed. Typical balloon inflation times were 15–20 seconds. Once PTA had been performed, the 5-F access site was used to selectively catheterize the CCA, and check angiography performed. If a satisfactory result was judged to have occurred, the 0.035-in. wire was removed and the procedure completed. If, however, the PTA result was considered to be poor, there were no dedicated stents available for the carotid bifurcation. The stents utilized in those circumstances were the balloon-expandable Palmaz™ or Palmaz-Shatz™ (Cordis, A Johnson and Johnson Company, Miami Lakes, Florida, U.S.A.) stents designed for the coronary circulation. If these were considered to be necessary, they were applied to the appropriate diameter balloon, and introduced through the 7-F sheath, over the 260-cm wire. The stent was advanced, without following it on the image intensifier (as this would result in loss of the roadmap), up to the carotid bifurcation, and placed at the stenosis.

Despite the obvious limitations in this technique, which appears crude in the modern era, the results of this technique were satisfactory (3), and provide the basis for the present technique.

ACCESS TO THE CAROTID TERRITORY

As a result of the technical limitations of PTA, and the perceived benefits of stenting (a better primary lumen result, less embolization, less problem with dissection and less restenosis) modern thinking is that the correct approach to endovascular carotid treatment is to place a dedicated carotid stent. To achieve this safely it may be necessary to predilate the lesion, prior to stent placement, but the primary intention, in the vast majority of cases, is to treat the lesion with a stent.

Modern carotid artery stenting (CAS) uses guiding catheters or long (80–100 cm) sheaths to act as a platform from which the procedure can take place. Assuming that appropriate imaging has been undertaken before an attempt at CAS, the operator should be familiar with the anatomy of the lesion and the vessels proximal and distal to it. It is imperative to the success of the remaining procedure that a safe and stable sheath/guiding catheter position is obtained in the CCA, and that this access is of an appropriate size. The entire standard dedicated CAS devices will pass through a 6-F sheath or an 8-F guiding catheter.

The majority of CAS procedures are performed from a femoral artery approach, as this is a large, superficially placed artery, and the pathway to the carotid territory is relatively straight. This considerably aids the technique.

The CCA on the side of the lesion to be treated is selectively catheterized, using a shaped catheter of the operators' choice. The precise shape will depend on individual preference, and upon the results of preprocedural imaging. In general it is advisable to use as simple a curve as the anatomy will allow, as this will make the remainder of the sheath positioning easier. Most cases can be performed with a simple 5-F Headhunter™ or Berenstein™ catheter, but occasionally more complex shapes, such as a Sidewinder™/Simmons™ may be needed.

Once selective catheterization has been achieved, precise images of the target lesion can be obtained, and a final plan formulated for treatment. In addition, the required measurements can be made (see below). The approach to the next stage may be altered by these images. If the external carotid artery (ECA) is patent, and the CCA not significantly diseased, then the ECA may be used for placement of a stiff 0.035-in. wire. If not, the intention is not to cross significant disease with the 0.035-in. devices.

If the ECA is available, the selective catheter is advanced (over a suitable wire) to allow the passage of a supportive 0.035-in. wire, which is placed in the ECA, under roadmap control. The supportive wire needs to be long enough to allow the diagnostic catheter to be removed and the selected sheath/guiding catheter replaced. This usually requires a 260-cm wire, as the selective catheters are usually 100 cm long, and the sheaths 80 to 100 cm long.

If the ECA or cranial CCA is diseased then the ECA cannot be used for anchoring the 0.035-in. wire; therefore the exchange for the sheath/guiding catheter needs to be performed caudal to the lesion (Fig. 1). This can be achieved by the use of a supportive wire with a short (1 cm) floppy tip. The diagnostic catheter is used to generate a roadmap, and the short tip wire advanced close to, but not across, the lesion in the CCA. The diagnostic catheter may then be

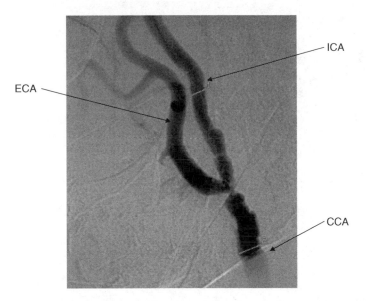

FIGURE 1 Significant disease is seen in the common and internal carotid arteries. This is particularly stenotic in the CCA, which should only be crossed once a stable proximal CCA position has been obtained. *Abbreviations*: CCA, common carotid artery; ECA, external carotid artery; ICA, internal carotid artery.

removed, and the sheath advanced to an appropriate site in the CCA. Alternatively, some sheaths are supplied with a central shaped catheter that acts as both the selective catheter and the stylet. Such a system may be used without the need to access the ECA.

Once an appropriately sized sheath or guiding catheter has been placed in the CCA, the 0.035-in. wire may be removed, and the platform for CAS achieved. Some operators, who prefer to use a guiding catheter, utilize a shaped guiding catheter, and use this alone to selectively catheterize the CCA. This technique, while clearly technically possible, runs the risk of the relatively large catheter dislodging any plaque material that may be in the aortic arch, or origin of the great vessel branches. This maneuver is contraindicated where there is any arch disease (see below).

In most cases a straight sheath or guiding catheter is appropriate, and has the benefit of simplicity. However, occasionally, tortuosity of the CCA results in the catheter tip lying up against the wall of the CCA, and this makes the remainder of the procedure difficult, and increases the risk of CCA dissection (Fig. 2). In such circumstances a curved sheath, such as a Multi-purpose A1 (MP-A1; Cordis) shape, may be helpful, and cause less distortion of the CCA.

The choice of sheath or guiding catheter is operator dependent. Each type of device has advantages and disadvantages, and personal experience/training will be relevant. Irrespective of personal preference, there are a number of features that need to be taken into account.

- Long (usually 80–100 cm) sheaths usually have a central stylet, which provides a smooth transition from the 0.035-in. wire to the 6-F sheath. As a result, if there is any atheromatous disease in the aortic arch, or proximal great vessel, then it is less likely to be disturbed by the positioning of the sheath. Indeed, to aid this positioning, shaped stylets can be used to facilitate this maneuver. Conversely, guiding catheters do not have dedicated stylets. As a result, at the origin of the arch vessel branch, when these track on the 0.035-in. wire their tip becomes deformed into an oval shape. A segment of this may then disturb disease in this region. Similarly as the guiding catheter is advanced in the CCA, the risk of CCA trauma and dissection is increased.
- A limited range of shaped sheaths is available, and these are usually simple shapes (such as the MP-A1 noted above). On the other hand guiding catheters are manufactured in a wide range of simple and complex curves. These shapes may enable selective catheterization

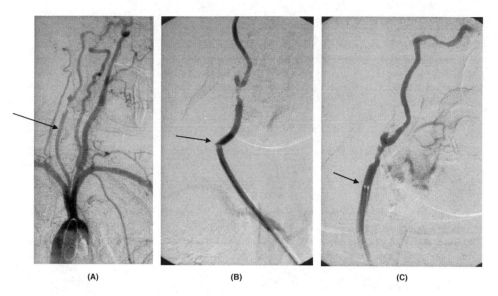

FIGURE 2 (**A**) Arch aortogram showing curvature of the index right CCA (*arrow*). (**B**) Tortuous CCA with straight Introducer Guide™ (Cordis, Miami Lakes, Florida, U.S.A.) tip pushing against the artery wall (*arrow*). (**C**) Same patient with a multi-purpose A1 Introducer Guide tip (*arrow*) in a much more satisfactory position.

of more complex curves at the aortic arch, and render previously unreachable lesions amenable to CAS. In addition, guiding catheters are designed to provide a stable platform in curved circumstances, and are generally sufficiently supportive to accommodate the CAS devices.

■ The devices that are manufactured for the external ends of sheaths and guiding catheters are different. Sheaths are usually manufactured with a hemostatic valve, which allows devices to be introduced over the wire that is in the sheath. They are simple to use, but may not be completely effective at preventing reflux of blood, particularly when 0.014-in. wire systems are in place. In addition there is a perception that if catheters are removed rapidly from such a closed system, then there is a risk that air may be introduced into the sheath. As it is routine practice to maintain a pressured flush through the sheath, this air may be pushed into the cerebral circulation. Therefore rapid catheter removal should be avoided. Guiding catheters have a Luer lock at their external end, to which can be attached either a rotating hemostatic valve (often packaged with the catheter) or a hemostatic valve. The rotating valve is more controllable by the operator, however, the sidearm design, along with the potential leakage when the valve is loose, makes it very difficult to ensure that flushing is fully effective.

In some circumstances approach to the carotid bifurcation from the femoral artery is not possible (e.g., aortoiliac occlusive disease or groin infections) and a brachial approach has been used for CAS. While it is possible to perform the procedure in this manner, the shape of the catheter route is much less advantageous than from the groin. This makes placement of the sheath difficult. This is particularly so if the ECA is not patent, and thus cannot be used for wire anchoring. In addition the caliber of the brachial artery is smaller than the femoral artery, and an unlicensed place for closure devices. It is, therefore, not recommended to attempt such cases except in unusual clinical circumstances, or once considerable experience has been obtained.

MEASUREMENTS

It is clearly important to ensure that the devices used for a particular patient are the appropriate size for that person. The dimensions that need to be measured are:

- Internal carotid artery (ICA) diameter
- CCA diameter
- Lesion length

These need to be known so that the protection device fits the ICA, the stent diameter is appropriate for both the ICA and CCA (assuming that most stents are placed from ICA to CCA), and that the stent will be long enough to cover the lesion as desired.

There are a number of methods that can be used to measure each of these dimensions, and if more than one can be used, then self-quality assurance can aid confidence in the values obtained.

- *Ultrasound*: Most patients with carotid artery disease will undergo duplex scanning to assess the bifurcation. These images can be used to measure the CCA with reliability. Unfortunately the section of ICA where protection filters or balloons may be placed is not usually visualized on ultrasound. However, a reliable CCA measurement can be very useful to confirm the calibration of angiography.
- *Magnetic resonance angiography (MRA)*: If MRA is used the axial images may be used to measure the ICA and the CCA. Sometimes, due to movement at the carotid bifurcation or low gradient power, the measurements may be difficult, but most times a reasonable measurement can be obtained. The lesion length may be obtained from reconstructed images.
- *Computed tomography angiography*: Like MRA, source computed tomography images and reconstructed images allow for accurate measurements.
- *Angiography*: The carotid bifurcation may be assessed by arch aortography or selective imaging. If arch aortography is used, then calibration is difficult, unless a rotational technique is used. If a rotational angiogram is obtained, and the patient placed in the isocenter, then back calibration can be performed, and measurements made. Unfortunately this technique has drawbacks, most notably that to obtain a rotational angiogram requires a large contrast bolus, which can flood the coronary circulation with contrast, which causes ischemia, and may result in dysrhythmias (17). When selective angiography is performed, usually during the CAS procedure, calibration is necessary. Some authors recommend the use of the sheath in the CCA for calibration. Unfortunately this is prone to errors for three reasons. Firstly the sheath tip may not be in the same plane as the bifurcation, and so there is a variable magnification factor that cannot be accounted for. Secondly if a sheath is used, the internal diameter of the sheath is known, but usually it is not the outer, which is used for measurements. If a guiding catheter is used, then this does not apply. Thirdly the diameter of the catheter is small, and the systematic error is high. However, if the CCA measurement correlates with the ultrasound measurement, then it seems reasonable to accept the ICA measurement.

Alternatively, if a larger measurement is used for calibration then the systematic errors can be reduced. This may be achieved in the following manner. If the imaging system is placed in anteroposterior and a thin metal disk of known diameter (e.g., a coin) is placed directly over the carotid bifurcation, then this disk lies in the same plane as the bifurcation. The imaging system can then be rotated 90° and centered between the coin and the bifurcation. The magnification factor is then the same for both the coin and the bifurcation. An imaging run in that position will allow the imaging chain to be calibrated from the coin. Again confirmation of the CCA values with the ultrasound imaging is reassuring. The ICA and lesion lengths can then be directly measured.

CEREBRAL PROTECTION DEVICES

It was noted above that the major concern limiting the adoption of CAS was the potential for particles to be liberated from the plaque at the time of carotid PTA and stent. Such an event would be likely to cause a stroke. A series of devices have been developed to attempt to prevent or limit this problem. These devices fall into the following three groups of "philosophy":

1. ICA occlusion by balloon
2. ICA filtration
3. ICA flow stasis or reversal

At present evidence would suggest that these devices do indeed achieve their intended benefit of reduced stroke risk; however their position remains to be proved (14). Not withstanding such data, most operators use some form of cerebral protection devices by default.

ICA balloon occlusion devices are integral to the guidewire that is used for the remainder of the CAS procedure. The wire tip may be shaped, and manipulated across the stenosis, usually under roadmap control, and advanced until the balloon markers are in an appropriate position (usually at least 1.5–2 cm distal to the lesion segment). The balloon may then be inflated to obtain the desired protection. However it should be remembered that once the protection has been activated it is not possible to obtain a new image of the index lesion, as the ICA flow will be stopped. Therefore an adequate roadmap must be produced before inflating the balloon, and the patient must be encouraged to maintain the same position. If the roadmap is lost, then the balloon must be deflated (after ICA aspiration) if another is required.

The ICA filters are again integral to the guidewire, with the exception of the EmboShield® (Abbott Laboratories, Abbott Park, Illinois, U.S.A.), which is loaded onto a specific guidewire after it has been used to cross the lesion. All of these devices have a guidewire with a malleable tip that can be shaped as required. The lesion is crossed with the wire, and the filter is introduced in a collapsed form. The filter is then released in the desired position in the ICA, and protection is in operation. As ICA blood flow should be uninterrupted, repeat roadmaps can be obtained if necessary. Once the stenting procedure has been completed (see below) the filter is captured, collapsed, and removed.

The flow stasis/reversal systems act by occluding the flow in the CCA and ECA. The difference in the stasis from the reversal system is that in the case of reversal the sheath lumen is connected to the low pressure femoral venous system (via a blood filter). These devices require that a short sheath (up to 10-F) be placed in the femoral artery to allow the devices to be introduced and placed. In view of the relative rigidity of these systems, a stable initial selective catheter position is essential in order that the 0.035-in. wire can be positioned to guarantee successful tracking of the device. In practical terms this means that the carotid bifurcation disease must be confined to the ICA, as if distal CCA disease is present the ECA cannot be used to anchor the wire, and also because the ECA balloon needs to be safely placed. If the CCA is diseased, then the placement of the ECA balloon may be problematic and subject the lesion to more manipulation than filter placement, prior to the inception of protection. A further technical issue that needs to be considered is that if, as is usually the case, the stent is placed from ICA to CCA, then the ECA balloon will need to be withdrawn between the expanded stent and the CCA wall. This is not usually a significant problem, but some stent designs may be potentially more likely to snag this process than others.

STENTING OF THE CAROTID BIFURCATION

Once a stable sheath position has been obtained, and protection has been established, attention can be transferred to the treatment of the index lesion. If a filter or ICA balloon occlusion system has been placed, then the lesion will already have a suitable wire across it. If a flow stasis/reversal system has been positioned, then the lesion may be crossed, using a 0.014-sin. wire of the operator's choice. The modern equipment used for CAS is almost all available on a Monorail/Rapid Exchange platform, and this includes balloons, stents and protection recovery. Therefore if a wire is not integral with the protection device, then this should be taken into account. If, on the other hand, over-the-wire devices are to be used, then a wire of sufficient length must be used as a part of, or in addition to, the protection device.

Once the lesion has been traversed, predilatation of the stenosis needs to be considered. As the stent delivery device profiles reduce in size (typically 5-F at present), and the tendency to treat less severe stenoses become more widely practiced, the need for predilatation has become less important. The intention of predilatation is to allow the smooth passage of the stent delivery system, while exposing the lesion to the minimum risk of embolization. If the protection device is completely effective, then it could be argued that predilatation is unnecessary. However it is clear that the devices are not completely effective and it would seem reasonable to try to keep the embolic load to a minimum (18–28). In addition, if a filter is used, a significant embolic load liberated during stent passage may fill the filter, resulting in flow stasis and potential filter malfunction. If predilatation is considered to be appropriate, a 3-mm balloon is usually sufficient to allow safe stent passage.

Once the lesion has been rendered suitable for stent placement, a stent needs to be selected, if not already decided upon. Whichever is considered, stents designed for the carotid territory are available, and approved, and only such devices should be considered. A number of factors need to be taken into account when choosing a stent:

- *ICA diameter*: This should be known from measurements (see above)
- *CCA diameter*: As above
- *Lesion length to be covered*: As above. If, as is usually the case, stenting from ICA to CCA is intended, then consideration should be paid to the choice of parallel-sided or a conical stent. There is no evidence to dictate that one type is superior to the other.
- *Vessel tortuosity*: Some stent designs tend to straighten the vessel anatomy at the bifurcation more than others (Fig. 3). In most cases this is not a significant issue; however in some this anatomical distortion may cause severe tortuosity in another position of the carotid artery, which potentially becomes flow limiting (with an increased risk of thrombosis). Clearly such a situation needs to be avoided, by appropriate stent selection (Fig. 4). In addition there may be abrupt changes in the caliber of the intended vessel lumen, which may be accommodated better by some stent designs.
- *Lesion characteristics*: There are data available that would indicate that the characteristics of the plaque alter the risk of embolization. In addition some stent designs may be more suited to fibrous calcified lesions (high radial force to resist the recoil) and others to softer plaque (smaller meshwork in the stent may more effectively exclude the plaque from the circulation, with less risk of material prolapse through the struts).

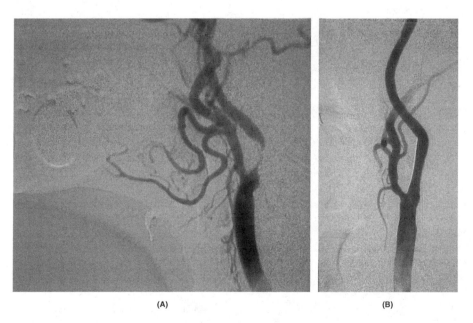

(A) (B)

FIGURE 3 (**A**) Carotid bifurcation lesion with some tortuosity above the stenosis. (**B**) The lesion has been successfully treated with a Carotid Wallstent™ (Boston Scientific, Natick, Massachusetts, U.S.A.), but the bifurcation orientation has been straightened by the stent.

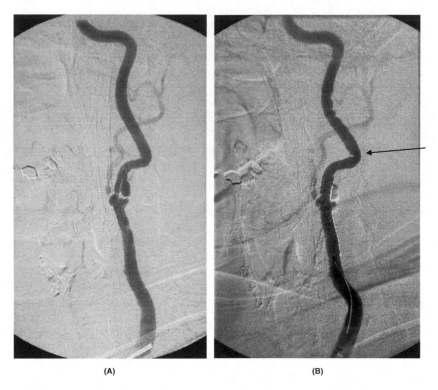

(A)   (B)

FIGURE 4   (**A**) A carotid bifurcation stenosis prior to treatment, with more acute curvature compared with Figure 3. (**B**) A Precise Rx® (Cordis, Miami Lakes, Florida, U.S.A.) stent has been used, as this generally causes minimal anatomical distortion. Despite this the internal carotid artery above the stent is tending toward a kink (*arrow*).

■ *Familiarity*: In common with other regions, there are a number of approved stents designed for the carotid bifurcation. Each stent design is slightly different, as is the delivery system for placing and deploying it. It is intended that the diseased segment covered by a stent, but with a minimum of stent necessary in the adjacent normal vessel. It is important to place the stent, of an appropriate length, accurately. Operator familiarity with the system should not be underestimated, as each delivery system has different features. Common sense would dictate that rather than try to be familiar with all of the systems, that the operator become familiar with a range that allows for treatment of most lesions. If a stent is wrongly placed, a second stent may need to be used, but often the placement of the second stent is rendered more problematic by the presence of the first stent. If this situation should occur it is recommended that the first stent be postdilated before attempting to place the second, as this will facilitate passage of the second device. Obviously this will prolong the procedure, and increase the amount of manipulation at the lesion, both of which are undesirable. If the lesion is of such a length that the use of two stents is inevitable, it is recommended that the cranial stent be placed first, so that the second delivery device does not need to be passed along the full length of the deployed stent.

DRUG THERAPY

All patients who are considered for carotid artery intervention should have their risk factors modified and such therapy should have been instituted at the time of diagnosis. This includes control of blood pressure, cholesterol lowering therapy, smoking cessation and antiplatelet medication. In an ideal world, this should all be instigated prior to considering CAS; however it is prudent to ensure that this is the case. In terms of the CAS procedure itself the following three areas of drug therapy need to be considered:

- Antiplatelet regime
- Anticholinergic treatment
- Anticoagulation

An appropriate antiplatelet regime is vital to maintaining a low event rate at CAS. Most patients will have been commenced on aspirin with or without the addition of dipyridamole. Evidence is available to show that a regime of aspirin and clopidogrel is effective at the time of CAS, and the patients need to be changed to this regime, and given time for this to be effective (29). Ideally the dual aspirin and clopidogrel (dipyridamole stopped) combination should be established approximately a week prior to CAS, and standard doses may be used (aspirin 75–325 mg daily, clopidogrel 75 mg daily). It is possible to give a loading dose of clopidogrel (recommendations vary between 300 and 600 mg) (30–35) but for this to be reliably active it must be given at least six hours before CAS. It is cautionary to understand that some patients do not respond to clopidogrel, and while it is not routine in most centers to test for this, it is possible, and may be a precaution that centers may adopt in the future.

Anticholinergic treatment is given prior to angioplasty and stenting of the carotid bifurcation. If the baroreceptors at the carotid bulb remain active, at the time of PTA or stenting, they will be stimulated and result in a reflex bradycardia and hypotension. This may be blocked by the use of either atropine (dose up to 1.2 mg) or glycopyrrolate (600 µg). This is usually given via a peripheral vein or directly into the carotid sheath. If the latter portal is used it must be remembered that it will result in differential pupil dilatation on the side of administration, which will persist for some hours. This may cause concern when nursing the patient post CAS, unless this situation is expected.

As the procedure takes in the region of 30 to 60 minutes, anticoagulation is used to prevent pericatheter thrombosis, and this is usually achieved by administration of heparin, as a bolus, with further doses should monitoring indicate that it is necessary. More recently there has been interest in the use of bivalirudin (36–38), as an alternative to heparin, but experience with this is limited. With the use of a combination of aspirin and clopidogrel there does not appear to be any benefit to continuing anticoagulation once the CAS procedure has been completed and the catheters removed.

LEARNING THE PROCEDURE

As with all endovascular and open surgical operations, the procedure needs to be learned, and the operator to be practiced in the use of the required equipment. Given that the ability to confer a benefit to the patient by carotid intervention is dependent upon keeping complications to a minimum, it is vital that CAS is learned properly (39–43). There does appear to be a "learning curve," which is likely to be different for an individual depending, among other issues, upon previous experience. A tool that may help in this process is Virtual Reality Simulation (44–47). In addition to this, attending one of the many training courses is useful, and the use of proctors/mentors is recommended by a number of research trials and statutory bodies. For the reasons above it is impossible to give dogmatic guidelines on training requirements; however it is vital that individual vanity does not impede the safe delivery of this and other procedures.

CONCLUSIONS

CAS is becoming a more accepted routine procedure, which can be offered either for patients at risk of stroke, for whom CEA is contraindicated, or as an alternative to CEA. It must be remembered that the procedure is being performed for stroke prevention, and for it to be effective CAS must be performed with an acceptable safety profile. It is therefore vital that CAS is performed with meticulous attention to the detail of the procedure, and with appropriate care and training. There are a number of devices that are specifically designed for use in CAS and the use of these should be familiar to those wishing to perform CAS.

REFERENCES

1. Coward LJ, Featherstone RL, Brown MM. Safety and efficacy of endovascular treatment of carotid artery stenosis compared with carotid endarterectomy: a Cochrane systematic review of the randomised evidence. Stroke 2005; 36:905–11.
2. Yadav JS, Wholey MH, Kuntz ME, et al. Protected carotid artery stenting versus endarterectomy in high-risk patients. N Engl J Med 2004; 351:1493–501.
3. Anonymous. Endovascular versus surgical treatment in patients with carotid stenosis in the Carotid and Vertebral Artery Transluminal Angioplasty Study (CAVATAS): a randomised trial. Lancet 2001; 357:1729–37.
4. Brooks WH, McClure RR, Jones MR, et al. Carotid angioplasty and stenting versus carotid endarterectomy: randomised trial in a community hospital. J Am Coll Cardiol 2001; 38:1589–95.
5. Brooks WH, McClure RR, Jones MR, et al. Carotid angioplasty and stenting versus carotid endarterectomy for treatment of asymptomatic carotid stenosis: a randomised trial in a community hospital. Neurosurgery 2004; 54:318–24.
6. Alberts MJ. Results of a multicentre prospective randomised trial of carotid artery stenting vs. carotid endarterectomy. Stroke 2001; 32:325.
7. Naylor AR, Bolia A, Abbott RJ, et al. Randomised study of carotid angioplasty and stenting versus carotid endarterectomy: a stopped trial. J Vasc Surg 1998; 28:326–34.
8. Wholey MH, Al-Mubarek N. Updated review of the global carotid artery stent registry. Catheter Cardiovasc Interv 2003; 60:259–66.
9. Zahn R, Roth E, Ischinger T, et al. Carotid artery stenting in clinical practice results from the carotid artery stenting registry of the Arbeitsgemeinschaft Leitende Kardiologische Krankenhausarzte (ALKK). Z Kardiologie 2005; 94(3):163–72.
10. Parodi JC, La Mura R, Ferreira LM, et al. Initial evaluation of carotid angioplasty and stenting with three different cerebral protection devices. J Vasc Surg 2000; 32(6):1127–36.
11. Castriota F, Cremonesi A, Manetti R, et al. Impact of cerebral protection devices on the early outcome of carotid stenting. J Endovasc Ther 2002; 9:786–92.
12. Macdonald S, McKevitt F, Venables GS, et al. Neurological outcomes after carotid stenting protected with the NeuroShield filter compared to unprotected stenting. J Endovasc Ther 2002; 9:777–85.
13. Al-Mubarak N, Colombo A, Gaines PA, et al. Multicenter evaluation of carotid artery stenting with a filter protection system. J Am Coll Card 2002; 39(5):841–6.
14. Kastrup A, Groschel K, Krapf H, et al. Early outcome of carotid artery angioplasty and stenting with and without cerebral protection devices: a systematic review of the literature. Stroke 2003; 34(3):813–9.
15. Casteneda-Zuniga WR, Formanek A, Tradavarthy M, et al. The mechanism of balloon angioplasty. Radiology 1980; 135(3):565–71.
16. Kumpa DA, Becker GJ, Percutaneous transluminal angioplasty and other endovascular techniques. In: Rutherford RB, ed. Vascular Surgery. 4th ed., Vol. 1. Philadelphia, Pennsylvania: W.B. Saunders Company, 1995:352–69.
17. Berczi V, Elfleet E, Turner D, et al. Adverse cardiac events as a result of high volume contrast injection during rotational arch aortography. JVIR 2005; 16(4):558–9.
18. Ohki T, Parodi J, Veith FJ, et al. Efficacy of a proximal occlusion balloon catheter with reversal of flow in the prevention of embolic events during carotid artery stenting: an experimental analysis. J Vasc Surg 2001; 33(3):504–9.
19. Ohki T, Marin ML, Lyon RT, et al. Humen ex-vivo carotid artery bifurcation stenting: correlation of lesion characteristics with embolic potential. J Vasc Surg 1998; 27:463–71.
20. Coggia M, Goeau-Brissonniere O, Duval JL, et al. Embolic risks of the different stages of carotid bifurcation balloon angioplasty: an experimental study. J Vasc Surg 2000; 31(3):550–7.
21. Ohki T, Roubin GS, Veith FJ, et al. Efficacy of a filter device in the prevention of embolic events during carotid angioplasty and stenting: an ex-vivo analysis. J Vasc Surg 1999; 30(6):1034–44.
22. Angelini A, Reimers B, Della Barbera M, et al. Cerebral protection during carotid artery stenting: collection and histopathological analysis of embolised debris. Stroke 2002; 33(2):456–61.
23. Al-Mubarak N, Vitek JJ, Iyer S, et al. Embolisation via collateral circulation during carotid stenting with the distal balloon protection system. J Endovasc Ther 2001; 8(4):354–7.
24. Muller-Hulsbeck S, Jahnke T, Liess C, et al. In vitro comparison of four cerebral protection filters for preventing human plaque embolization during carotid interventions. J Endovasc Ther 2002; 9:793–802.

25. Jaeger H, Mathias K, Drescher R, et al. Clinical results of cerebral protection with a filter device during stent implantation of the carotid artery. CVIR 2001; 24(4):249–56.
26. Albuquerque FC, Teitelbaum GP, Lavine SD, et al. Balloon protected carotid angioplasty. Neurosurgery 2000; 46(4):918–21.
27. Ohki T, Veith FJ, Grenall S, et al. Initial experience with cerebral protection devices to prevent embolisation during carotid artery stenting. J Vasc Surg 2002; 36(6):1175–85.
28. Terada T, Tsuura M, Matsumoto H, et al. Results of endovascular treatment of internal carotid artery stenoses with a newly developed balloon protection catheter. Neurosurgery 2003; 53(3):617–23.
29. McKevitt FM, Randall MS, Cleveland TJ, et al. The benefits of combined anti-platelet treatment in carotid artery stenting. Eur J Vasc Endovas Surg 2005; 29(5):522–7.
30. Kastrati A, von Beckerath N, Joost A, et al. Loading with 600 mg clopidogrel in patients with coronary artery disease with and without chronic clopidogrel therapy. Circulation 2004; 110(14):1916–9.
31. Gurbel PA, Bliden KP, Hayes KM, et al. The relation of dosing to clopidogrel responsiveness and the incidence of high post-treatment platelet aggregation in patients undergoing coronary stenting. J Am Coll Cardiol 2005; 45(9):1392–6.
32. Angiolillo DJ, Fernandez-Ortiz A, Bernardo E, et al. Identification of low responders to a 300-mg clopidogrel loading dose in patients undergoing coronary stenting. Thromb Res 2005; 115(1–2):101–8.
33. Angiolillo DJ, Fernandez-Ortiz A, Bernardo E, et al. High clopidogrel loading dose during coronary stenting: effects on drug response and interindividual variability. Eur Heart J 2004; 25(21):1903–10.
34. Matsagas M, Jagroop IA, Geroulakos G, et al. The effect of a loading dose (300 mg) of clopidogrel on platelet function in patients with peripheral arterial disease. Clin Appl Thromb Hemost 2003; 9(2):115–20.
35. Bhatt DL, Kapadia SR, Bajzer CT, et al. Dual antiplatelet therapy with clopidogrel and aspirin after carotid artery stenting. J Invasive Cardiol 2001; 13(12):767–71.
36. Allie DE, Hall P, Shammas NW, et al. The Angiomax Peripheral Procedure Registry of Vascular Events trial (APPROVE): in hospital and 30 day results. J Invasive Cardiol 2004; 16:651–6.
37. Gurm HS, Rajagopal V, Fathi R, et al. Effectiveness and safety of bivalirudin during percutaneous coronary intervention in a single medical center. Am J Cardiol 2005; 95(6):716–21.
38. Dnagas G, Lasic Z, Mahran R, et al. Effectiveness of the concomitant use of bivalirudin and drug-eluting stents [from the prospective multicenter BivAlirudin and Drug-Eluting Stents (ADEST) study]. Am J Cardiol 2005; 96(5):659–63.
39. Rosenfield K, Society for Cardiovascular Angiography and Interventions, Society for Vascular Medicine and Biology, et al. Clinical competence statement on carotid stenting: training and credentialing for carotid stenting-multispeciality consensus recommendations. Catheter Cardiovasc Interv 2005; 64(1):1–11.
40. Sacks D, Connors J. Carotid stenting, stroke prevention, and training. J Vasc Interv Radiol 2004; 15(12):1381–4.
41. SCAI/SVMB/SVS Writing Committee. SCAI/SVMB/SVS clinical competence statement on carotid stenting: training and credentialing for carotid stenting- multispecialty consensus recommendations. Vasc Med 2005; 10(1):65–75.
42. Connors J, Sacks D, Furlan AJ, et al. Training, competency, and credentialing standards for diagnostic cervicocerebral angiography, carotid stenting, and cerebrovascular intervention: a joint statement from the American Academy of Neurology, the American Association of Neurological Surgeons, the American Society of Interventional and Therapeutic Neuroradiology, the Congress of Neurological Surgeons, the AANS/CNS Cerebrovascular Section, and the Society of Interventional Radiology. Neurology 2005; 64(2):190–8.
43. Rosenfield K, Babb JD, Cates CU, et al. Clinical competence statement on carotid stenting-multi-specialty consensus recommendations: a report of the SCAI/SVMB/SVS Writing Committee to develop a clinical competence statement on carotid interventions. J Am Coll Cardiol 2005; 45(1):165–74.
44. Issenberg SB, McGaghie WC, Hart IR, et al. Simnlation technology for healthcare professional skills training and assessment. JAMA 1999; 282:861–6.
45. Hsu JH, Younan D, Pandalai S, et al. Use of computer simulation for determining endovascular skill levels in a carotid stenting model. J Vasc Surg 2004; 40:1118–25.
46. Dayal R, Faries PL, Lin SC, et al. Computer simulation as a component of catheter-based training. J Vasc Surg 2004; 40:1112–7.
47. Gallagher AG, Cates CU. Virtual reality training for the operating room and cardiac catheterization laboratory. Lancet 2004; 364:1538–40.

18 | Management of Complications During and After Carotid Angioplasty and Stenting

Marc R. H. M. van Sambeek, Johanna M. Hendriks, and Lukas C. van Dijk
Department of Vascular Surgery and Department of Radiology, Erasmus University Medical Center, Rotterdam, The Netherlands

INTRODUCTION

In effort to minimize interventions, in the last decade carotid artery stenting (CAS) has been suggested as an alternative to surgical endarterectomy for patients with symptomatic and asymptomatic extra cranial carotid artery obstructive disease. Acceptable technical success and complication rates have shown promise for the procedure. In major publications, there has been much description of the technique and its technical success, but only brief overview of complications and the management of neurological complications.

This chapter will address complications and management of these complications in the following areas:

■ embolic complications
■ hemodynamic complications
■ thrombotic complications
■ hyperperfusion syndrome

When a (neurological) complication occurs during or after the procedure, the patient should be promptly evaluated by a neurologist for signs of true neurological event as opposed to a drug reaction.

EMBOLIC COMPLICATIONS

Despite the improvements in technical skills and materials, embolic complications remain a major unpredictable clinical event. Atherosclerotic material or thrombus can be dislodged either by the guidewire or percutaneous transluminal angioplasty balloon and may embolize to the cerebral circulation and result in cerebral ischemia and infarction. Using Transcranial Doppler (TCD) monitoring, Jordan et al. (1) detected eight times more emboli during angioplasty when compared to surgery. Jaeger et al. (2) performed diffusion-weighted magnetic resonance imaging in 67 patients with 70 high-grade stenosis, before and 24 hours after carotid stenting. The neurological status was unchanged in 69 of the 70 procedures. Nevertheless, new ipsilateral lesions were found in 20 patients (29%) and new contralateral lesions in 6 patients (9%). In all patients except one, the new lesions were clinically asymptomatic. Flach et al. (3) treated 44 patients (23 CEA, 21 CAS) with a significant symptomatic carotid stenosis. In the operated group two patients had new lesions (9%) compared to nine patients in the stented group (43%). The importance of silent cerebral infarction after carotid stenting remains undefined.

Whether embolic complications are symptomatic or asymptomatic, it is considered an adverse event and it is generally appreciated that embolic protection devices (EPD) might play an important role in the prevention of these emboli.

Embolic Protection Devices

Protection devices such as occlusion balloons, filters and reversed flow devices are currently undergoing clinical evaluation.

Distal balloon occlusion was the first described of all protection devices. The balloon is inflated in the internal carotid artery (ICA), distal to the stenosis, and temporarily occludes the flow during the critical phases of the procedure. After stent placement and post-dilatation the arterial segment from carotid bifurcation to distal balloon is cleared from debris by suction.

The principle of a distal filter is that it collects debris during the procedure while preserving the flow in the ICA. The filter device is passed beyond the lesion and deployed in a suitable segment of the ICA distal from the lesion. After the procedure the filter device is retrieved by a specially designed retrieval catheter.

Proximal balloon occlusion is designed to reverse the flow in the ICA before treatment of the lesion. A guiding catheter is positioned in the common carotid artery. Through this guiding catheter a small and low profile balloon is positioned and inflated in the external carotid artery. After inflation of the balloon at the tip of the guiding catheter in the common carotid artery, obstruction of flow is created. Reversal of flow can be achieved by suction on the guiding catheter or connection of this guiding catheter with a sheath in the common femoral vein.

All the devices have their own strengths and weaknesses (4). Okhi et al. (5) and Parodi et al. (6) tested the three different devices and concluded that all devices can be used safely. Cremonesi et al. (7) published the results of protected CAS in 442 patients. In-hospital stroke/death and 30-day ipsilateral stroke/death rate was 1.1%. The overall complication rate was 3.4%. The cerebral protection device-related complications were 0.9%. Reimers et al. (8) evaluated, in a multicenter study, the short-term outcome of 753 patients who underwent carotid stenting with the routine use of EPDs. The 30-day incidence of stroke and death was 3.3%. Protection device-related vascular complications, none of which led to neurological complications, occurred in 1.1% of the cases. Many of these noncomparative studies led some authors to suggest that the use of EPD should be mandatory.

In an attempt to provide some substantive evidence, a nonrandomized study compared the clinical outcome in 75 patients treated with Neuroshield (MedNova™) protection device with 75 patients who were treated unprotected (9). No statistically difference in cerebral outcome was observed. Recently Vos et al. (10) compared protected and unprotected CAS by measuring emboli with TCD. Patients were divided in three groups: 161 patients treated before EPDs had become available, 151 patients treated with filtering EPDs, and 197 patients without EPD after EPDs had become available. They measured a higher number of micro emboli during filter-protected CAS than during unprotected CAS. Macro emboli occurred only in the unprotected groups but only during the first 186 procedures. Of the eight patients with a macro embolus five patients were symptomatic.

Although there is consensus among opinion leaders that a protection device should be used to prevent embolic complications (11), evidence either for or against the use of cerebral protection is still lacking. Only a large randomized multicenter trial can solve this dilemma.

Complications and Side-Effects Related to EPD

Some patients do not tolerate flow obstruction or reversal of flow. In case of neurological symptoms during occlusion it is generally advisable to deflate the balloon and use a filter device.

Transient spasm of the distal segment of the carotid artery is occasionally related to the EPD (Fig. 1). Spasm can be prevented by minimal manipulations, to prevent excessive movement of the EPD and avoiding any significant over sizing of the EPD. If the spasm is mild a conservative approach is justified. Severe spasm with obvious flow obstruction can be resolved by administration of intra-carotid nitroglycerin (200–400 µg) and/or EPD removal.

During the procedure, massive embolization of atherothrombotic material can cause filter thrombosis. When angiography is performed during this complication, obstructed flow can be observed. The risk for filter thrombosis may be decreased, but not completely abolished by adequate intra operative anticoagulation. Once filter occlusion occurs there are several options

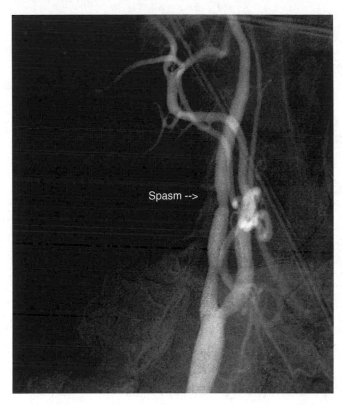

FIGURE 1 Spasm in the extracranial internal carotid artery at the distal end of the stent.

to resolve this complication. Some interventionists advise retrieval of the filter without closing it. Thrombosuction and/or thrombolysis are used by others. An alternative is to introduce a protection device based on flow reversal followed by a combination of thrombolysis and thrombosuction (12).

Intracranial Embolic Complications

When significant intracranial embolization occurs it can be recognized by TCD monitoring. The patient will usually develop neurological symptoms. If a preoperative intracranial angiogram is not performed, it may be difficult to recognize the obstructed vessel segment. Therefore it is advisable to perform an intracranial angiogram at the start of the procedure and after completion (Fig. 2).

Once an intracranial embolus and/or thrombosis is recognized, several options are possible. If the neurological deficit is only limited, the risk of an intracranial procedure should be weighed against the symptoms. Sometimes a conservative strategy is justified. In general super-selective catheterization of the obstructed vessel segment is performed. Thrombolysis and/or thrombosuction can then be utilized. If this is not successful some interventionists perform a balloon dilatation with a coronary balloon to recover flow. Some dedicated clot removal devices are on the market to treat intracranial embolization. These devices range from basket-shaped wires to specially designed corkscrew shaped wires. In general it is advised to administer platelet glycoprotein IIb/IIIa receptor inhibitors (abciximab) immediately at the onset of symptoms caused by intracranial embolization.

HEMODYNAMIC COMPLICATIONS

Cerebral autoregulation is the major mechanism to ensure a stable cerebral blood flow (CBF) despite fluctuations in cerebral perfusion pressure (CPP). If CPP changes, CBF can be kept

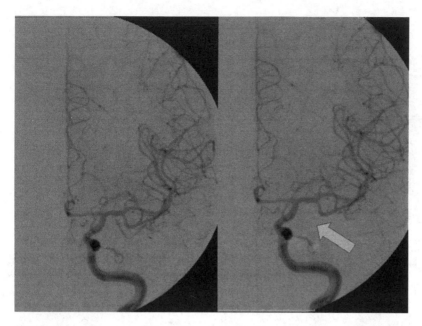

FIGURE 2   Preoperative and postoperative intracranial angiography showing an acute embolization and obstruction.

constant by changes in cerebral vascular resistance. In certain circumstances (obstructive carotid disease or critical perfusion) the cerebral autoregulation mechanism is compromised and in these situations, changes in blood flow can lead to a significant decrease in the CBF.

Hemodynamic changes may complicate the stent procedure. Stents or balloons distend the carotid sinus, thereby activating stretch-sensitive mechanoreceptors that connect with the brain stem. This reflex may trigger a reduction of sympathetic tone in peripheral blood vessels thus decreasing blood pressure. Impulses from the carotid sinus may also enhance para-sympathetic stimulation of the heart, causing bradycardia.

Several authors have reported both bradycardia and hypotension during carotid stenting (13,14) which may be associated with neurological complications. A retrospective analysis (15) of 471 patients showed that 7% of patients had severe hypotension or bradycardia despite prophylactic atropine and adequate fluid balance. Neurological complications were 7% in the hemodynamically stable group compared with 12% in the unstable group. This difference was not statistically significant. Howell et al. (16) concluded that patients with a severely elevated systolic blood (>180 mmHg) may be at higher risk for hemodynamic instability. It has been observed that the greater the change in systolic blood pressure the more severe the neurological event, as there were no neurological events in patients with a <50 mmHg change in systolic blood pressure.

Different techniques have been used to prevent hemodynamic instability. Most interven-tionists will use prophylactic atropin to prevent hemodynamic instability. Some interventionists prefer prophylactic beta-adrenergic agonists that stimulate both heart rate and contractility. Others (17) use a temporary pacemaker, although this is another invasive procedure. More research has to be done to evaluate the hemodynamic changes during angioplasty and stenting.

THROMBOTIC COMPLICATIONS

At the inception of endovascular carotid intervention, patients with a significant carotid artery stenosis were treated with balloon angioplasty alone (18–21). Initial reports observed rates of periprocedural stroke and death that were of concern. In patients undergoing percutaneous coronary intervention, the clinical and angiographic outcomes were improved in patients who received a stent (22). As a consequence of this observation, angioplasty and stenting became standard for carotid endovascular intervention and is hypothesized to be safer, because recoil, dissection and occlusion of the carotid artery are less likely to occur (23,24).

The clinical utility of intracoronary stent implantation was initially limited by a 3.5% incidence of subacute stent thrombosis (22,25). The development of improved stent implantation and the use of ticlopidine and aspirin reduced the occurrence of stent thrombosis in these specific interventions. Clopidogrel was approved for clinical use by the Food and Drug Administration in 1998 and subsequently has rapidly replaced ticlopidine as part of combination antiplatelet therapy following coronary stenting (26,27). Clopidogrel offers potential advantages compared with ticlopidine with better tolerance, lower cost, reduced risk of neutropenia and lower incidence of thrombotic thrombocytopenic purpura. In coronary stenting clopidogrel with aspirin is the regimen of choice to prevent stent thrombosis although the optimal dosing regimen is still a subject of research (28–31).

The role of antithrombotic therapy in carotid stenting has not been fully characterized. Bhatt et al. (32) showed in a small group of patients, that dual antiplatelet therapy with clopidogrel plus aspirin in patients receiving carotid artery stents was associated with a low rate of ischemic events. Clopidogrel appeared to be superior to ticlopidine in this study. McKevitt et al. (33) published a randomized controlled trial which compared aspirin and 24-hour heparin with aspirin and clopidogrel for patients undergoing CAS. Bleeding complications occurred in 17% of the heparin and 9% of the clopidogrel group ($p=0.35$). The neurological complication rate in the 24-hour heparin group was 25% compared to 0% in the clopidogrel group ($p=0.02$), whilst the 30-day 50% to 100% stenosis rates were 26% in the heparin group and 5% in the clopidogrel group ($p=0.10$).

Most centers now give a combination of aspirin and clopidogrel at the time of stenting to reduce the risk of in-stent thrombosis and treatment related stroke.

Acute carotid artery closure after carotid stenting can manifest with significant neurological symptoms. A duplex ultrasound should be performed in these cases to diagnose acute stent thrombosis. Because acute carotid stent thrombosis is an uncommon phenomenon, there is only limited experience in its treatment. Setacci et al. (34) reported on three cases of acute stent thrombosis treated by surgical management (stent removal and complete endarterectomy in two patients and embolectomy in one patient). Some authors have reported successful treatment of acute carotid stent thrombosis by combination therapy using percutaneous mechanical thrombectomy and adjunctive GP IIb IIIa receptor inhibitors (35,36). Despite good results in the literature with this combination technique, there are concerns about the possibility of thrombus embolization during treatment. The intraluminal manipulation with guidewires and catheters in association with thrombosuction and/or thrombolysis may cause fragmentation of clot. The risk of distal embolization might be limited if reversal of flow was instituted with a cerebral protection device before manipulation commenced (12).

HYPERPERFUSION SYNDROME

Hyperperfusion syndrome consists of a triad of ipsilateral throbbing headache (with or without nausea), seizures and focal neurological symptoms. In the extreme form it may present as intracerebral hemorrhage. Originally, hyperperfusion syndrome was described in patients undergoing carotid endarterectomy for severe carotid stenosis, but more recently it has been described following carotid stenting. It is not yet known if the risk for a hyperperfusion syndrome is comparable between carotid endarterectomy and carotid stenting (1–3%). Hypertension, the severity of the treated stenosis, and the presence of a contralateral stenosis or occlusion are identified as potential risk factors for hyperperfusion syndrome.

Hyperperfusion is a well-recognized complication, caused by increased CBF in combination with impaired cerebral autoregulation. The chronic low-flow state induced by severe carotid disease, may result in a compensatory dilatation of cerebral vessels, which impairs the

TABLE 1 Management of Complications with Carotid Stenting

Complications	Prevention	Treatment
Embolic complications		
Intolerance to flow obstruction	Use of filter device	Deflate balloon and use filter device
Spasm of internal carotid artery	Gentle technique, no over-sizing of embolic protection devices	Expectative/intracarotid nitroglycerin
Filter thrombosis	Rapid procedure and adequate anticoagulation	Retrieve filter/thrombosuction or thrombolysis
Intracranial embolization	Rapid procedure and adequate anticoagulation	Abciximab/thrombosuction or thrombolysis or balloon dilatation or clot removal
Hemodynamic complications		
Hypotension and bradycardia	Adequate fluid balance/β-adrenergic agonists/temporary pacemaker	Fluid administration and β-adrenergic agonists
Thrombotic complications		
Acute stent thrombosis	Dual treatment (aspirin and clopidogrel)	Stent removal/mechanical thrombectomy/thrombolysis
Hyperperfusion	Monitoring and control of blood pressure	Withhold antiplatelet/antihypertensive medication

ability to autoregulate vascular resistance in response to changes in blood pressure. This impaired autoregulation may manifest in increased CBF after recanalization. Symptoms of hyperperfusion usually occur between the second and fifth postoperative day. TCD may be able to predict which patients are at increased risk of hyperperfusion syndrome by measuring increased mean flow velocities in the ipsilateral middle cerebral artery (37).

Prevention of hyperperfusion is critical. The most important component of preoperative management is vigilant monitoring and control of systemic blood pressure. Additional efforts to reduce the risk of hyperperfusion may include limiting the duration of balloon inflation and employing EPD (38). If patients develop clinical symptoms suggestive of hyperperfusion or if patients have a documented elevation of the middle cerebral artery blood flow velocities it is suggested to withhold antiplatelet agents and administer antihypertensive medication until symptoms have resolved and the blood pressure is optimally controlled (Table 1).

CONSIDERATIONS

CAS is a promising technique. Evidence is still lacking and there is some concern about the long-term value of CAS. However, major improvements have been made in technique and materials, which make carotid stenting safer. Perhaps the most important component of periprocedural risk reduction on this moment is understanding, which patients and lesions can be treated safely with this technology.

REFERENCES

1. Jordan WD, Voellinger DC, Doblar DD, Plyushsheva NP, Fisher WS, Mc Dowell HA. Microemboli detected by transcranial Doppler monitoring in patients during carotid angioplasty versus carotid endarterectomy. Cardiovasc Surg 1999; 7:33–8.
2. Jaeger HJ, Mathias KD, Hauth E, et al. Cerebral ischemia detected with diffusion-weighted MR imaging after stent implantation in the carotid artery. Am J Neuroradiol 2002; 23:200–7.
3. Flach HZ, Ouhlous M, Hendriks JM, et al. Cerebral ischemia after carotid intervention. J Endovasc Ther 2004; 11:251–7.
4. Hendriks JM, Zindler JD, van Dijk LC, van Sambeek MR. Cerebral protection during percutaneous carotid intervention: which device should be used? Acta Chir Belg 2004; 104:300–3.
5. Ohki T, Veith FJ, Grenell S, et al. Initial experience with cerebral protection devices to prevent embolisation during carotid artery stenting. J Vasc Surg 2002; 36:1175–85.
6. Parodi JC, La Mura R, Ferreira LM, et al. Initial evaluation of carotid angioplasty and stenting with three different cerebral protection devices. J Vasc Surg 2000; 32:1127–36.

7. Cremonesi A, Manetti R, Setacci F, Setacci C, Castriota F. Protected carotid stenting: clinical advantages and complications in 442 consecutive patients. Stroke 2003; 34:1936–41.
8. Reimers B, Schluter M, Castriota F, et al. Routine use of cerebral protection during carotid artery stenting: results of a multicenter registry of 753 patients. Am J Med 2004; 116:217–22.
9. Macdonald S, Mckevitt F, Venables GS, Cleveland TJ, Gaines PA. Neurological outcomes after carotid stenting protected with neuroshield filter compared to unprotected stenting. J Endovasc Ther 2002; 9:777–85.
10. Vos JA, van den Berg JC, Ernst SM, et al. Carotid angioplasty and stent placement: comparison of transcranial Doppler U.S. data and clinical outcome with and without filtering cerebral protection devices in 509 patients. Radiology 2005; 234:493–9.
11. Veith FJ, Amor M, Ohki T, et al. Current status of carotid bifurcation angioplasty and stenting based on a consensus of opinion leaders. J Vasc Surg 2001; 33:S111–6.
12. Parodi JC, Rubin BG, Azizzadeh A, Batoli M, Sicari GA. Endovascular treatment of an internal carotid artery thrombus using reversal of flow: a case report. J Vasc Surg 2005; 41:146–50.
13. Qureshi AI, Luft AR, Sharma M, et al. Frequency and determinants of postprocedural hemodynamic instability after carotid angioplasty and stenting. Stroke 1999; 30:2086–93.
14. Mendelsohn FO, Wiessman NJ, Lederman RJ, et al. Acute hemodynamic changes during carotid artery stenting. Am J Cardiol 1998; 82:1077–81.
15. Mlekusch W, Schillinger M, Sabeti S, et al. Hypotension and bradycardia after elective carotid stenting: frequency and risk factors. J Endovasc Ther 2003; 10:851–9.
16. Howell M, Krajcer Z, Dougherty K, et al. Correlation of periprocedural systolic blood pressure changes with neurological events in high-risk patients. J Endovasc Ther 2002; 9:810–6.
17. Harrop JS, Sharan AD, Benitez RP, Armanda R, Thomas J, Rosenwasser RH. Prevention of carotid angioplasty-induced bradycardia and hypotension with temporary venous pacemaker. Neurosurgery 2001; 49:814–22.
18. Bockenheimer S, Mathias K. Percutaneous transluminal angioplasty in atherosclerotic internal carotid artery disease. AJNR Am J Neuroradiol 1983; 4:791–2.
19. Tsai F, Matovich V, Hieshima G, et al. Percutaneous transluminal angioplasty of the carotid artery. ANJR AM J Neuroradiol 1986; 7:349–58.
20. Becker G, Katzen B, Dake M. Noncoronary angioplasty. Radiology 1989; 170:921–40.
21. Kachel R. Results of balloon angioplasty in the carotid arteries. J Endovasc Surg 1996; 3:22–30.
22. Serruys PW, de Jaegere P, Kiemeneij F, et al. A comparison of balloon-expandable-stent implantation with balloon angioplasty in patients with coronary artery disease. Benestent Study Group. N Engl J Med 1994; 331:489–95.
23. Roubin GS, New G, Iyer SS, et al. Immediate and late clinical outcomes of carotid artery stenting in patients with symptomatic and asymptomatic carotid artery stenosis. A 5-year prospective analysis. Circulation 2001; 103:532–7.
24. Diethrich EB, Ndiaye M, Reid DB. Stenting in the carotid artery: initial experience in 110 patients. J Endovasc Surg 1996; 3:42–6.
25. Fischman DL, Leon MB, Baim DS, et al. A randomized comparison of coronary-stent placement and balloon angioplasty in the treatment of coronary artery disease. N Engl J Med 1994; 331:496–501.
26. Bertrand ME, Rupprecht HJ, Urban P, Gershlick AH. Double-blind study of the safety of clopidogrel with and without a loading dose in combination with aspirin compared with ticlopidine in combination with aspirin after coronary stenting: the clopidogrel aspirin stent international cooperative study (CLASSICS). Circulation 2000; 102:624–9.
27. Taniuchi M, Kurz HI, Lasala JM. Randomized comparison of ticlpidine and clopidogrel after intracoronary stent implantation in a broad patient population. Circulation 2001; 104:539–43.
28. Bennett CL, Davidson CJ, Raisch DW, Weinberg PD, Bennett RH, Feldman MD. Thrombotic thrombocytopenic purpura associated with ticlopidine in the setting of coronary artery stents and stroke prevention. Arch Intern Med 1991; 159:2524–8.
29. Gurbel PA, Cummings CC, Bell CR, Alford AB, Meister AF, Serebruany VL. Onset and extent of platelet inhibition by clopidogrel loading in patients undergoing elective coronary stenting: the Plavix Reduction Of New Thrombus Occurrence (PRONTO) trial. Am Heart J 2003; 145:239–347.
30. Serebruany VL, Steinhubl SR, Berger PB, Malinin AI, Bhatt DL, Topol EJ. Variability in platelet responsiveness to clopidogrel among 544 individuals. J Am Coll Cardiol 2005; 45:246–51.
31. Gurbel PA, Bliden KP, Zaman KA, Yoho JA, Hayes KM, Tantry US. Clopidigrel loading with eptifibatide to arrest the reactivity of platelets: results of the clopidogrel loading with eptifibatide to arrest the reactivity of platelets (CLEAR PLATELETS) study. Circulation 2005; 111:1153–9.
32. Bhatt BL, Kapadia SR, Bajzer CT, et al. Dual antiplatelet therapy with clopidogrel and aspirin after carotid artery stenting. J Invasive Cardiol 2001; 13:767–71.
33. Mc Kevitt FM, Randall MS, Cleveland TJ, Gaines PA, Tan KT, Venables GS. The benefits of combined anti-platelet treatment in carotid artery stenting. Eur J Vasc Endovasc Surg 2005; 29:522–7.
34. Setacci C, de Donato G, Setacci F, et al. Surgical management of acute carotid thrombosis after carotid stenting: a report of three cases. J Vasc Surg 2005; 42:993–6.

35. Bush RL, Bhama JK, Lin PH, Lumsden AB. Transient ischemic attack due to early carotid stent thrombosis: successful rescue with rheolytic thrombectomy and systemic abciximab. J Endovasc Ther 2003; 10:870–4.
36. Tong FC, Cloft HJ, Joseph GJ, Samuels OB, Dion JE. Abciximab rescue in acute carotid stent thrombosis. AJNR Am J Neuroradiol 2000; 21:1750–2.
37. Jansen C, Sprengers AM, Moll FL, et al. Prediction of intracerebral haemorrhage after carotid endarterectomy by clinical criteria and intraoperative transcranial Doppler monitoring: results of 233 operations. Eur J Vasc Surg 1994; 8:220–5.
38. Abou-Chebl A, Yadav JS, Reginelly JP, Bajzer C, Bhatt D, krieger DW. Intracranial hemmorrhage and hyperperfusion syndrome following carotid artery stenting. J Am Coll Cardiol 2004; 43:1596–601.

19 | Vertebral Artery Occlusive Disease (Indications for Intervention, Technical Aspects, Troubleshooting and Current Results)

Andrew G. Clifton
Department of Neuroradiology, St. George's Hospital, London, U.K.

INTRODUCTION

Approximately 25% of ischemic strokes involve the posterior or vertebrobasilar circulation (1,2). The anatomy and imaging of this region are important for treatment and have been extensively reviewed by Cloud and Markus (3). Doppler ultrasound, digital subtraction angiography (DSA), computed tomography angiography (CTA) and contrast enhanced magnetic resonance angiography (MRA) can all be used to assess the vertebrobasilar circulation. Imaging of the posterior circulation should include detailed views of the vertebral artery origins. In this location, duplex ultrasonography may be limited as this modality is able to image the origin in only 60% of subjects. CTA and MRA are more accurate in assessment of the vertebral origins although MRA may over estimate stenosis, and for these reasons the current gold standard remains DSA.

Stenotic lesions, particularly at the origin of the vertebral artery are not uncommon. Studies (4,5) have demonstrated a degree of proximal extracranial stenosis in 18% of right vertebral arteries and 22% on the left. The management of vertebral artery stenosis both at the vertebral artery origin, more distally and intracranially is poorly defined at the present time. Until recently intracranial atherosclerotic disease has not been amenable to intervention as the surgical options were unviable.

Rothwell et al. (6) reviewed the perception of vertebrobasilar transient ischemic attacks and minor stroke. They reported that vertebrobasilar territory TIAs were perceived to have a better prognosis than carotid territory events, and were therefore managed less aggressively. This philosophy appeared to stem from a few small studies in the 1960s and 1970s. Rothwell et al. (6) also reviewed the available world literature and found no evidence that patients presenting with vertebrobasilar events had a lower risk of subsequent stroke or death compared with patients presenting with carotid territory TIAs. Patients with vertebrobasilar TIAs were demonstrated to be at increased risk of stroke in the acute phase, particularly in the first seven days after presenting symptoms, compared to patients presenting with anterior circulation symptoms.

Surgery for vertebrobasilar ischemia is a relatively rare procedure in most centers. Surgery for these lesions is often technically difficult due to the position of the vertebral artery origin, although vertebral endarterectomy and transposition are well described. Surgical access to the bony or intracranial segment of the vertebral artery is prohibitive. In reported series, complication rates of surgery are relatively low (7). An analysis of 369 extracranial vertebral reconstructions reported a procedural stroke or death rate of 5.1% in 215 patients treated prior to 1991 and 1.9% in 154 patients treated since 1991, with 92% patency at 10 years.

MEDICAL TREATMENT

Medical treatment has traditionally assumed the major therapeutic role for posterior circulation stroke and has been previously reviewed (3). There have been no randomized trials of the use of different antiplatelet therapies or anticoagulation against antiplatelet therapies in extracranial artery disease. With respect to intracranial atherosclerosis, there have been two studies comparing warfarin and aspirin for symptomatic intracranial disease covering both anterior and posterior circulation stenoses (8,9). In the initial study symptomatic patients with intracranial large artery stenosis (greater than 50%) were treated with either aspirin or warfarin and evaluated for the success of medical therapy. At a follow-up of approximately 14.7 months there was an 8.4% stroke or death rate in the warfarin group and with a follow-up of 19.3 months, an 18.1% rate of major stroke or death in the aspirin group. In a subset of patients with posterior circulation stenoses, the annualized stroke rate in the territory of a stenotic basilar artery was 10.7% and in a vertebral artery 7.8%.

The second study, following on from this earlier investigation, was the National Institutes of Health–sponsored warfarin/aspirin symptomatic intracranial disease trail (WASID) performed from 1998 to 2003. This was a double blind randomized trail and patients with symptomatic angiographic verified stenosis greater than 50% of a major intracranial artery were randomized to receive either warfarin or aspirin. The trial was prematurely halted because of concerns about the safety of the patients who had been assigned to receive warfarin. In aspirin-treated patients, ischemic stroke in the same vascular territory was 12% at one year and in warfarin-treated patients 11%. Death occurred in 4.3% of the aspirin group and 9.7% in the warfarin group, whilst major hemorrhage was reported in 3.2% of the aspirin group and 8.3% of the warfarin group. Similarly, myocardial infarction or sudden death was revealed in 2.9% of the aspirin group and 7.3% in the warfarin group. The conclusion was that aspirin should be used rather than warfarin for patients with intracranial arterial stenosis because of the severe hemorrhage rate in those patients treated with warfarin.

ENDOVASCULAR TREATMENT

With increasing realization of the poor prognosis of vertebrobasilar disease and the advances in endovascular techniques, interventional intraluminal techniques have become more common (Figs. 1 and 2). The literature for extracranial and intracranial cerebral artery stenting and angioplasty will be reviewed separately.

Extracranial Vertebral Artery Stenting

There has been only one completed randomized trial comparing vertebral artery stenting with best medical therapy. The data derive from a subset of patients within the Carotid and Vertebral Artery Transluminal Angioplasty Study (10,11). In this study, 16 patients were randomized, 8 patients to endovascular treatment in association with best medical therapy and 8 to medical care alone. All patients had symptoms attributable to their vertebral artery stenosis with the

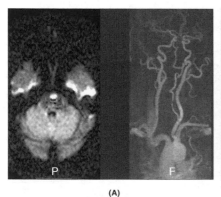 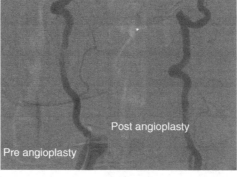

(A)   (B)

FIGURE 1   **(A)** (*Left*) Diffusion weighted MRI showing an acute pontine infarction in a 57-year-old man with recurrent posterior circulation strokes. *(Right)* CEMRA showing occlusion of the right vertebral artery and tight stenosis of the proximal left cervical vertebral artery. **(B)** Same patient appearances pre- and post-angioplasty.

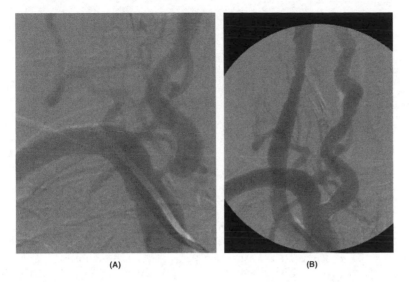

(A)   (B)

FIGURE 2 **(A)** Tight stenosis of right vertebral artery origin, pre-stent. **(B)** Post-stent.

vast majority symptomatic in the six months prior to randomization. Endovascular treatment was technically successful in all eight patients but TIAs occurred in the posterior circulation in two patients within 30 days of the procedure. There were no strokes in any arterial territory or deaths in either group within 30 days of randomization or treatment. Patients were followed up for a mean of 4.5 years in the endovascular group and 4.9 years in the medical group. There were no further vertebrobasilar territory strokes in either group during this time. Five of the patients had angioplasty alone and three were treated by stenting. Clearly only very limited conclusions can be drawn from such a small sample.

Early reports of treatment of vertebral origin stenoses used percutaneous transluminal angioplasty (PTA) alone, but were associated with marked incidence of restenosis which led to the use of primary stenting (12–15). There have been many published series detailing primary deployment of stents to stenotic lesions of 50% or more in the extracranial vertebral arteries, including the origins. Cloud et al. (14) reported 14 patients who underwent vertebral PTA and stenting, all but one symptomatic with recurrent symptoms despite maximal antiplatelet therapy. All stenoses were treated successfully, but complications included two posterior circulation TIAs. In the four patients treated with primary angioplasty, all four restenosed and one was symptomatic with a TIA at 18 months which was retreated with a primary stent procedure. All 11 primary stenting patients had no further symptoms at follow-up. No significant restenosis was seen at follow-up.

The rate of restenosis after endovascular treatment of vertebral artery stenosis varies between series. Storey et al. (13), reported that all three patients who underwent vertebral PTA developed symptomatic restenosis within three months. Stenting was subsequently undertaken and follow-up catheter angiography in two of these patients showed no restenosis three months and one year after stent insertion. Higashida (16), used a combination of Doppler ultrasound, MRA and catheter angiography to follow up patients after proximal vertebral PTA and showed restenosis in only 3 of 34 patients (9%). Chastain et al. (17), have followed up the largest reported series of patients after extracranial vertebral artery stent placement for the treatment of symptomatic vertebral artery stenosis. Out of 49 patients, 44 underwent angiographic follow up at six months and 48 of 55 vessels treated (87%) had involvement of the origin or proximal extracranial vertebral artery. A moderate degree of restenosis was reported in 10% of treated vessels.

The results of these, albeit limited, case series suggest that from a technical view point primary stenting of vertebral artery atherosclerotic stenosis at the vessel origin has a high success rate, an acceptable complication rate, and a low rate of restenosis. However, in the light of the advances of secondary preventative treatment for stroke patients over the past decade with antiplatelet, antilipid, and antihypertensive medication in particular, data from well designed, randomized clinical trials are required to compare the outcome after endovascular treatment with best medical care alone in this patient population.

Intracranial Vertebral Artery Stenosis

Since the advent of endovascular therapy over the past 10 to 20 years there have been many individual case reports, as well two prospective multi-center trials looking at intracranial angioplasty and stenting for patients with severe intracranial atherosclerotic stenosis of both the anterior and posterior circulations. Conners and Wojak (18) treated 70 patients over nine years. They modified their technique and in their last 50 patients described a slow inflation of an undersized balloon relative to the vessel diameter. Using the newer technique no abrupt vessel occlusions or strokes were experienced. Complications included angiographic vessel dissection 14%, vessel thrombosis requiring fibrinolysis in 4%, and one death. Good clinical outcome and good angiographic outcome was achieved in 98%. Kim et al. (19), treated 17 patients with stent-assisted angioplasty for medically refractory vertebrobasilar artery stenosis. Out of 17, 13 lesions were of the intracranial vertebral artery with a mean degree of stenosis decreased from 76% to 14% after the procedure. Acute in-stent thrombosis developed in one case which was successfully treated with thrombolytics and angioplasty. No symptoms related to the vertebrobasilar territory were seen at follow-up ranging from 6 to 24 months.

The Stenting of Symptomatic Atherosclerotic Lesions in the Vertebral or Intracranial Arteries (20) trial reported a success rate of 95% in 61 cases. Strokes after stent placement occurred in 2 of 22 intracranial cases (14%) during a one-year follow-up period. The 30-day complication rate reported a 6.6% stroke rate.

The WingSpan study, investigated the treatment of intracranial atherosclerotic stenoses with balloon dilatation and a self-expanding stent (WingSpan™, Boston Scientific, Natick, Massachusetts, U.S.A.) in 15 patients (21). Anatomically and clinically adequate results were achieved in all patients. The initial degree of stenosis was 72%, balloon dilatation resulted in a mean residual stenosis of 54%, reduced further to 38% after stent deployment. All patients were either stable or improved four weeks after the treatment.

Conclusion

Recommendations for endovascular treatment of vertebrobasilar stenoses are difficult in the light of the poor evidence base. A position statement was recently published by the American Society of Interventional Therapeutic Neuroradiology, the Society of Interventional Radiology and the American Society of Neuroradiology (22). It was suggested that symptomatic patients with a greater than 50% intracranial stenosis who have failed medical therapy could be considered for balloon angioplasty with or without stenting. The statement suggests that similar to revascularization for extracranial artery stenosis (23), patient benefit from revascularization for symptomatic intracranial arterial stenosis is critically dependent on a low periprocedural stroke and death rate, and should only be performed by experienced interventionalists.

However a more realistic view is given in an editorial by Barnett (24) who suggests that randomized trials will be necessary to define the position of interventional procedures for vertebrobasilar stenoses. Barnett states that the widespread practice of intracranial stenting is premature and asks stroke neurologists to unite in wrestling another stroke prevention strategy from the gloom of uncertainty, bringing possibly dangerous conventional wisdom to the level of reality by supporting a proposed trial of posterior circulation stenting versus medical therapy. He states that such trials will only succeed if they gain support from international neurologists and committed, experienced interventionalists. Only a large international trial will solve the conundrum as to whether increasingly better medical treatment is equal to or better than new, rapidly developing endovascular treatments.

TECHNICAL ASPECTS

Extracranial Vertebral Origin and Extracranial Vertebral Stenosis

The patient should receive dual antiplatelet therapy, aspirin 75 mg and clopidogrel 75 mg a day for at least five days or given loading doses of 600 mg of both the day before the procedure. Intervention is performed under local anesthesia with anesthetic supervision. A standard femoral approach is used, and angiography utilized to visualize both vertebral origins and the vertebrobasilar circulation. After intravenous injection of 5000 U Heparin to increase the activated clotting time to two to three times normal, an exchange catheter is placed in the appropriate subclavian artery. The stenosis is crossed, either with a 0.14- or 0.18-in. wire depending on the type of stent being used. The stenosis is then crossed using a balloon mounted stent and the balloon inflated to deploy the stent across the stenosis. Stent of 1 to 2 mm are placed within the subclavian artery so that the full thickness of the stenosis is treated. The balloon is deflated; angiography performed and provided the appearances are angiographically adequate, the balloon is removed. If necessary a further balloon dilatation is performed. The wire and guiding catheter are removed and a sealant device used to seal the groin puncture site. The patient remains on dual antiplatelet therapy for one month and then aspirin for life. As a variation on the technique, if the vessels are very tortuous and it is difficult to achieve a stable position of the catheter, a 7-F guiding catheter may be required. The guiding catheter is stabilized using a second 0.35-in. wire, through the guiding catheter into the subclavian artery.

Intracranial Stenting and Angioplasty

These interventions are usually performed under general anesthesia. As with extracranial stenting the patients are placed on dual antiplatelet therapy. Standard percutaneous access is obtained using a 6- or 7-F sheath via one of the femoral arteries, and angiography is performed. After full heparinization, a guiding catheter is exchanged into the appropriate vertebral artery. Stenoses can be treated with primary angioplasty using a coronary balloon, with pre-dilation and stenting or with primary stenting using a coronary stent. Some operators undersize the stent, others dilate to the size of the vessel (25). An alternative treatment uses a new self-expanding stent (WingSpan™) (21). In this technique, a dilation balloon is chosen so that at its nominal pressure the diameter would not exceed 80% of the vessel proximal or distal to the stenosis. The balloon is then dilated using a slow dilation for 90 seconds. The balloon is removed and the self-expanding stent introduced and deployed with the diameter of the stent slightly larger than the diameter of the balloon.

CONCLUSION

The natural history of symptomatic vertebral artery stenosis, particularly that resistant to medical therapy, is poor and it does not seem unreasonable to treat these stenoses endovascularly. For intracranial disease this position is supported by the recent position statement of the American Societies (22). However, appropriate randomized, controlled trials are required to clarify indications and results of endoluminal intervention in the vertebrobasilar circulation.

REFERENCES

1. Bamford J, Sandercock P, Dennis M, et al. Classification and natural history of clinically identifiable subtypes of cerebral infarction. Lancet 1991; 337:1521–6.
2. Bogousslavsky J, Van Melle G, Regli F. The Lausanne Stroke Registry: analysis of 1000 consecutive patients with first stroke. Stroke 1988; 19:1083–92.
3. Cloud GC, Markus HS. Diagnosis and management of vertebral artery stenosis. Q J Med 2003; 96:27–54.
4. Crawley F, Clifton A, Brown MM. Treatable lesions demonstrated on vertebral angiography for posterior circulation ischaemic events. Br J Radiol 1998; 71:1266–70.
5. Hass WK, Fields WS, North RR, Kircheff II, et al. Joint study of extracranial arterial occlusion. II. Arteriography, techniques, sites and complications. J Am Med Assoc 1968; 203:961–8.

6. Flossman E, Rothwell P. Prognosis of vertebrobasilar transient ischaemic attack and minor stroke. Brain 2003; 126:1940–54.
7. Berguer R, Flynn LM, Kline RA, et al. Surgical reconstruction of the extracranial vertebral artery: management and outcome. J Vasc Surg 2000; 31:9–18.
8. Chimowitz MI, Kokkinos J, Strong J, et al. The warfarin–aspirin symptomatic intracranial disease study. Neurology 1995; 45:1488–93.
9. Chimowitz MI, Lynn MJ, Howlett-Smith H, et al. Comparison of warfarin and aspirin for symptomatic intracranial arterial stenosis. N Engl J Med 2005; 352:1305–16.
10. CAVATAS Investigators. Endovascular versus surgical treatment inpatients with carotid stenosis in the Carotid and Vertebral Artery Transluminal Angioplasty Study (CAVATAS): a randomised trial. Lancet 2001; 357:1729–37.
11. Coward LJ, Featherstone RL, Brown MM. Percutaneous transluminal angioplasty and stenting for vertebral artery stenosis. Stroke 2005; 36:2047–8.
12. Crawley F, Brown MM, Clifton AG. Angioplasty and stenting in the carotid and vertebral arteries. Postgrad Med J 1998; 74:7–10.
13. Storey GS, Marks MP, Dake M, et al. Vertebral artery stenting following percutaneous transluminal angioplasty: technical note. J Neurosurg 1996; 84:883–7.
14. Cloud GC, Crawley F, Clifton A, McCabe DJH. Vertebral artery origin angioplasty and primary stenting: safety and restenosis rates in a prospective series. J Neurol Neurosurg Psychiatr 2003; 74:586–91.
15. Roubin GS, Cannon AD, Agrawal SK, et al. Intracoronary stenting for acute and threatened closure complicating percutaneous transluminal coronary angioplasty. Circulation 1992; 85:916–27.
16. Higashida RT, Tsai FY, Halbach VV, et al. Transluminal angioplasty for atherosclerotic disease of the vertebral and basilar arteries. J Neurosurg 1993; 78:192–8.
17. Chastain HD, II, Campbell MS, Iyer S, et al. Extracranial vertebral artery stent placement in hospital and follow up results. J Neurosurg 1999; 91:547–52.
18. Conners JJ, III, Wojak JC. Percutaneous transluminal angioplasty for intracranial atherosclerotic lesions: evolution of technique and short term results. J Neurosurg 1999; 91:415–23.
19. Kim DJ, Lee BH, Kim DI, et al. Stent assisted angioplasty of symptomatic intracranial vertebrobasilar artery stenosis: feasibility and follow up results. Am J Neuroradiol 2005; 26:1381–8.
20. SSYLVIA Study Investigators. Stenting of Symptomatic Atherosclerotic Lesions in the Vertebral or Intracranial Arteries (SSYLVIA): study results. Stroke 2004; 35:1388–92.
21. Henkes H, Miloslavski E, Lowens S, et al. Treatment of intracranial atherosclerotic stenoses with balloon dilatation and self expanding stent deployment (WingSpan). Neuroradiology 2005; 47:222–8.
22. Higashida RT, Meyers PM, Connors JJ, et al. Intracranial angioplasty and stenting for cerebral atherosclerosis: a position statement of the American Society of Interventional and Therapeutic Neuroradiology, Society of Interventional Radiology and the American Society of Neuroradiology. Am J Neuroradiol 2005; 26:2323–7.
23. Biller J, Feinberg WM, Castaldo JE, et al. Guidelines for carotid endarterectomy: a statement for healthcare professionals from a special writing group of the Stroke Council, American Heart Association. Stroke 1998; 29:554–62.
24. Barnett HJ. Conventional wisdom versus reality in stroke prevention. Neurology 2005; 64:1122–4.
25. Yu W, Smith WS, Singh V, et al. Long term out come of endovascular stenting for symptomatic basilar artery stenosis. Neurology 2005; 64:1055–7.

20 | Renal and Visceral Angioplasty and Stent Placement

Nick Chalmers
Department of Radiology, Manchester Royal Infirmary, Manchester, U.K.

INTRODUCTION

Renal artery angioplasty and stent placement have been performed worldwide for many years despite limited good quality scientific evidence in support of any worthwhile benefit. Visceral (celiac and superior mesenteric) endovascular intervention, on the other hand, has received relatively little attention, and the published data are limited to a few small case series.

RENAL ARTERY INTERVENTION

Renal Artery Pathology

Several pathological processes may affect the renal artery including atherosclerosis, fibromuscular disease (FMD) and vasculitis. By far the commonest cause of renal artery stenosis (RAS) in western society is atherosclerotic renovascular disease (ARVD). ARVD most commonly affects the renal artery ostium (defined as within 10 mm of the aortic lumen). The underlying disease is mainly atherosclerotic plaque in the aorta encroaching on the renal artery ostium (1). ARVD is predominantly found in the middle-aged and elderly population, usually in association with other manifestations of vascular disease, and in association with the well-known risk factors such as hypertension, smoking and hypercholesterolaemia (Fig. 1A).

FMD is relatively uncommon. FMD is found predominantly in young and middle-aged females. The commonest and most typical pattern is that of medial fibroplasia which probably has a genetic origin. This gives rise to multiple web-like stenoses and focal dilatations, which are usually seen in the main renal artery (non-ostial) and in the intrarenal branches (Fig. 2). The less common intimal form of FMD produces a smooth non-ostial stenosis resulting from diffuse intimal hypertrophy. This pattern occurs as a primary disease of unknown etiology, but may also occur as the result of previous intimal injury.

Several syndromes are associated with developmental fibromuscular stenoses involving the renal arteries and sometimes the aorta also. These include neurofibromatosis (Fig. 3), the "middle aortic syndrome" and William's syndrome. Takayasu's arteritis causes aortic and RAS in its later stages. It has a particular geographical distribution, occurring most commonly in the Far East and the Indian Subcontinent. Takayasu's arteritis is predominantly seen in young females and usually occurs in association with disease involving the aortic arch and supra-aortic arteries (2).

Hypertension is the most frequent clinical consequence of RAS. The pathophysiological mechanism of renovascular hypertension mediated by the renin-angiotensin system is well known. Unfortunately, correcting the stenosis does not automatically result in a cure of hypertension. Other clinical manifestations of RAS include impairment of renal function, reduction in renal size and proteinuria. FMD is often associated with hypertension, but rarely with renal impairment. ARVD, in contrast, is a relatively common cause of impaired renal

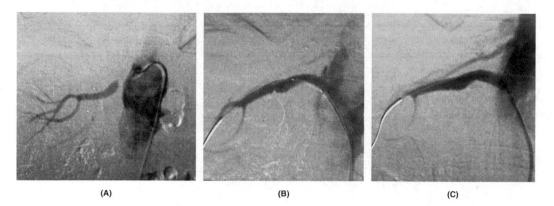

(A)   (B)   (C)

FIGURE 1 Atherosclerotic right renal artery stenosis with contralateral occlusion. (**A**) The ostial stenosis is due to bulky aortic plaque. A reverse curve (shepherd's hook) catheter is used to select the renal artery ostium. (**B**) After balloon dilatation, the stent is carefully positioned prior to deployment. Accurate profiling of the renal artery ostium is required. (**C**) Following deployment, the stent should protrude slightly into the aortic lumen to prevent restenosis at the ostium.

function, particularly in the elderly. It is the cause of end-stage renal failure in 25% of patients aged more than 60 years (3). ARVD is associated with high mortality due to cardiovascular disease.

Surgical treatments for renal artery disease have been undertaken for many years, but have declined in recent years due to the increased acceptance of angioplasty and stenting. Percutaneous treatment is obviously less invasive, although by no means without risk. Currently, good evidence in favor of percutaneous treatment versus surgery or versus conservative management is lacking.

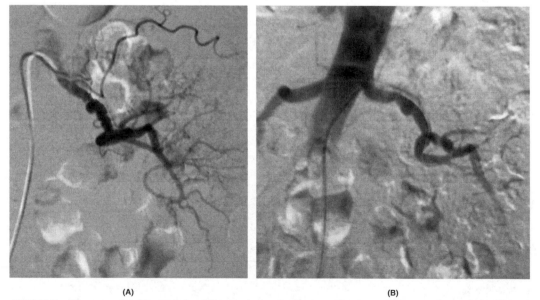

(A)   (B)

FIGURE 2 Fibromuscular disease: intimal fibroplasia causing hypertension in a middle-aged female. (**A**) The typical beaded appearance, non-ostial, of the main renal artery. (**B**) Following balloon angioplasty, some irregularity of the arterial wall persists. Stent placement is not generally required.

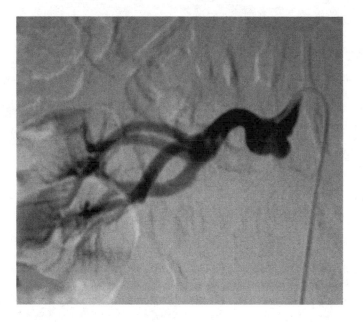

FIGURE 3 Neurofibromatosis with hypertension. There is tight ostial stenosis associated with aneurysmal dilatation of the main renal artery. This stenosis proved resistant to balloon dilatation; marked waisting persisted at maximum inflation pressure.

Techniques

The underlying principles of renal artery intervention differ slightly from those of peripheral arterial intervention. The basic concept of passing a guidewire across a stenosis followed by dilatation with an angioplasty balloon [i.e., percutaneous transluminal angioplasty (PTA)] are similar. The use of stents in the peripheral vascular system is usually reserved for cases in which balloon angioplasty gives an unsatisfactory result. In the renal arteries, however, there is good evidence that stent placement in ostial stenoses results in improved long-term patency compared with balloon angioplasty alone (4). In the periphery, angioplasty techniques are frequently used to recannalize long-standing arterial occlusions. Long-standing total occlusions in the renal arteries are seldom suitable for revascularization: Alhadad et al. reviewed their series of 34 patients undergoing attempted revascularization of renal artery occlusion. There was technical success in 24 patients and failure to recannalize the occlusion in 10 patients. Improvement in blood pressure control was seen equally in both groups suggesting that factors other than the intervention itself were responsible for the improvement (5). Reversal of dialysis dependency has been reported following revascularization of total occlusions in small series of patients. Factors which seem to favor improvement in renal function are the recent onset of the occlusion and the presence on scintigraphy or other imaging modalities of viable renal tissue (6,7).

Renal artery angioplasty is usually performed from a femoral approach. The only disadvantage of the femoral approach is the common downward trajectory of the renal artery relative to the aorta. This may cause difficulty in selective cannulation and subsequent intervention from the femoral approach in some individuals. If the renal arteries are at approximately 90° to the aorta, a cobra catheter may be appropriate to cannulate the renal artery. If the renal artery slopes inferiorly, a catheter with a reverse curve such as a Sidewinder catheter (Cordis, Johnson & Johnson, New Jersey) or a SOS Omni catheter (Angiodynamics, Queensbury, New York) is more useful for engaging the renal artery ostium (Fig. 1B). The catheter tip may sometimes be advanced through the stenosis by traction on the catheter hub. This may not be possible if the stenosis is tight or angulated, in which case the stenosis must first be crossed with a hydrophilic guidewire. These manoeuvres require care and finesse to avoid dissecting the vessel. If a dissection is created in the renal artery by inadvertent force during cannulation of the stenosis, catheterizing the true lumen is usually very difficult and often impossible.

If the downward angulation of the renal artery makes selective catheterization from the femoral artery impossible, it may be possible to cannulate the renal artery from the arm. The radial artery, brachial artery or axillary artery may be used as an access artery for renal artery intervention. Traditionally the axillary artery route has been used. The axillary artery is relatively large and close to the aorta, compared with alternatives such as brachial and radial, so equipment of standard calibre and length can be used. The main disadvantage of the axillary approach is the difficulty of achieving good compression post-procedure. A relatively small hematoma may compromise the nerves of the brachial plexus, which accompany the artery in a fascial sheath. This can result in permanent neurological sequelae in the upper limb. The radial artery provides a potentially safer alternative to the axillary. It is widely used by cardiologists for both diagnostic and interventional coronary procedures. The radial artery will accommodate a 6F sheath in the majority of patients. It can easily be controlled by external compression after sheath withdrawal and usually remains patent, such that it can be reused for future access in 95%. The disadvantage of the radial approach for renal artery intervention is the distance from access to target, necessitating long catheters and wires, with loss of torque control and stability as a result. Nevertheless, the radial approach has been used successfully (8). Whichever, upper limb access artery is chosen, the catheter of choice to cannulate the renal artery is the multipurpose catheter which has hockey-stick shape, well suited for catheterization of renal arteries from the arm. A general problem with upper extremity access for renal artery intervention is the necessity to use longer catheters than are required via the femoral route. Departments need to keep a stock of these longer selective catheters, and there is no doubt that longer catheters are more difficult to use because they have reduced torque control and are more difficult to track across narrow stenoses.

Having achieved catheterization, a guidewire of suitable stiffness is required to give adequate support to the balloon and stent. Renal artery PTA/stenting can be performed with either 0.035- or 0.018-in. balloon/stent/guidewire systems. Most interventionalists have moved from the 0.035- to 0.018-in. systems. Whichever system is used, a stiff guidewire with a floppy, atraumatic tip is required. The wire must be advanced into an intrarenal branch so that the stiff portion is across the stenosis and can provide adequate support for passage of the balloon or stent across the stenosis. The tip of the guidewire must be advanced with care. It is actually possible for the wire to be advanced through the renal parenchyma and capsule, which can result in major retroperitoneal hemorrhage (Fig. 4). It is important that the image intensifier

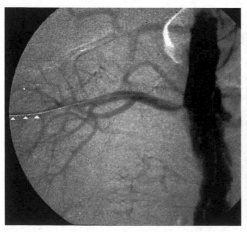 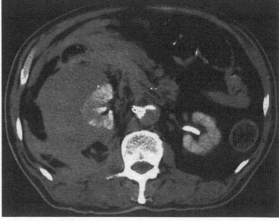

(A)   (B)

FIGURE 4 Retroperitoneal hemorrhage due to guidewire perforation of the renal capsule. Even the small capsular perforation caused by the guidewire can cause considerable bleeding. (**A**) During the procedure, the guidewire tip is inadvertently advanced out of the field of view, through the renal parenchyma. (**B**) Post-procedure computed tomography scan showing extensive peri-renal hematoma.

field of view is large enough to keep the guidewire tip in view at all times during the intervention.

Atherosclerotic RAS

The great majority of renal artery interventions involve atherosclerotic disease at the arterial ostium. PTA alone has historically resulted in poor patency rates for ostial RAS. Convincing randomized trial evidence (4) indicates that stents give significantly improved patency compared with PTA for ostial RAS. Balloon-expandable stents are preferred to self-expanding stents. A typical renal artery requires a 6 mm diameter stent of 15 mm length. The stent requires careful positioning so that the renal artery ostium is covered and the stent protrudes 2 to 3 mm into the aortic lumen (Fig. 1B,C). If the stent does not protrude by a few millimetres into the aorta, restenosis by encroachment of aortic plaque over the end of the stent will occur. Accurate positioning of the stent requires an understanding of the angle of origin of the renal artery from the aorta in the axial plane, and oblique screening at the appropriate angle to view the renal artery ostium in profile. A computed tomography scan, if available, is useful to select the optimum obliquity for visualization of the renal artery.

Intervention in Non-Atherosclerotic Renal Artery Disease

Although there is evidence to support the use of stents in ARVD, the same is not true of FMD. Medial fibroplasia is associated with multiple fine web-like stenoses and a characteristic "string of beads" appearance. These stenoses are more difficult to traverse with a guidewire than the initial angiographic appearances would suggest: each web behaves like a closed curtain through which the guidewire must be manipulated. Having traversed the abnormal segment, balloon dilatation is generally effective. Stents are rarely used or necessary. Angioplasty may not totally obliterate the beaded appearance; however, the obstructing webs are obliterated by the balloon (Fig. 2).

Neurofibromatosis, middle-aortic syndrome, Takayasu's arteritis and intimal FMD are more challenging to treat by PTA. Here, the difficulty is not usually the crossing of the lesion. Rather, it is the resistance of the stenosis to dilatation. In many cases, a waist persists on the balloon despite the use of maximal dilatation pressure. This reflects the underlying tough fibrous nature of the stenosis. Stent placement is not appropriate if the stenosis is resistant to high balloon pressure. Other endovascular treatment options are described in small numbers only and include the use of high pressure balloons (up to 30 atmospheres) and cutting balloons. These are angioplasty balloons which incorporate three or four fine sharp blades arranged radially. When the balloon is inflated, these produced a controlled incision in the vessel wall of 0.15 mm depth. In theory this incision overcomes the resistance to dilatation of the resistant stenosis. Evidence in support of their use in this situation is limited to small case series (9,10). On the other hand, several case reports of renal artery rupture and false aneurysm formation have been published in recent years so their use cannot be recommended without reservation (11–13). Cutting balloons have also been used to treating in-stent restenosis in the renal arteries as in the coronary arteries (14).

Outcomes after Renal Artery Intervention

Clinical effectiveness of renal artery intervention has been addressed in several series. Most series have not been controlled. A meta-analysis in 1990 concluded that PTA for FMD disease appeared to be worthwhile, whereas the benefits for atherosclerotic lesions were small (15). The benefits in FMD appear to be durable, particularly when disease is confined to the main renal artery (16). A recent series from India suggests that PTA can also produce sustained benefit in Takayasu's disease (17).

Most uncontrolled series have generally given optimistic assessments of the effects of PTA on renal function. For example, Martin and colleagues reported a significant and sustained drop in serum creatinine in 43% of patients following renal PTA (18). Canzanello, on the other hand, showed that renal function declined in 48% of patients over two years despite a good angiographic result (19). These conflicting opinions emphasize the importance of a control group.

Published randomized controlled trials are few and have included fewer than 200 patients in total (20–22). They include only atherosclerotic RAS and were all primarily concerned with hypertension, rather than renal function, as an outcome measure. A meta-analysis of the controlled trials has concluded that there is evidence for only minimal effect on blood pressure and that there is no evidence of benefit in renal function (23). The published trials were performed before the current widespread use of stents and therefore the intervention was PTA alone, which we now know to be inferior to stenting in terms of patency in ARVD. Weibull and colleagues published a randomized trial in 1993 which compared PTA with surgical reconstruction (24). They demonstrated that surgery achieved superior primary patency; however, since this was before the days of stents, this no longer reflects the state of the art in endovascular technique. Randomized trial data relating to renal artery stenting are rudimentary: Van de Ven showed no difference in clinical outcomes between patients randomized to stents and PTA in a trial of 85 patients despite superior patency in the stent group (4).

Stenting or PTA for RAS seems to be useful in the setting of the clinical syndrome of "flash pulmonary edema." Flash pulmonary edema refers to a clinical condition of recurrent bouts of pulmonary edema which occurs despite relatively well preserved left ventricular function. It is associated with severe, usually bilateral RAS resulting in hypertension and avid salt and water retention. Following successful renal revascularization, there is frequently a marked diuresis, with resolution of the pulmonary edema. Flash pulmonary edema is generally considered to be a good indication for intervention, although the evidence is limited to a few small case series (25,26). Occasionally it is possible to restore kidney function in patients presenting with anuria (6,7). These are usually patients with known vascular disease, who present with acute onset of anuria, but whose kidneys are near-normal in size. These cases are few, and in general attempts to revascularize chronically occluded renal arteries, or arteries to shrunken kidneys (less than 7 cm in length) are futile.

Ongoing Controlled Trials

Although revascularization may not produce dramatic improvement in renal function, there remains the possibility that a progressive decline to end-stage renal failure may be retarded. This could have obvious public health benefits as ARVD is the cause of end-stage renal failure in 25% of patients over 60 years starting renal replacement programmes in Europe (3). Harden et al. undertook a longitudinal study of patients after renal artery stenting and showed that the rate of decline in renal function was greater before intervention than after (27). However, it is possible that factors other than the intervention itself might be responsible. The clinical effectiveness of renal artery stent placement is currently the subject of two large randomized trials. The ASTRAL trial is a U.K. based multicenter randomized trial of renal artery stent placement versus conservative therapy and is nearing its target of 750 patients. The main outcome measure is the rate of decline in renal function. The trial organizers hope to identify whether intervention can produce a relatively small but clinically worthwhile reduction in the rate of decline of renal function. The CORAL trial is based in the U.S.A. with a recruitment target of 1000 patients. The target group is hypertensive patients with RAS. The primary endpoint is a composite of a range of cardiovascular and renal events (28).

Complications of Renal Artery Intervention

Renal artery intervention is associated with a significant complication rate. Beek et al. reported a 10% severe and a 10% mild clinical complication rate in addition to 16% technical complications without clinical sequelae (29). Dissection (Fig. 5) and capsular perforation (Fig. 4) are infrequent complications and have been mentioned previously. Cholesterol embolization (CE) is more common and is seen in up to 10% of patients (29). This complication can cause persistent deterioration in renal function following intervention despite an apparently satisfactory angiographic result. Although CE may occur spontaneously, it is particularly likely during renal artery interventions, which inevitably involves disruption of aortic plaques. The disrupted plaque may continue to leak cholesterol crystals into the renal artery for an indefinite period, sometimes weeks after intervention. These crystals lodge in small arteries and excite a foreign

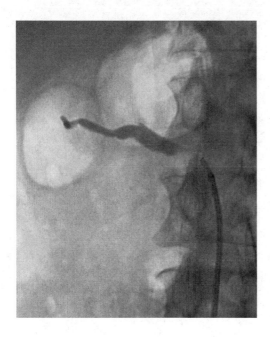

FIGURE 5 Guidewire-induced dissection. Following attempted traverse of a tight ostial stenosis with a guidewire, injection of contrast reveals stasis within a subintimal dissection in the main renal artery. It is unlikely to be possible to regain the true lumen with the wire.

body reaction. Evidence of CE to the lower limbs may be apparent with patchy blue discoloration of the skin and painful superficial ulcers. The resulting renal impairment may be sudden or progressive in onset. There are no effective treatments for CE and efforts are aimed towards prevention. This involves minimizing trauma to the aortic wall by catheter manipulation and avoidance of unnecessary disruption of aortic plaque. This may be very difficult if catheterization of the RAS is technically very difficult. Recently, interest has grown in the use of embolic protection devices analogous to those used in the carotid artery. The Angioguard device (Cordis) is an umbrella like device with a porous membrane which captures embolic material released during angioplasty and is collapsed and retrieved after the procedure. Its use in the renal artery is more difficult than in the carotid artery because there is usually less room to deploy it in the main stem renal artery distal to the stenosis. Despite this, it is possible to deploy it in many cases, and debris (which presumably might have occluded distal renal branches) can often be extracted from the filter. Clearly, the filter does not reduce the continuing CE that occurs after the procedure (30,31). Embolization of thrombus may occlude the renal artery or its branches after intervention. This may be treatable by aspiration through a large bore catheter, or by local thrombolysis. However, some degree of renal impairment is likely, even if renal artery patency can be restored.

Complications resulting in partial or total loss of the function of a kidney are reported in 4%. Puncture site complications were reported in 4% (29), although the modern use of smaller calibre systems should reduce this figure (32). Misplacement of a stent may be treated by extracting the stent through a groin sheath (if it has not already been expanded) (Fig. 6) or by deploying the stent in the external iliac artery.

Further complications are associated with the use of iodinated contrast media. Risk factors include preexisting renal impairment, diabetes and multiple procedures involving use of contrast medium over a short time interval. The risk of contrast medium induced nephrotoxicity can be reduced by adequate hydration and by the use of a non-ionic dimer (iodixanol) as opposed to a monomer (33,34). Minimizing contrast medium dose is important: it should be possible to complete a renal stent procedure with substantially less than 50 mL of contrast medium in most cases. Carbon dioxide is a useful alternative contrast agent. It carries no risk of nephrotoxicity, but requires special imaging software for optimal results (8).

The risk of complications in the individual depends to a large extent on the anatomy of the aorta and renal artery. The experienced operator can differentiate the angiographic

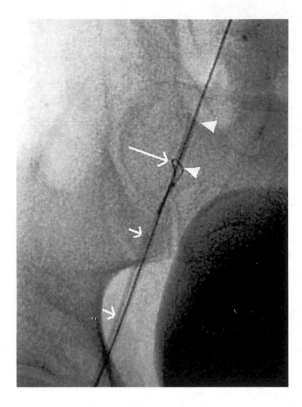

FIGURE 6 Retrieval of an undeployed stent using a gooseneck snare. The stent became dislodged from the balloon during attempted positioning in the renal artery. Because it had not been deployed, it was possible to retrieve it through the groin sheath using a snare. If it had been partially deployed, it could have been "parked" in the external iliac artery.

appearances of the straightforward and safe procedure from the complex and high risk intervention. In view of the absence of convincing data for the benefits of intervention, there is a reasonable argument for avoiding interventions in high-risk lesions (Fig. 7).

VISCERAL ARTERY INTERVENTION

Clinical Features

Compared with the renal artery, there is limited published experience of endovascular interventions for occlusive disease of the visceral arteries (i.e., the celiac and mesenteric

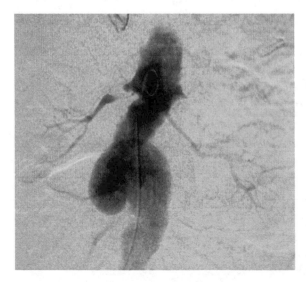

FIGURE 7 A markedly eccentric severe stenosis of the right renal artery associated with severe aortic atheroma and aneurysm and occlusion of the main left renal artery. This is a "high risk" case, to be avoided if possible.

arteries). Visceral artery stenosis and occlusion are less common than renal artery disease. Furthermore, there is extensive collateral circulation between all of the visceral vessels so that occlusion of one or more of these is usually subclinical. Symptoms generally occur when there is severe stenotic or occlusive disease of two out of the three arteries—usually the celiac and the superior mesenteric arteries (SMAs). The clinical presentation of mesenteric angina is non-specific, and diagnosis involves exclusion of other more common conditions. The typical presentation is with severe abdominal pain, after eating, and often associated with weight loss, and a fear of large meals. Patients are frequently cachectic at presentation and usually have evidence of widespread vascular disease. There may be abdominal bruits and a high velocity jet may be detected on Doppler ultrasound of the celiac and SMA origins.

Pathology

Stenosis of SMA and inferior mesenteric artery (IMA) is almost always due to atherosclerosis, and, as in the renal arteries, almost always involves the origin of the artery (Fig. 8). Stenosis of the celiac artery may be due to atherosclerosis. The commonest cause of isolated celiac artery stenosis is median arcuate ligament compression. The median arcuate ligament of the diaphragm forms a loop around the aorta. Median arcuate ligament compression causes a characteristic indentation on its superior surface about 1 cm from its origin (Fig. 9). This may result in significant narrowing, so that the celiac territory is supplied mainly through collaterals from the SMA. Celiac artery stenosis, due to median arcuate ligament compression, occurs in 7.3% of asymptomatic individuals (35). It varies with respiration and is more pronounced in expiration (36). Occasionally it appears to be the cause of ischemic symptoms, which have been successfully relieved by division of the median arcuate ligament. Balloon angioplasty is predictably ineffective (37).

Visceral Artery Intervention Techniques

Many aspects of revascularization technique in the visceral vessels are similar to the renal arteries. The visceral vessels usually arise from the aorta at an acute angle and slope

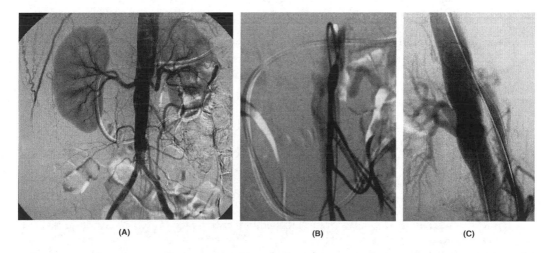

(A)   (B)   (C)

FIGURE 8 Atherosclerotic stenosis of the superior mesenteric artery (SMA) origin. Celiac axis is occluded. There is severe inferior mesenteric artery (IMA) stenosis. (**A**) The aortogram shows very little opacification of visceral vessels. The liver is supplied by intercostal collaterals. A naso-jejunal feeding tube is in situ. (**B**) A selective angiogram shows a severe stenosis of SMA ostium. (**C**) From an axillary approach the SMA has been catheterized using a multi-purpose catheter. A self-expanding Wallstent (Boston Scientific, Natick, MA, U.S.A.) has been deployed in the SMA. *Abbreviations*: IMA, inferior mesenteric artery; SMA, superior mesenteric artery.

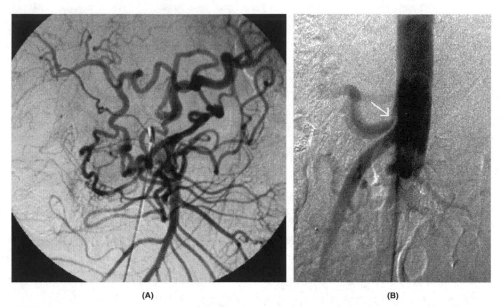

(A)   (B)

FIGURE 9   Median arcuate ligament compression. (**A**) Superior mesenteric artery angiogram shows that the celiac territory is supplied through collateral circulation. The increased flow may result in aneurysm formation (not shown). (**B**) Lateral aortogram showing the characteristic indentation on the superior aspect of the celiac axis by the median arcuate ligament.

downwards, which gives rise to similar technical difficulties experienced in catheterization of the renal arteries. From a femoral approach, a sidewinder type catheter is required (Fig. 10). Catheterization of the SMA is sometimes easier from the axillary or brachial approach, however this is associated with the problems described earlier (Fig. 9) (38). The transradial approach has also been described (39). Most series deal with stenotic disease only: reports of successful endovascular treatment of complete occlusions are few (40,41).

There are no data to indicate whether visceral artery lesions should be treated by PTA or stents, or whether balloon expandable stents should be used in preference to self-expanding stents. Early series involved PTA alone (42,43). More recent series have used stents either exclusively (41,44,45) or selectively (37,38). These have not shown convincing superiority of stents over angioplasty, but there are no large series and certainly no controlled trials. Reintervention seems to be required in about 50% of cases that are followed up (44,45). Whereas balloon expandable stents are preferred in the renal arteries by virtue of being relatively easy to place accurately, other criteria apply in the visceral arteries. SMA stenoses may involve a longer segment of vessel and therefore may require a longer stent than those designed for the renal arteries. Hence a self-expanding stent may be preferred for visceral artery stenoses, although, anecdotally, either type is satisfactory (Figs. 8 and 10). Compression of the celiac axis by the median arcuate ligament could result in deformation of a stent. A balloon expandable stent could be permanently deformed, whereas a self-expanding stent usually reverts to its predetermined shape when the pressure relaxes.

The IMA is frequently totally occluded in these patients with severe aortic atheroma. This does not usually have clinical sequelae, the IMA territory being supplied by collaterals from SMA and internal iliacs. IMA revascularization is therefore rarely performed, and published experience is limited to a few case reports. The durability of stent placement in the IMA is unknown. The IMA is a small vessel, measuring only 3 to 4 mm diameter. By analogy with renal vessels, one would expect a lower long-term patency rate in the smaller caliber vessel. Isolated case reports exist of IMA intervention as the only option to revascularize the gut in the presence of celiac and SMA occlusion (46,47).

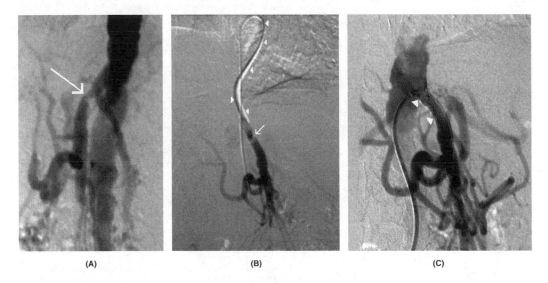

(A)   (B)   (C)

FIGURE 10   Superior mesenteric artery (SMA) stent placement from a femoral approach. (**A**) Lateral aortogram shows severe ostial stenosis of the SMA. (**B**) The SMA is catheterized using a sidewinder catheter from the groin. (**C**) A Palmaz Genesis balloon expandable stent has been deployed. The hairpin bend is technically challenging, but is partially straightened by the stiff 0.018-in. SV-5 wire. *Abbreviation*: SMA, superior mesenteric artery.

Clinical Effectiveness

Satisfactory clinical improvement with resolution of pain and weight gain is achieved in the short term in about 80% to 90% of patients following revascularization. The relative efficacy of endovascular intervention versus conventional surgical bypass is unknown. The consensus is that the endovascular approach carries less operative risk, but inferior durability compared with surgery (45). Repeat intervention is frequently required to maintain patency following angioplasty or stent placement: Landis and colleagues reported an average of 1.9 interventions per patient (48). However, bearing in mind that these patients are typically severely malnourished, and have widespread vascular comorbidity, the lower risk strategy is attractive. The percutaneous approach is not without risk: brachial hematoma (38), CE (49) and flow-limiting dissection (48) have been reported. Restenosis of a visceral stent may result in thrombosis, which could cause infarction of the gut with probably fatal consequences (45). Endovascular treatment may be used as a bridge to more definitive treatment: surgical bypass can be performed more safely after a suitable interval, once the patient has regained weight (45,50).

CONCLUSION

Renal artery intervention appears to be effective in the management of hypertension due to FMD, but of doubtful value when the etiology is atherosclerosis. In atherosclerosis, improved patency can be achieved with the use of stents compared with balloon angioplasty alone. Renal artery stenting can produce dramatic clinical improvement, such as the recovery of renal function in patients on dialysis, and in patients with flash pulmonary edema, although such cases are uncommon. In most cases, however, the value of renal artery intervention in the preservation of renal function is uncertain. On-going large scale randomized trials will hopefully provide important information in this respect.

Visceral artery intervention for the treatment of mesenteric ischemia is less commonly undertaken. When successful there is a high probability that symptoms will be improved. However, recurrence of stenosis is not uncommon and repeat intervention is frequently required whether or not stents are used. Surgical treatment for visceral artery stenosis appears more durable albeit with higher operative risk.

REFERENCES

1. Kaatee R, Beek FJA, Verschuyl EJ, et al. Atherosclerotic renal artery stenosis: ostial or truncal? Radiology 1996; 199:637–40.
2. Rathod KR, Deshmukh HL, Garg AI, et al. Spectrum of angiographic findings in aortoarteritis. Clin Radiol 2005; 60:746–55.
3. Mailloux LU, Bellucci AG, Napolitano B, et al. Survival estimates for 683 patients starting dialysis from 1970 through 1989: identification of risk factors for survival. Clin Nephrol 1994; 42:127–35.
4. Van de Ven PJG, Kaatee JJ, Beek FJA, et al. Arterial stening and balloon angioplasty in ostial atherosclerotic renovascular disease: a randomised trial. Lancet 1999; 353:282–6.
5. Alhadad A, Mattiasson I, Ivancev K, et al. Sustained beneficial effects on blood pressure during long time retrospective follow-up after endovascular treatment of renal artery occlusion. J Hum Hypertens 2004; 18:739–44.
6. Dwyer KM, Vrazas JI, Lodge RS, et al. Treatment of acute renal failure caused by renal artery occlusion with renal artery angioplasty. Am J Kidney Dis 2002; 40:189–94.
7. Boyer L, Ravel A, Boissier A, et al. Percuatneous recanalization of recent renal artery occlusions: report of 10 cases. Cardiovasc Intervent Radiol 1994; 17:258–63.
8. Kessel DO, Robertson I, Edward JT, Patel JV. Renal stenting from the radial artery: a novel approach. Cardiovasc Intervent Radiol 2003; 26:146–9.
9. Tanemoto M, Abe T, Chaki T, et al. Cutting balloon angioplasty of resistant renal artery stenosis caused by fibromuscular dysplasia. J Vasc Surg 2005; 41:898–901.
10. Haas NA, Ocker V, Knirsch W, et al. Successful management of a resistant renal artery stenosis in an child using a 4 mm cutting balloon catheter. Catheter Cardiovasc Interv 2002; 56:227–31.
11. Oquzkurt L, Tercan F, Gulcan O, et al. Rupture of the renal artery after cutting balloon angioplasty in a young woman with fibromuscular dyplasia. Cardiovasc Intervent Radiol 2005; 28:360–3.
12. Caramella T, Lahoche A, Negaiwi Z, et al. False aneurysm formation following cutting balloon angioplasty in the renal artery of a child. J Endovasc Ther 2005; 12:746–9.
13. Lupattelli T, Nano G, Inglese L. Regarding cutting balloon angioplasty of renal fibromuscular dysplasia: a word of caution. J Vasc Surg 2005; 42:1038–9.
14. Munneke GJ, Engelke C, Morgan RA, Belli A-M. Cutting balloon angioplasty for resistant renal artery in-stent restenosis. J Vasc Interv Radiol 2002; 13:327–31.
15. Ramsay LE, Waller PC. Blood pressure response to percutaneous transluminal angioplasty for renovascular hypertension: an overview of published series. Br Med J 1990; 300:569–72.
16. Alhadad A, Mattiasson I, Ivancev K, et al. Revascularisation of renal artery stenosis caused by fibromuscular dysplasia: effects on blood pressure during 7-year follow-up are influenced by duration of hypertension and branch artery stenosis. J Hum Hypertens 2005; 19:761–7.
17. Tyagi S, Singh B, Kaul UA, et al. Balloon angioplasty for renovascular hypertension in Takayasu's arteritis. Am Heart J 1993; 125:1386–93.
18. Martin LG, Casarella WJ, Gaylord GM. Azotemia caused by renal artery stenosis: treatment by percutaneous angioplasty. AJR 1988; 150:839–44.
19. Canzanello VJ, Millan VG, Spiegel JE, et al. Percutaneous renal angioplasty in the management of atherosclerotic renovascular hypertension: results in 100 patients. Hypertension 1989; 13:163–72.
20. Van Jaarsveld BC, Krijnen P, Pieterman H, et al. The effect of balloon angioplasty on hypertension in atherosclerotic renal-artery stenosis. N Engl J Med 2000; 342:1007–14.
21. Webster J, Marshall F, Abdalla M, et al. Randomised comparison of percutaneous angioplasty vs continued medical therapy for hypertensive patients with atheromatous renal artery stenosis. J Hum Hypertens 1998; 12:329–35.
22. Plouin PF, Chatelier G, Darné B, Raynaud A. Blood pressure outcome of angioplasty in atherosclerotic renal artery stenosis: a randomized trial. Hypertension 1998; 31:823–9.
23. Ives NJ, Wheatley K, Stowe RL, et al. Continuing uncertainty about the value or percutaneous revascularisation in atherosclerotic renovascular disease: a meta-analysis of randomized trials. Nephrol Dial Transplant 2003; 18:298–304.
24. Weibull H, Bergqvist D, Bergentz S-E, et al. Percutaneous transluminal renal angioplasty versus surgical reconstruction of atherosclerotic renal artery stenosis: a prospective randomized study. J Vasc Surg 1993; 18:841–52.
25. Pickering TG, Devereux RB, James GD, et al. Recurrent pulmonary oedema in hypertension due to bilateral renal artery stenosis: treatment by angioplasty or surgical revascularisation. Lancet 1988; ii:551–2.
26. Missouris CG, Buckenham T, Vallance PJT, MacGregor GA. Renal artery stenosis masquerading as congestive heart failure. Lancet 1993; 341:1521–2.

27. Harden PN, MacLeod MJ, Rodger RSC, et al. Effect of renal-artery stenting on progression of renovascular renal failure. Lancet 1997; 349:1133–6.
28. Murphy TP, Cooper CJ, Dworkin LD, et al. The cardiovascular outcomes with renal atherosclerotic lesions (CORAL) study: rationale and methods. J Vasc Interv Radiol 2005; 16:1295–300.
29. Beek FJ, Kaatee R, Beutler JJ, et al. Complications during renal artery stent placement for atherosclerotic ostial stenosis. Cardiovasc Intervent Radiol 1997; 20:184–90.
30. Henry M, Henry I, Klonaris C, et al. Renal angioplasty and stenting under protection: the way for the future? Catheter Cardiovasc Interv 2003; 60:299–312.
31. Hagspiel KD, Stone JR, Leung DA. Renal angioplasty and stent placement with distal protection: preliminary experience with the FilterWire EX. J Vasc Interv Radiol 2005; 16:125–31.
32. Sapoval M, Zähringer M, Pattynama P, et al. Low-profile stent system for treatment of atherosclerotic renal artery stenosis: the GREAT trial. J Vasc Interv Radiol 2005; 16:1195–202.
33. Chalmers N, Jackson RW. Comparison of iodixanol and iohexol in renal impairment. Br J Radiol 1999; 72:701–3.
34. Aspelin P, Aubry P, Fransson S-G, et al. Nephrotoxic effects in high-risk patients undergoing angiography. N Engl J Med 2003; 348:491–9.
35. Park CM, Chung JW, Kim HB, et al. Celiac axis stenosis: incidence and etiologies in asymptomatic individuals. Korean J Radiol 2001; 2:8–13.
36. Lee VS, Morgan JN, Tan AGS, et al. Celiac artery compression by the median arcuate ligament: a pitfall of end-expiratory MR imaging. Radiology 2003; 228:437–42.
37. Matsumoto AH, Angle JF, Spinosa DJ, et al. Percutaneous transluminal angioplasty and stenting in the treatment of chronic mesenteric ischemia: results and longterm followup. J Am Coll Surg 2002; 194:S22–31.
38. Tamam C, Agaaicha A, Biard M, et al. Endovascular treatment of chronic mesenteric ischemia: results in 14 patients. Cardiovasc Interv Radiol 2004; 27:637–42.
39. Raghu C, Louvard Y. Transradial approach for percutaneous transluminal angioplasty and stenting in the treatment of chronic mesenteric ischaemia. Catheter Cardiovasc Interv 2004; 61:450–4.
40. Maleux G, Wilms G, Stockx L, et al. Percutaneous recanalization and stent placement in chronic proximal superior mesenteric artery occlusion. Eur Radiol 1997; 7:1228–30.
41. Sheeran SR, Murphy TP, Khwaja A, et al. Stent placement for treatment of mesenteric artery stenoses or occlusions. J Vasc Interv Radiol 1999; 10:861–7.
42. Matsumoto AH, Tegtmeyer CJ, Fitzcharles EK, et al. Percutaneous transluminal angioplasty of visceral arterial stenoses: results and long-term clinical follow-up. J Vasc Interv Radiol 1995; 6:165–74.
43. Maspes F, Mazzetti-di-Pietralata G, Gandini R, et al. Percutaneous transluminal angioplasty in the treatment of chronic mesenteric ischemia: results and 3 years of follow-up in 23 patients. Abdom Imaging 1998; 23:358 63.
44. Resch T, Lindh M, Dias N, et al. Endovascular recanalisation in occlusive mesenteric ischemia—feasibility and early results. Eur J Vasc Endovasc Surg 2005; 29:199–203.
45. Brown DJ, Schermerhorn ML, Powell RJ, et al. Mesenteric stenting for chronic mesenteric ischemia. J Vasc Surg 2005; 42:268–74.
46. Alam A, Uberoi R. Chronic mesenteric ischaemia treated by isolated angioplasty of the inferior mesenteric artery. Cardiovasc Intervent Radiol 2005; 28:536–8.
47. Akpinar E, Cil BE, Arat A, et al. Spontaneous recanalization of superior mesenteric artery occlusion following angioplasty and stenting of inferior mesenteric artery. Cardiovasc Intervent Radiol 2006; 29:137–9.
48. Landis MS, Rajan DK, Simons ME, et al. Percutaneous management of chronic mesenteric ischemia: outcomes after intervention. J Vasc Interv Radiol 2005; 16:1319–25.
49. Rose SC, Quigley TM, Raker EJ. Revascularization for chronic mesenteric ischemia: comparison of operative arterial bypass grafting and percutaneous transluminal angioplasty. J Vasc Interv Radiol 1995; 6:339–49.
50. Biebl M, Oldenburg WA, Paz-Fumagalli R, et al. Endovascular treatment as a bridge to successful surgical revascularization for chronic mesenteric ischemia. Am Surg 2004; 70:994–8.

21 Thoracic Aneurysms (Classification, Natural History, Indications for Open Repair, and Results of Surgery)

Anthony L. Estrera, Charles C. Miller III, Ali Azizzadeh, and Hazim J. Safi
Department of Cardiothoracic and Vascular Surgery, University of Texas at Houston Medical School, Memorial Hermann Heart and Vascular Institute, Houston, Texas, U.S.A.

CLASSIFICATION

In the mid-1950s, the first thoracoabdominal aortic aneurysm (TAAA) repairs were performed, initially with a homograft in 1955 then using a Dacron® (Invista, Wichita, Kansas, U.S.A.) tube graft in 1956. In the following decades, results of TAAA and descending thoracic aortic aneurysm (DTAA) repair varied tremendously from center to center. This was probably due to the lack of coherent methods of reporting and classifying these aneurysms.

This chapter describes the rationale for classification of DTAA and TAAA. In the last decade, our group began classifying descending thoracic aneurysms based upon whether they affected the upper half, lower half, or entire thoracic aorta, known as Extents A, B, and C, respectively (Fig. 1) (1). Type A involves the upper half, Type B involves the sixth intercostal space to T12, and Type C comprises the entire thoracic aorta. This classification system became meaningful when we demonstrated a significant association between the extent of the aneurysm and the neurologic injury during repair (2). This has obvious implications with regard to complete coverage during endovascular repairs of the descending thoracic aorta.

TAAA is an extensive aneurysm involving the thoracic aorta and varying degrees of the abdominal aorta. These are categorized by the modified "Crawford classification" (Fig. 2). Extent I is from the left subclavian to above the renal arteries. Extent II is from the left subclavian artery to below the renal arteries, and Extent III is from the sixth intercostal space to below the renal arteries. Extent IV involves the total abdominal aorta from T12 to below the renal arteries. Extent V, which has been described most recently, is from the sixth intercostal space to the suprarenal abdominal aorta. In the past, we found that the extent of the aneurysm correlated with a high incidence of neurological deficit, the highest being in Extent II and then Extents I, III, and IV. In the era of the clamp-and-sew technique, the clamp time and the extent of the aneurysm correlated to neurologic deficit. In Extent II, the overall incidence of neurological deficit was 31% with the clamp-and-sew technique (3).

INCIDENCE

Ruptured aortic aneurysm remains the 13th leading cause of death in the Western world with an increasing prevalence (4). This may be attributable to improved imaging techniques, increasing mean age of the population, and overall heightened awareness (5). The incidence of ruptured abdominal aortic aneurysm is estimated to be 9.2 cases per 100,000 person-years (6–8). The incidence of rupture thoracic aortic aneurysms (TAAs) and acute aortic dissection is estimated to be 2.7 and 3.0 cases per 100,000 person-years, respectively (9–12). The mean age of this population is between 59 and 69 years with a male-to-female ratio of 3:1 (9).

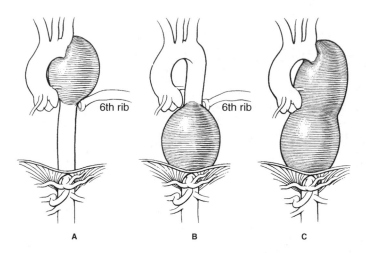

FIGURE 1 Descending thoracic aortic aneurysms are classified as: Type A, left subclavian artery to T6; Type B, T6 to the diaphragm; and Type C, left subclavian artery to the diaphragm.

ETIOLOGY

Arteriosclerosis has long been associated with aortic aneurysms. Atherosclerosis mainly affects the intima, causing occlusive disease, while aortic aneurysm is a disease of the media and adventitia. They are distinct conditions that nonetheless often occur together. An aortic aneurysm is typically characterized by a thinning of the media and destruction of smooth muscle cells and elastin as well as infiltration of inflammatory cells. The infiltrate consists of macrophages as well as lymphocytes T and B, which excrete proteases and elastases causing wall degradation (13). In both clinical and experimental studies, metalloproteinases, a most

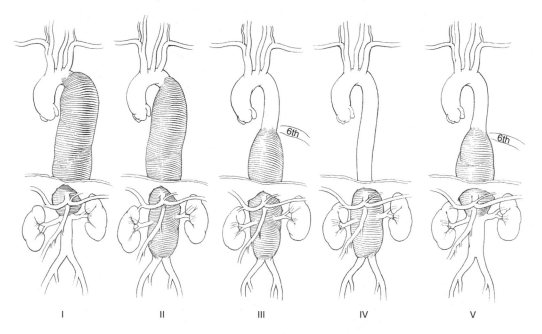

FIGURE 2 Thoracoabdominal aortic aneurysm classification. Extent I, distal to the left subclavian artery to above the renal arteries; Extent II, distal to the left subclavian artery to the below the renal arteries; Extent III, from the sixth intercostal space to below the renal arteries; Extent IV, the 12th intercostal space to the iliac bifurcation (total abdominal aortic aneurysm); and Extent V, below the sixth intercostal space to just above the renal arteries.

prominent group of elastases, have emerged as playing a role in the development of aortic aneurysms (13–16).

Familial clustering of aortic aneurysms is evident as up to 20% of patients have one or more first-degree relatives who have also suffered from the disease (17–19). Genetic mapping studies have recently identified a number of chromosomal loci that are responsible for familial thoracic aneurysms and dissections. A mutation in transforming growth factor-β receptor type II is responsible for approximately 5% of familial aneurysms and dissections (20). Future studies may further elucidate the role of genetics in this disease process.

Marfan syndrome, a connective tissue disorder causing skeletal, ocular, and cardiovascular abnormalities, is the disorder most commonly associated with TAAA, as well as aortic dissection. It occurs in approximately 1 in 5000 people worldwide. Aortic dilation in individuals with Marfan syndrome has been linked to a mutation in fibrillin-1. Other such disorders include Ehlers–Danlos syndrome, Turner syndrome, polycystic kidney disease, as well as other not yet identified familial disorders (21). In the majority of these families, the phenotypes for TAAA and dissection are inherited in an autosomal dominant manner with a marked variability in age and decreased penetrance (21).

At times, an aneurysm may be caused by an extrinsic factor, such as infection (mycotic aneurysm—see chap. 23) or trauma (pseudoaneurysm—see chap. 29). A mycotic aneurysm is caused by bacteria or septic emboli that seed the aortic wall. It can also result from a contiguous spread from empyema or adjacent infected lymph node. Though any organism can be the cause of a mycotic aneurysm, the most commonly described are the following: *Salmonella, Haemophilus influenza, Staphylococcus,* and *Treponema pallidum spirochetes* species (22,23).

There is also a connection between TAAA and aortic dissection. One-fourth of TAAA are associated with aortic dissection, and 24% of patients with an aortic dissection will develop TAAA within two to five years (17–19). Persistent patency of the false lumen has been shown to be a significant predictor for aneurysm formation, though neither dissection nor false lumen have been linked to higher risk of rupture (24–27).

NATURAL HISTORY

The survival rate for patients with untreated TAAs is dismal, estimated to be between 13% and 39% at five years (9,28–30). The lifetime probability of rupture in untreated thoracic aneurysms and TAA is between 75% and 80% (9,28). The most common cause of death is rupture (31). Moreover, the few patients who survive the operation for rupture sustain significant morbidity, prolonged hospital course, and, ultimately, a poor quality of life.

The time that elapses between aneurysm formation and rupture is influenced by aneurysm size and growth rate, hypertension, smoking, history of chronic obstructive pulmonary disease, presence of pain, etiology, and age. The size of the aortic aneurysm remains the single most important determinant of the likelihood of rupture. Rupture is more likely to occur in TAAs exceeding 5 cm in diameter with the likelihood increasing significantly as the aneurysm enlarges (28,32–35). Growth rate is a component in formulating the rate of rupture or indication for surgical intervention (32,36). The rate of growth is exponential with larger aneurysms growing at greater rates; at 0.12 cm/yr for aneurysms greater than 5.2 cm in diameter (36,37).

Hypertension and subsequent increased aortic wall tension play a significant role in aneurysm formation. Though systemic hypertension is widely recognized as a risk factor for aneurysm formation, it is diastolic blood pressure that has been specifically correlated with aneurysm rupture. Multiple reports have noted an association of increased diastolic blood pressure (greater than 100 mmHg) with rupture of both abdominal and TAAs (32,36,38). As was demonstrated by Wheat in his work on aortic dissections, decreasing the force of myocardial contraction or dp/dt may decrease the progression of disease and the likelihood of rupture (39). Consequently, many recommend that beta-adrenergic blocking agents be included in the antihypertensive treatment regimen for patients with known aortic aneurysms.

Although smoking has been implicated as a risk factor for rupture in abdominal aortic aneurysms (40,41), a stronger association with chronic obstructive pulmonary disease has been identified (32,36). In one study, chronic obstructive pulmonary disease was defined as a forced expiratory volume in one second of less than 50% of the predicted (41). This correlation may be related to the increased collagenase activity seen in smokers (42). It is theorized that the proteolytic activity may weaken the aortic wall of those patients who are susceptible (43). Patients with chronic obstructive pulmonary disease have demonstrated a connective tissue intolerance to smoke-related toxicity, which may be seen as an indicator of susceptibility (44). In addition, it has been documented that patients with a history of smoking have a more rapid expansion of thoracic aneurysms (36,45). This evidence further justifies the cessation of smoking in the presence of an aortic aneurysm.

Further implicated in the increased likelihood of aortic rupture are pain, chronic dissection and age. Vague or uncharacteristic pain in the presence of TAA has been significantly associated with subsequent rupture (32). Generally, the etiology of TAA has been attributed to a degenerative process. It has also been suggested that rupture is associated with chronic dissection, but the evidence is not compelling (9,46). In a prospective study by Juvonen et al. aneurysms associated with chronic dissection were observed to be smaller (median diameter of 5.4 cm) than degenerative aneurysms (median diameter of 5.8 cm) (26). Significant alterations in the structure of the aortic wall occur with aging that are distinct from the formation of aneurysms. However, age in TAA patients has been associated with increased risk of rupture (11). Furthermore, Juvonen et al. demonstrated that the relative risk for rupture increased by a factor of 2.6 for every decade of age (11).

The natural course of the majority of aortic aneurysms is rupture and death. Aneurysm size and growth rate, patient age, medical history and symptoms must be carefully weighed when considering when to intervene surgically. Elective surgery for TAA repair has been demonstrated to improve long-term survival (30). Methods have been devised to attempt to predict the risks of surgical repair for TAAs (32,36). Although these formulas may allow one to preoperatively stratify the risks of surgery for a patient, the decision to operate still remains with the clinician based upon clinical evaluation and the patient preference.

RESULTS

During the clamp-and-sew era, aortic cross-clamp time was the principal predictor of immediate postoperative neurologic deficit during repairs of the thoracic and thoracoabdominal aorta. In Crawford's experience with 1509 patients, aortic cross-clamp time greater than 60 minutes was associated with an overall incidence of paraplegia of 27% (3). The incidence of paraplegia in patients whose aortic cross-clamp time was less than 30 minutes was still significant at 8% (3). Our group reported similar findings when the clamp-and-go technique was used (47). The incidence of neurologic deficit ultimately led to the adoption of the combined adjuncts of distal aortic perfusion and cerebrospinal fluid (CSF) drainage.

Encouraged by the work of Hollier et al. with CSF drainage and Connolly's report using distal aortic perfusion for TAA repairs (48,49), it was hypothesized that by increasing distal aortic perfusion pressure, using left heart bypass in combination with decreasing CSF pressure with drainage, spinal cord perfusion could be improved. In the last 15 years, our group settled on the adjunct consisting of three elements: distal aortic perfusion, in which oxygenated blood is taken from the left atrium directly to the femoral artery via the left lower pulmonary vein using the centrifugal pump, CSF drainage, and moderate passive hypothermia, in which core temperature is allowed to drift to 33°C to 34°C.

Using this adjunct our group performed 1887 operations for ascending/arch or DTAA/TAAAs up until 2005. Seven hundred eighty-one of these cases involved the proximal aorta (ascending and transverse arch). The 30-day mortality in this group of patients was 11.5% (90/781). The stroke rate was 2.1% (16/781). During the same period, our group performed 1106 operations for repair of the distal aorta (DTAAs, $n=305$; TAAAs, $n=801$). The 30-day mortality rate was 14.5% with an immediate neurological deficit rate of 3.2%. It is important to emphasize that the mortality rate highly correlates with preoperative renal function as determined by calculated glomerular filtration rate (GFR). Patients with a GFR greater than

90 mL/min per 1.73 m^2 had a mortality rate of 5.6% compared to a rate of 27.8% in patients with a GFR less than 49 mL/min per 1.73 m^2 (50).

Aortic cross-clamp times have increased significantly (34 sec/yr) since 1991. Despite this increase in cross-clamp time, neurologic deficit rates have declined during this period. This decrease in neurologic deficit is most pronounced with the Extent II TAAAs (21.1 to 3.3%). The use of the adjunct (CSF drainage and distal aortic perfusion) increased the cross-clamp time by a mean of 12 minutes, but was associated with a significant protective effect against neurologic deficit. Although other previously established risk factors remained significantly associated with neurologic deficit, cross-clamp time is no longer significant (51). The use of the adjunct appears to blunt the effect of the cross-clamp time and may provide the surgeon the ability to operate without being hurried. Because cross-clamp time has been effectively eliminated as a risk factor with the use of the adjunct, using this variable to construct risk models becomes irrelevant in our experience.

In repairs of DTAAs, the incidence of neurologic deficit after all repairs was 2.3%. The incidence of neurologic deficit (immediate and delayed) in the adjunct group was 1.3%, and in the nonadjunct group was 6.5%. One case of delayed paraplegia occurred in each group. All neurologic deficits occurred in patients with aneurysmal involvement of the entire descending thoracic aorta. Statistically significant predictors for neurologic deficit were the use of the adjunct, previous repaired abdominal aortic aneurysm, type C aneurysm, and cerebrovascular disease history. Significant multivariate predictors of 30-day mortality were preoperative renal dysfunction and female gender.

Remarkable progress in the treatment of TAAAs has been achieved in the last decade. Morbidity and mortality have declined which has been attributed to the adoption of the adjuncts distal aortic perfusion and CSF drainage as well as the evolution of surgical techniques to include sequential aortic cross-clamp, intercostal artery reattachment and moderate hypothermia. Currently, the overall incidence of neurological deficit in DTAA is 0.8% and mortality rate in patients with normal renal function is 5%.

The introduction of endovascular repair has added a new approach to the armamentarium of surgeons treating this disease. Currently available technology is limited by patients' anatomical criteria. Future advances will widen the availability of this approach to a larger group of patients.

For now, aortic surgeons need to maintain expertise in both open and endovascular approaches. Regardless of the technique, we believe complex aortic aneurysms should be treated in centers with the capability and experience necessary to manage this challenging group of patients.

REFERENCES

1. Estrera AL, Rubenstein FS, Miller CC, III, et al. Descending thoracic aortic aneurysm: surgical approach and treatment using the adjuncts cerebrospinal fluid drainage and distal aortic perfusion. Ann Thorac Surg 2001; 72(2):481–6.
2. Estrera AL, Miller CC, III, Chen EP, et al. Descending thoracic aortic aneurysm repair: 12-year experience using distal aortic perfusion and cerebrospinal fluid drainage. Ann Thorac Surg 2005; 80(4):1290–6 (Discussion 1296).
3. Svensson LG, Crawford ES, Hess KR, et al. Experience with 1509 patients undergoing thoracoabdominal aortic operations. J Vasc Surg 1993; 17(2):357–68 (Discussion 368–70).
4. Coady MA, Rizzo JA, Goldstein LJ, et al. Natural history, pathogenesis, and etiology of thoracic aortic aneurysms and dissections. Cardiol Clin 1999; 17(4):615–35 (vii).
5. LaRoy LL, Cormier PJ, Matalon TA, et al. Imaging of abdominal aortic aneurysms. AJR Am J Roentgenol 1989; 152(4):785–92.
6. Svensjo S, Bengtsson H, Bergqvist D. Thoracic and thoracoabdominal aortic aneurysm and dissection: an investigation based on autopsy. Br J Surg 1996; 83(1):68–71.
7. Bickerstaff LK, Hollier LH, Van Peenen HJ, et al. Abdominal aortic aneurysms: the changing natural history. J Vasc Surg 1984; 1(1):6–12.
8. Choksy SA, Wilmink AB, Quick CR. Ruptured abdominal aortic aneurysm in the Huntingdon district: a 10-year experience. Ann R Coll Surg Engl 1999; 81(1):27–31.
9. Bickerstaff LK, Pairolero PC, Hollier LH, et al. Thoracic aortic aneurysms: a population-based study. Surgery 1982; 92(6):1103–8.

10. Clouse WD, Hallett JW, Jr., Schaff HV, et al. Acute aortic dissection: population-based incidence compared with degenerative aortic aneurysm rupture. Mayo Clin Proc 2004; 79(2):176–80.
11. Johansson G, Markstrom U, Swedenborg J. Ruptured thoracic aortic aneurysms: a study of incidence and mortality rates. J Vasc Surg 1995; 21(6):985–8.
12. Meszaros I, Morocz J, Szlavi J, et al. Epidemiology and clinicopathology of aortic dissection. Chest 2000; 117(5):1271–8.
13. Ailawadi G, Eliason JL, Upchurch GR, Jr. Current concepts in the pathogenesis of abdominal aortic aneurysm. J Vasc Surg 2003; 38(3):584–8.
14. Longo GM, Xiong W, Greiner TC, et al. Matrix metalloproteinases 2 and 9 work in concert to produce aortic aneurysms. J Clin Invest 2002; 110(5):625–32.
15. Annabi B, Shedid D, Ghosn P, et al. Differential regulation of matrix metalloproteinase activities in abdominal aortic aneurysms. J Vasc Surg 2002; 35(3):539–46.
16. McMillan WD, Pearce WH. Increased plasma levels of metalloproteinase-9 are associated with abdominal aortic aneurysms. J Vasc Surg 1999; 29(1):122–7 (Discussion 127–9).
17. Biddinger A, Rocklin M, Coselli J, et al. Familial thoracic aortic dilatations and dissections: a case control study. J Vasc Surg 1997; 25(3):506–11.
18. Coady MA, Davies RR, Roberts M, et al. Familial patterns of thoracic aortic aneurysms. Arch Surg 1999; 134(4):361–7.
19. Hasham SN, Willing MC, Guo DC, et al. Mapping a locus for familial thoracic aortic aneurysms and dissections (TAAD2) to 3p24-25. Circulation 2003; 107(25):3184–90.
20. Pannu H, Fadulu VT, Chang J, et al. Mutations in transforming growth factor-beta receptor type II cause familial thoracic aortic aneurysms and dissections. Circulation 2005; 112(4):513–20.
21. Milewicz DM, Chen H, Park ES, et al. Reduced penetrance and variable expressivity of familial thoracic aortic aneurysms/dissections. Am J Cardiol 1998; 82(4):474–9.
22. Jarrett F, Darling RC, Mundth ED, et al. Experience with infected aneurysms of the abdominal aorta. Arch Surg 1975; 110(11):1281–6.
23. Bakker-de Wekker P, Alfieri O, Vermeulen F, et al. Surgical treatment of infected pseudoaneurysms after replacement of the ascending aorta. J Thorac Cardiovasc Surg 1984; 88(3):447–51.
24. Bernard Y, Zimmermann H, Chocron S, et al. False lumen patency as a predictor of late outcome in aortic dissection. Am J Cardiol 2001; 87(12):1378–82.
25. Marui A, Mochizuki T, Mitsui N, et al. Toward the best treatment for uncomplicated patients with type B acute aortic dissection: A consideration for sound surgical indication. Circulation 1999; 100(19):II275–80.
26. Juvonen T, Ergin MA, Galla JD, et al. Risk factors for rupture of chronic type B dissections. J Thorac Cardiovasc Surg 1999; 117(4):776–86.
27. Sueyoshi E, Sakamoto I, Hayashi K, et al. Growth rate of aortic diameter in patients with type B aortic dissection during the chronic phase. Circulation 2004; 110(11 Suppl. 1):II256–61.
28. Perko MJ, Norgaard M, Herzog TM, et al. Unoperated aortic aneurysm: a survey of 170 patients. Ann Thorac Surg 1995; 59(5):1204–9.
29. Pressler V, McNamara JJ. Thoracic aortic aneurysm: natural history and treatment. J Thorac Cardiovasc Surg 1980; 79(4):489–98.
30. Crawford ES, DeNatale RW. Thoracoabdominal aortic aneurysm: observations regarding the natural course of the disease. J Vasc Surg 1986; 3(4):578–82.
31. Bonser RS, Pagano D, Lewis ME, et al. Clinical and patho-anatomical factors affecting expansion of thoracic aortic aneurysms. Heart 2000; 84(3):277–83.
32. Juvonen T, Ergin MA, Galla JD, et al. Prospective study of the natural history of thoracic aortic aneurysms. Ann Thorac Surg 1997; 63(6):1533–45.
33. Lobato AC, Puech-Leao P. Predictive factors for rupture of thoracoabdominal aortic aneurysm. J Vasc Surg 1998; 27(3):446–53.
34. Elefteriades JA, Hartleroad J, Gusberg RJ, et al. Long-term experience with descending aortic dissection: the complication-specific approach. Ann Thorac Surg 1992; 53(1):11–20 (Discussion 20–1).
35. Cambria RA, Gloviczki P, Stanson AW, et al. Outcome and expansion rate of 57 thoracoabdominal aortic aneurysms managed nonoperatively. Am J Surg 1995; 170(2):213–7.
36. Dapunt OE, Galla JD, Sadeghi AM, et al. The natural history of thoracic aortic aneurysms. J Thorac Cardiovasc Surg 1994; 107(5):1323–32 (Discussion 1332–3).
37. Rizzo JA, Coady MA, Elefteriades JA. Procedures for estimating growth rates in thoracic aortic aneurysms. J Clin Epidemiol 1998; 51(9):747–54.
38. Szilagyi DE, Smith RF, DeRusso FJ, et al. Contribution of abdominal aortic aneurysmectomy to prolongation of life. Ann Surg 1966; 164(4):678–99.
39. Palmer RF, Wheat MW. Management of impending rupture of the aorta with dissection. Adv Intern Med 1971; 17:409–23.
40. Strachan DP. Predictors of death from aortic aneurysm among middle-aged men: the Whitehall study. Br J Surg 1991; 78(4):401–4.

41. Cronenwett JL, Murphy TF, Zelenock GB, et al. Actuarial analysis of variables associated with rupture of small abdominal aortic aneurysms. Surgery 1985; 98(3):472–83.
42. Cannon DJ, Read RC. Blood elastolytic activity in patients with aortic aneurysm. Ann Thorac Surg 1982; 34(1):10–5.
43. Busuttil RW, Abou-Zamzam AM, Machleder HI. Collagenase activity of the human aorta: a comparison of patients with and without abdominal aortic aneurysms. Arch Surg 1980; 115(11):1373–8.
44. Ergin MA, Spielvogel D, Apaydin A, et al. Surgical treatment of the dilated ascending aorta: when and how? Ann Thorac Surg 1999; 67(6):1834–9 (Discussion 1853–6).
45. Lindholt JS, Jorgensen B, Fasting H, et al. Plasma levels of plasmin–antiplasmin-complexes are predictive for small abdominal aortic aneurysms expanding to operation-recommendable sizes. J Vasc Surg 2001; 34(4):611–5.
46. Pitt MP, Bonser RS. The natural history of thoracic aortic aneurysm disease: an overview. J Card Surg 1997; 12(2):270–8.
47. Safi HJ, Bartoli S, Hess KR, et al. Neurologic deficit in patients at high risk with thoracoabdominal aortic aneurysms: the role of cerebral spinal fluid drainage and distal aortic perfusion. J Vasc Surg 1994; 20(3):434–44 (Discussion 442–3).
48. Hollier LH, Money SR, Naslund TC, et al. Risk of spinal cord dysfunction in patients undergoing thoracoabdominal aortic replacement. Am J Surg 1992; 164(3):210–3 (Discussion 213–4).
49. Connolly JE, Wakabayashi A, German JC, et al. Clinical experience with pulsatile left heart bypass without anticoagulation for thoracic aneurysms. J Thorac Cardiovasc Surg 1971; 62(4):568–76.
50. Huynh TT, van Eps RG, Miller CC, III, et al. Glomerular filtration rate is superior to serum creatinine for prediction of mortality after thoracoabdominal aortic surgery. J Vasc Surg 2005; 42(2):206–12.
51. Safi HJ, Estrera AL, Miller CC, et al. Evolution of risk for neurologic deficit after descending and thoracoabdominal aortic repair. Ann Thorac Surg 2005; 80(6):2173–9 (Discussion 2179).

22 | Thoracic Aneurysms (Endovascular Repair)

Adam Howard
Department of Vascular and Endovascular Surgery, St. George's Healthcare NHS Trust, London, U.K.

Ian M. Loftus
St. George's Vascular Institute, St. George's Hospital, London, U.K.

INDICATIONS FOR ENDOVASCULAR REPAIR

Patients with degenerative thoracic aortic aneurysms (TAAs) have a reduced life expectancy when compared to an age-matched disease-free population. Five-year survival rates if untreated range from 13% to 39%, the principle cause of death being rupture (1–3). The true incidence and prevalence of TAAs is difficult to ascertain due to the silent nature of the condition, and estimates are derived largely from post-mortem studies. Epidemiological studies suggest an incidence of 10.4 per 100,000 patient years, though this is increasing with rising life expectancy and improved cross-sectional imaging (4). The natural history involves progressive expansion, eventually leading to aneurysm rupture which is usually fatal. Expansion is strongly associated with maximal diameter, increasing exponentially with increasing aneurysm size (1–3,5). Other factors related to TAA expansion are location in the descending aorta and the presence of thrombus (6,7). Patient factors thought to influence expansion include age, hypertension, smoking, and chronic obstructive pulmonary disease (8–10).

Intervention is indicated in the presence of symptoms, rapid dilatation, significant compression of surrounding structures and rupture. The diameter threshold for intervention varies from 50 to 70 mm depending on the patient population, coexisting comorbidity, and anatomical complexity. The timing of intervention is based on the balance of risk of rupture and of the procedure, in terms of mortality and morbidity. Open thoracoabdominal aortic aneurysms repair is complex and confers significant potential morbidity, including cardio-respiratory compromise, stroke and paraplegia rates, and renal impairment. The mortality rate is reported to be as high as 30%, with one- and five-year survival rates of 75% to 82% and 50% to 60% respectively in large-volume specialized centers (5,6,11–15). The risks increase further with emergency surgery.

Conversely thoracic endovascular aneurysm repair (TEVAR) offers significant potential advantages over open repair, reflected by apparent reductions in mortality and morbidity. The cause of this effect is multifactorial, related to preservation of aortic blood flow during deployment, avoiding thoracotomy with associated extensive dissection, left lung collapse, and aortic cross-clamping. With the first-generation stent grafts, respective one- and five-year survival rates of 93% and 78% were reported (16). As TEVAR has become more established and further generations of devices developed, a number of series have reported encouraging short- and mid-term results (17–19). Advances in stent-graft technology and the use of aortic debranching-procedures to extend landing zones, have increased the proportion of descending thoracic aneurysms anatomically suitable for TEVAR to 70% to 80% (20).

Due to the lack of clinical equipoise, randomized controlled trials for TAA similar to those performed for abdominal aortic aneurysms (21–23) have not been performed. The trials that have been performed have often been undertaken for regulatory purposes with restricted anatomical criteria, and do not reflect everyday clinical practice. Outcome data rely on individual series and registries, though these are difficult to compare with historical data for open repairs as the patient populations and patho-morphologies are not homogeneous.

The published data regarding TEVAR generally comprise mixed aortic pathology and includes patients unfit for open surgery. Results may also be influenced by learning curves and developments in endovascular techniques and devices.

Together with the apparent benefits in mortality, there are obvious clinical advantages. TEVAR can be performed under regional or local anesthesia. Cardiovascular stability during the procedure is better, and there seems to be a reduced incidence of spinal cord ischemia (SCI) and subsequent paraplegia. Postoperative recovery is quicker, mirrored by a reduced length of hospital stay.

As a consequence of these promising results, TEVAR has become the first line treatment modality for a wide variety of thoracic aortic pathologies. It is now increasingly common practice to treat TAA with unfavorable anatomy, perform hybrid procedures for the aortic arch and thoraco-abdominal aneurysms and repair ruptured thoracic aneurysms using endovascular techniques.

Some thoracic aortic pathologies have less well-defined indications for intervention, in particular chronic type B dissections (CTBD). Most clinicians accept that intervention is warranted in the presence of intractable pain, aneurysmal expansion to greater than 5.5 cm, side branch complications and rupture. Successful stent-graft placement with closure of entry tears and subsequent thrombosis of the false lumen leads to aortic remodeling. Other indications are less clear, particularly for stable dissections. The treatment of persistent and dilating false lumens is complex. There is evidence to suggest that persistent perfusion of the false lumen predisposes to aneurysmal dilatation and consequent risk of rupture. The endovasular management and results for TAA and CTBD will be discussed in this chapter.

PREOPERATIVE IMAGING

Computed Tomography

Post-imaging processing using specific vascular protocols can provide an array of three-dimensional reconstructions and simulations of conventional angiography. A large number of axial images taken during the "arterial phase" combined with multiplanar reconstructions can provide computed tomographic angiography. The extent and nature of the aortic disease can then be accurately evaluated and measured for stent-graft repair. Computed tomography (CT) can delineate aneurismal dilatation, intraluminal thrombus, aortic wall calcification and compression of peri-aortic structures such as the left main bronchus and pulmonary artery. The disadvantages of CT include the contrast load and radiation exposure (the equivalent of 3 to 400 chest X-rays per thoracoabdominal CT). Patients with abnormal renal function should be well hydrated with intravenous fluids prior to the scan, but the prophylactic use of N-acetylcysteine is controversial.

Angiography

Conventional aortography has largely been replaced by CT angiography, though may still be useful for detailed anatomical measurements of landing zones and assessment of side branches. Three-dimensional reconstructions are possible with improvements in rotational angiography. In addition, standard angiography is sometimes required to assess diseased access vessels. Angiography has the disadvantage of being invasive and requiring an intra-arterial injection of contrast media.

Duplex Ultrasound

Ultrasound is not routinely used in the thorax because the air content of the lungs generates a poor image quality. However, Duplex ultrasound is an important part of the preoperative assessment to evaluate the carotid and vertebral circulation, the left subclavian artery (LSA), and the iliac arteries for stent-graft access. In the presence of significant carotid disease imaging of the circle of Willis is indicated with magnetic resonance angiography (MRA) to establish the status of the cerebral collateral circulation.

Magnetic Resonance

MRA is performed with intravenously injected paramagnetic contrast such as gadolinium. High performance gradient systems and high resolution three-dimensional imaging can chase a single contrast bolus throughout the whole body for MRA, albeit in 45 minutes. MRA in the arterial phase only demonstrates the aortic lumen with aneurysm morphology provided by post-contrast images. MRA is not suitable in some patients due to the time required to complete the scan, though it is preferable in patients with renal impairment or with contrast allergy.

Transesophageal Echocardiography

Transesophageal echocardiography (TOE) can provide short axis (axial) and long axis images of the descending aorta to the level of the stomach. Atherosclerosis of the aorta can be assessed and graded. The benefits of TOE include the absence of contrast, though many patients find the test uncomfortable. In addition the quality of the images are operator dependent and the service is not readily available in some centers. Incidentally, trans-thoracic echocardiography is commonly performed in patients as part of the optimization process prior to TEVAR.

MORPHOLOGICAL REQUIREMENTS

Thoracic stent grafts were originally modified designs of abdominal aortic endoprotheses. However, thoracic aortic pathology confers specific challenges including the ability of a stent graft to conform to the aortic arch, the ability to track and deploy the device around the aortic arch, and gain secure and accurate fixation. More recent third-generation thoracic devices have adapted to the specific challenges posed by thoracic aortic pathology by extensive stent graft and delivery device modifications. These have led to significant shifts in the anatomical suitability for TEVAR including the ability to treat aneurysms in tortuous aortas, with limited proximal and distal fixation zones, and pathologies of the aortic arch and thoracoabdominal aorta (24–26).

There remain a number of anatomical parameters that are required to enable successful TEVAR. The aortic diameter at the level of the proximal landing zone needs to less than 40 mm because the largest commercially available stent is 46 mm, though it is possible to order larger customized stents. In order to achieve an adequate seal a proximal landing zone of 20 mm on the lesser curve of the aortic arch is usually required (Fig. 1). The proximal end of the stent graft will sit perpendicular to this landing zone and may cover the left subclavian or left common carotid arteries. The landing zone cannot include an acutely angled arch as the stent may lie proud over the angle and not form a tight circumferential seal. The LSA can be covered by the stent graft and the subsequent incidence of left arm ischemia is low. The role of LSA revascularization, by carotid–subclavian bypass or subclavian–carotid transposition, is controversial. There is some evidence that the incidence of spinal ischemia and left posterior circulation compromise is higher in patients who do not undergo revascularization (27–30). This will be discussed further.

If a landing zone is required more proximally, covering the origin of the left common carotid artery, more extensive debranching procedures are required; such as a right-to-left carotid–carotid and carotid–subclavian bypass (Fig. 2).

The tortuosity of the descending aorta may cause difficulties with endograft placement and fixation, though the latest generation devices have improved tracking capability, flexibility and kink resistance (24–26). A horizontal section of the aorta distal to the aneurysm may appear angiographically favorable for the distal landing zone, but has the potential to undergo continued dilatation and subsequent poor long-term distal fixation. At least 15 mm of normal aorta is required for the distal landing zone. If the only suitable distal landing zone is within the infrarenal aorta then a hybrid procedure with mesenteric and renal revascularization may be considered. Unless the aneurysm is very localized, it is preferable to stent the whole of the descending thoracic aorta (Figs. 3 and 4). To increase the distal landing zone without celiac revascularization, there are reports of uncomplicated stenting over the origin of

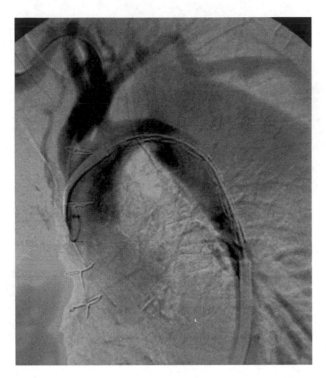

FIGURE 1 Proximal landing zone within the distal aortic arch.

the celiac trunk in selected patients with a proven collateral circulation to the superior mesenteric artery (31). This technique requires further evaluation and cannot be recommended for routine practice. Another technique used to lengthen the distal landing zone is to use a reversed "open web" thoracic stent graft (Fig. 5) to seal around the celiac trunk without covering the origin which in selected high-risk cases may negate the need for visceral revascularization.

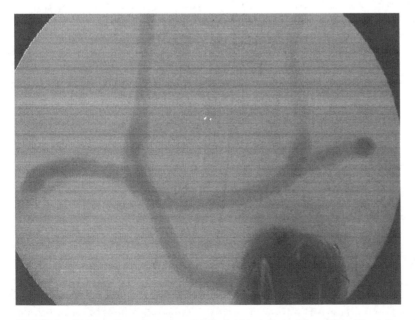

FIGURE 2 Distal aortic arch stent graft with right-to-left carotid–carotid with a left carotid to left subclavian bypass.

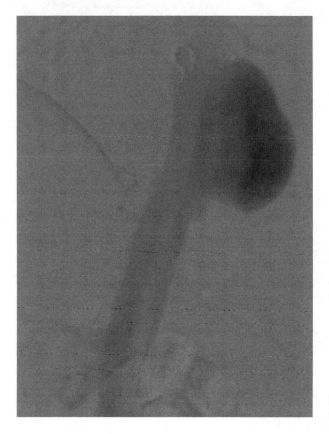

FIGURE 3 Stent grafting of a localized descending thoracic aneurysm.

Other anatomical considerations include the diameter and tortuosity of the iliac arteries, and the presence of extensive calcification. For most of the commercially available devices, a minimum iliac diameter of 7 mm in the absence of significant calcification, is required for stent graft delivery. If the iliac vessels are too small or heavily calcified, alternative access may be required. An iliac conduit may be used, or access gained through the carotid or subclavian arteries. If simultaneous open infrarenal repair is required, this can be used for access.

RESULTS: MORTALITY AND MORBIDITY

Degenerative Distal Arch and Descending TAAs

TEVAR has been successfully used in the emergency setting to treat acute aortic syndromes and aortic transections, and electively to treat degenerative aneurysmal disease and chronic dissection.

The European Collaborators on Stent/Graft Techniques for Aortic Aneurysm Repair (EUROSTAR) and U.K. Thoracic Registries reported a multicenter experience of 443 patients who underwent TEVAR; consisting of degenerative aneurysms ($n=249$), aortic dissections ($n=131$), false aneurysms ($n=13$) and traumatic injuries ($n=50$) (17). The initial ($n=443$) and one-year ($n=195$) outcomes were recorded. In the "degenerative aneurysm group" 69% were elective, 24% emergency and 7% unclassified. The anatomical and procedural details are shown in Table 1. The majority of stents were placed in the proximal and mid-thoracic aorta for TAA with a primary success rate of 87%. The origin of the LSA was covered in 17% of patients; half undergoing left subclavian revascularization.

The 30 day mortality rates for the TAA group was 10% (5.3% and 27.9% for elective and emergency procedures respectively). The cumulative one-year survival rate was 80%, with a 1% late rupture rate. The one year outcomes are summarized in Table 2.

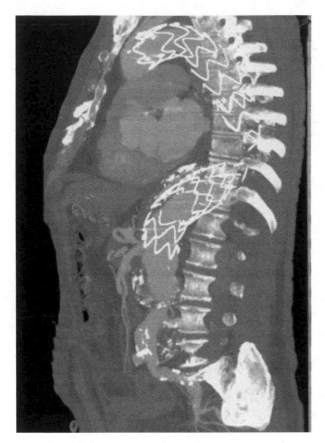

FIGURE 4 Stent grafting of a descending thoracic aneurysm to the celiac trunk.

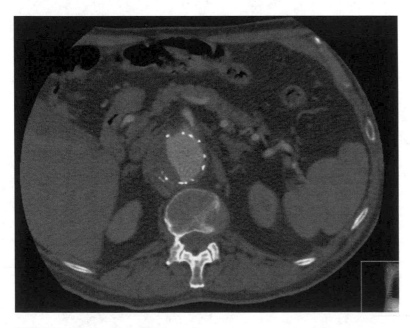

FIGURE 5 Reverse stent graft.

TABLE 1 Anatomical and Procedural Details of Patients with Degenerative TAA

	Percentage of patients ($n=249$)
Location of TAA	
Ascending aorta	0
Aortic arch	13.9
Proximal descending thoracic aorta	51.9
Mid-descending thoracic aorta	50.3
Distal descending thoracic aorta	37.4
Regional or local anesthesia	15.2
Access artery	
Femoral artery	78.8
Iliac artery	11.2
Abdominal aorta	5.2
Number of stents used	
1 stent only	34.1
2 stents	36.5
$\geq$3 stents	25.7
Additional procedures	
Endovascular	23.3
Surgical	26.4

Abbreviation: TAA, thoracic aortic aneurysms.
Source: Modified from Ref. 17.

The Talent Thoracic Retrospective Registry reported the results from 457 consecutive patients who underwent TEVAR (344 elective and 113 emergency) with the Talent™ (Medtronic Ave Inc., Santa Rosa, California, U.S.A.) stent graft. The interventions were for a spectrum of aortic diseases, predominantly aortic dissections (39.4%) and degenerative TAA (30%). The results were presented for the entire cohort and not for individual pathologies. The in-hospital mortality rate was 5.1% (4.1% and 7.9% for elective and emergency respectively). The most frequent in-hospital complications were stroke (3.7%) and local vascular injury during the

TABLE 2 Thirty-Day and One-Year Complications after Thoracic Aortic Aneurysms Endovascular Repair

	Percentage of patients ($n=249$)
Complications after 30 days	
Intraoperative complications	
Device related	15.7
Arterial	2.4
In-hospital complications	
Paraplegia or paresis	4
Stroke	2.8
Systemic	28.8
Endoleak	
Proximal	4.8
Midgraft	1.6
Distal	1.2
Perfusion from side branches	1.6
Complications after 1 year	
Endoleak	4.2
Migration	0
Aneurysm expansion	14.6
Late intervention	5.2
Late rupture	1

Source: Modified from Ref. 17.

procedure (3.3%). The paraplegia and paraparesis rate was 1.7% (eight patients), equally distributed between TAA and type B dissections, and significantly associated with stenting more than 20 cm of aortic length. The mean duration of follow up was 24 months with a late mortality rate of 8.5%, one-third of which were aortic-related. The late endoleak (type I and III) rate was 10% (18).

Recent smaller series have demonstrated similar morbidity and mortality rates. Bavaria et al. used the Gore TAG™ Thoracic Endograft (W.L. Gore & Associates Inc., Flagstaff, Arizona, U.S.A.) in 140 patients with descending TAA and compared the results to a cohort of 94 patients who underwent open surgical repair. The perioperative mortality was significantly lower in the stent group (2.1% vs. 11.7% in the "open" group). In the endovascular group there was significantly less SCI (3% vs. 14%), respiratory failure (4% vs. 20%) and renal impairment (1% vs. 13%), but more peripheral vascular complications (14% vs. 4%). At two years there was no overall difference in mortality (32).

Czerny and coworkers prospectively followed 79 patients who underwent TEVAR between 1996 and 2006 to a mean of 42 months. The in-hospital mortality rate was 6.5% and overall survival was 96%, 86% and 69% at one, three and five years respectively. The early type I and III endoleak rate was 29% and the late endoleak (I and III) rate was 21%. The presence of a short proximal landing zone and a high number of stent grafts were independent risk factors for endoleak (33). Stone et al. compared a cohort of 105 patients who underwent TEVAR with 93 open surgical repairs. The perioperative mortality for TEVAR was favorable (7.6% vs. 15% for open repair) as was the paraplegia rate (6.7% vs. 8.6%) (34). The results from these studies need to be interpreted with some caution due to the nature of the study designs and restricted anatomical criteria.

The later generation stent grafts have in general delivered better results than the earlier generation stent grafts. In 99 patients who underwent stenting of descending TAA with first and second-generation stents between 1999 and 2005, the overall in-hospital mortality was 5% and spinal ischemia rate was 2%. The second-generation stent grafts had less perioperative peripheral vascular complications (23% vs. 42%, $p=0.069$) and lower early endoleak rates (15% vs. 46%, $p=0.001$) than the earlier generation devices (35). Recent reports of thoracic aortic endografting with third-generation devices, used in patients with high American Society of Anesthesiologists (ASA) grades and challenging anatomy (many requiring carotid reconstructions), demonstrated promising early results (24,25).

The difference between device specific mortality rates and complications is hard to evaluate due to a lack of homogeneous data. Different characteristics of specific stent grafts are used to counteract morphological differences, particularly with regard to landing zones and access vessels, to achieve optimal results. Any comparisons must take into account case-mix complexity in terms of anatomy, pathology and comorbidity.

The results for the Medtronic Talent and Valiant thoracic devices have been discussed previously. The patients in these studies had a spectrum of thoracic pathologies, mainly TAA and CTBD (18,24,25). Many had significant comorbidities and increasingly complex morphologies which makes comparisons of outcome data difficult. The Gore TAG Thoracic Endoprothesis was used to treat descending thoracic pathologies, mainly degenerative TAA, again in high-risk patients. This device achieved a 30-day mortality rate of 3.8% in 158 patients, an endoleak rate of 11.5% and 2.5% of patients experienced symptoms of SCI (36). Twenty percent of patients required LSA revascularizations to create adequate proximal landing zones. The Zenith® TX1 device (Cook Medical Inc., Bloomington, Indiana, U.S.A.) was used in 45 consecutive patients (38 with degenerative TAA) who suffered no in-hospital deaths or strokes, one transient paraplegia (2%) and two endoleaks (type I and II) (37). These results were achieved despite involvement of the aortic arch in 17 patients and 10 patients who underwent hybrid open/endovascular procedures. Although the data are not homogeneous, the results for the Cook, Gore and Medtronic thoracic endoprostheses seem to be similar. The literature will undoubtedly provide further information on device specific efficacies and complications as the available data increases (38). The EUROSTAR and U.K. Registries will continue to collate endograft outcomes and a number of new registries will provide addition data on specific stent grafts and specific pathologies, including the VIRTUE study for acute dissection and VALOR II study for TAA.

Chronic Type B Dissection

The aim of endovascular treatment of chronic aortic dissection is to seal off entry tears, re-establish normal blood flow in the true lumen and achieve thrombosis of the false lumen. This may lead to remodeling of the aortic wall and/or stabilization of the dilated aorta. The common indications for endovascular treatment of CTBD are persistent pain, uncontrollable hypertension, aortic expansion to 5.5 cm, side branch ischemia and rupture. A more controversial issue is the management of asymptomatic stable CTBD to prevent late aneurysmal dilatation, thought to occur in 30% to 40% of cases. In a recent Swedish multicenter study of 129 patients who underwent TEVAR for CTBD, 80% demonstrated thrombosis of the false lumen adjacent to the stent but 50% remained patent distally. Despite this, only 5% identified peri-stent aortic dilatation if the entry tear was adequately sealed and only 16% showed signs of dilatation of the distal uncovered aorta (39). Most centers would delay intervention, preferring serial CT surveillance. The presence of progressive dilatation of the false lumen may increase the risk of rupture and endovascular treatment of entry tears; significant fenestrations and endoleaks should be considered. Hybrid revascularization procedures may need to be considered if the aortic arch or suprarenal aorta requires endografting to prevent flow in the false lumen. Patients that have undergone TEVAR should be entered in to an endograft surveillance program to monitor aortic diameter, false lumen filling and stent position.

The Talent Thoracic Registry comprised 217 patients with CTBD of a total 457 patients. Thirty-seven were classified as acute and 180 chronic. The overall in-hospital mortality was 5.1% and the endoleak rate was 9.6%. After moderate-term follow up there were a further 36 deaths (8.5%), including seven ruptured aneurysms, of which six were primary dissections. All patients with late rupture demonstrated persistent type I endoleaks and anuerysmal expansion (18).

The EUROSTAR and U.K. Registry demonstrated a more favorable outcome for dissections compared to TAA (17). Of the 443 procedures in the Registry, 131 were for dissections. They had comparable ASA grades and associated comorbidities, but were on average 10 years younger. All had descending thoracic aortic dissection, 12% with arch involvement. Most were asymptomatic. The primary success rate was 89%, with failures due to inadequate coverage of the entry tear, lack of false lumen thrombosis, endoleaks and failed expansion of the true lumen. The elective 30-day and late mortality rates was 6.5% and 1.5% respectively. The early and one-year endoleak rates were 1.5% and 2.8% respectively. In addition, the rate of paraplegia in the dissection group was significantly lower (0.8%) than in the degenerative TAA group (4%). This may be related to the number of stents deployed. In the dissection group, 63% required a single stent whereas two or more stents were deployed in 66% of the TAA group (17).

A meta-analysis of 39 studies of endovascular treatment of aortic dissection demonstrated a procedural success rate of 98%. Perioperative stroke and paraplegia occurred in 1.9% and 0.8% respectively. The mortality (10% vs. 3%) and complication rates (21% vs. 9%) were significantly greater in patients with acute dissection than with chronic dissection (40). The encouraging results for CTBD have led to further studies which should help to further define the role of endovascular intervention in the management of chronic dissection (41).

SPECIFIC COMPLICATIONS AND THEIR PREVENTION

Spinal Cord Ischemia

Endovascular thoracic and thoracoabdominal aortic repair has a reduced rate of SCI compared to open repair. The reasons for this are complex. SCI is related to direct loss of spinal perfusion, perioperative hypotension, reperfusion injury and spinal edema. It is possible that the lack of aortic cross-clamping, reduced spinal reperfusion injury and the maintenance of the distal aortic blood flow may contribute to the lower incidence of spinal complications. The incidence of SCI ranges in the reported series between 0% and 5% for endovascular thoracic repair. The risk of ischemia increases with the proportion of aorta involved, previous abdominal aortic aneurysm repair, perioperative mean arterial pressure of less than 70 mmHg, lack of spinal cord collateral circulation and occlusion of the LSA without revascularization (42–47). The preventative use of neurophysiological monitoring has been investigated. Transcranial motor-evoked potentials (tcMEP), somatosensory-evoked potentials (SSEP), and constant cerebrospinal fluid (CSF) pressure monitoring with vital parameter measurements have proved useful for intraoperative prediction of SCI. The role of CSF drainage has not been clearly defined, though it has been recommended when there is a loss of tcMEP and SSEP, and a CSF pressure increase to greater than 15 mmHg (47). Other protective measures reportedly used to prevent or reverse SCI are pharmacological correction of arterial pressure, steroid administration and the use of a temporary "retrievable stent" with spinal cord monitoring before definitive device deployment (27,46,48).

If intraoperative monitoring is not used, the development of post-procedure lower limb neurological deficit should prompt urgent CSF drainage. A CSF pressure of 10 mmHg or less and the maintenance of mean arterial pressure greater than 90 mmHg is thought to be optimal. In a series of 75 patients with descending TAA treated by stent grafting, five patients developed SCI, four of which made a full recovery and one patient a near complete recovery with CSF drainage (46). Safi and colleagues demonstrated threefold reduction of SCI with spinal cord drainage and distal aortic perfusion in open thoracic aortic repair (28).

Routine spinal cord drainage carries the inherent risk of catheter complications in patients at relatively low risk of SCI. Conversely, drain placement can be selective in patients who are deemed high risk. In our unit, spinal cord drainage is used if a patient requires prolonged postoperative intubation, if there is significant perioperative hypotension or if symptoms of lower limb neurological deficit develop after TEVAR. A catheter is inserted into the third or fourth lumbar spinal space and the systolic blood pressure kept above 100 mmHg. The CSF is drained at a rate in order to keep the CSF pressure below 10 mmHg, but no more than 30 mL of CSF per hour. Drainage is normally maintained for three days. The role of LSA revascularization will be discussed later in this chapter.

Retrograde Type A Dissection

Iatrogenic acute retrograde type A dissection of the aortic arch has been described, necessitating urgent endovascular or surgical treatment. If unrecognized this can cause devastating complications including stroke, coronary ischemia, pericardial tamponade and death. Most reports are associated with treatment of acute or CTBD. Other predisposing factors may include guidewire manipulation or proximal stent fixation with springs or barbs, creating an iatrogenic false lumen (49–51).

Cerebrovascular Accident and the Role of Cerebral Protection

The rate of stroke after TEVAR varies in the literature from 3% to 5% (17,18,28,30). Stenting of the aorta involves the manipulation of stiff wires in the aortic arch with the inherent risk of embolic strokes. Wires should be introduced carefully and manipulation kept to a minimum. Strokes are also associated with the extent of stent grafting around the aortic arch (52) related to increased proximal instrumentation and complications of supraaortic debranching procedures. Debranching aortic arch vessel bypasses for hybrid endovascular repairs have reported stroke rates of up to 4% (53–56). Cerebral protection can be implemented if the risk of embolization is deemed high, either using a distal embolic filter device (usually introduced via the left brachial artery) or proximal branch ligation after revascularization.

Endoleaks

The type I endoleak rate is related to the morphological complexity of the proximal landing zone. The primary type I leak rate is 0% to 5% with a similar incidence of secondary leaks (17,18,33). A short proximal landing zone and a high number of stent grafts have been shown to be independent risk factors for a reported combined early type I and III endoleak rate of 29% and late endoleak rate of 21% (30). The force of the cardiac output can push the stent graft distally during deployment, so the device must be held firmly by the operator to achieve accurate deployment. Extending the length of the proximal landing zone by deliberate overstenting of the LSA has proven beneficial in the prevention of type I endoleaks, though clearly may predispose to type II leaks (20,52).

Endograft designs have varied proximal fixation devices, including bare springs that exert radial forces to achieve a seal (Valiant®, Medtronic Ave Inc., Santa Rosa, California, U.S.A.), and barbs to anchor the proximal stent to the aortic wall (Cook TX2™, Cook Medical Inc., Bloomington, Indiana, U.S.A.). The Gore TAG device relies on radial force in the absence of bare springs or barbs. As discussed previously, there are no comparative data to recommend a particular design. Clinicians choose the design most appropriate for a particular pathology.

The Role of Carotid–Subclavian Bypass

Overstenting of the LSA can significantly increase the proximal landing zone to reduce the risk of type I endoleak. Revascularization is achieved by either left carotid to subclavian bypass (with coil embolization or ligation proximal to the left vertebral artery origin) or subclavian to left common carotid artery transposition. Some authors recommend an expectant approach, while others routinely revascularize the LSA (52,53,57). The literature regarding the relative advantages and disadvantages of LSA overstenting is scarce and conflicting. Left arm claudication or critical ischemia occurs in up to 20% of cases but this is rarely a significant problem. In some reports, the incidence of spinal ischemia, endoleak and left posterior cerebral circulation compromise is increased in those without reconstruction when compared to patients with LSA revascularization (52–57). The Talent Thoracic Registry reported 17 patients who developed strokes, significantly associated with non-revascularized LSA occlusion (17). It is not fully understood whether these are embolic as a result of increased aortic arch instrumentation, or primarily hemodynamic, but it seems likely that both factors are involved. The long-term patency rates for supra-aortic bypasses are excellent; approaching 90% at 10 to 15 years (58). Further studies regarding the role of LSA revascularization are clearly needed.

CONCLUSIONS

The results from registries and small cohort studies suggest that there are benefits with stent grafting in terms of perioperative mortality, SCI, respiratory failure, renal impairment, intensive care requirements and length of hospital stay. These advantages are offset by more peripheral vascular complications with TEVAR and similar late all-cause mortality rates (16–19). There still seems to be a significant risk of SCI associated with the extent of the pathology, previous abdominal aortic aneurysm repair, perioperative hypotension, poor spinal cord collateral circulation and occlusion of the LSA without revascularization (17,40–48). The use of neurophysiological and CSF pressure monitoring has a role in predicting SCI, though further work is required to establish evidence based protocols.

The endovascular stent designs are improving, but patient cohorts are potentially more challenging and the indications for endovascular interventions are changing. The largest published registry series were reported in 2004 and 2006, but for procedures performed between 1997 and 2003 and 1996 and 2004. Since then, the results may have improved with the advent of third-generation endografts. Reports indicate that the second-generation stent grafts had less perioperative peripheral vascular complications and lower early endoleak rates than the earlier generation devices (29). The presence of a short proximal landing zone and a high number of stent grafts were independent risk factors for type I endoleak (26). A trend exists for more favorable short-term results for stent grafting of CTBD than with degenerative TAA (17). There is minimal literature regarding the third-generation stents and more recent studies comprise an increasingly complex case mix (24,25). Differences between device specific mortality and morbidity rates are hard to evaluate due to the lack of homogeneous data.

Areas of focus for future work include reducing the risk of iatrogenic stroke, paraplegia and type A retrograde dissection. Long-term follow-up in terms of mortality, morbidity and durability of second and third-generation endoprostheses is required to fully assess this rapidly advancing technology (59). The management of CTBD is complex and the role of endovascular intervention requires further clarification.

REFERENCES

1. Bickerstaff LK, Pairolero PC, Hollier LH, et al. Thoracic aortic aneurysms: a population-based study. Surgery 1982; 92:1103–8.
2. Pressler V, McNamara JJ. Aneurysm of thoracic aorta. Review of 260 cases. J Thorac Cardiovasc Surg 1985; 89:50–4.
3. Perko MJ, Norgaard M, Herzog TM, et al. Unoperated aortic aneurysm: survey of 170 patients. Ann Thorac Surg 1995; 59:1204–9.
4. Clouse WD, Hallett JW, Jr., Schaff HV, et al. Improved prognosis of thoracic aortic aneurysms: a population-based study. JAMA 1998; 280:1926–9.
5. Crawford ES, Cohen ES. Aortic aneurysm: a multifocal disease. Arch Surg 1982; 117:1393–400.
6. Elefteriades JA. Natural history of thoracic aortic aneurysms: indications for surgery, and surgical versus nonsurgical risks. Ann Thorac Surg 2002; 74:S1877–80.
7. Bonser RS, Pagano D, Lewis ME, et al. Clinical and patho-anatomical factors affecting expansion of thoracic aortic aneurysms. Heart 2000; 84:277–83.
8. DaPunt OE, Galla JD, Sadeghi AM, et al. The natural history of thoracic aortic aneurysms. J Thorac Cardiovasc Surg 1994; 107:1323–32.
9. Strachen DP. Predictors of death from aortic aneurysm among middle-aged men: the Whitehall study. Br J Surg 1991; 78:401–4.
10. MacSweeney ST, Ellis M, Worrell PC, Greenhalgh RM, Powell JT. Smoking and growth rate of small abdominal aortic aneurysms. Lancet 1994; 344:651–2.
11. The Society of Cardiothoracic Surgeons of Great Britain and Ireland. National Adult Cardiac Surgical Database Report 2000–2001. Berkshire Dendrite Clinical Systems, Reading, U.K., 2002.
12. Coselli JS, LeMaire SA, Miller CC, III, et al. Mortality and paraplegia after thoracoabdominal aneurysm repair: a risk factor analysis. Ann Thorac Surg 2000; 69:409–14.
13. Svensson LG, Crawford ES, Hess KR, et al. Experience with 1509 patients undergoing thoracoabdominal aortic operations. J Vasc Surg 1993; 17:357–68 (Discussion 368–70).
14. Moreno-Cabral CE, Miller DC, Mitchell RS, et al. Degenerative and degenerative aneurysms of the thoracic aorta. Determinants of early and late surgical outcome. J Thorac Cardiovasc Surg 1984; 88:1020–32.
15. Svensson LG, Crawford ES, Hess KR, et al. Variables predictive of outcome in 832 patients undergoing repairs of the descending thoracic aorta. Chest 1993; 104:1248–53.
16. Demeres P, Miller D, Mitchell R, et al. Midterm results of endovascular repair of descending thoracic aortic aneurysms with first generation stent grafts. J Thorac Cardiovasc Surg 2004; 127:664–73.
17. Leurs LJ, Bell R, Dgrieck Y, et al. Endovascular treatment of thoracic aortic diseases: combined experience from the EUROSTAR and United Kingdom Thoracic Endograft registries. J Vasc Surg 2004; 40:670–80.
18. Fattori R, Nienaber CA, Rousseau H, et al. Results of endovascular repair of the thoracic aorta with the Talent Thoracic stent graft: the Talent Thoracic Retrospective Registry. J Thorac Cardiovasc Surg 2006; 132:332–9.
19. Aasland J, Lundbom J, Eide TO, et al. Recovery following treatment of descending thoracic aortic disease. A comparison between endovascular repair and open surgery. Int Angiol 2005; 24:231–7.
20. Riesenman PJ, Farber MA, Mendes RR, et al. Coverage of the left subclavian artery during thoracic endovascular aortic repair. J Vacs Surg 2007; 45:90–4.
21. EVAR Trial Participants. Endovascular aneurysm repair versus open repair in patients with abdominal aortic aneurysm (EVAR trial 1): randomised controlled trial. Lancet 2005; 365:2179–86.
22. EVAR Trial Participants. Endovascular aneurysm repair and outcome in patients unfit for open repair of abdominal aortic aneurysm (EVAR trial 2): randomised controlled trial. Lancet 2005; 365:2187–92.
23. Prince M, Verhoeven EL, Buth J, et al. A randomised trial comparing conventional and endovascular repair of abdominal aortic aneurysms. N Engl J Med 2004; 11:1607–18.
24. Brooks M, Loftus I, Morgan R, Thompson M. The Valiant thoracic endograft. J Cardiovasc Surg 2006; 47:269–78.
25. Thompson MM, Ivaz S, Morgan R, Loftus I. European experience with the Medtronic Valiant thoracic endograft. Endovascular Today, March 2007:11–15.
26. Makaroun MS, Dillavou ED, Kee ST, et al. Endovascular treatment of thoracic aortic aneurysms: results of the phase II multicentre trial of GORE-TAG thoracic endoprosthesis. J Vasc Surg 2005; 41:1–9.
27. Gravereaux EC, Faries PL, Burks JA, et al. Risk of spinal cord ischaemia after endograft repair of thoracic aortic aneurysms. J Vasc Surg 2001; 34:997–1003.
28. Safi HJ, Miller CC, Azizzadeh A, et al. Neurological deficit in patients at high risk with thoracoabdominal aortic aneurysms: the role of cerebral spinal fluid drainage and distal aortic perfusion. J Vasc Surg 1994; 20:434–44.
29. Scharrer-Palmer R, Kotis T, Kapfer X, et al. Complications after endovascular treatment of thoracic aortic aneurysms. J Endovasc Ther 2003; 10:711–8.

30. Melissano G, Civilini E, Bertoglio L, et al. Results of endografting of the aortic arch in different landing zones. Eur J Vasc Endovasc Surg 2007; 33:561–6 (Epub ahead of print).

31. Vaddinemi SK, Taylor SM, Patterson MA, Jordan WD, Jr. Outcome after celiac artery coverage during endovascular thoracic aortic aneurysm repair: preliminary results. J Vasc Surg 2007; 45:467–71.

32. Bavaria JE, Appoo JJ, Makaroun MS, et al. Endovascular stent grafting versus open surgical repair of descending thoracic aortic aneurysms in low-risk patients: a multicenter comparative trial. J Thorac Cardiovasc Surg 2007; 133:369–77.

33. Czerny M, Grimm M, Zimpfer D, et al. Results after endovascular stent graft placement in atherosclerotic aneurysms involving the descending aorta. Ann Thorac Surg 2007; 83:450–5.

34. Stone DH, Brewster DC, Kwolek CJ, et al. Stent-graft versus open-surgical repair of the thoracic aorta: mid-term results. J Vasc Surg 2006; 44:1188–97.

35. Appoo JJ, Moser WG, Fairman RM, et al. Thoracic aortic stent grafting: improving results with newer generation investigational devices. J Thorac Cardiovasc Surg 2006; 131:1087–94.

36. Wheatley GH, Gurbuz AT, Rodriguez-Lopez JA, et al. Midterm outcome in 158 consecutive Gore TAG thoracic endoprotheses: single centre experience. Ann Thorac Surg 2006; 81:1570–7.

37. Melissano G, Civilini E, de Moura MR, Calliari F, Chiesa R. Single center experience with a new commercially available thoracic endovascular graft. Eur J Vasc Endovasc Surg 2005; 29:579–85.

38. Hassoun HT, Matsumara JS. The Cook TX2 thoracic stent graft: preliminary experience and trial design. Semin Vasc Surg 2006; 19:32–9.

39. Resch TA, Delle M, Falkenburg M, et al. Remodelling of the thoracic aorta after stent-grafting of type B dissection: a Swedish multicentre study. J Cardiovasc Surg (Torino) 2006; 47:503–8.

40. Eggebrecht H, Nienaber CA, Neuhauser M, et al. Endovascular stent-graft placement in aortic dissection: a meta-analysis. Eur Heart J 2006; 27(4):489–98.

41. Nienaber CA, Zannetti S, Barbieri B, et al. Investigation of stent grafts in patients with type B aortic dissection: design of the INSTEAD trial—a prospective multicentre European randomized trial. Am Heart J 2005; 149:592–9.

42. Sunder-Plassmann L, Orend KH. Stentgrafting of the thoracic aorta—complications. J Cardiovasc Surg (Torino) 2005; 46:121–30.

43. Kawaharada N, Morishita K, Kurimoto Y, et al. Spinal cord ischaemia after elective endovascular stent-graft repair of the thoracic aorta. Eur J Cardiothorac Surg 2007; 31:998–1003 (Epub ahead of print).

44. Schurink GW, Nijenhuis RJ, Backes WH, et al. Assessment of spinal cord circulation and function in endovascular treatment of thoracic aortic aneurysms. Ann Thorac Surg 2007; 83:S877–81.

45. Cheung AT, Pochettino A, McGarvey ML, et al. Strategies to manage paraplegia risk after endovascular stent repair of descending thoracic aortic aneurysms. Ann Thorac Surg 2005; 80:1280–8.

46. Chiesa R, Melissano G, Marrocco-Trischitta MM, et al. Spinal cord ischaemia after elective stent-graft repair of the thoracic aorta. J Vasc Surg 2005; 42:11–7.

47. Weigang E, Hartert M, Siegenthaler MP, et al. Neurophysiological monitoring during thoracoabdominal aortic endovascular stent graft implantation. Eur J Cardiothorac Surg 2006; 29:392–6.

48. Ishimaru S, Kawaguchi S, Koizumi N, et al. Preliminary report on prediction of spinal cord ischaemia in endovascular stent graft repair of thoracic aortic aneurysm by retrievable stent graft. J Thorac Cardiovasc Surg 1998; 115:811–8.

49. Zhang R, Kofidis T, Baus S, Klima U. Iatrogenic type A dissection after attempted stenting of a descending aortic aneurysm. Ann Thorac Surg 2006; 82(4):1523–5.

50. Misfeld M, Notzold A, Geist V, Richardt G, Sievers HH. Retrograde type A dissection after endovascular stent grafting of type B dissection. Z Kardiol 2002; 91(3):274–7.

51. Neuhauser B, Czermak BV, Fish J, et al. Type A dissection following endovascular thoracic aortic stent-graft repair. J Endovasc Ther 2005; 12(1):74–81.

52. Woo EY, Bavaria JE, Pochettino A, et al. Techniques for preserving vertebral artery perfusion during thoracic aorta stent grafting requiring aortic arch landing. Vasc Endovascular Surg 2006; 40:367–73.

53. Schumacher H, Von Tengg-Kobligk H, Ostovic M, et al. Hybrid aortic procedures for endoluminal arch replacement in thoracic aneurysms and type B dissections. J Cardiovasc Surg (Torino) 2006; 47:509–17.

54. Jackson BM, Carpenter JP, Fairman RM, et al. Anatomical exclusion from endovascular repair of thoracic aortic aneurysms. J Vasc Surg 2007; 45:662–6.

55. Caronno R, Piffaretti G, Tozzi M, et al. Intentional coverage of the left subclavian artery during endovascular stent graft repair for thoracic aortic disease. Surg Endosc 2006; 20:915–8.

56. Weigang E, Lehr M, Harloff A, et al. Incidence of neurological complications following overstenting of the left subclavian artery. Eur J Cardiothorac Surg 2007; 31:628–36.

57. Peterson BG, Eskandari MK, Gleason TG, Morasch MD. Utility of left subclavian artery revascularisation in association with endoluminal repair of acute and chronic thoracic aortic pathology. J Vasc Surg 2006; 43:433–9.

58. Uurto IT, Lautamatti V, Zeitlin R, Salenius JP. Long-term outcome of surgical revascularisation of supraaortic vessels. World J Surg 2002; 26:1503–6.

59. Greenberg RK, O'Neill S, Walker E, et al. Endovascular repair of thoracic aortic lesions with Zenith TX1 and TX2 thoracic grafts: intermediate-term results. J Vasc Surg 2005; 41:589–96.

23 | Endovascular Treatment in the Management of Mycotic Aortic Aneurysms

P. R. Taylor and Y. C. Chan
Department of Vascular and Endovascular Surgery, Guy's and St. Thomas' NHS Foundation Trust, London, U.K.

INDICATIONS FOR ENDOVASCULAR TREATMENT OF MYCOTIC ANEURYSMS

Mycotic aneurysms are rare, accounting for only 0.65% to 1.3% of all aortic aneurysms (1–3). The natural history of mycotic aortic aneurysms is associated with significant mortality and morbidity, which are due to delay in diagnosis, recurrent septic emboli, sudden expansion and rupture with exsanguination. In addition any in situ prosthesis used to repair the aneurysm may become secondarily infected, compounding the problem (Figs. 1A,B and 2).

The pathogenesis of mycotic aneurysms is complex. They are most commonly caused by organisms arising in a distant septic focus, such as the heart (e.g., subacute bacterial endocarditis), the gastrointestinal tract or the urinary tract. These organisms settle on atherosclerotic plaques which behave as a culture medium, resulting in weakening of the arterial wall with the subsequent formation of mycotic aneurysm (5). The septic emboli usually lodge in diseased areas of the descending thoracic aorta and at the origins of mesenteric vessels and may be multiple in nature. In a series of 31 patients with mycotic aneurysms diagnosed at the Mayo Clinic, less than a third (10 of 31) were infrarenal. The majority of cases involves the thoracic or abdominal aorta at or above the renal arteries (6). Rarely a local extravascular infectious focus, such as osteomyelitis of the spine, may extend directly into the aorta, where the local suppurative process weakens the arterial wall (7). Immunosuppressed or malnourished patients have an increased risk of developing mycotic aneurysms. This group includes those with chronic diseases, concomitant malignancy and intravenous drug users (8).

The diagnosis may be difficult, as mycotic aneurysms can present with nonspecific symptoms such as fever and night sweats associated with leucocytosis and raised inflammatory markers. This may be diagnosed as a "pyrexia of unknown origin" with no clinical imperative to perform further investigations especially in the absence of localizing symptoms. Early commencement of broad-spectrum antibiotics with no samples taken for culture makes the subsequent isolation of microbes difficult if not impossible, and is a practice that must be avoided. A low threshold for performing imaging of the aorta can help make an early diagnosis particularly when the patient complains of localizing symptoms such as back pain, hemoptysis or hematemesis in association with a pyrexia of unknown origin. Computed tomography (CT) or magnetic resonance angiography will readily identify any mycotic aortic aneurysm. Emergency surgical or endovascular intervention is essential for survival, in order to prevent the complications of rupture, fistula formation and exsanguination.

Conventional open surgery on mycotic aortic aneurysms carries a high perioperative mortality ranging from 27% to 36% (2,3,9). The most important determinants of outcome are aneurysm location (thus determining the magnitude and complexity of aortic surgery), the size of the aneurysm (which correlates with the risk of rupture), the presence of significant cardiac, pulmonary, and renal comorbidity, and the virulence of the infecting organism. The bacteria responsible include *Salmonella* species, *Bacteroides fragilis*, *Staphylococcus aureus*, and *Pseudomonas aeruginosa*. These organisms accounted for all deaths, ruptures, and suprarenal aneurysm infections in 10 of 13 aneurysms in one series (2).

Open surgery can be performed in a number of ways, and may involve excision of the mycotic aneurysm with oversewing of the aorta proximal and distal to the aneurysm with

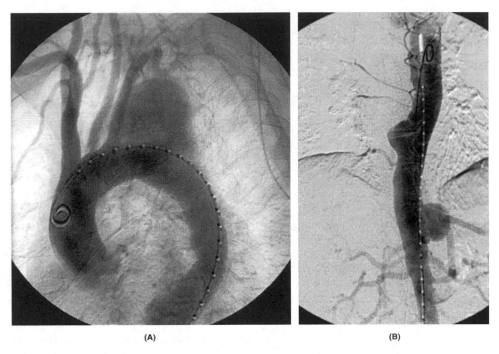

(A)   (B)

FIGURE 1 (**A**, **B**) Intra-arterial digital subtraction angiography demonstrating three mycotic aneurysms in the descending thoracic aorta. *Source*: From Ref. 4.

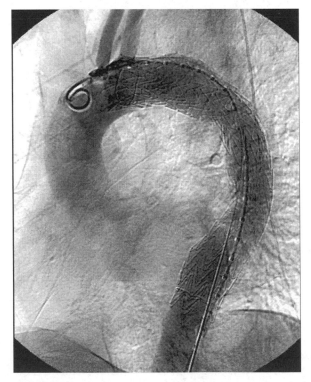

FIGURE 2 Intra-arterial digital subtraction angiography showing stent graft successfully excluding the mycotic aneurysm distal to the left subclavian artery. *Source*: From Ref. 4.

extra-anatomic reconstruction. This carries the risk of aortic stump rupture, graft thrombosis and sepsis. The alternative is in situ replacement with either antibiotic-soaked synthetic grafts, homografts, or autologous deep veins from the leg. However, in situ replacement is associated with an early mortality of 27% (9,10), and up to 20% of patients require further surgery because of infection or thrombosis of the in situ graft (10).

Over the past decade, endovascular treatment of atherosclerotic aneurysms of the thoracic and abdominal aorta has become established as an alternative to open surgery with low perioperative mortality (11–13). Stent grafts have a role in the treatment of mycotic aneurysms either as a temporizing treatment in a difficult clinical situation prior to definitive open surgical repair, or they may be the only therapeutic option in frail unfit patients. Placement of a prosthetic stent graft in the septic environment of a mycotic aneurysm clearly contravenes the principles of conventional open surgery, as the infected aorta and surrounding septic tissue is not excised or debrided, and the septic field cannot be irrigated (14–17).

TECHNICAL ASPECTS OF ENDOVASCULAR TREATMENT OF MYCOTIC ANEURYSMS

The benefits of endovascular repair include the avoidance of general anesthesia, thoracotomy, aortic cross-clamping and cardiopulmonary bypass. Endoluminal repair also lessens the requirement for intensive care or high dependency care and reduces the length of stay in hospital, resulting in an earlier return to activities of daily living and consequent improvement in the quality of life (18).

Antibiotic therapy is an important adjunct to endoluminal treatment. However, it may be very difficult to isolate the causative organisms, as patients may not have positive blood cultures, probably as a result of treatment with antibiotics before or after admission to hospital. Ideally multiple blood cultures should be taken before antibiotics are commenced. *S. aureus*, *Streptococcus*, and *Salmonella* species are the most common organisms; with *Staphylococcus* being responsible for more than a third of cases in the world's literature (19). *Methicillin-resistant S. aureus* is a common pathogen, in patients who are critically ill, have prolonged hospital stay, or who undergo invasive procedures (20). *S. aureus* is overtaking *Salmonella* as the most common causative organism of suprarenal aortic mycotic aneurysms since the 1990s. Certain bacteria notably *S. aureus*, *Salmonella*, *B. fragilis*, and *P. aeruginosa* are associated with a high risk of rupture (2). Mycotic aneurysms may also be caused by *Mycobacterium tuberculosis*, although tuberculous mycotic aneurysm of the aorta is exceedingly rare (21), and may be difficult to diagnose.

If no organisms are cultured, then broad-spectrum antibiotics should be started after discussion with microbiologists. The duration of antibiotic treatment is controversial, although six to eight weeks seem sufficient to avoid relapses after successful open surgery (22). After endoluminal treatment, some authors suggest that the duration of antibiotic treatment should be determined by monitoring the patient's temperature, erythrocyte sedimentation rate (ESR) and C-reactive protein. Once these markers return to normal there is no further benefit to be gained in continuing antibiotics. Others recommend that antibiotics should be continued for life, or for as long as the patient can tolerate them (18). There is always the potential for late stent-graft infection. The use of antibiotic-soaked grafts or silver-impregnated grafts has not been proven to be useful in randomized trials.

Multislice and three-dimensional reconstructed CT angiography is now the preoperative investigation of choice. The CT findings suggestive of aortic infection include hazy periaortic tissue, retroperitoneal para-aortic stranding, and periaortic gas and fluid collections (23,24). In the early stages, subtle periaortic changes may be difficult to detect and can be overlooked. The presence of gas is rarely seen in the early stages unless there is gas-forming inflammation around the aneurysm (25). In some circumstances, it may be possible to aspirate periaortic fluid for microbiological analysis, in order to determine the most appropriate antibiotic treatment. Magnetic resonance angiography is also used to detect mycotic aneurysms and the coexistence of para-aortic abnormalities and vertebral involvement, although its use is less widespread than CT (26,27). Radio-labeled leucocyte scintigraphy or positron emission tomography may be a useful adjunct in certain cases where the infective nature of the aneurysm is uncertain particularly when it is correlated with the findings on CT or magnetic resonance angiography (28,29).

Not all mycotic aneurysms of the aorta are suitable for endovascular treatment as commercially available devices have anatomical limitations. It is important to have a proximal and distal portion of normal aorta (the so called "landing zone") in order to secure satisfactory exclusion of the mycotic aneurysm. The proximal and distal neck should ideally be more than 2 cm in length. Aneurysms with shorter landing zones can be treated endovascularly, but the risks of failure are higher. The development of branched and fenestrated stent grafts allows the treatment of aneurysms which involve the origins of the great vessels and the visceral and renal arteries. However, experience in this technique is limited to a few centers and the technology is still being developed. The device is oversized by 10% to 15% relative to the diameter of the normal aorta at the landing zones in order to achieve an adequate seal and to prevent migration. Some devices also use hooks and barbs to prevent migration. Wide discrepancies between the proximal and distal landing zone diameters can be dealt with by using a tapered device or a tromboning device of different diameters.

Currently there is poor long-term follow-up data on endovascular treatment of mycotic aneurysm. Lifelong clinical and radiological follow-up is essential. Serial CT and measurement of inflammatory markers at 3, 6, and 12 months and then annually thereafter are advised. These tests ensure that the aneurysm remains successfully excluded and recurrent sepsis is identified.

TROUBLESHOOTING IN ENDOVASCULAR TREATMENT OF MYCOTIC ANEURYSMS

Problems with Access

The large size of devices used for treating mycotic aneurysms of the thoracic aorta may require angioplasty of significant stenoses of the access arteries, usually the iliac arteries. Extensive iliac disease may require access procedures in order to introduce the device into the aorta. Prosthetic grafts can be sutured to either the common iliac or infrarenal aorta to act as a conduit. Suturing grafts to the external iliac artery is rarely required as this artery has a similar diameter to the common femoral artery.

Short Landing Zones

The landing zones may be inadequate to secure the device and prevent endoleaks. Bypass grafts or transposition of the arch vessels can be performed prior to insertion of the stent graft. Right-to-left carotid–carotid bypass and carotid subclavian bypass can allow the origins of the left common carotid and left subclavian arteries to be covered. A duplex scan of the carotid bifurcations to exclude significant internal carotid artery stenoses is essential. The caliber and direction of flow in the vertebral arteries should also be assessed. Covering the origin of the left subclavian artery in a patient who has a dominant left vertebral artery may result in a posterior cerebral circulation stroke. The vertebral artery is also an important blood supply to the proximal spinal cord, so that paraplegia may also result from occlusion of the subclavian artery. Both of these catastrophic complications could be avoided by a carotid subclavian bypass or carotid subclavian transposition. Reconstruction of the left subclavian artery prior to deployment of a device which covers only the origin of this vessel remains a contentious issue. Any resulting ischemia of the arm usually improves with time. However, patients who develop rest pain should have reconstructive surgery.

The distal landing zone can be compromised by the proximity of the visceral and renal arteries. Branched and fenestrated endoluminal devices are available and provide an elegant solution to this problem. The alternative in fit patients is to revascularize the visceral and renal arteries with bypass grafts from either the infrarenal aorta or iliac arteries. This hybrid procedure using extra-anatomical reconstruction together with an endoluminal device has been associated with good results, but most series are small and the follow-up is short (see chap. 26).

Secondary Infection of the Endoprosthesis

The various antibiotic treatments have already been discussed. If there is a successful outcome, the aneurysm sac should shrink with diminution of periaortic gas, fluid collection and stranding (Fig. 3). This is associated with a fall in the ESR and C-reactive protein to normal levels. If the treatment is unsuccessful these indices will either fail to normalize or increase. Cross-sectional imaging may show a rapidly expanding, lobulated saccular aneurysm with the development of adjacent fluid collections (8). When the endoprosthesis becomes infected, this will inevitably perpetuate the problem by affecting a greater length of aorta including previously normal landing zones, and this may cause delayed rupture of the fragile vessel because of the necessary oversizing used to hold the device in place. The use of further stents to seal any leak may be successful in the short term but these are likely to become infected with time. Antibiotic therapy for life is mandatory in this clinical scenario, although this recommendation is not based on any evidence. Consideration should also be given to removal of the infected grafts if the patient is well enough. Surgical removal of the infected prosthesis together with excision of the infected tissue is technically difficult, and a major undertaking, even for medically fit patients.

CURRENT RESULTS OF ENDOVASCULAR TREATMENT OF MYCOTIC ANEURYSMS

Endoluminal treatment of mycotic aneurysms is not without risks and is associated with a significant in-hospital mortality of up to 40% (30–38). As mycotic aneurysms are rare, randomized controlled trials comparing open surgery versus endoluminal treatment are very difficult to conduct. Most of the reports in the literature are of single cases, or of small single-center case series (39). A number of commercially available devices have been used with good results, with mid-term follow-up in excess of three years (40,41). The current literature shows that stent grafts are becoming a successful alternative to open surgery for the treatment

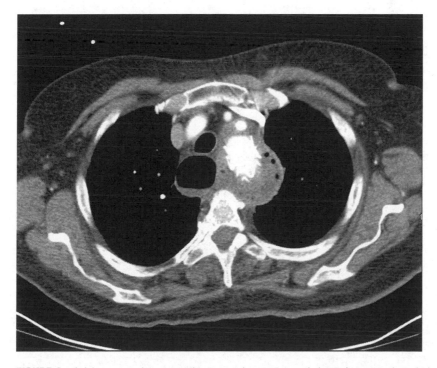

FIGURE 3 Axial computed tomography scan taken one month later demonstrating air bubbles surrounding the stent graft.

of mycotic aneurysms involving the descending thoracic and abdominal aorta especially as a temporizing measure in patients unfit for open surgery.

Despite these initial encouraging reports, long-term results are still lacking. It is logical to presume that endovascular treatment is only successful when active microbes in the mycotic aneurysms are successfully controlled or eradicated, especially at the time of stent-graft deployment. This may have been achieved by the use of broad-spectrum antibiotics given on an empirical basis to treat a pyrexia of unknown origin. Future success will rely on new technology and the manufacture of graft materials which provide surface characteristics to resist microbes and incorporate antimicrobial substances within their structure. There are now new methods of chemically binding antibiotics such as gentamicin or rifampin to vascular prostheses and these are bacteriostatic to *Escherichia coli*, *P. aeruginosa* and *S. aureus* strains (42,43).

REFERENCES

1. Chan FY, Crawford ES, Coselli JS, Safi HJ, Williams TW. In situ prosthetic graft replacement for mycotic aneurysm of the aorta. Ann Thorac Surg 1989; 47:193–203.
2. Reddy DJ, Shepard AD, Evans JR, Wright DJ, Smith RF, Ernst CB. Management of infected aortoiliac aneurysms. Arch Surg 1991; 126:873–9.
3. Muller BT, Wegener OR, Grabitz K, Pillny M, Thomas L, Sandmann W. Mycotic aneurysms of the thoracic and abdominal aorta and iliac arteries: experience with anatomic and extra-anatomic repair in 33 cases. J Vasc Surg 2001; 33:106–13.
4. Chan YC, Morales JP, Taylor PR. The management of mycotic aortic aneurysms: is there a role for endovascular treatment? Acta Chirurgica Belgica 2005; 105(6):580–7.
5. Reddy DJ. Aortic aneurysm infections. Ann Vasc Surg 1988; 2:98.
6. Macedo TA, Stanson AW, Oderich GS, Johnson CM, Panneton JM, Tie ML. Infected aortic aneurysms: imaging findings. Radiology 2004; 231:250–7.
7. Rubery PT, Smith MD, Cammisa FP, Silane M. Mycotic aortic aneurysm in patients who have lumbar vertebral osteomyelitis. A report of two cases. J Bone Joint Surg Am 1995; 77:1729–32.
8. Bogers AJ, van't Wout JW, Cats VM, Quaegebeur JM, Huysmans HA. Mediastinal rupture of a thoracoabdominal mycotic aneurysm caused by Salmonella typhimurium in an immunocompromised patient. Eur J Cardiothorac Surg 1987; 1:116–8.
9. Kyriakides C, Kan Y, Kerle M, Cheshire NJ, Mansfield AO, Wolfe JHN. 11-year experience with anatomical and extra-anatomical repair of mycotic aortic aneurysms. Eur J Vasc Endovasc Surg 2004; 27:585–9.
10. Alonso M, Caeiro S, Cachaldora J, Segura R. Infected abdominal aortic aneurysm: in situ replacement with cryopreserved arterial homograft. J Cardiovasc Surg 1997; 38:371–5.
11. Mitchell RS, Miller DC, Dake MD. Stent-graft repair of thoracic aortic aneurysms. Semin Vasc Surg 1997; 10:257–71.
12. Demers P, Miller DC, Mitchell RS, Kee ST, Chagonjian L, Dake MD. Stent-graft repair of penetrating atherosclerotic ulcers in the descending thoracic aorta: mid-term results. Ann Thorac Surg 2004; 77:81–6.
13. Greenhalgh RM, Brown LC, Kwong GP, Powell JT, Thompson SG, EVAR Trial Participants. Comparison of endovascular aneurysm repair with open repair in patients with abdominal aortic aneurysm (EVAR trial 1), 30-day operative mortality results: randomised controlled trial. Lancet 2004; 364:843–8.
14. Hsu RB, Chen RJ, Wang SS, Chu SH. Infected aortic aneurysms: clinical outcome and risk factor analysis. J Vasc Surg 2004; 40:30–5.
15. Strachan CJ, Newsom SW, Ashton TR. The clinical use of an antibiotic-bonded graft. Eur J Vasc Surg 1991; 5:627–32.
16. Haverich A, Hirt S, Karck M, Siclari F, Wahlig H. Prevention of graft infection by bonding of gentamycin to Dacron prostheses. J Vasc Surg 1992; 15:187–93.
17. Strachan CJ, Avramovic J. In situ replacement of infected vascular prostheses with rifampin-soaked vascular grafts. J Vasc Surg 1993; 18:1075.
18. Smith JJ, Taylor PR. Endovascular treatment of mycotic aneurysms of the thoracic and abdominal aorta: the need for level I evidence. Eur J Vasc Endovasc Surg 2004; 27:569–70.
19. Schrander-vd Meer AM, Guit GL, van Bockel JH, van Dorp WT. Mycotic aneurysm of the suprarenal abdominal aorta. Neth J Med 1994; 44(1):23–5.
20. Nishimoto M, Hasegawa S, Asada K, Tsunemi K, Sasaki S. Stent-graft placement for mycotic aneurysm of the thoracic aorta: report of a case. Circ J 2004; 68:88–90.
21. Long R, Guzman R, Greenberg H, Safneck J, Hershfield E. Tuberculous mycotic aneurysm of the aorta: review of published medical and surgical experience. Chest 1999; 115(2):522–31.

22. Fernandez Guerrero ML, Aguado JM, Arribas A, Lumbreras C, de Gorgolas M. The spectrum of cardiovascular infections due to *Salmonella* enterica: a review of clinical features and factors determining outcome. Medicine (Baltimore) 2004; 83:123–38.

23. Vogelzang RL, Sohaey R. Infected aortic aneurysms: CT appearance. J Comput Assist Tomogr 1988; 12:109–12.

24. Lee MH, Chan P, Chiou HJ, Cheung WK. Diagnostic imaging of *Salmonella*-related mycotic aneurysm of aorta by CT. Clin Imaging 1996; 20:26–30.

25. Gonda RL, Jr., Gutierrez OH, Azodo MV. Mycotic aneurysms of the aorta: radiologic features. Radiology 1988; 168:343–6.

26. Moriarty JA, Edelman RR, Tumeh SS. CT and MRI of mycotic aneurysms of the abdominal aorta. J Comput Assist Tomogr 1992; 16:941–3.

27. Walsh DW, Ho VB, Haggerty MF. Mycotic aneurysm of the aorta: MRI and MRA features. J Magn Reson Imaging 1997; 7:312–5.

28. Seabold JE, Binet EF, Schaefer RF. Mycotic aortic aneurysm diagnosed by In-111 leukocyte scintigraphy and computed tomography. Clin Nucl Med 1983; 8:486–7.

29. Bell D, Jackson MH, Stevenson AJ, Nicoll JJ. Intrathoracic mycotic aneurysm detected by indium-111 labelled autologous neutrophils with single photon emission computed tomography. Thorax 1987; 42:397–8.

30. Semba CP, Sakai T, Slonim SM, et al. Mycotic aneurysms of the thoracic aorta: repair with use of endovascular stent-grafts. J Vasc Interv Radiol 1998; 9:33–40.

31. Lagatolla NRF, Baghai M, Biswas S, et al. Tuberculous false aneurysm of the femoral artery treated by endoluminal stent graft insertion. Eur J Vasc Endovasc Surg 2000; 19:440–2.

32. Madhaven P, McDonnell CO, Dowd MO, et al. Suprarenal mycotic aneurysm exclusion using a stent with a partial autologous covering. J Endovasc Ther 2000; 7:404–9.

33. Kinney EV, Kaebnick HW, Mitchell RA, Jung MT. Repair of mycotic paravisceral aneurysm with a fenestrated stent-graft. J Endovasc Ther 2000; 7:192–7.

34. Liu WC, Kwak BK, Kim KN, et al. Tuberculous aneurysm of the abdominal aorta: endovascular repair using stent grafts in two cases. Korean J Radiol 2000; 1:215–8.

35. Bond SE, McGuinness CL, Reidy JF, Taylor PR. Repair of secondary aortoesophageal fistula by endoluminal stent-grafting. J Endovasc Ther 2001; 8:597–601.

36. Bell RE, Taylor PR, Aukett M, Evans GH, Reidy JF. Successful endoluminal repair of an infected thoracic pseudoaneurysm caused by methicillin-resistant *Staphylococcus aureus*. J Endovasc Ther 2003; 10:29–32.

37. Berchtold C, Eibl C, Seelig MH, Jakob P, Schonleben K. Endovascular treatment and complete regression of an infected abdominal aortic aneurysm. J Endovasc Ther 2002; 9:543–8.

38. Bell RE, Taylor PR, Aukett M, Sabharwal T, Reidy JF. Results of urgent and emergency thoracic procedures treated by endoluminal repair. Eur J Vasc Endovasc Surg 2003; 25:527–31.

39. Stanley BM, Semmens JB, Lawrence-Brown MM, Denton M, Grosser D. Endoluminal repair of mycotic thoracic aneurysms. J Endovasc Ther 2003; 10:511–5.

40. Krohg-Sorensen K, Hafsahl G, Fosse E, Geiran OR. Acceptable short-term results after endovascular repair of diseases of the thoracic aorta in high risk patients. Eur J Cardiothorac Surg 2003; 24:379–87.

41. Jones KG, Bell RE, Sabharwal T, Aukett M, Reidy JF, Taylor PR. Treatment of mycotic aortic aneurysms with endoluminal grafts. Eur J Vasc Endovasc Surg 2005; 29:139–44.

42. Ginalska G, Kowalczuk D, Osinska M. A chemical method of gentamicin bonding to gelatine-sealed prosthetic vascular grafts. Int J Pharm 2005; 288:131–40.

43. Ginalska G, Osinska M, Uryniak A, et al. Antibacterial activity of gentamicin-bonded gelatin-sealed polyethylene terephthalate vascular prostheses. Eur J Vasc Endovasc Surg 2005; 29:419–24.

24 | Current Endografts for Endovascular Repair of the Thoracic Aorta

Robert A. Morgan and Graham J. Munneke
Department of Radiology, St. George's Hospital, London, U.K.

INTRODUCTION

It is almost two decades since the first reports of the treatment of thoracic aortic aneurysms using homemade endografts (1,2). In the intervening years, the efforts of the endograft companies have been directed at producing the perfect endograft for use in the thoracic aorta. The ideal endograft would have the following features: durable graft and stent material, ease of deployment, accuracy of deployment, adequate radial force to maintain the aortic lumen, a low-profile delivery system, conformability for the curves of the aortic arch and tortuous thoracic aortas, availability in a wide variety of diameters and lengths to treat all sizes of aortic lesions in patients of all ages, and different designs of endografts to treat a variety of aortic pathologies.

The early devices were custom made by the operators themselves, on the bench from a combination of surgical graft material and Gianturco-Z™ stents attached at the proximal and distal ends of the graft by surgical sutures to provide fixation between the stents and the graft material. After construction, the homemade grafts were compressed into a long sheath prior to insertion. Once at the desired site in the aorta, deployment of the devices was achieved by pushing the endograft out of the end of the sheath by a pusher at the desired location. The body of the device was not supported by stents and if fixation failed or the device migrated it was prone to collapse into the aneurysm sac.

A few years after the first published reports using homemade devices, a handful of companies (e.g., W.L. Gore, Flagstaff, Arizona; World Medical, Sunnybrook Florida, U.S.A.) started to produce factory-made endografts. The first generation commercial endografts were superior to custom-made devices in two ways. Firstly, they consisted of graft material supported along the entire length by nitinol stents which produced far superior column strength compared with devices with stents placed only at each end. Secondly, the devices were mounted in sophisticated delivery sheaths which facilitated the smooth passage of the stent to the landing zone and its accurate deployment at the desired location. The most commonly used first generation devices were the TAG™ endograft (W.L. Gore, Flagstaff, Arizona, U.S.A.) and the Talent™ endograft (World Medical, currently produced by Medtronic Corp., Santa Rosa, California, U.S.A.).

These early devices were a vast improvement on the previous homemade iterations and facilitated the increased use of endografts to treat aortic pathology in the thorax worldwide (3–6). However, neither graft could be considered to be the "finished article." One of the problems with these early devices was fracture of the longitudinal struts placed to give the devices columnar strength. Reports appeared in the literature of cases where the longitudinal struts were observed to have fractured on follow-up plain radiographs. Although there were no reports of clinical harm arising from this occurrence, fracture of the longitudinal struts might have had the potential for tearing of the graft material or erosion by the fractured struts through the aortic wall (6). As a result of this possibility, the Gore™ device was withdrawn from the market temporarily. The updated Gore TAG was released a few years later without the longitudinal strut and with modifications to the graft and stent structure to compensate for the absence of the longitudinal strut. The Talent device was also modified and the new

Medtronic device was released in 2005 as the Valiant™ device (Medtronic, Santa Rosa, California, U.S.A.). The main thoracic endografts currently on the market are the Valiant endograft, the Gore TAG endograft and the Cook TX2™ endograft (William Cook Europe, Bjaerverkov, Denmark). These three devices will be described in detail below.

VALIANT™ ENDOGRAFT

The Valiant device, like the Talent endograft is constructed of an external skeleton of Nitinol™ stents sewn to thin-walled polyester graft material by nonabsorbable sutures. The absence of a longitudinal supporting strut produces enhanced flexibility and allows the endograft to conform better to tortuous aortic arches (Fig. 1A). The device is available in three

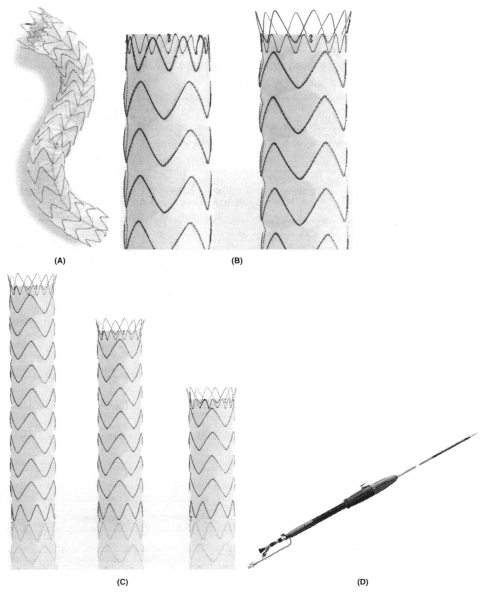

(A)   (B)

(C)   (D)

FIGURE 1   The Valiant™ (Medtronic, Santa Rosa, California, U.S.A.) endograft. (**A**) Note the flexibility. (**B**) Bare spring and closed web versions. (**C**) Available in three different lengths. (**D**) The Xcelerant delivery system.

configurations: (*i*) proximal bare spring (FreeFlo™ device), (*ii*) no bare spring (Closed web™ device), and (*iii*) distal bare spring (Fig. 1B). The Closed web design is available as a straight or tapered device. The FreeFlo device should be used if it is the first (or only) device to be deployed in the thoracic aorta. The Closed web device should be used if a second, third or more devices are required—the rationale being that placement of a second device with a bare spring (instead of a Closed web device) might traumatize the graft material of the first device. The distal bare spring device is useful if the distal landing zone is very close to the celiac artery, because the bare spring can be deployed over the origin of the celiac artery which gives slightly increased stability to the graft when deploying it in this location.

The endograft has radiopaque markers to facilitate accurate deployment and the placement of more than one overlapping endograft. Proximal figure of 8 markers and distal 0 markers identify the extent of the graft material. Figure of 8 markers placed approximately 5 cm above the proximal end of the graft indicates the minimal length of graft for overlap when placing a second device.

The Valiant device is available in a good range of lengths and diameters (Fig. 1C). In particular the availability of the longer lengths is a marked improvement on the Talent device which was only available in a single, relatively short, length of 130 mm. The device is available in diameters from 24 to 46 mm in 2-mm intervals and in three lengths. The exact length measurements differ slightly depending on the diameter of the device. However, broadly speaking the available lengths are 11, 16 and 21 cm of covered graft, excluding the bare springs (see below).

The device is mounted on the Xcelerant delivery system, which is also used to carry the same company's abdominal aortic endograft (Fig. 1D). The Xcelerant delivery system is notable for having two methods to release the endograft: (*i*) a screw mechanism which releases the graft slowly and in a controlled manner by rotating the handle and (*ii*) a trigger mechanism which when retracted releases the graft rapidly. The mechanical advantage produced by the delivery system removes the need for excessive operator force to withdraw the sheath, which was a feature of the Talent endograft. Now the device can be released from its sheath with ease even around a curved aortic arch. The delivery system has a lubricious outer coating enabling it to pass through narrow iliac arteries and can be passed around the vast majority of even the most tortuous aortas. The delivery system varies from 22 to 25 F depending on the diameter of stent graft used.

Device Deployment

The device should be advanced about a centimeter more proximal to its desired final site of deployment. After angiography to confirm this position, the proximal end of the endograft should be released by rotating the blue handle counterclockwise which slowly retracts the covering outer sheath. The device might move forward a few millimeters during the initial process of release which is counteracted by gentle traction on the delivery system. Once two or three of the stent components of the endograft have been released, angiography should be performed. The delivery system and partially released endograft should be withdrawn until they are in the ideal location. After this, the remainder of the endograft can be released by one of the following: (*i*) further rotation of the handle until all of the device is released, (*ii*) by further rotation of the handle to release a few more stents, followed by rapid release of the remainder of the device using the trigger mechanism, or (*iii*) by rapid release of the device using the trigger mechanism. Pharmacologically induced hypotension should be employed (to a mean arterial pressure of 80–100 mm Hg) to avoid a wind sock effect occurring during partial release of the endograft.

Pros

The device represents a significant step forward compared with the previous Talent device. The Xcelerant delivery system enables easy, controlled and accurate deployment which is useful particularly in the aortic arch. The device conforms very well to the aortic arch and at the present time is probably the best device available for patients with marked angulation at the junction of the arch and descending aorta. The Valiant endograft has the widest range of lengths and diameters among its competitors. The delivery system is very flexible and can be advanced up challenging diseased iliac arteries easier than some of the other devices.

Cons

A range of smaller sizes for younger patients are desirable and the production of a smaller delivery system would be beneficial.

TAG™ ENDOGRAFT

The Gore TAG device replaced the first generation Gore endograft. The TAG graft consists of non porous expanded polytetrafluoroethylene (PTFE) heat sealed to a nitinol stent exoskeleton. This avoids the use of sutures and the possibility of graft leaks through suture holes. Sealing cuffs are positioned at both ends and the ends of the stent are crenulated (Fig. 2A). Radiopaque gold markers at the bases of the crenulations are located 1 cm from the ends of the endoprosthesis. There is no longitudinal supporting strut which was removed when the previous Gore graft was modified. The TAG endograft is available in diameters of 26 to 40 mm enabling the treatment of patients with landing zone diameters of between 23 and 37 mm. The graft is supplied in three lengths: 10, 15 and 20 cm and similar to the Valiant device, several overlapping grafts may be deployed to treat longer lesions.

The endograft is mounted on the end of a delivery catheter constrained within an expanded PTFE sleeve (20–24 F; Fig. 2B). However, this relatively small delivery catheter must be inserted through an introducer sheath, 30 cm long (20–24 F inner diameter, 23–27 F outer diameter). The delivery catheter itself is relatively low profile and is easily trackable around the aortic arch.

Device Deployment

The endograft is deployed using Gore's SIM-PULL™ release system. Once the endograft is deemed to be in a satisfactory position, it is released by pulling a cord emanating from the proximal side arm of the delivery catheter, which unzips the restraining sleeve. The endograft deploys from its center outward in less than one second (Fig. 2C,D). This reduces the possibility of the cardiac output causing stent malposition during deployment. Therefore the windsock effect alluded to in the section on the Valiant™ device is not a concern with the TAG endograft and the systolic blood pressure does not need to be reduced when implanting the TAG endograft.

Pros

The TAG endograft is a very good device. It is extremely easy to position and deploy. Its ease of use and rapid delivery definitely has obvious advantages in situations such as aortic rupture, when speed of deployment and rapid exclusion of the aortic tear are paramount. Although the device needs to be inserted through a relatively large delivery catheter, if the iliac arteries are very narrow, the delivery catheter can be inserted on its own (the so-called "bareback" insertion) through an arteriotomy, although there are drawbacks with this option in terms of bleeding at the access site and potential trauma to the endograft itself by the diseased iliac arteries as it is passed through them.

Cons

Although deployment of the device is very rapid, the "all or nothing" nature of the delivery system is also its major disadvantage. Occasionally, the endograft may move forward or backward a little during release. If this happens, there is no way to reposition it, except by attempting to drag it back with a balloon. For this reason, if accuracy of deployment is very important, for example when the landing zones are close to the supra-aortic arteries or the celiac artery, precise location of the deployed endograft cannot be guaranteed, and for this reason, we do not use the device if accurate positioning is essential.

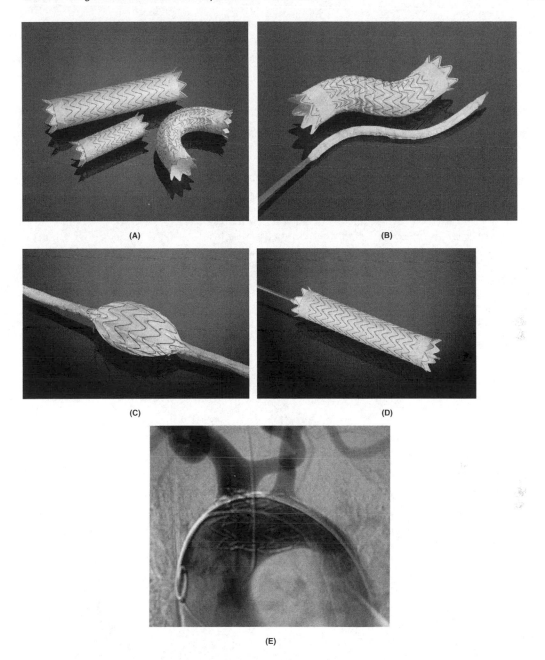

(A)   (B)

(C)   (D)

(E)

FIGURE 2 (**A**) The TAG™ endograft (W.L. Gore, Flagstaff, Arizona, U.S.A.). (**B**) The deployed endograft and the endograft constrained on its delivery sheath. (**C**) The SIM-PULL™ system releases the endograft from the center outward. (**D**) The graft is fully deployed in less than a second. (**E**) The graft may not conform well to an angulated aortic arch. *Source*: Photos courtesy of W.L. Gore & Associates, Inc.

Although there is no longitudinal supporting strut, the device does not conform as well around acutely angulated aortic arches as the Valiant device. In young patients, who have this arch morphology, the proximal end of the endograft may sit up in the arch which may give rise to the potential for collapse of the proximal end of the graft by cardiac output (Fig. 2E).

One other important drawback of the system is the requirement of an introducer sheath. Operators should be aware that the sheath diameters quoted by the manufacturers refer to the inner rather than the outer diameters. For example, the 24-F sheath required by the 37- and 40-mm diameter grafts actually has an outer diameter of 9.1 mm corresponding to a sheath size of 27 F. The large sheath sizes for the Gore device should be taken into consideration when the iliac arteries are of borderline caliber.

ZENITH TX2™ ENDOGRAFT

The current Cook TX2 is similar in construction and delivery to their existing abdominal endograft. It is available in two configurations: (*i*) a single-piece design and (*ii*) as a two-piece modular configuration (Fig. 3A). In practice, the single-piece endograft is seldom used and most patients treated with the TX2 endograft receive the two-part configuration, which enables long segments of thoracic aorta to be treated. The endograft is constructed of stainless steel Z stents sutured to a polyester fabric graft. In both configurations, fixation is enhanced by 5 mm long caudally orientated barbs which protrude through the fabric at the proximal end. At the distal end, an uncovered stent with cranially orientated barbs is present (Fig. 3B). The TX2 proximal and distal components fit into each other with a two-stent overlap, although the degree of overlap can be increased if necessary.

The single-piece endograft is rather short (81–85 mm long) and may be used in some patients with short lesions such as aortic transactions, although most operators are more comfortable with a slightly longer device for this indication.

The two-piece device is available in a much wider range of sizes. The range of diameters is from 22 up to 42 mm. The 22 mm device is the smallest thoracic endograft available and is

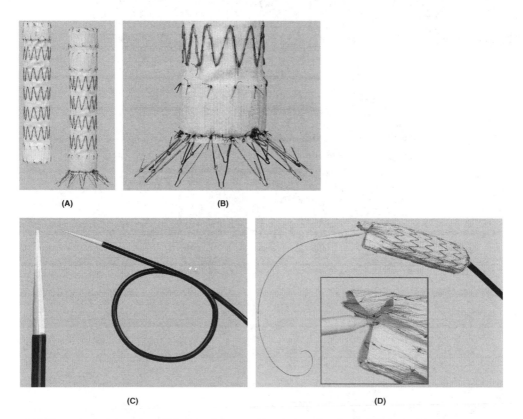

FIGURE 3 The TX2™ device (William Cook Europe, Bjaeverskov, Denmark). (**A**) The proximal and distal components. The distal component has the bare spring. (**B**) The lower end of the distal component with the bare spring. Note the barbs. (**C**) The delivery sheath. Note the tapered tip, the flexibility of the sheath and the hydrophilic coating which enables good trackability through narrow tortuous vessels. (**D**) The proximal device has been partially released but is still not fully expanded because of the retaining ties.

therefore suited to younger patients with aortic transactions. The proximal component is available in a tapered and straight configuration. The tapered device reduces in size by 4 mm from the top to the bottom. Both the straight and tapered components are available in at least two lengths for each diameter ranging from 108 to 216 mm. Proximal and distal extensions are available if required.

The delivery system for the TX2 is not dissimilar to the Zenith™ (William Cook Europe, Bjaeverskov, Denmark) abdominal endograft delivery system. It allows accurate positioning and keeps the graft stable during deployment. The stent graft is mounted on a central nitinol core within a braided sheath. The inner nitinol core provides increased flexibility compared with the previous Cook device. The sheath has a hydrophilic coating to facilitate introduction (Fig. 3C). Trigger wires hold the device in position even when the sheath has been retracted. The proximal stent is pinched-in toward the central core allowing blood to pass around the stent and making proximal repositioning a possibility. Once a satisfactory position has been achieved, two trigger wires release the proximal and distal stent attachments and allow the delivery system to be withdrawn. The device has the lowest profile sheath, and is only 20 F for endograft diameters up to 34 mm, and 22 F for the larger size endografts.

Device Deployment

With the sheathed endograft in position, the sheath is retracted exposing the endograft which partially expands, but is prevented from attaining its maximum diameter by the presence of the trigger wires. Even when the whole of the device has been uncovered by the outer sheath, it is possible to move the device to achieve the optimal position (Fig. 3D). Once the device is deemed to be in the best location, the proximal restraining trigger wire is released. The final step in the procedure is the release of the distal bare spring.

Pros

The presence of the trigger wires that prevent full expansion of the endograft provides additional control when accuracy of placement is paramount. Therefore, the endograft is well suited for patients when the landing zones are close to the supra-aortic vessels and celiac artery. Anecdotal reports suggest that the TX2 is particularly useful when the landing zone is close to the celiac artery. The delivery system is the lowest profile of the three main thoracic endografts which provides a potential advantage when the access vessels are narrow.

Cons

The device does not conform to curves as well as one would like. Therefore, we choose not to use this device if the aorta is very angulated. The range of sizes is wide, although there is a need for endografts wider than 42 mm. Finally, although the proximal fixation barbs prevent migration they may make the endograft less suitable for patients with thoracic dissection because of the potential for trauma to the fragile intima, producing further dissection. However this has not as yet been seen in clinical practice.

Other Thoracic Endografts

There are several other devices currently available undergoing evaluation. The published experience with these devices is low and only a brief description of the devices is included.

RELAY™

The endograft graft consists of nitinol stents stitched to surgical graft material with an uncovered proximal bare stent. The proximal fixation and sealing zone has an independent "freeflex" articulation with the body of the stent graft that is said to make it very conformable around the aortic arch. The endograft is mounted within a dual sheath delivery system. A rigid outer sheath facilitates device insertion into the abdominal aorta. The stent graft is advanced to the thoracic aorta inside the inner sheath. Deployment is achieved by withdrawing the inner sheath. The proximal bare stent is held closed within an apex grip allowing forward and backward repositioning in the semi-deployed situation, which has similarities to the TX2 endograft. The endograft is available in a good range of sizes (diameters of 22–46 mm, the availability of tapered devices, and lengths of 9–20 cm).

ENDOFIT™ ENDOGRAFT

This is the modified version of the first generation Endofit™ (LeMaitre Vascular, Germany) graft, which was withdrawn in 2005 because of issues with the proximal bare spring. The device consists of nitinol stents encapsulated in two layers of PTFE without the need for sutures. There is an uncovered stent at the proximal end of the device to aid fixation. Each stent, except the proximal bare stent, is separated from the others. The endograft is inserted into the aorta through a hydrophilic delivery sheath which provides trackability and is deployed simply by retracting the sheath and uncovering the endograft. The device is available in diameters of 30 to 42 mm and in lengths of 12 to 20 cm. Similar to the Relay™ device (Bolton Medical, Sunrise, Florida, U.S.A.), there is little published experience and therefore data on the advantages and disadvantages of these devices are limited.

THE ZENITH DISSECTION DEVICE (TX-D™)

At the time of writing, this device was undergoing clinical evaluation. The device is designed for placement in patients with acute dissection as a second device to stent open the true lumen after closure of the main communication in the thorax with a covered endograft (TX2).

It is a one-piece cylindrical device constructed from self-expanding stainless steel Cook-Z® (William Cook Europe, Bjaerverskov, Denmark) stent segments sewn together with polyester suture. The stents are uncovered to avoid blockage of dominant spinal cord intercostal arteries and allow for deployment of the stents across branch vessel origins as needed to treat the dissection. The device is available in multiple lengths (four, six or eight stent segments). At the present time, due to relative uniformity in radial force over the intended range of treatment diameters (24–38 mm), the TX-D™ (William Cook, Bjaerverskov, Denmark) is available in only one diameter (46 mm). As a result of this, the overall device length will vary in vivo with vessel diameter (Fig. 4).

We have used this device in two patients with acute dissection. In both cases, the follow-up computed tomography scan at two months has shown completion abolition of the false lumen in the thorax. Whether this encouraging early clinical experience is translated into similar results in larger numbers of patients will be seen with time.

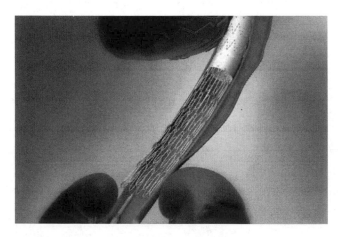

FIGURE 4 An illustration of the Zenith dissection device (TX-D™; William Cook, Bjaerverskov, Denmark). A covered TX-2 endograft has been placed across the main entry site into the false lumen in the upper thorax. The uncovered TX-D has been placed below the covered device, partially overlapping the covered device.

SUMMARY

There have been substantial improvements in the standard of thoracic endografts since the first implantations using homemade devices. The main devices available at this time are easy to use and provide good technical results in patients with a wide variety of pathologies involving the thoracic aorta. However, none of the endografts currently available are ideal in every respect. We can expect further developments in endograft technology to continue to be a feature of this exciting area of endovascular therapy in the future.

REFERENCES

1. Parodi JC, Palmaz JC, Barone HD. Transfemoral intraluminal graft implantation for abdominal aortic aneurysms. Ann Vasc Surg 1991; 5:491–9.
2. Volodos NL, Karpovich IP, Troyan VI, et al. Clinical experience of the use of self-fixing synthetic prostheses for remote endoprosthetics of the thoracic and the abdominal aorta and iliac arteries through the femoral artery and as intraoperative endoprosthesis for aorta reconstruction. Vasa Suppl 1991; 33:93–5.
3. Matravers P, Morgan R, Belli A. The use of stent grafts for the treatment of aneurysms and dissections of the thoracic aorta: a single centre experience. Eur J Vasc Endovasc Surg 2003; 26(6):587–95.
4. Sayed S, Thompson MM. Endovascular repair of the descending thoracic aorta: evidence for the change in clinical practice. Vascular 2005; 13(3):148–57.
5. Brandt M, Hussel K, Walluscheck KP, et al. Early and long-term results of replacement of the descending aorta. Eur J Vasc Endovasc Surg 2005; 30(4):365–9.
6. Ellozy SH, Carroccio A, Minor M, et al. Challenges of endovascular tube graft repair of thoracic aortic aneurysm: midterm follow-up and lessons learned. J Vasc Surg 2003; 38(4):676–83.

25 | Branch Endograft Technology for Endovascular Procedures on the Thoracic Aorta and Aortic Arch (Current and Future Applications)

Robert J. Hinchliffe and Krassi Ivancev
Endovascular Department, University Hospital, Malmo, Sweden

INTRODUCTION

The first thoracic stent grafts were used in the mid-1990s. They significantly reduced the perioperative morbidity and mortality of selected patients with thoracic aortic pathology. However, first and second generation stent-graft technology had significant limitations. Until recently, endovascular procedures have almost exclusively been restricted to pathology distal to the left subclavian artery. Recent attention has focussed on endovascular methods to deal with pathology in the arch of the aorta. This chapter addresses the technical considerations of stent-grafting in the aortic arch with particular reference to branch endograft technology.

MORPHOLOGY OF THE AORTIC ARCH

The morphology of the aortic arch is not well described. Conveniently, some authors have arbitrarily divided the arch of the aorta into zones dependent upon the site of the major arch branches (1).

Dake assessed the proportion of patients suitable for endovascular repair of thoracic aortic aneurysm in a study over a 19-month period (2). During this time 155 patients with thoracic aortic aneurysms were assessed. Using morphologic criteria suitable for first generation devices he found only 8% of all thoracic aneurysms were suitable for endovascular repair. Isolated descending thoracic aneurysms were most likely to be suitable for endovascular repair (37%). Further analysis found that 26% of patients with descending thoracic or thoracoabdominal aneurysms would be suitable. Inadequate access vessels or an aneurysm neck that was too short or too wide accounted for the majority of those who were unsuitable.

In an angiographic study of blunt thoracic aortic injury (transection), Carter and colleagues demonstrated that 46% (42/91) of injuries commenced less than 1 cm from the left subclavian artery (3). Interestingly, those injuries commencing less than 1 cm from the left subclavian artery were associated with a significantly higher mortality rate following attempted conventional surgical repair (43% vs. 22%). These might just be the group of patients who might benefit the most from endovascular branch stent-graft technology. One method of increasing the numbers of patients treatable by the endovascular technique is by covering the left subclavian artery. Some authors have found that coverage of the left subclavian artery increases the length of proximal landing zone by at least 2 cm (extending the landing zone to the left common carotid artery origin) (4).

ENDOVASCULAR CHALLENGES IN THE AORTIC ARCH

Endovascular surgery of the aortic arch is more challenging than the infrarenal aorta at every stage from preoperative planning, through intraoperative imaging and deployment to postoperative complications.

Significant discrepancies may arise in the measurement of length between those calculated by the centerlines of the computed tomography (CT) reformat, and that which is taken by a calibration angiographic catheter. The two techniques produce significantly different results in very large aneurysms or tortuous vessels (5). In the arch any discrepancy may have disastrous results. Modular stent-graft systems are particularly helpful in this situation because they have a degree of length adjustment to accommodate any discrepancy in length assessment.

Generally speaking, thoracic aortic stent grafts are more difficult to deploy than their infrarenal counterparts. Intraoperative visualization of thoracic endovascular stent grafts is made difficult because of tortuosity of the arch. To improve visualization, some authors have advocated transesophageal echocardiography in order to aid deployment (6). This technique is particularly useful to identify true and false lumens of a dissection and aortic side branches.

The movement of the aortic arch and forces placed upon stent grafts within it are high. The surgeon is further hampered by reduced torqueability and pushability of the stent-graft system. It is difficult to rotate and advance the sheath once positioned in the aortic arch. This is because the system is a long way from the access site and there are multiple angles between the two points. Fortunately, stent grafts generally orientate themselves in such a way as to lie around the outer curvature of the arch of the aorta. A stent graft that is orientated around the outer curve of the arch facilitates the deployment sequence.

The high endoleak rates associated with thoracic stent grafts (7–20%) are due to poor alignment of the stent grafts in the region of the aortic arch (7). Conventional stent grafts do not conform easily to the angles in the arch. In vitro analysis suggests that most stent grafts permit perigraft flow (endoleak) at angles less than 30° (8). The size of the endoleak increases with the degree of vessel angulation. One way to address this problem is to push the stent graft further around the arch, thus improving alignment. However, there is no guarantee that extending the proximal landing zone and improving alignment will ensure adequate seal. In one study in which all left subclavian arteries were overstented, the primary proximal (type I) endoleak rate was 17% (4/23) (4).

There are other complications that occur as a result of poor stent-graft alignment in the aortic arch. These include complete stent-graft collapse with acute thoracic aortic occlusion (9). Reports of retrograde type A dissection have emerged following endovascular treatment of type B dissection and aneurysms (10). Others have described the erosion of uncovered stents through the aortic arch and from true-to-false lumens (7). The use of proximal bare stents in the arch of the aorta, an inadequate coverage of the primary intimal tear of a type B dissection or excessive ballooning of the proximal stent graft may also contribute to these complications.

BRANCH VESSEL REPERFUSION

Stent-grafting in the aortic arch requires attention to branch vessel perfusion. While it would not be possible to occlude other the left common carotid artery or brachiocephalic trunks, many surgeons routinely cover the origin of the left subclavian artery without performing a bypass procedure. In a paper combining the U.K. RETA and the EUROSTAR Registries of thoracic stent-grafting it was necessary to overstent the left subclavian artery in 17% (42/249) of patients with aneurysmal disease and 28% (37/131) of patients with type B dissection (11).

There are some important considerations before blindly overstenting the left subclavian artery. These include congenital anomalies of the left vertebral artery, contributions to the cerebral and spinal cord circulation and left upper limb ischemia.

First, it is important to recognize congenital abnormalities of the left vertebral artery and vertebrobasilar system. The left vertebral artery is usually the dominant artery in 60% of individuals and arises from an anomalous location in up to 5% (12). Anomalous left vertebral arteries most frequently arise from the aortic arch between the left common carotid artery and the left subclavian artery and are visible on CT (13). A study by Tsuchida found that 13% (4/30) of patients have inadequate vertebrobasilar communications on preoperative cerebral angiography (14). In 7% (2/30) the left vertebral artery supplied a large area of the posterior fossa. And a hypoplastic vertebral artery is observed in 10% to 40% of normal angiograms (15,16).

Preoperative investigation of the cerebral circulation can be adequately assessed with either intracerebral CT angiography or magnetic resonance angiography.

In addition to the posterior cerebral circulation, the vertebrobasilar system makes important contributions to the spinal cord. The anterior spinal artery arises from one vertebral artery in 21% of cases, with approximately equal incidence from each side (17).

One should also be aware of patients who have had coronary bypass grafting using a left internal mammary artery conduit. Failure to do so may result in sudden death from coronary bypass graft occlusion. If the patient survives, a coronary steal phenomenon is another possibility (18).

There are few long-term data on the effects of subclavian artery occlusion following stent-graft repair of the thoracic aorta. Some patients may suffer delayed complications. Any long-term sequelae are likely to depend upon the development of collateral circulation and the patient's level of physical activity. Coverage of the left subclavian artery with a stent graft is likely to result in a significant fall in mean arterial pressure in the left arm (mean 48 mmHg) (4). In one study, three of eight (37%) patients who were initially asymptomatic postoperatively developed subclavian steal syndrome with vertigo and rest pain or claudication of their left arm during follow-up (19). Rehders suggested in his study that 32% of patients developed symptoms after left subclavian coverage but that none required intervention a mean of 24 months postoperatively (20). Another important factor not to be overlooked is the potential of backbleeding from an overstented left subclavian artery to the thoracic aneurysm sac (type II endoleak).

One way to prevent the complications of overstenting the left subclavian artery is to perform a preoperative extra-anatomic bypass (carotid–subclavian). However, this technique is not without complications. In the recently published results of the GORE TAG phase II multicenter trial, where all patients with an inadequate proximal sealing zone had preemptive open subclavian revascularization the stroke rate was 4% (5/139) (21). Carotid–subclavian bypass did not appear to offer any protection from stroke. Of the 28 (20%) who underwent carotid–subclavian bypass, four (14%) suffered a stroke. Overall, 80% of strokes occurred in those who underwent preoperative bypass. The reasons for this are not clear but may reflect more proximal aneurysm disease or stroke in the carotid territory rather than the vertebral.

STENT-GRAFT DESIGN

Modular Stent Grafts (Fenestrations/Scallops)

Stent grafts with fenestrations/scallops offer the advantage of providing an improved hemostatic seal while maintaining the patency of the target vessels toward which the fenestrations/scallops are oriented. This is particularly true in patients with aneurysms involving the inner curve of the aortic arch or with type B dissections where the main entry site tear is situated adjacent to the origin of the left subclavian artery. In both situations a standard thoracic stent graft would fail due to lack of sufficient implantation zone. In addition, the stent graft may perform poorly in the curved portion of the aortic arch because of unsatisfactory alignment. This has led to a compromise, which involves placement of a standard stent graft across the left subclavian artery, deploying it immediately after the origin of the left common carotid artery. Such a compromise carries the risk for inadvertent partial coverage of the left common carotid artery, thus jeopardizing flow in the anterior cerebral circulation and risking stroke.

Addressing these problems, Chinese endovascular specialists have reported the use of a branched stent graft for the left subclavian artery, achieving encouraging results in the treatment of patients with type B dissections (22). They have used a device with a branch stent graft–oriented cephalad. The branch is pulled into the left subclavian artery as the stent graft is advanced. Although they reported excellent results other groups have found the use of such a device cumbersome due to the angulation of the aortic arch at the origin of the left subclavian artery. There are further difficulties involved in bringing a side branch of the stent graft into the subclavian artery.

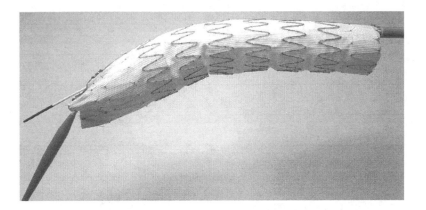

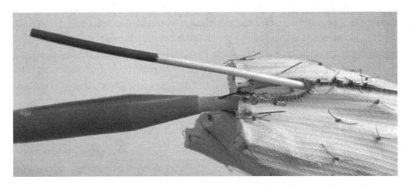

FIGURE 1 5-F catheter preloaded through scallop allowing for easy target vessel catheterization.

Because of this our group (Malmo, Sweden) has employed fenestrations/scallops in this situation. In order to facilitate the orientation of the device we have been using a 5-F catheter with a 0.035-in. guidewire preloaded through the fenestration/scallop. In this way, when the stent graft is only partially deployed, the target vessel can be catheterized allowing for correct orientation of the stent graft (Fig. 1). Orientation is the most problematic part of stent-graft treatment in the aortic arch. Though it appears that the wire preloaded into the catheter through the fenestration/scallop can easily be grasped with a snare from the target vessel (left subclavian artery, left common carotid artery or brachiocephalic trunk), there is a significant risk that this may result in inadvertent wrapping of the wire and catheter around the main stent graft. This complication is more likely in the aortic arch due to its tortuous nature and large lumen. Therefore it is preferable to catheterize the target vessels first and then grasp the wire with a snare, establishing a through-and-through position of the guidewire, ensuring correct orientation of the stent graft.

Once this is accomplished the procedure is continued with the placement of a stent graft through the fenestration, resulting in a modular type of branch (Fig. 2). An alternative technique is to use a large scallop, identified with radiopaque markers. This permits orientation of the scallop toward the target vessels. This potentially provides target vessel patency with a reduced embolic risk (Fig. 3A–C).

Inner sleeves may help address the problem with the orientation of stent grafts in the arch (Fig. 4A,B). These branches are reinforced with nitinol rings on the inside of the stent graft. Internal sleeves can be oriented cephalad or caudad and may also be preloaded with a catheter and wire facilitating catheterization of target vessels. It is possible to use a combination of fenestrations and inner sleeves. Once the fenestration is properly oriented, it necessarily follows that the inner sleeve is correctly orientated. Both the inner sleeve and fenestration would then be an implantation site for the placement of covered stents as branch stent grafts from the target vessel (Fig. 5A,B).

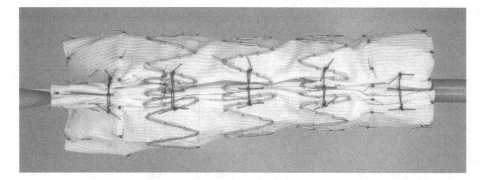

FIGURE 2 Placement of stent graft through fenestration resulting in modular type of branch.

While using this technique in the arch, the risk for incidental stroke is significant. This may be minimized either by the so-called "debranching" of the arch, performing extra-anatomic bypasses to the cervical vessels such as subclavian–carotid or carotid–carotid bypass, or the use of embolic protection such as filters in the internal carotid artery. Although these additional steps may further complicate an already complex procedure, the risk of stroke is considered high enough to justify such a precaution.

When there is no landing zone for implanting a stent graft in the aortic arch, despite the use of fenestrations/scallops and inner sleeves, there is a possibility of placing the stent graft further into the ascending thoracic aorta. This technique was developed by Chuter (23–25). It includes the placement of a bifurcated stent graft from the right common carotid artery. The cerebral flow is maintained by performing a left subclavian-to-left carotid bypass and a left carotid-to-right carotid bypass prior to introduction of the stent graft.

Once cerebral perfusion is secured the stent graft is orientated and deployed in the ascending aorta. Induction of temporary asystole with adenosine is helpful to aid deployment. The main body of the stent-graft system is similar to the modular bifurcated devices used in the infrarenal abdominal aorta. The smaller limb of the bifurcated device is deployed into the brachiocephalic trunk and the larger limb is deployed into the proximal portion of the aortic arch (Fig. 6). Once this is accomplished the flow to the right common carotid artery is reestablished. The second part of the stent graft is then introduced transfemorally and connected to the large limb of the bifurcated device in the aortic arch, thus reconstructing the whole arch with the two stent grafts (Fig. 7 and Figs. 8A–C).

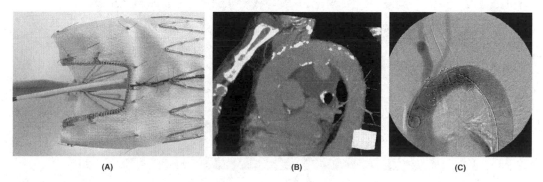

| (A) | (B) | (C) |

FIGURE 3 (**A**) Large scallop for preservation of arch branch. (**B**) Preoperative computed tomograph of aortic arch aneurysm. (**C**) Successfully excluded aneurysm with preservation of left common carotid artery with large scallop on intraoperative angiography.

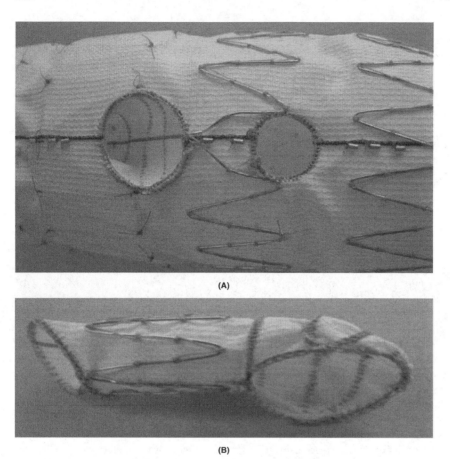

(A)

(B)

FIGURE 4 (**A**) Stent graft demonstrating inner sleeve stent-graft orientation adjacent to a graft fenestration. (**B**) Inner sleeve (during manufacture prior to being sutured to inside of stent graft).

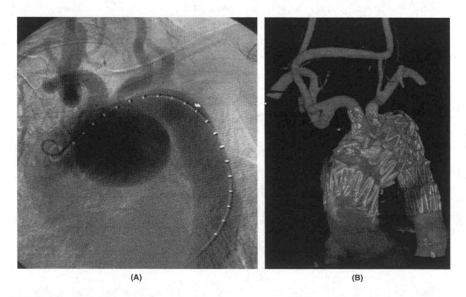

(A)   (B)

FIGURE 5 (**A**) Arch aortography demonstrating aneurysm. (**B**) Three-dimensional computed tomography reconstruction of aortic arch following branched stent-graft repair.

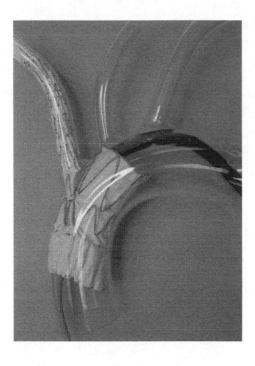

FIGURE 6 Bifurcated arch branch stent graft deployed in glass model prior to insertion of aortic arch limb.

In Situ Stent-Graft Fenestration

The feasibility of in situ fenestration of stent grafts was reported by McWilliams et al. in 2003 (26). Following in vitro and animal testing this group performed fenestration of a Zenith thoracic stent graft in a single patient to allow perfusion of a left subclavian artery (27).

The technique involves fenestration of the stent graft from the target vessel. A guidewire punctures the graft retrogradely and a cutting angioplasty balloon fenestrates the deployed stent graft. After serial dilatations a balloon-expandable stent graft is placed from the thoracic stent graft into the left subclavian artery.

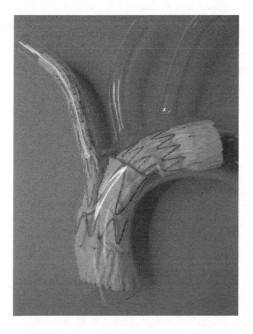

FIGURE 7 Fully deployed modular arch branch stent graft in glass model.

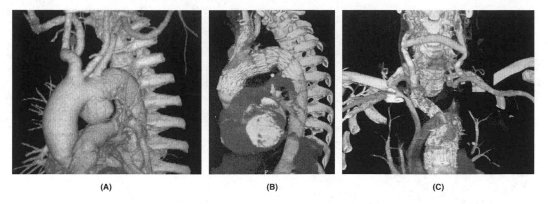

(A)   (B)   (C)

FIGURE 8   (**A**) Three-dimensional computed tomography reconstruction of aortic arch aneurysm. (**B,C**) Successful aneurysm exclusion with modular stent graft introduced via the brachiocephalic trunk.

This is an attractive technique because it does not require a preloaded customized stent graft. There are a number of drawbacks. It is possible that the orientation of the stents in the main graft may preclude satisfactory fenestration. In addition, there are concerns regarding the consequences of an uncontrolled graft fabric tear created in situ with the cutting balloons.

There have been no further publications on this technique following the first successful case report. It remains to be seen whether this technique can be applied to the left common carotid or brachiocephalic artery (either singly or in combination), which may not tolerate significant occlusion times.

Branched Stent Grafts (Unitary System)

The Inoue branched stent graft was first reported in 1996 in a patient with a type B aortic dissection. Since then there have been a number of reports on its use (28).

The stent graft is a unitary (one-piece) design and made from polyester supported by a ringed nickel titanium wire. In the early reports only one branch was used but subsequently a stent graft with three branches has been successfully implanted.

The stent graft is advanced into the thoracic aorta constrained by diameter restricting ties. Using preloaded traction wires and a snare from the target vessel (left subclavian, left common carotid, brachiocephalic) it is pulled into position in the target vessel. The stent graft is then deployed.

In their second report of 17 patients (1999–2004) only the single branched stent graft was included (29). Stent-graft implantation was successful in all patients. Complete exclusion of the aneurysm was achieved in 14 of 17 patients on postoperative CT (three type I endoleaks). There were no deaths, one paraparesis and three local groin complications. During follow-up (mean 26 months) two of the three endoleaks were successfully treated by endovascular extensions. The other patient was too frail for any intervention. Two deaths occurred, neither was aneurysm related.

The Inoue system is unitary and does not allow for any intraoperative customization of length. It should be noted that unitary stent grafts have largely been discarded in the infrarenal aorta because they are difficult to deploy. The aortic arch is more challenging, and may be better suited to a modular stent-graft system. An additional drawback of the uritary system is the high risk of generating emboli. The risk is high because of the multiple wires used and the high degree of endovascular manipulation required. The technique of pulling branches of the stent graft into the target vessels is of major concern.

CONCLUSIONS

Endovascular repair has significantly reduced the morbidity and mortality from procedures on the thoracic aorta. The aortic arch is more challenging due to the degree of angulation and the presence of critical side branches.

The first steps taken to deal with more complex thoracic aortic morphology involved deploying stent grafts further around the arch. This improved stent-graft conformity at the expense of overstenting the left subclavian artery. Occlusion of the left subclavian artery is not without complications; however, preservation of the left subclavian artery is now perfectly possible using scallops and fenestrations.

Greater understanding and improving technology have recently allowed the first few successful endovascular stent-graft procedures to be performed further around the arch.

This represents a new era for endovascular surgery. Endovascular procedures on the aortic arch are likely to become routine in much the same way as they have become in the infrarenal aorta. It is perfectly feasible that such procedures could be combined with endovascular aortic valve replacement, significantly reducing the need for open surgery.

REFERENCES

1. Criado FJ, Barnatan MF, Rizk Y, Clark NS, Wang CF. Technical strategies to expand stent-graft applicability in the aortic arch and proximal descending thoracic aorta. J Endovasc Ther 2002; 9:II32–8.
2. Dake MD, Miller DC, Semba CP, Mitchell RS, Walker PJ, Liddell RP. Transluminal placement of endovascular stent-grafts for the treatment of descending thoracic aortic aneurysms. N Engl J Med 1994; 331:1729–34.
3. Carter Y, Meissner M, Bulger E, et al. Anatomical considerations in the surgical management of blunt thoracic aortic injury. J Vasc Surg 2001; 34:628–33.
4. Gorich J, Asquan Y, Seifarth H, et al. Initial experience with intentional stent-graft coverage of the subclavian artery during endovascular thoracic aortic repairs. J Endovasc Ther 2002; 9(Suppl. 2):II39–43.
5. Armon MP, Whitaker SC, Gregson RH, Wenham PW, Hopkinson BR. Spiral CT angiography versus aortography in the assessment of aortoiliac length in patients undergoing endovascular abdominal aortic aneurysm repair. J Endovasc Surg 1998; 5:222–7.
6. Rocchi G, Lofiego C, Biagini E, et al. Transesophageal echocardiography-guided algorithm for stent-graft implantation in aortic dissection. J Vasc Surg 2004; 40.880–5.
7. Sunder-Plassmann L, Orend KH. Stent-grafting of the thoracic aorta—complications. J Cardiovasc Surg 2005; 46:121–30.
8. Albertini JN, Demasi MA, Macierewicz J, et al. Aorfix stent graft for abdominal aortic aneurysms reduces the risk of proximal type 1 endoleak in angulated necks: bench-test study. Vascular 2005; 13:321–6.
9. Hinchliffe RJ, Krasznai A, SchultzeKool L, et al. Observations on the failure of stent-grafts in the aortic arch Europ J Vascular Endovasc Surg (in press).
10. Neuhauser B, Czermak BV, Fish J, et al. Type A dissection following aortic stent-graft repair. J Endovasc Ther 2005; 12:74–81.
11. Leurs LJ, Bell R, Degrieck Y, et al. Endovascular treatment of thoracic aortic diseases: combined experience from the EUROSTAR and United Kingdom Thoracic Endograft Registries. J Vasc Surg 2004; 40:670–9.
12. Shrontz C, Dujovny M, Ausman JI, et al. Surgical anatomy of the arteries of the posterior fossa. J Neurosurg 1986; 65:540–4.
13. Vorster W, du Plooy PT, Meiring JH. Abnormal origin of internal thoracic and vertebral arteries. Clin Anat 1998; 11:33–7.
14. Tsuchida K, Hashimoto A, Aomi S, Hirayama T, Endo M, Koyanagi H. Prevention of cerebral complications during thoracic aortic aneurysms operation: study of preoperative selective cerebral arteriography. Kyobu Geka (Japanese) 1991; 44:380–3.
15. Matula C, Trattnig S, Tschabitscher M, Day JD, Koos WT. The course of the prevertebral segment of the vertebral artery: anatomy and clinical significance. Surg Neurol 1997; 48:125–31.
16. Davis WLJJ. Cerebral vasculature: normal anatomy and pathology. In: Osborn AG, ed. Diagnostic Neuroradiology. St Louis: Mosby, 1994:117–53.
17. Wollschlaeger G, Wollschlaeger PB, Lucas FV, Lopez VF. Experience and result with postmortem cerebral angiography performed as routine procedure of the autopsy. Am J Roentgenol Radium Ther Nucl Med 1967; 101:68–87.

18. Bicknell CD, Subramanian A, Wolfe JH. Coronary subclavian steal syndrome. Eur J Vasc Endovasc Surg 2004; 27:220–1.
19. Tiesenhausen K, Hausegger KA, Oberwalder P, et al. Left subclavian artery management in endovascular repair of thoracic aortic aneurysms and aortic dissections. J Card Surg 2003; 18:429–35.
20. Rehders TC, Petzsch M, Ince H, et al. Intentional occlusion of the left subclavian artery during stent-graft inplantation in the thoracic aorta: risk and relevance. J Endovasc Ther 2004; 11:659–66.
21. Makaroun MS, Dillavou ED, Kee ST, et al. Endovascular treatment of thoracic aortic aneurysms: results of the phase II multicenter trial of the GORE TAG thoracic endoprosthesis. J Vasc Surg. 2005; 41:1–9.
22. Wang ZG, Li C. Single-branch endograft for treating stanford type B aortic dissections with entry tears in proximity to the left subclavian artery. J Endovasc Ther 2005; 12:588–93.
23. Schneider DB, Curry TK, Reilly LM, Kang JW, Messina LM, Chuter TA. Branched endovascular repair of aortic arch aneurysm with a modular stent-graft system. J Vasc Surg 2003; 38:855.
24. Chuter TA, Buck DG, Schneider DB, Reilly LM, Messina LM. Development of a branched stent-graft for endovascular repair of aortic arch aneurysms. J Endovasc Ther 2003; 10:940–5.
25. Chuter TA, Schneider DB, Reilly LM, Lobo EP, Messina LM. Modular branched stent graft for endovascular repair of aortic arch aneurysm and dissection. J Vasc Surg 2003; 38:859–63.
26. McWilliams RG, Fearn SJ, Harris P L, et al. Retrograde fenestration of endoluminal grafts from target vessels: feasibility, technique and potential usage. J Endovasc Ther 2003; 10:946–52.
27. McWilliams RG, Murphy M, Hartley D, Lawrence-Brown MM, Harris PL. In situ stent-graft fenestration to preserve the left subclavian artery. J Endovasc Ther 2004; 11:170–4.
28. Inoue K, Sato M, Iwase T, et al. Clinical endovascular placement of branched graft for type B aortic dissection. J Thorac Cardiovasc Surg 1996; 112:1111–3.
29. Saito N, Kimura T, Odashiro K, et al. Feasibility of the Inoue single-branched stent-graft implantation for thoracic aortic aneurysm or dissection involving the left subclavian artery: short- to medium-term results in 17 patients. J Vasc Surg 2005; 41:206–12.

26 | Hybrid Surgical Procedures for Thoracic Pathology (Great Vessel Transposition and Bypass, Mesenteric and Visceral Revascularization)

Robert E. Brightwell and Nicholas J. W. Cheshire
Division of Surgery, Oncology, Reproductive Biology and Anaesthetics, Imperial College London, St. Mary's Hospital, London, U.K.

INTRODUCTION

As a direct evolutionary step from stenting abdominal aortic aneurysms, endovascular techniques have been successfully used to treat a variety of lesions in the thoracic aorta, including aneurysms, dissections, penetrating ulcers, aorto-visceral fistulas, acute transections, coarctations and complications of previous aortic repair (1–8). The early results of a minimally invasive, endoluminal approach have been favorable, with reduced blood loss, a lower rate of spinal cord injuries, shorter intensive therapy unit (ITU) and hospital stays, and a reduced recovery time for the patient.

Whilst the possible benefits of endovascular surgery are patent, the increasing complexity and severity of thoracic aortic pathology encountered frequently demands that standard techniques are modified: hybrid procedures (combining open and endovascular surgery) are often mandatory to effectively and safely treat complex pathologies such as aneurysm and dissection, and are now described in more detail (9–12).

HYBRID APPROACHES TO TREAT THORACOABDOMINAL ANEURYSM

A thoracoabdominal aortic aneurysm (TAAA) is defined by involvement of the origins of the celiac, superior mesenteric and renal arteries. Crawford's classification system is universally accepted (Fig. 1) (13).

TAAA have a high mortality and morbidity when treated by open techniques (14,15). These risks persist despite advances in operative technique (including left heart bypass, spinal cord protection, hypothermic cardiopulmonary arrest, and selective visceral perfusion) and higher standards of perioperative care.

The use of endovascular stents for the treatment of TAAA showed significant early promise, a number of centers published encouraging early use of endovascular stents limited to the thoracic segment (16). This was due to the limitations imposed by the involvement of the origin of the visceral arteries. Combining endovascular techniques with an open abdominal procedure to revascularize the visceral and renal arteries is attractive as it avoids thoracotomy, left heart bypass, extensive tissue dissection, excessive blood loss, and supra-celiac aortic cross clamp (Fig. 2).

Early Experience of Visceral Hybrid Repair

The first case describing a combined open and endovascular approach to treat a TAAA was in 1999 by Quinones-Baldrich et al. (17). In this instance prior abdominal surgery and

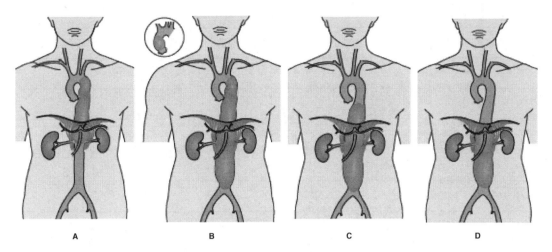

FIGURE 1 Crawford's classification of thoracoabdominal aortic aneurysms. *Source*: From Ref. 13.

aneurysms of the visceral arteries precluded open repair. Subsequent to this report nine further individual cases/small series using a hybrid approach in the treatment of TAAA were published (18–26). The results of these individual cases were encouraging, despite the extremely complex nature of the disease and significant comorbidity of the patients being treated. It is worth highlighting that no standard technique was employed, and a variety of stent-grafts deployed.

Of the 20 patients reported in these series, only one (5%) died within a median period of follow up of 13 months. Spinal ischemia appeared to be rare (it was not reported in a single case), other complications were greatly reduced, and intensive care stay declined compared with open surgery.

Institutional Technique of Hybrid TAAA Stent Grafting and Visceral Bypass

The patient is placed in a supine position under general and epidural anesthesia, with routine cerebrospinal fluid (CSF) drainage. We routinely use cell salvage techniques (with rapid infusers available) and invasive monitoring with arterial and central venous lines, urethral catheterization, and transoesophageal echocardiography.

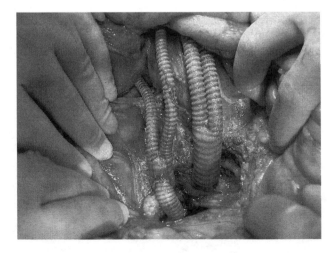

FIGURE 2 Operative picture of visceral and renal arteries bypass. In this case a fifth limb has been tunneled to the femoral artery to improve access for the thoracoabdominal stent.

A midline laparotomy allows for adequate exposure of the abdominal aorta, the origin of each renal artery, the celiac axis, and the superior mesenteric artery (SMA). The inflow site for visceral bypass grafting is determined by previous abdominal aortic surgery and distal extent of aneurysmal disease. Where a previous infra-renal repair has been undertaken the bypass grafts are anastomosed in an end-to-side fashion to the existing graft. Where an infra-renal repair is possible, this is completed first and bypass grafts are subsequently sutured as above. If the infra renal aorta is normal an arteriotomy is performed and the bypass grafts anastomosed in an end-to-side fashion to the native aorta: when aneurysmal disease extends to the bifurcation, one external iliac artery provides the inflow sites.

Most often two inverted (14 by 7 mm or 16 by 8 mm) Dacron grafts function as the conduits. The renal arteries are sequentially anastomosed in an end-to-side or end to end fashion. The two remaining graft limbs are routed along the base of the small bowel mesentery to the celiac axis (via a retropancreatic tunnel) and SMA in an end-to-side fashion. If Doppler signals are satisfactory in the bypass grafts (with the origins of the native vessel clamped) they are subsequently suture-ligated to prevent retrograde flow into the aneurysm sac (termed Type II endoleak).

Following successful visceral and renal bypass a suitable access site is chosen for endovascular stent deployment: usually a dedicated conduit attached to the common iliac artery or the abdominal aorta. An angiography catheter is introduced on the contra-lateral side and the stents are deployed in a sequential fashion from the left subclavian artery through the thoracic aorta to the landing zone. Our unit prefers this technique for Crawford Type I, II, and III TAAA, while an open approach with medial visceral rotation is used for Crawford Type IV aneurysms.

Results of Visceral Hybrid Graft

The current results from our unit include hybrid surgery for 47 patients, 27 elective, 15 urgent, and 5 emergency. The lesion morphology included Crawford Type I (5), Type II (21), Type III (16), Type IV (1) and Complex (4). A completed procedure was given for 43 patients (91%), with the median ischemic time being 15 minutes (range 13–27 minutes) for each anastomosis. There were two cases of paraplegia (4%) within 30 days, and the elective mortality was 13%. There were 16 endoleaks in the perioperative period; Type I (9), Type II (6), Type III (1). At a median follow-up of 13 months 94% of visceral grafts were patent

ADVANTAGES OF HYBRID APPROACH TO THORACIC AORTIC ANEURYSM REPAIR

The authors perceive several advantages of this approach over standard, open techniques:

- Avoidance of thoracotomy
  - Potentially fewer pulmonary complications
  - Fewer cardiac arrhythmias
  - Less pain
- Reduced hypothermia with subsequent reduction in:
  - Coagulopathy
  - Cardiovascular instability
- Reduced rate of spinal ischemia
- Reduced duration of mesenteric and visceral ischemia with reduction in:
  - Acidosis and associated problems
  - Gut bacteria translocation/sepsis
  - Renal failure/use of renal replacement therapy
- Less blood loss/reduced transfusion requirement
- Reduced hospital stay
  - ITU
  - Absolute
- More patients can be treated where comorbidity previously excluded them

FUTURE OF TAAA MANAGEMENT

The hybrid approach to TAAA may be a bridging measure until the technology of branched endovascular stent grafts (EVSG) becomes established (see chap. 39). Endovascular repair of juxtarenal and suprarenal abdominal aortic aneurysms with preservation of visceral perfusion by fenestrated (28,29) or branched (30) EVSG has been shown to be feasible, and, using similar technology, several authors have described total endovascular repair of complex thoracic aortic disease (31,32). Until recently Chuter et al. were the only authors to report total endovascular repair of a TAAA with preservation of all four visceral vessels in a single patient (33). Anderson et al. reported a series of four patients treated in this way: 12 out of 13 target vessels were revascularized, with no endoleaks. three of the patients required further procedures to correct bleeding from access vessels, and one patient died from multi-organ dysfunction syndrome after such a procedure. Computed tomography at 12 months confirmed antegrade perfusion in all 10 target vessels (34).

Further improvement of, and access to, such devices, and correct patient selection [in light of the endovascular aneurysm repair trial 2 results (35)] may see a reduction in the numbers of visceral hybrid procedures being performed for TAAA. In the meantime, and in cases not suitable for repair using fenestrated/branched EVSG, the hybrid approach provides an adaptable and robust method of treating this complex disease.

HYBRID APPROACH TO TREAT ARCH/THORACIC ANEURSYMS

Standard endoluminal stent grafting techniques cannot be used to treat the cerebral vessel-bearing areas of the arch, and a variety of methods have been described to overcome this problem.

In April 2005, Bergeron et al. reported their experience of using great vessel transposition/bypass followed by endovascular exclusion (36). Twenty-nine patients presented with acute thoracic aortic pathologies involving the aortic arch and were treated by endovascular exclusion. A synopsis of pathologies follows: atherosclerotic aneurysms of the descending thoracic aorta in 15 cases, acute Stanford Type A dissections in six cases, Stanford Type B dissections in seven cases (one acute), and one false aneurysm of the ascending aorta.

Total-arch transpositions of all supra-aortic vessels (aortic "debranching") to the ascending aorta were completed in 11 cases through a standard median sternotomy. Carotido-carotid bypass (hemi-arch transposition) was performed in 16 patients by neck incision. Secondary to surgical transpositions, EVSG were placed in all but two patients for final exclusion, the two remaining were planned to have endovascular exclusion later. The Talent™ (Medtronic, Santa Rosa, California, U.S.A.), Excluder® (W.L. Gore and Associates, Inc., Flagstaff, Arizona, U.S.A.), TAG® (W.L. Gore and Associates, Inc., Flagstaff, Arizona, U.S.A.) and Zenith® (Cook Inc., Bloomington Indiana, U.S.A.) stent grafts were used in 12, 3, 1 and 4 cases, respectively. An aortic banding technique was used as an adjunctive procedure in some cases.

All surgical transpositions were successful although one led to a minor stroke (1/29=3.5%); this worsened to major stroke after endovascular exclusion. Endovascular procedures were performed in all but one case (26/27=96.3%). Two patients (2/26=7.7%) died from catheterization related complications after endovascular exclusion (iliac rupture and left ventricle perforation). One patient had a delayed minor stroke (1/26=3.8%). Recirculation was found in 13.3% (2/15) of aneurysms and 27.3% of thoracic false channels. During a mean follow-up of 15.7 months (13 days to 45.5 months), one patient (1/26=3.8%) who had preoperative chronic pulmonary failure died at six months from respiratory failure. The authors observed one case (3.8%) of unilateral limb palsy unrelated to cerebral ischemia, which was successfully treated by CSF drainage. No stent-related complication was noted. One new Type I endoleak appeared at 12 months in a patient treated for an aneurysm; this resolved after stent graft extension. Three thoracic dissection false channels remained patent during follow-up, of which one was retrograde originating distally in the descending aorta.

It was concluded that secondary endovascular exclusion of thoracic aortic diseases involving the arch in high risk patients is made technically possible using the described aortic debranching procedures. Total-arch transposition was suggested to be of greater interest and importance in cases of proximal neck length uncertainty, and where there is a greater risk of embolization from the diseased aortic arch. There is no doubt that carotid–carotid bypass may be successfully used to expand the number of patients suitable for endovascular repair of thoracic pathology (Fig. 3).

Most recently Matalanis et al. described an elegant technique of aortic arch branch transposition and antegrade stent deployment for complete arch repair in a 77-year-old man with lifestyle-limiting airways disease (37). Through a median sternotomy and the application of a side-biting clamp, the common trunk of a bifurcation Dacron graft was anastomosed to the ascending aorta, and a conduit for introducing the stent grafts anastomosed to that. The limbs of the graft were anastomosed to the innominate and left common carotid arteries, respectively. The left subclavian artery was ligated and not revascularized. Two endoluminal stent grafts were deployed via the side arm in the Dacron graft, covering the distal ascending aorta, the whole arch, and the proximal descending aorta (Fig. 4).

An extra-anatomic technique had been described previously where a left-to-right carotid crossover graft is run across the midline of the neck, and then onto the left subclavian artery (38). This, however, renders cerebral inflow entirely dependent on the brachiocephalic trunk. In addition, it allows only partial coverage of the arch, but does not necessitate median sternotomy. Akasaka et al. also used an endovascular stent to cover the arch following extra-anatomical bypass grafting of the arch vessels (39). Their technique was more complicated–using left heart bypass and selective cerebral perfusion.

A similar technique to that described by Matalanis was developed by Kato et al. (40). However, this group did not transpose the brachiocephalic trunk; instead, they bypassed the left carotid and left subclavian arteries–meaning they could only cover the mid and distal arch. Also, in Kato's technique, the endovascular graft was inserted directly into the common trunk of the bifurcation graft rather than via a dedicated side limb.

Elephant Trunk Procedure

The treatment of thoracic aneurysms that affect the arch and proximal descending thoracic aorta often requires a two-stage repair that requires a proximal elephant trunk graft placement and later completion of thoracic or thoracoabdominal repair.

The two-stage approach first requires a median sternotomy then, under hypothermic circulatory arrest, placement of an elephant trunk graft with or without arch repair. The second-stage procedure (completion operation) traditionally requires a left thoracotomy or thoracoabdominal approach to extend the elephant trunk graft to the healthy distal aorta, with possible reimplantation of intercostal or visceral vessels. The morbidity and mortality risks

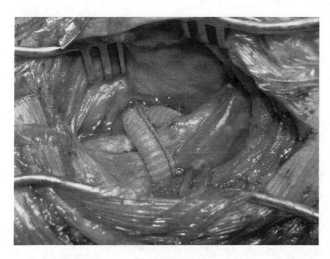

FIGURE 3 Operative picture of a retropharyngeal carotid–carotid bypass with an additional graft to left subclavian bypass.

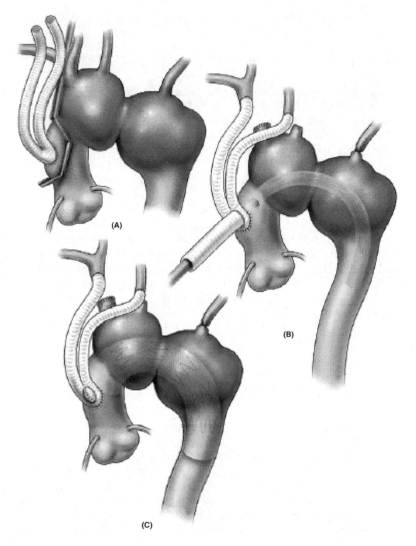

FIGURE 4 (**A**) The bifurcation graft is sewn onto the ascending aorta; (**B**) two endovascular stent grafts deployed via the side arm in the bifurcation graft; (**C**) complete coverage of the arch aneurysms. *Source*: From Ref. 37.

associated with the open two-stage approach remain substantial and have been reported previously (41–43). Some surgeons have explored the use of endovascular stent graft technologies to complete elephant trunk graft repairs and thus avoid the requisite thoracotomy or thoracoabdominal incision.

In a recent report of their institutional experience using this hybrid technique, Greenberg et al. describe the results in 22 patients who required elephant trunk and endovascular completion (Fig. 5) (44). Three patients underwent mesenteric bypass in addition to their proximal repairs. Mean follow-up was 10 months (range 1–42 months). Technical success was achieved in all patients, no ruptures were reported, and all patients returned for follow-up. The 1-, 12-, and 24-month mortality rates (by Kaplan–Meier analysis) were 4.5%, 15.8%, and 15.8%, respectively. Caudal migration of the endograft occurred in one patient, and all but two aneurysms decreased or remained stable in size. The two patients with growth included a Type III endoleak (which resolved after treatment) and pressurization through an expanded polytetrafluoroethylene stent graft. Three cases of transient paraparesis occurred (all in patients requiring mesenteric bypass or abdominal aortic aneurysm repair), and there were no paraplegias or strokes.

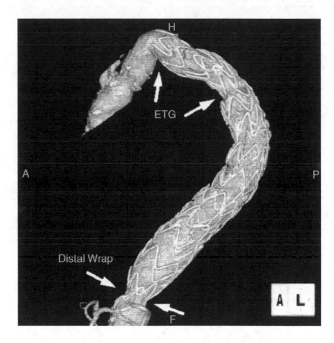

FIGURE 5 A Talent stent graft is located within an ETG proximally, and distally a seal is created between the stent graft and a supraceliac aortic band (aortic banding) that was placed during the first-stage procedure through a posterior pericardial approach. *Abbreviations*: ETG, elephant trunk graft; A, anterior; L, lateral. *Source*: From Ref. 44.

The authors concluded that this approach showed great promise in terms of feasibility and results—even in a group of patients with significant comorbidity. They did warn however, of the need for meticulous postoperative imaging to detect persistent aneurysm sac pressurization.

Development of Hybrid Endograft

In current practice a two-step surgical approach is often required to treat patients with coexisting pathologies affecting the ascending thoracic aorta, arch, and descending thoracic aorta. Such diseases include Stanford Type A aortic dissections and aneurysms of multiple thoracic aortic segments.

The same is true for patients who require surgery involving the ascending aorta, such as coronary artery bypass grafting (CABG) or aortic valve replacement (AVR), and have multiple aneurysms or dissections of the aortic arch and descending aorta. In patients with Type A aortic dissections, the proximal aorta is initially replaced with or without the "elephant trunk" technique, followed by subsequent completion surgery via a thoracotomy, as described previously.

In 2005, Chavan et al. reported their early experiences using a hybrid endograft that enables such treatment during a single operation (45). The hybrid endograft (Chavan–Haverich endograft; Curative GmbH, Dresden, Germany) consisted of a woven Dacron vascular prosthesis with stainless-steel stents affixed to the inner aspect at its distal end (Fig. 6). The stents had a length of 22 mm each; a gap of 5 mm between adjacent stents provided flexibility to the system—very necessary given the profile of the aortic arch and descending thoracic aorta. The distance between the stents was maintained with the help of two longitudinally oriented stainless-steel wires. The proximal portion of the endograft contained no stent and consisted only of a Dacron sleeve that could be sutured surgically to the aortic wall or a proximal vascular prosthesis. The median diameter of the hybrid endograft was 36 mm (range, 30–46 mm). The total lengths of the endografts varied between 200 and 365 mm (median, 276 mm). The number of stents varied between two and four (median of three). The delivery system was flexible, could be advanced into the descending aorta over a 0.035-in. super stiff guide wire (Back-up Meier; Boston Scientific, Watertown, MA), and possessed a "sheath-in-sheath" design. It consisted of a 39-F outer sheath, a 34-F inner sheath, and a central pusher. Withdrawal of the outer sheath while

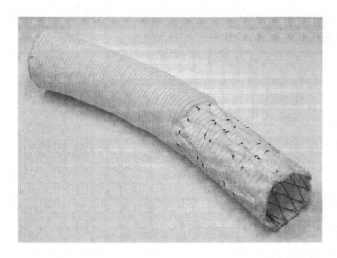

FIGURE 6 Chavan–Haverich hybrid endograft consisting of a woven Dacron vascular graft with stainless-steel stents at its distal end. The proximal portion does not contain stents. *Source*: From Ref. 45.

holding the inner sheath and the pusher steady released the stent-containing portion of the endograft. The proximal Dacron tube could then be released by pulling back both the sheaths simultaneously steady.

After median sternotomy, extracorporeal circulation was established by cannulating the ascending while holding the pusheraorta and right atrium. Core cooling to 25°C was attained and during hypothermic circulatory arrest, selective antegrade cerebral cold blood–brain perfusion was initiated. The aortic arch was subsequently opened for implantation of the hybrid endograft in the descending aorta. The authors report that in the first five patients, implantation of the endograft was performed over only an antegradely placed super-stiff guide wire: after perforating the aortic wall with the introducer system in one patient with a tortuous descending aorta, a through-and-through guide wire technique was employed in the subsequent patients. The guide wire was placed via a femoral artery and drawn out proximally after the aortic arch was opened. Manipulation at both ends of the guide wire was used to facilitate easy introduction of the endograft system. The distal landing site of the stent graft was at or above the level of the tenth thoracic vertebra. Choosing this level was a consequence of the pathologic anatomy present in the patients; possible reduction in the incidence of paraplegia was a secondary consideration. Anchoring further distally was not deemed necessary in the sub-group of patients with atherosclerotic aneurysms. In patients with dissections, the anchoring was more proximal in accordance with the recommendation made by Svensson and colleagues to keep the distal "elephant trunk" shorter than 10 to 15 cm—thus reducing the risk of paraplegia (46). After deployment, the stent-containing portion of the endograft was manipulated using a balloon catheter and the non-stent-containing Dacron graft segment was sutured circumferentially to the aorta distal to the origin of the left subclavian artery. The proximal Dacron portion was used to reconstruct the aortic arch or was sutured onto a previously placed ascending aortic graft. Additional procedures on the heart or the proximal aorta (e.g., AVR, CABG, ascending aortic graft) were performed before or after endograft implantation. Twenty-two consecutive patients with multisegment disease of the proximal and descending thoracic aorta were treated. Thirteen (59.1%) patients were men and nine (40.9%) were women. The median age was 64 years (range, 47–77 years). The patients belonged to three broad groups: those with atherosclerotic aneurysms (7–32%); those with Type A dissections (11–50%); and those with Type B dissections (4–18%). Additional disease such as aortic incompetence and coronary artery disease requiring ancillary procedures such as AVR or CABG was present in 11 patients.

Endograft implantation was successful in all but one patient (95%). The time required for stent-graft deployment varied between 7 and 26 minutes (median, 12 minutes). There was one in-hospital death as a result of hemorrhage from an iatrogenic arterial injury (30-day mortality rate, 4.5%). Major clinical complications occurred in a total of 18% of patients and consisted of one stroke (4.5%), one case of paraplegia (4.5%), and two cases of vocal chord paralysis (9%). Eighteen percent of the patients experienced minor complications. Repeat thoracotomy for bleeding was necessary in two patients.

CONCLUSIONS

Hybrid techniques have expanded the applications of endovascular stent-graft technologies. As a result, patients affected by most aortic pathologies have benefited from the minimally-invasive approach such procedures offer. With such operations becoming safer, more and more patients considered otherwise unfit for surgical intervention are now able to be treated effectively with acceptable risk.

It must be understood that the endovascular revolution moves on at an increased pace, with further advances in technology and application announced frequently. While branched and fenestrated endovascular grafts are now available their cost, and inherent delay in manufacture of bespoke grafts, makes them generally unavailable. As such their widespread use will not increase until costs and availability improve. In the meantime a hybrid approach to many diseases of the thoracic aorta will continue to offer patients and their surgeons a minimally-invasive, cost-effective option to treat such complex diseases.

REFERENCES

1. Thompson CS, Rodriguez JA, Ramaiah VG, et al. Acute traumatic rupture of the thoracic aorta treated with endoluminal stent-grafts. J Trauma 2002; 52:1173–7.
2. Thompson CS, Goxotte VD, Rodriguez JA, et al. Endoluminal stent grafting of the thoracic aorta: initial experience with the Gore Excluder. J Vasc Surg 2002; 35:1163–70.
3. Ramaiah VG, Rodriguez-Lopez J, Dietrich EB. Endografting of the thoracic aorta. J Card Surg 2003; 18:444–54.
4. Rodriguez JA, Olsen DM, Diethrich EB. Thoracic aortic dissections: unpredictable lesions that may be treated using endovascular techniques. J Card Surg 2003; 18:334–50.
5. Diethrich EB. Endovascular thoracic aortic repairs: greater experience brings rewards…and new problems to challenge us. J Endovasc Ther 2004; 11:168–9.
6. Nathanson DR, Rodriguez-Lopez JA, Ramaiah VG, et al. Endoluminal stent-graft stabilization for thoracic aortic dissection. J Endovasc Ther 2005; 12:354–9.
7. Wheatley GH, Gurbuz AT, Rodriguez-Lopez JA, et al. Midterm outcome in 158 consecutive Gore TAG thoracic endoprostheses: a single-centre experience. Ann Thorac Surg (in press).
8. Carrel TP, Berdat PA, Baumgartner I, et al. Combined surgical and endovascular approach to treat a complex aortic coarctation without extracorporeal circulation. Ann Thorac Surg 2004; 78:1462–5.
9. Kato M, Kuratani T, Kaneko M, et al. The results of total arch graft implantation with open stent-graft placement for type A dissection. J Thorac Cardiovasc Surg 2002; 124:531–40.
10. Schumacher H, Bockler D, Bardenheuer H, et al. Endovascular aortic arch reconstruction with supra-aortic transposition for symptomatic contained rupture and dissection: early experience in 8 high-risk patients. J Endovasc Ther 2003; 10:1066–74.
11. Naganuma J, Ninomiya M, Miyairi T, et al. Total aortic arch aneurysm repair using a stent graft without cardiac or cerebral ischemia. Jpn J Thorac Cardiovasc Surg 2002; 50:298–301.
12. Melissano G, Civilini E, Maisano F, et al. Off-pump endovascular treatment of aortic arch aneuysms (in Italian). Ital Heart J Suppl 2004; 5:727–34.
13. Crawford ES, Crawford JL, Safi HJ, et al. Thoracoabdominal aortic aneurysms: preoperative and intraoperative factors determining immediate and long-term results of operations in 605 patients. J Vasc Surg 1986; 3:389–404.
14. Svensson LG, Crawford ES, Hess KR, et al. Experience with 1509 patients undergoing thoracoab-dominal aortic operations. J Vasc Surg 1993; 17:357–70.
15. Svensson LG, Crawford ES, Hess KR, et al. Dissection of the aorta and dissecting aortic aneurysms: improving early and long-term surgical results. Circulation 1990; 82:IV24–38.
16. Dake MD, Miller DC, Mitchell RS, et al. The "first generation" of endovascular stent-grafts for patients with aneurysms of the descending thoracic aorta. J Thorac Cardiovasc Surg 1991; 111:689–703.
17. Quinones-Baldrich WJ, Panetta TF, Vescera CL, et al. Repair of type IV thoracoabdominal aneurysm with a combined endovascular and surgical approach. J Vasc Surg 1999; 30:555–60.
18. Macierewicz JA, Jameel MM, Whitaker SC, et al. Endovascular repair of perisplanchnic abdominal aortic aneurysm with visceral vessel transposition. J Endovasc Ther 2000; 7(5):410–4.

19. Juvonen T, Biancari F, Ylönen K, et al. Combined surgical and endovascular treatment of pseudoaneurysms of the visceral arteries and of the left iliac arteries after thoracoabdominal aortic surgery. Eur J Vasc Endovasc Surg 2001; 22:275–7.

20. Watanabe Y, Ishimaru S, Kawaguchi S, et al. Successful endografting with simultaneous visceral artery bypass grafting for severely calcified thoracoabdominal aortic aneurysm. J Vasc Surg 2002; 35:397–9.

21. Khoury M. Endovascular repair of recurrent thoracoabdominal aortic aneurysm. J Endovasc Ther 2002; 9:II 106–111.

22. Agostinelli A, Saccani S, Budillon AM, et al. Repair of coexistent infrarenal and thoracoabdominal aortic aneurysm: combined endovascular and open surgical procedure with visceral vessel relocation. J Thorac Cardiovasc Surg 2002; 124:184–5.

23. Saccani S, Nicolini F, Beghi C, et al. Thoracic aortic stents: a combined solution for complex cases. Eur J Vasc Endovasc Surg 2002; 24:423–7.

24. Fleck TM, Hutschala D, Tschernich H, et al. Stent graft placement of the thoracoabdominal aorta in a patient with Marfan syndrome. J Thorac Cardiovasc Surg 2003; 125:1541–3.

25. Rimmer J, Wolfe JHN. Type III thoracoabdominal aortic aneurysm repair: a combined surgical and endovascular approach. Eur J Vasc Endovasc Surg 2003; 26:677–9.

26. Flye MW, Choi ET, Sanchez LA, et al. Retrograde visceral vessel revascularisation followed by endovascular aneurysm exclusion as an alternative to open surgical repair of thoracoabdominal aortic aneurysm. J Vasc Surg 2004; 39:454–8.

27. Black SA, Wolfe JHN, Clark M, et al. Complex thoraco-abdominal aortic aneurysms: endovascular exclusion with visceral revascularization. In: Vascular Annual Meeting 2005, Chicago, IL, U.S.A., Scientific Program 2005 (Abstract S16; 58).

28. Greenberg RK, Haulon S, O'Neill S, et al. Primary endovascular repair of juxtarenal aneurysms with fenestrated endovascular grafting. Eur J Vasc Endovasc Surg 2004; 27:484–91.

29. Verhoeven ELG, Prins TR, Tielliu IFJ, et al. Treatment of short-necked infrarenal aortic aneurysms with fenestrated stent-grafts: short-term results. Eur J Vasc Endovasc Surg 2004; 27:477–83.

30. Hosokawa H, Iwase T, Sato M, et al. Successful endovascular repair of juxtarenal and suprarenal aortic aneurysms with a branched stent graft. J Vasc Surg 2001; 33:1087–92.

31. Inoue K, Iwase T, Sato M, et al. Transluminal endovascular branched graft placement for a pseudoaneurysm: reconstruction of the descending thoracic aorta including the celiac axis. J Thorac Cardiovasc Surg 1997; 114:859–61.

32. Bleyn J, Schol F, Vanhandenhove I, et al. Side-branch modular endograft system for thoracoabdominal aortic aneurysm repair. J Endovasc Ther 2002; 9:838–41.

33. Chuter TAM, Gordon RL, Reilly LM, et al. An endovascular system for thoracoabdominal aortic aneurysm. J Endovasc Ther 2001; 8:25–33.

34. Anderson JL, Adam DJ, Berce M, et al. Repair of thoracoabdominal aneurysms with fenestrated and branched endovascular stent grafts. J Vasc Surg 2005; 42:600–7.

35. EVAR Trial Participants. Endovascular aneurysm repair and outcome in patients unfit for open repair of abdominal aortic aneurysm (EVAR trial 2): randomised controlled trial. Lancet 2005; 365:2187–92.

36. Bergeron P, Coulon P, De Chaumaray T, et al. Great vessels transposition and aortic arch exclusion. J Cardiovasc Surg 2005; 46:141–7.

37. Matalanis G, Durairaj M, Brook M. A hybrid technique of aortic arch transposition and antegrade stent graft deployment for complete arch repair without cardiopulmonary bypass. Eur J Cardiothorac Surg 2006; 29:611–2.

38. Bergeron P, De Chaumaray T, Gay J, et al. Endovascular treatment of thoracic aortic aneursysms. J Cardiovasc Surg (Torino) 2003; 44:349–61.

39. Akasaka J, Tabayashi K, Saiki Y, et al. Stent grafting technique using Matsui–Kitamura (MK) stent for patients with aortic arch aneurysm. Eur J Cardiothorac Surg 2005; 27(4):649–53.

40. Kato M, Kaneko M, Kuratani T, et al. New operative method for distal aortic arch aneurysm: combined cervical branch bypass and endovascular stent graft implantation. J Thorac Cardiovasc Surg 1999; 117:832–4.

41. Safi HJ, Miller CC, III, Estrera AL, et al. Staged repair of extensive aortic aneurysms: long-term experience with the elephant trunk technique. Ann Surg 2004; 240:677–84.

42. Svensson LG, Crawford ES, Hess KR, et al. Experience with 1509 patients undergoing thoracoabdominal aortic operations. J Vasc Surg 1993; 17:357–68.

43. Safi HJ, Miller CC, III, Estrera AL, et al. Staged repair of extensive aortic aneurysms: morbidity and mortality in the elephant trunk technique. Circulation 2001; 104:2938–42.

44. Greenberg RK, Haddad F, Svensson L, et al. Hybrid approaches to thoracic aortic aneurysms: the role of endovascular elephant trunk completion. Circulation 2005; 112:2619–26.

45. Chavan A, Karck M, Hagl C, et al. Hybrid endograft for one-step treatment of multisegment disease of the thoracic aorta. J Vasc Interv Radiol 2005; 16:823–9.

46. Svensson LG, Kim KH, Blackstone EH, et al. Elephant trunk procedure: newer indications and uses. Ann Thorac Surg 2004; 78:109–16.

27 | Thoracic Dissection (Classification of Spectrum of Disease, Natural History, Indications for Intervention)

Rachel Bell
Department of General and Vascular Surgery, Guy's and St. Thomas' Hospital, London, U.K.

INTRODUCTION

Aortic dissection is the commonest aortic emergency affecting 10 to 20 people per million population (1). The mortality associated with dissection is high if no treatment is given, with mortality ranging from 36% to 72% (2). Mortality from dissection is approximately 1% per hour for the first 48 hours with a higher mortality when the ascending aorta is involved (2). Death results from rupture into the pericardial cavity causing tamponade, or from rupture into the mediastinum, the pleura or the abdomen. Serious complications arise from ischemia of the branch vessels resulting in myocardial infarction, stroke, limb ischemia, paraplegia, visceral and renal ischemia.

CLASSIFICATION OF AORTIC DISSECTION

Aortic dissections are classified according the time from first symptoms (acute or chronic), from the site of the primary entry tear (Stanford), the part of the aorta affected (DeBakey) and whether there is evidence of end organ ischemia or rupture (uncomplicated versus complicated). Aortic dissection has also been reclassified by the European Society of Cardiologists to include penetrating ulcer, intramural hematoma and traumatic dissection (3).

ACUTE OR CHRONIC DISSECTION

■ Acute dissection: if less than 14 days since onset of symptoms
■ Chronic dissection: if beyond 14 days since onset of symptoms

The reason for this distinction is that the risk of life threatening complications is greatest in the first days following dissection (4). In acute dissection the fragility of the intimal flap has implications for management as it is very easily torn and the aortic wall does not hold sutures well.

DEBAKEY CLASSIFICATION

The DeBakey classification of aortic dissection has three groups: Type I affects both the ascending and descending aorta; Type II is localized to the ascending aorta and Type III affects the descending thoracic aorta and is divided into IIIa which affects the aorta above the level of the diaphragm and IIIb which affects the aorta to a level below the diaphragm.

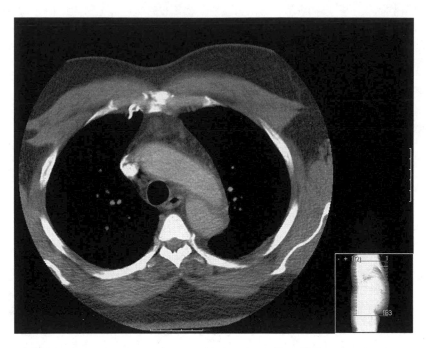

FIGURE 1 Computed tomography scan showing classic Type B dissection with patent true and false lumens.

STANFORD CLASSIFICATION

The Stanford classification has two groups depending on the site of the primary tear: Type A where the primary entry tear is in the ascending aorta and Type B where the primary entry tear is not in the ascending aorta. The primary entry tear for Type B dissection is usually found just distal to the origin of the left subclavian artery in the descending thoracic aorta.

INTERNATIONAL REGISTRY OF AORTIC DISSECTION

The International Registry for Acute Aortic Dissection (IRAD) classification describes five types of aortic dissection. Type I is the traditional dissection with true and false lumens separated by an intimal flap (Fig. 1). Type II is where there is disruption of the media with intramural hemorrhage (Fig. 2) or hematoma. Type III is called discrete or subtle dissection where there is a bulge at the tear site with no hematoma. In Type IV the underlying problem is rupture of a plaque or a penetrating ulcer (Fig. 3). Type V is caused either by trauma or is iatrogenic. This classification may be helpful as to deciding which types are suitable for endovascular treatment. Clearly those with a localized entry point such as Type III, IV and V are more suited to endovascular treatment. Type II may not have a clearly defined entry tear on imaging, and Type I may have either single or multiple entry tears.

PATHOPHYSIOLOGY

Most aortic dissections are caused by a tear in the intima, which allows blood to track between the intima and media. Alternatively, the blood may originate from rupture of the vasa vasorum on the outside of the vessel. The blood in the wall may thrombose causing an intramural hematoma. Intramural hematoma is a radiological diagnosis of blood within the aortic wall without communication with the aortic lumen. Penetrating ulcers develop at the edge of atherosclerotic aortic plaques and can give the appearance of a localized dissection. The intramural blood may not thrombose creating a second or "false" lumen, which can extend in an antegrade or retrograde fashion. Painful, deep ulcers with adjacent hematoma are

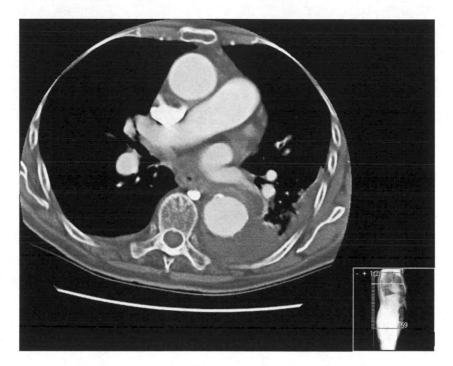

FIGURE 2   Computed tomography scan illustrating intramural hematoma.

more prone to rupture (5). Aortic branches may be compromised at their origin by blood in the false lumen, so-called static obstruction. Aortic branches may also be occluded by movement of the dissection flap during systole/diastole which is dynamic obstruction.

Aortic dissection is associated with cystic medial necrosis. Inherited conditions such as Marfan syndrome, Ehlers–Danlos syndrome, bicuspid aortic valve and aortic coarctation

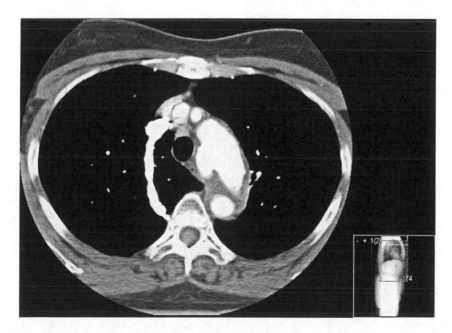

FIGURE 3   Computed tomography scan illustrating penetrating aortic ulcer.

predispose to aortic dissection. In addition acquired conditions such as Bechet's disease, Takakyasu's arteritis and cocaine abuse also increase the risk of developing aortic dissection.

CLINICAL PRESENTATION

Aortic dissection is a great clinical mimic. The common presenting symptoms and signs include:

■ Severe "ripping/tearing" chest pain radiating to the back
■ Back pain
■ Syncope
■ Congestive cardiac failure
■ Acute limb ischemia
■ Stroke
■ Paraplegia
■ Severe abdominal pain—mesenteric ischemia
■ Acute renal failure

   On examination hypertension is common due to either preexisting hypertensive disease or increased sympathetic drive. Hypotension affects 25% of patients and is due to acute aortic regurgitation, cardiac tamponade or left ventricular failure (3). Differences in pulse and blood pressure between the two arms are seen in 40% of patients (3). Carotid, subclavian and femoral bruits may be heard on auscultation.

DIAGNOSIS AND IMAGING

The early diagnosis of aortic dissection is crucial if the correct treatment is to be instituted, however, delay in diagnosis is not unusual due to the protean nature of presentation which can mimic many other acute and more common conditions. The delay in diagnosis has catastrophic consequences particularly for Stanford Type A dissection (mortality during the first 48 hours greater than 1% per hour) (2). A high index of clinical suspicion is therefore necessary to diagnose aortic dissection.

Computerized Tomography

Multi-slice computed tomography (CT) scan with intravenous contrast is the commonest initial investigation and is used to confirm the diagnosis and define the type and extent of the dissection. It can also identify the relationship of the main aortic branches to the true and false lumen. Three-dimensional image reconstructions (multi-planar reformatting) are useful in delineating the extent of the dissection and are almost comparable to conventional angiography. The disadvantages of this technique are the relatively high x-ray dose and the nephrotoxic effects of the contrast medium.

Magnetic Resonance Angiography

Contrast-enhanced magnetic resonance angiography provides useful information about flow in the true and false lumen. Importantly it involves no radiation and provides cross-sectional imaging, which can be reconstructed in any plane. Unfortunately it is less readily available than CT, particularly "out of hours" and it is not suitable for unstable patients.

TRANSESOPHAGEAL ECHOCARDIOGRAPHY

Transesophageal echocardiography is considered to be the initial investigation of choice in patients with acute dissection with sensitivity and specificity rates above 95%, however, certain artifacts can mimic the intimal flap (6). This technique requires skilled operators which may not be readily available in all hospitals. Transesophageal echocardiography can be very helpful in localizing the primary entry tear in aortic dissection and provides information regarding the extent and type of dissection and also the status of the aortic valve and left ventricular function.

Angiography

Conventional angiography has largely been superseded in recent years by other imaging techniques. However centers performing endovascular treatment have continued to use this modality as part of the preprocedural work-up. It is possible to locate the primary entry tear and to define the relationship of the aortic branches with the true or false lumen. A calibrated catheter can be used to measure length if endovascular repair is being contemplated. It is important to remember that arch angiography carries a small risk of stroke (7).

Intravascular Ultrasound

Intravascular ultrasound can be useful in aortic dissection as it is good at identifying the true and false lumens and the associated reentry tears. The technique has been used to aid percutaneous fenestration procedures of the dissection flap (8).

NATURAL HISTORY

Acute Type A aortic dissection has a mortality of 24% at 24 hours, 29% by 48 hours, and 49% by two weeks (9). Type A dissections can extend retrogradely and cause myocardial ischemia, aortic valve regurgitation and cardiac tamponade. Antegrade extension of Type A dissection can cause stroke and acute limb ischemia, paraplegia, and visceral ischemia.

Uncomplicated acute Type B aortic dissection has a lower mortality as with medical treatment 90% of patients will survive one month, 60% to 80% will survive five years and 40% to 45% survive 10 years (10,11). However patients with complicated Type B dissection with rupture or end organ ischemia have a mortality approaching that of Type A dissections, up to 25% by 48 hours, despite surgical intervention (12,13). If the aortic diameter is greater than 4 cm at presentation more than 70% will go on to develop aneurysms at five years. Persistence of flow in the false lumen appears to increase the risk of late complications and spontaneous thrombosis of the false lumen is rare (9,14,15).

ENDOVASCULAR INTERVENTION

Type A Aortic Dissection

The accepted treatment of choice for acute Type A dissection is immediate open surgical repair. Open surgery concentrates on repairing the ascending aorta and this usually leaves the distal dissection flap. High flow in the distal false lumen is associated with a late mortality (43%) (16). For this reason some groups advocate the use of a combination of open surgical repair (elephant-trunk) and endovascular repair of the distal dissection (17). Endovascular repair of a primary entry tear in the ascending aorta is very difficult because the coronary ostia are often involved in the dissection. The only role for endovascular treatment in the management of Type A dissection is when the primary entry tear is in the descending aorta and there is retrograde extension (18).

Type B Dissection

Currently the preferred treatment for uncomplicated acute Type B aortic dissection is medical management, the aim is to relieve pain and prevent extension or rupture of the dissection with a combination of anti-hypertensive agents and opiates. This is based on reports of survival rates of only 50% for open surgery compared with 80% for medical treatment alone (19). Emergency surgery or endovascular intervention is currently reserved for on-going pain, refractory hypertension, localized false aneurysm, end organ ischemia and rupture, all of which occur in 30% to 40% of patients (20,21). Recently the IRAD showed that mortality for patients with Type B dissection treated medically was 11% compared with 31% for those who required surgery (3). Renal and mesenteric ischemia carries a surgical mortality of 50% and 88%, respectively (21).

Endovascular treatment of complicated Type B dissection includes covering the primary entry tear with a stent graft, percutaneous fenestration of the intimal flap (see chap. 28) and stenting of obstructed aortic side-branches. Endovascular treatment has also been recommended for penetrating ulcers and intramural hematomas of the descending aorta, which have been identified as precursors of dissection (3).

The endovascular techniques used to treat Type B dissection are:

1. Placing a covered stent graft over the primary entry tear to obliterate the flow into the false lumen.
2. Percutaneous fenestration of the intimal flap.
3. Stenting the aortic side-branches.

The aims of treatment are to cause thrombosis of the false lumen and relieve end organ ischemia. Thrombosis of the false lumen has been shown to decrease the risk of aneurysm formation (10).

Stent Grafts to Cover the Primary Tear

Dissection can compromise flow into aortic side branches by one of two mechanisms. In static obstruction, the dissection continues into the aortic branch and expansion of the false lumen within the branch occludes the vessel. In dynamic obstruction the aortic intimal flap bows into the origin of the vessel effectively occluding it (Fig. 4). The endoluminal treatment of aortic dissection is aimed at sealing the primary entry tear with a covered stent (Fig. 5). This decreases the pressure in the false lumen by obliterating flow through it and encourages thrombosis. Covering the primary tear can also be an effective treatment for dynamic and static obstruction of aortic side branches.

In 2004, EUROSTAR reported the outcome of 131 patients (43% symptomatic) with Type B aortic dissection that were treated endovascularly. Technical success was achieved in 89%, with low rates of paraplegia (0.8%) and mortality (6.5% elective and 12% emergency) (22). In the published literature there is a failure to differentiate between complicated acute and chronic dissection and those patients who were treated for uncomplicated Type B dissection. Table 1

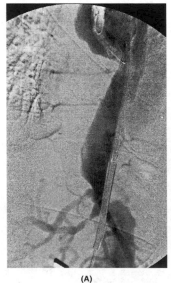
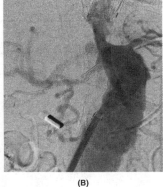
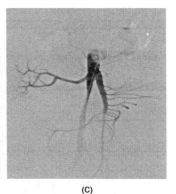

(A)   (B)   (C)

FIGURE 4 (**A,B**) Patient who presented with renal ischemia following and acute Type B dissection. Renal perfusion did not improve after closure of the entry tear and renal stenting was required. (**C**) Patient with dynamic visceral ischemia following acute Type B dissection—hanging viscera sign.

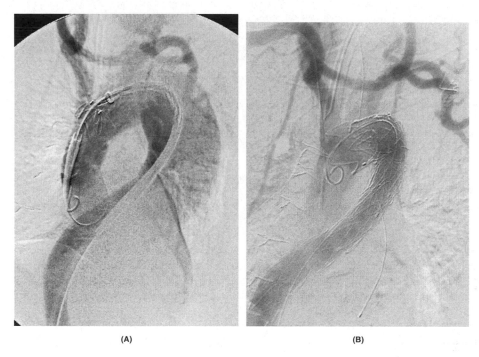

(A)   (B)

FIGURE 5 Endovascular repair of a chronic Type B dissection. A carotid–carotid bypass has been performed to increase the landing zone.

summarizes the case series reporting the results of endovascular repair for Type B dissection. In the majority of the series endovascular treatment was reserved for patients with complicated acute Type B dissection. It is to be noted that no series was consecutive and exclusions were common due to unfavorable anatomy, complex anatomy and dissected iliacs.

The end points for endovascular repair of aortic dissection are 30 days or in-hospital mortality and thrombosis of the false lumen in the thorax, which may be complete or partial. Primary technical success for closure of the primary entry tear is achieved in 90% to 100%. The mortality ranges from 0% to 16% and the majority of patients completely thrombose the false lumen. However, between 7% and 21% of patients achieve only partial thrombosis of the false lumen.

There is one case-control study of endovascular repair for thoracic aortic dissection. Twelve patients had endovascular repair of chronic Type B dissections and were compared to

TABLE 1 Published Case Series of Endovascular Repair of Acute and Chronic Type B Dissection

Author	Year	N	Technical success	30-day mortality (%)	Follow-up (months)	Late survival (%)
Nienaber (23)	2003	11	100	0	15	100
Dake (24)	1999	19	100	16	13	84.2
Nienaber (25)	1999	12	100	0	3	100
Won (26)	2001	12	91	0	12	91
Bortone (27)	2002	12	71	8	10	91.7
Shimono (28)	2002	37	94	3	24	97.3
Buffolo (29)	2002	181	91	2	2	87.4
Lopera (30)	2003	10	90	0	30	80
Lonn (31)	2003	20	100	15	13	85
Bortone (32)	2004	43	96	7	20	83.7
Dialetto (33)	2005	28	100	3	18	73.7
Eggebrecht (34)	2005	38	100	3	15	87.5

historical matched controls undergoing open surgery. There were no deaths or complications in the patients treated with endoluminal repair. However there were four deaths and five serious complications in the open surgical group (25). This study was repeated for acute Type B dissection, with 11 patients treated with endovascular repair and 11 historical controls. For patients treated with endoluminal repair there were no deaths or complications out to a follow-up of 15 months. In the open surgical historical controls there were three early deaths and one late death from aortic rupture (23). We await the results of the INSTEAD trial (INvestigation of STEnt grafts in Aortic Dissection) and the Gore Thoracic Aortic Graft trial for uncomplicated Type B aortic dissection treated with endovascular repair when compared with best medical treatment.

The Endoluminal Treatment of Dissection with Branch Vessel Ischemia

The use of stent grafts to cover the primary tear allows the successful revascularization of 67% to 95% of compromised side branches (24,35,36). Fenestration procedures and stents placed in the origin of compromised branches have been very effective in treating end organ ischemia (37). The mortality in such patients is much less than open surgical repair ranging from 16% to 25%. Fenestration of the intimal flap can be performed by puncturing the intimal flap with a needle to allow passage of a guidewire. Balloon angioplasty on its own is often successful in acute cases, but placement of a stent may be required if the fenestration does not stay open (which often occurs in chronic dissections). Some authorities suggest that stents should be placed in the orifices of important compromised branches, such as the renal and visceral arteries, before the stent graft is used to cover the primary tear. They cite the difficulties in crossing such branches once the stent graft has been successfully deployed. They also suggest that preprocedure dialysis is useful in order to avoid the huge backwash of metabolites into the circulation from ischemic organs. The delay this may cause in the definitive management of these seriously ill patients has to be balanced against the benefits.

Uncovered Stents

Residual static obstruction of aortic branches after stenting across the primary entry tear can occur. In these circumstances an uncovered stent can be placed in the true lumen of the aortic branch to relieve the obstruction. Stents can also be placed from the false lumen of the aorta to restore flow to the true lumen of the branch vessel. Deployment of an infrarenal stent graft in the true lumen of the abdominal aorta can be used to treat limb ischemia.

At present there is no evidence as to how to treat such patients who do not completely thrombose the false lumen. The majority are treated expectantly, but in theory, the use of bare stents would encourage thrombosis of the false lumen without occluding important branches such as the intercostal, visceral or renal arteries. The fragility of the intimal flap in the acute stage mitigates against the use of bare stents, but they could be useful in the chronic phase of the dissection if the false lumen is not thrombosed.

Percutaneous Fenestration

This technique can be used in cases of true lumen collapse in order to allow blood flow into the true lumen, decrease the pressure in the false lumen and to allow reperfusion of aortic branches which have been isolated by the dissection (see chap. 28). Sometimes fenestration alone does not provide adequate reperfusion and adjunctive procedures may be required (37). In acute dissection the intimal flap is fragile and tears easily and the fenestrations remain patent. For chronic dissection the intimal flap is stiffer and deployment of a bridging stent across the fenestration has been used to ensure adequate distal flow. In cases of true lumen collapse in the iliac arteries placing guidewires in the true and false lumens and advancing a single introducer sheath over both wires causes a longitudinal tear in the intimal flap leading to reperfusion of the ischemic limb. However the technique is difficult and not widely practiced. Fenestration is contraindicated in the presence of partial or complete thrombosis of either lumen due to the risk of distal embolization.

TECHNICAL CONSIDERATIONS

There are some important technical points in treating patients with dissection. The stent graft should be sized according to the normal aorta proximal to the dissection. The stent graft is usually oversized by 10% to 15% relative to this diameter. Excessive oversizing may result in poor application of the stent graft to the aortic wall resulting in proximal endoleak. The fabric of the stent graft must be positioned at least 2 cm proximal to the primary tear to allow sufficient length for fixation to the normal diameter aorta. Some authorities suggest that the most dependable part of the thoracic aorta is that between the left common carotid artery and the left subclavian artery. Therefore the stent graft should be deployed close to the origin of the left subclavian, covering it if necessary.

The majority of left subclavian arteries can be covered with little or no clinical sequelae. Some patients develop a cold left hand, but this usually improves with time. However, in certain patients the left subclavian artery provides an essential blood supply either to the spinal cord or the brain. Preoperative carotid duplex is essential to determine whether the left vertebral artery is the dominant part of the posterior circulation to the brain.

The use of bare stents to fix the stent graft to the aorta has been associated with aortic rupture, particularly if the stent graft is fairly rigid and does not conform to the bend of the aortic arch. Bare stents adjacent to the intimal flap are almost certain to tear it in the acute phase and are therefore not recommended.

Deaths have been reported by the conversion of Stanford Type B dissections into Type A. The retrograde extension of the dissection can cause death from myocardial ischemia and cardiac tamponade and must be avoided. Balloon dilatation to fix the stent graft in position should not be employed as this can cause dissection at the most proximal level of the stent graft. Self-expanding stent grafts are therefore used exclusively in the treatment of dissections. Conversion to Type A dissection has also occurred with the placement of stent grafts in a collapsed true lumen distal to the primary entry tear. The sudden increase in pressure in the false lumen distally results in proximal extension of the dissection at the entry site. Therefore the first procedure is to place a stent graft to adequately cover the primary tear. Excessive force should never be used to place a stent graft, as this may cause intimal damage resulting in a more proximal dissection (Fig. 6).

IMPROVING STENT GRAFT DESIGN

There is no perfect stent graft to treat acute aortic dissection, although several companies are striving towards that goal. The forces acting on the thoracic aorta involve a spiral flow which needs to be taken into account in new stent graft designs. A graft that is too flexible may not be durable and may not fix adequately to the aorta. It may also have insufficient radial strength to compress the false lumen. A graft that is too stiff may be unable to negotiate tortuous anatomy, and may tear the fragile intimal flap or, worse, the aortic wall. Grafts with the flexibility to accommodate the geometry of the aortic arch may require different degrees of flexibility throughout their length, being strong and inflexible at the proximal fixation and more pliable distally where the stent is in contact with the intimal flap. However, some strength is required distally to help to occlude the false lumen. The development of branched and fenestrated stent grafts may have an important role in the future endoluminal treatment of acute aortic dissection.

CONCLUSION

Current recommendations are that endovascular repair can be used to treat acute complications of Type B dissection such as: rupture, end organ ischemia, ongoing pain and false lumen expansion. The dilated aortic arch (>38 mm) is a contraindication for endovascular repair as none of the current devices are large enough. Endovascular repair can also be used to treat patients with expanding intramural hemtomas or complicated penetrating ulcers. In addition stent grafts can be used to manage the distal dissection in conjunction with open ascending or arch repair in Type A dissection.

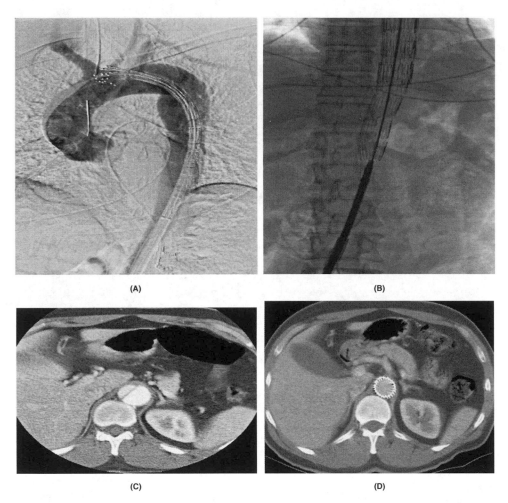

(A)   (B)

(C)   (D)

FIGURE 6   Patient with acute Type B dissection and visceral ischemia. (**A,B**) Primary entry tear covered with a stent graft and bare metal stent in the true lumen of the peri-visceral aorta. (**C**) Pre-stent and (**D**) Post-stent showing remodeling of the aorta.

The case series published suggest that that the morbidity and mortality are highest when stenting is performed in the acute setting (34,38). There is a suggestion that early intervention within the first six months to a year, is associated with aortic remodeling and might be the optimal time for intervention to avoid the early complications (39). The INSTEAD trial, a multicenter European randomized trial is being performed to investigate the role of endovascular intervention in this area (40). Published results of this trial have not yet been released but preliminary presentations suggest that early stenting of asymptomatic Type B dissections does not confer any immediate survival benefit.

For uncomplicated Type B dissection in patients treated medically at presentation have a 30% to 40% risk of aneurysm formation during follow-up. Treatment is advised if the aneurysm becomes symptomatic or more than 5.5 to 6 cm in diameter (14,41). Aneurysms related to previous dissection have a high risk of rupture and appear to rupture at a smaller diameter than degenerative aneurysms (41).

The long-term durability of stent grafts is also a cause for concern, particularly if they are used in young patients. The role of stent grafts in the treatment of patients with Marfan syndrome is also controversial. These patients often have multiple entry tears which are not suitable for stent grafts and endoluminal repair carries a higher risk of paraplegia. They also tend to have a fragile aorta which tears more easily than a normal aorta with endoluminal manipulation.

Endovascular repair can be used to treat both complicated acute and chronic Type B dissection. There is a suggestion that the use of covered stent grafts may alter the natural history of uncomplicated acute Type B dissection and therefore prevent late complications and dissection-related deaths.

REFERENCES

1. Pate JW, Richardson RL, Eastridge CE. Acute aortic dissections. Am Surg 1976; 42(6):395–404.
2. Anagnostopoulos CE, Prabhakar MJ, Kittle CF. Aortic dissections and dissecting aneurysms. Am J Cardiol 1972; 30(3):263–73.
3. Hagan PG, Nienaber CA, Isselbacher EM. The International Registry of Acute Aortic Dissection (IRAD)—new insights into an old disease. JAMA 2000; 283:897–903.
4. Hirst AE, Jr., Johns VJ, Jr., Kime SW, Jr. Dissecting aneurysm of the aorta: a review of 505 cases. Medicine (Baltimore) 1958; 37(3):217–79.
5. von Kodolitsch Y, Nienaber CA. Ulcer of the thoracic aorta: diagnosis, therapy and prognosis. Z Kardiol 1998; 87(12):917–27.
6. Vignon P, Spencer KT, Rambaud G, et al. Differential transesophageal echocardiographic diagnosis between linear artifacts and intraluminal flap of aortic dissection or disruption. Chest 2001; 119(6):1778–90.
7. Mayberg MR, Winn HR. Endarterectomy for asymptomatic carotid artery stenosis. Executive Committee for the Asymptomatic Carotid Atherosclerosis Study. JAMA 1995; 273(18):1421–8.
8. Manninen HI, Rasanen H. Intravascular ultrasound in interventional radiology. Eur Radiol 2000; 10(11):1754–62.
9. Erbel R, Alfonso F, Boileau C, et al. Diagnosis and management of aortic dissection. Eur Heart J 2001; 22(18):1642–81.
10. Bernard Y, Zimmermann H, Chocron S, et al. False lumen patency as a predictor of late outcome in aortic dissection. Am J Cardiol 2001; 87(12):1378–82.
11. Umana JP, Lai DT, Mitchell RS, et al. Is medical therapy still the optimal treatment strategy for patients with acute type B aortic dissections? J Thorac Cardiovasc Surg 2002; 124(5):896–910.
12. Bogaert J, Meyns B, Rademakers FE, et al. Follow-up of aortic dissection: contribution of MR angiography for evaluation of the abdominal aorta and its branches. Eur Radiol 1997; 7(5):695–702.
13. Meszaros I, Morocz J, Szlavi J, et al. Epidemiology and clinicopathology of aortic dissection. Chest 2000; 117(5):1271–8.
14. Juvonen T, Ergin MA, Galla JD, et al. Risk factors for rupture of chronic type B dissections. J Thorac Cardiovasc Surg 1999; 117(4):776–86.
15. Kozai Y, Watanabe S, Yonezawa M, et al. Long term prognosis of acute aortic dissection with medical treatment: a survey of 263 unoperated patients. Jpn Circ J 2001; 65(5):359–63.
16. Erbel R, Oelert H, Meyer J, et al. Effect of medical and surgical therapy on aortic dissection evaluated by transesophageal echocardiography. Implications for prognosis and therapy. The European Cooperative Study Group on Echocardiography. Circulation 1993; 87(5):1604–15.
17. Palma JH, Almeida DR, Carvalho AC, Andrade JC, Buffolo E. Surgical treatment of acute type B aortic dissection using an endoprosthesis (elephant trunk). Ann Thorac Surg 1997; 63(4):1081–4.
18. Kato N, Shimono T, Hirano T, Ishida M, Yada I, Takeda K. Transluminal placement of endovascular stent-grafts for the treatment of type A aortic dissection with an entry tear in the descending thoracic aorta. J Vasc Surg 2001; 34(6):1023–8.
19. Wheat MW, Jr. Acute dissecting aneurysms of the aorta: diagnosis and treatment—1979. Am Heart J 1980; 99(3):373–87.
20. Fann JI, Sarris GE, Mitchell RS, et al. Treatment of patients with aortic dissection presenting with peripheral vascular complications. Ann Surg 1990; 212(6):705–13.
21. Cambria RP, Brewster DC, Gertler J, et al. Vascular complications associated with spontaneous aortic dissection. J Vasc Surg 1988; 7(2):199–209.
22. Leurs LJ, Bell R, Degrieck Y, Thomas S, Hobo R, Lundbom J. Endovascular treatment of thoracic aortic diseases: combined experience from the EUROSTAR and United Kingdom Thoracic Endograft registries. J Vasc Surg 2004; 40(4):670–9 (Discussion 679–80).
23. Nienaber CA, Ince H, Weber F, et al. Emergency stent-graft placement in thoracic aortic dissection and evolving rupture. J Card Surg 2003; 18(5):464–70.
24. Dake MD, Kato N, Mitchell RS, et al. Endovascular stent-graft placement for the treatment of acute aortic dissection. N Engl J Med 1999; 340(20):1546–52.
25. Nienaber CA, Fattori R, Lund G, et al. Nonsurgical reconstruction of thoracic aortic dissection by stent-graft placement. N Engl J Med 1999; 340(20):1539–45.
26. Won JY, Lee DY, Shim WH, et al. Elective endovascular treatment of descending thoracic aortic aneurysms and chronic dissections with stent-grafts. J Vasc Interv Radiol 2001; 12(5):575–82.

27. Bortone AS, Schena S, D'Agostino D, et al. Immediate versus delayed endovascular treatment of post-traumatic aortic pseudoaneurysms and type B dissections: retrospective analysis and premises to the upcoming European trial. Circulation 2002; 106(12 Suppl. 1):I234–40.

28. Shimono T, Kato N, Yasuda F, et al. Transluminal stent-graft placements for the treatments of acute onset and chronic aortic dissections. Circulation 2002; 106(12 Suppl. 1):I241–7.

29. Buffolo E, da Fonseca JH, de Souza JA, Alves CM. Revolutionary treatment of aneurysms and dissections of descending aorta: the endovascular approach. Ann Thorac Surg 2002; 74(5):S1815–7 (Discussion S1825–32).

30. Lopera J, Patino JH, Urbina C, et al. Endovascular treatment of complicated type-B aortic dissection with stent-grafts: midterm results. J Vasc Interv Radiol 2003; 14(2 Pt 1):195–203.

31. Lonn L, Delle M, Falkenberg M, et al. Endovascular treatment of type B thoracic aortic dissections. J Card Surg 2003; 18(6):539–44.

32. Bortone AS, De Cillis E, D'Agostino D, Schinosa Lde L. Stent graft treatment of thoracic aortic disease. Surg Technol Int 2004; 12:189–93.

33. Dialetto G, Covino FE, Scognamiglio G, et al. Treatment of type B aortic dissection: endoluminal repair or conventional medical therapy? Eur J Cardiothorac Surg 2005; 27(5):826–30.

34. Eggebrecht H, Schmermund A, Herold U, et al. Endovascular stent-graft placement for acute and contained rupture of the descending thoracic aorta. Catheter Cardiovasc Interv 2005; 66(4):474–82.

35. Mitchell RS, Miller DC, Dake MD, Semba CP, Moore KA, Sakai T. Thoracic aortic aneurysm repair with an endovascular stent graft: the "first generation". Ann Thorac Surg 1999; 67(6):1971–4 (Discussion 1979–80).

36. Eggebrecht H, Nienaber CA, Neuhauser M, et al. Endovascular stent-graft placement in aortic dissection: a meta-analysis. Eur Heart J 2006; 27(4):489–98.

37. Slonim SM, Miller DC, Mitchell RS, Semba CP, Razavi MK, Dake MD. Percutaneous balloon fenestration and stenting for life-threatening ischemic complications in patients with acute aortic dissection. J Thorac Cardiovasc Surg 1999; 117(6):1118–26.

38. Kato N, Hirano T, Shimono T, et al. Treatment of chronic aortic dissection by transluminal endovascular stent-graft placement: preliminary results. J Vasc Interv Radiol 2001; 12(7):835–40.

39. Kato M, Matsuda T, Kaneko M, et al. Outcomes of stent-graft treatment of false lumen in aortic dissection. Circulation 1998; 98(19 Suppl.):II305–11 (Discussion II311–2).

40. Nienaber CA, Zannetti S, Barbieri B, Kische S, Schareck W, Rehders TC. INvestigation of STEnt grafts in patients with type B aortic dissection: design of the INSTEAD trial—a prospective, multicenter, European randomized trial. Am Heart J 2005; 149(4):592–9.

41. Griepp RB, Ergin MA, Galla JD, et al. Natural history of descending thoracic and thoracoabdominal aneurysms. Ann Thorac Surg 1999; 67(6):1927–30 (Discussion 1953–8).

28 Fenestration for Aortic Disease (Indications and Technique)

Jean-Paul Beregi
Cardio-Vascular Radiological and Imaging Unit, Service de Radiologie et d'Imagerie Cardio-Vasculaire, Hôpital Cardiologique, Lille, France
Mohamad Koussa
Vascular Surgery Unit, Hôpital Cardiologique, Lille, France
Philippe Asseman
Cardiac Intensive Care Unit, Hôpital Cardiologique, Lille, France
Virginia Gaxotte, Christophe Lions, Ziad Negaiwi, and Serge Willoteaux
Cardio-Vascular Radiological and Imaging Unit, Hôpital Cardiologique, Lille, France
Alain Prat
Cardiac and Thoracic Surgery Unit, Hôpital Cardiologique, Lille, France

INTRODUCTION

Fenestration is one of the classical techniques used to treat acute malperfusion syndrome (1–3) secondary to aortic dissection. Surgical fenestration was first described in 1935 and the endovascular approach in 1990 (4). In this chapter, the indications and technique of endovascular fenestration will be reviewed (5–7). The number of cases requiring acute fenestration has diminished in recent years with the advent of endovascular graft placement to close the entry site in acute dissections (see chap. 27). Endovascular fenestration remains an essential part of the armamentarium for treating acute aortic dissection.

INDICATIONS

Management of Aortic Dissection

Acute aortic dissection is a medical emergency (8,9). Dissection of the ascending aorta almost invariably requires emergency surgical replacement. When the ascending aorta is not involved (Type B dissection), the condition is primarily treated medically, unless complications arise (10). Aortic fenestration is indicated for acute malperfusion and end organ ischemia.

Clinical Indications for Fenestration: Acute Malperfusion Syndrome

Malperfusion can involve the heart, brain, and spinal cord if the proximal aorta is involved, and the digestive tract, kidneys, and lower limbs when the dissection extends distally. Malperfusion exacerbates the high morbidity and mortality associated with acute aortic dissection (11,12). Several mechanisms may be responsible for malperfusion, and the indication for endovascular treatment is dependent on these mechanisms.

 The symptoms observed in the acute phase of an aortic dissection will suggest malperfusion of the various end arteries (renal, celiac, superior mesenteric artery or iliac), and if present must be treated rapidly. In some cases, treatment of malperfusion may be performed before the ascending thoracic aorta can be repaired in the case of a Type A aortic dissection (Fig. 1) (13,14).

Morphological Indications for Fenestration

Malperfusion can be treated by several endovascular techniques; implantation of arterial stents in the branches of the abdominal aorta, deployment of a thoracic aortic stent graft to close

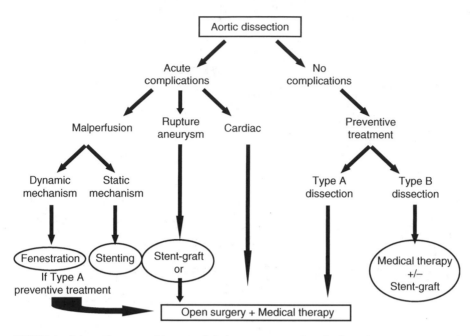

FIGURE 1 Schematic proposal for new clinical management of aortic dissection.

the proximal entry site and improve true lumen perfusion and aortic fenestration. In order to choose the appropriate treatment modality, it is important to understand the morphology of aortic dissection.

Williams et al. (15) reported the mechanisms of visceral malperfusion in acute aortic dissection. The authors proposed a system that classifies malperfusion as static or dynamic. Static lesions are analagous to classic atheromatous lesions that narrow the diameter of the artery with a fixed obstruction. Dynamic lesions result from compression of the true arterial lumen by a false lumen secondary to high pressure in the latter. However, this classification system does not describe all possible cases and it is often difficult to link symptoms with mechanisms. In fact, it is reasonable to argue that all lesions are dynamic. Static lesions result from an extension of the dissection into a blind ending visceral artery. This extension leads to a narrowing in the true channel by compression of the false channel, where the blood enters but cannot exit. This artery then tends to thrombose, giving rise to the diagnosis of a static lesion.

Our group classified the morphological lesions that result in malperfusion in a study of 61 patients (Fig. 2). It is suggested (16) that Type 1c and 1d lesions with malperfusion may be treated with fenestration (Fig. 2), whereas Type 2a, 2b, 2c, and 3c lesions are better treated with a stent into the affected artery (Fig. 3). However, many patients with dynamic malperfusion from Type B dissections could be successfully treated with an endovascular stent graft to close the proximal entry point, depressurize the false lumen and increase perfusion in the true lumen. This option is not available in Type A dissection where fenestration may be the only therapeutic maneuvre available prior to emergency surgery.

Technique of Fenestration

Prior to fenestration, a diagnosis of aortic dissection with dynamic obstruction causing malperfusion must be made.

Imaging

The objectives of imaging in cases of suspected aortic dissection include:

- Verification of the diagnosis of aortic dissection or intramural hematoma
- Staging the level of the extension into the aorta (ascending, arch, descending)

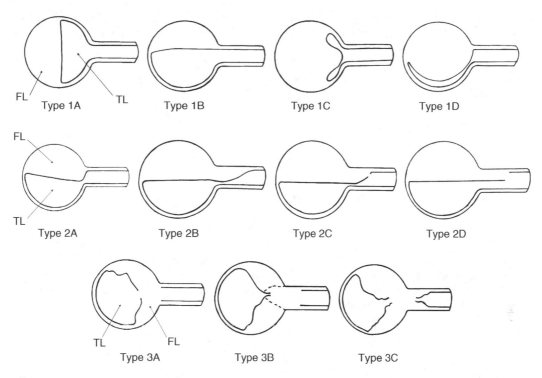

FIGURE 2 Morphologic evaluation of the position of the intimal flap in the aorta, extension into branches and ostial disconnection. *Abbreviations*: FL, false lumen; TL, true lumen.

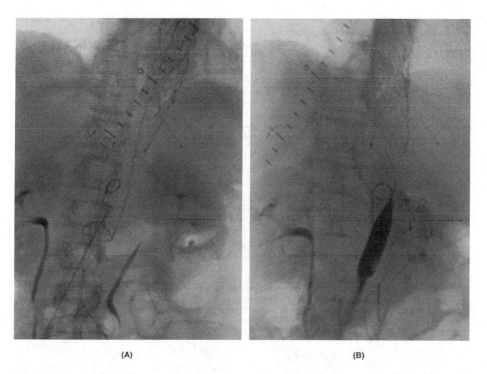

FIGURE 3 (**A**) Catheter passed from true to false lumens by use of membrane perforation and snare. (**B**) Fenestration enlarged by a balloon.

- Analyzing the trajectory of the true and false lumens throughout the entire aorta and to evaluate the position of the intimal flap (degree of compression of the true lumen)
- Detecting the number and location of entry tears
- Diagnosing thoracic complications of the aortic dissection
- Analysing possible extension into branches of the aorta and disconnection of the origin; to look for ischemic signs in the organs supplied by; supra-aortic vessels; visceral arteries (kidneys and bowel ischemia); iliac arteries (lower limb ischemia)
- Evaluating the tortuosity, calcification and diameter of iliac and common femoral arteries for possible endovascular treatments

The diagnostic imaging techniques include transthoracic echocardiography (TTE), transesophageal echocardiography (TOE), computed tomography (CT) angiography, magnetic resonance imaging (MRI) and diagnostic arteriography. TOE, CT angiogram and MRI display high, identical levels of sensitivity (>90%) in the diagnosis of aortic dissection (9,17–19).

The performance of CT angiography in the evaluation of aortic dissection has been well established (20–22). The essential objectives cited above can be achieved using this technique. The data acquisition techniques for axial sections are variable and depend on the performance of the equipment used. This technology has allowed more extensive investigation and thorough comprehension of malperfusion. It is also the preferred technique for detecting and analysing malperfusion on a practical level.

Endovascular Fenestration

Endovascular fenestration is specific to the treatment of aortic dissections. This technique is utilized whenever malperfusion is associated with a dynamic mechanism that cannot be resolved with closure of the entry site. The principle of fenestration entails creating a wide orifice of communication between the true and false channels or in increasing the passage of blood between these two channels (23,24). This may be achieved by perforating the intimal flap, from the true channel towards the false channel, using a trans-septal needle. The technique is facilitated by the use of an endovascular ultrasound probe, which can locate the position of the intimal flap and guide perforation (25). Once the aperture has been made in the flap, it is enlarged by angioplasty with a balloon measuring over 12 mm in diameter (Fig. 2). Occasionally a stent may be placed to maintain the fenestration.

An alternative approach, termed the scissor technique (26), involves the introduction of a rigid guide into the true channel and another into the false channel, both using the same sheathed introducers (8 F minimum, 45 cm long) installed by the femoral route. A fixed point on the guides allows a tear to be made in the aortic membrane (Fig. 4). The flap can then be unfolded by inflating a large-diameter balloon (over 12 mm) inside the thoracic aorta and retracting it as far as the iliac junction, with the balloon inflated.

The risk of a torn flap folding back in itself must be taken into account as this can induce ischemia in the lower limbs (27). It is also important to stent the flap beneath the fenestration site if the false channel is perfused without an exit as there is a risk of aortic rupture due to high pressure in the false channel. The scissor fenestration technique does not need to be extensively long, a fenestration of 3 to 5 cm seems sufficient. This length of fenestration lowers the pressure in the false channel, reduces compression of the true lumen, and relieves the ischemia linked to dynamic obstruction.

Endovascular treatment of aortic dissection should be combined with medical treatment (9). Blood pressure must be controlled, even if this requires the intravenous administration of several antihypertensive drugs. Our group utilizes anticoagulant treatment with intravenous heparin in cases of malperfusion in order to combat organ ischemia. After fenestration, regardless of whether a stent was deployed in the visceral branches or a stent graft used, anticoagulant treatment is continued until malperfusion is relieved and the symptoms disappear.

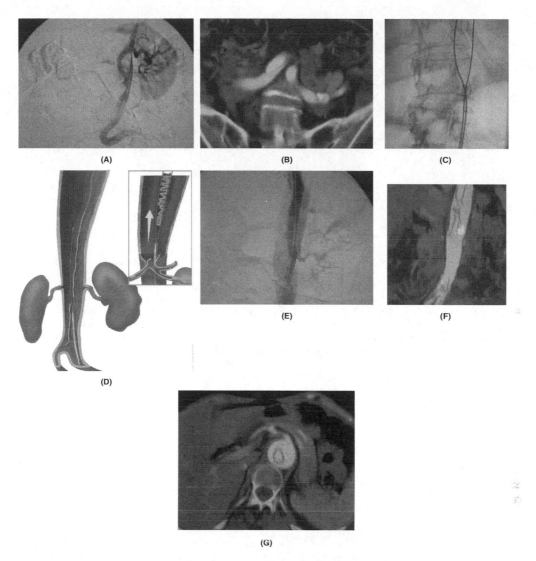

FIGURE 4 (**A**) Arteriogram of the aorta in a woman with anuria and lower limb ischemia after Type B aortic dissection, showing compression of the true lumen that perfuses the left renal artery and left iliac artery. (**B**) Axial view of the CT scan indicating entry tears at the level of right iliac artery. (**C**) X ray of the two guidewires inserted through the same sheath, one in the true and one in the false lumen. (**D**) Schematic representation of the dissection with the guidewire in place. (**E**) Arteriogram after fenestration up to the renal arteries after injection of contrast media into the true lumen. (**F**) Multiplanar reconstruction view of the CT scan six months after fenestration showing the intimal flap in the center of the aorta at the level of renal arteries (one was stented) without any obstruction, then the absence of flap in the abdominal aorta and an intimal flap in the distal aorta and iliac arteries. (**G**) Axial CT view showing a complete "endarterectomy" after endovascular fenestration. *Abbreviation*: CT, computed tomography.

REFERENCES

1. Hartnell GG, Gates J. Aortic fenestration: a why, when, and how-to guide. Radiographics 2005; 25:175–89.
2. Vedantham S, Picus D, Sanchez LA, et al. Percutaneous management of ischemic complications in patients with type-B aortic dissection. J Vasc Interv Radiol 2003; 14:181–94.
3. Williams DM, Lee DY, Hamilton BH, et al. The dissected aorta: percutaneous treatment of ischemic complications—principles and results. J Vasc Interv Radiol 1997; 8:605–25.
4. Williams DM, Brothers TE, Messina LM. Relief of mesenteric ischemia in type III aortic dissection with percutaneaous fenestration of the aortic septum. Radiology 1990; 174:450–2.

5. Reber D, Aebert H, Manke M, Birnbaum DE. Percutaneous fenestration of the aortic dissection membrane in malperfusion syndrome. Eur J Cardiothorac Surg 1999; 15:91.

6. Walker PJ, Dake MD, Mitchell RS, Miller DC. The use of endovascular techniques for the treatment of complications of aortic dissection. J Vasc Surg 1993; 18:1042–51.

7. Williams DM, Andrews JC, Marx MV, Abrams GD. Creation of reentry tears in aortic dissection by means of percutaneous balloon fenestration: gross anatomic and histologic considerations. J Vasc Interv Radiol 1993; 4:75–83.

8. Wolf JE, Eicher JC, Rezaizadeh-Bourdariat K. Dissection aortique. Rev Prat 2002; 52:1084–8.

9. Erbel R, Alfonso F, Boileau C, et al. Diagnosis and management of aortic dissection: Task Force on Aortic Dissection, European Society of Cardiology. Eur Heart J 2001; 22:1642–81.

10. Kouchoukos NT, Dougenis D. Surgery of the thoracic aorta. N Engl J Med 1997; 336:1876–88.

11. Cambria RP, Brewster DC, Gertler J, et al. Vascular complications associated with spontaneous aortic dissection. J Vasc Surg 1988; 7:199–209.

12. Mehta RH, Suzuki T, Hagan PG, et al. Predicting death in patients with acute type A aortic dissection. Circulation 2002; 105:200–6.

13. Fabre O, Vincentelli A, Willoteaux S, Beregi JP, Prat A. Preoperative fenestration for type A acute aortic dissection with mesenteric malperfusion. Ann Thorac Surg 2002; 73:950–1.

14. Deeb GM, Williams DM, Bolling SF, et al. Surgical delay for acute type A dissection with malperfusion. Ann Thorac Surg 1997; 64:1669–75.

15. Williams DM, Lee DY, Hamilton BH, et al. The dissected aorta: part III. Anatomy and radiologic diagnosis of branch-vessel compromise. Radiology 1997; 203:37–44.

16. Gaxotte V, Cocheteux B, Haulon S, et al. Relationship of intimal flap position to endovascular treatment of malperfusion syndromes in aortic dissection. J Endovasc Ther 2003; 10:719–27.

17. Chemla P, Rousseau H, Otal P, Chabbert V, Joffre F. Imagerie de l'aorte. Rev Prat 2002; 52:1066–72.

18. Rousseau H, Otal P, Soula P, Colombier D, Joffre F. Diagnostic et traitement endovasculaire de la pathologie aortique thoracique. J Radiol 1999; 80:1064–79.

19. Sommer T, Fehske W, Holzknecht N, et al. Aortic dissection: a comparative study of diagnosis with spiral CT, multiplanar transesophageal echocardiography, and MR imaging. Radiology 1996; 199:347–52.

20. Ledbetter S, Stuk JL, Kaufman JA. Helical (spiral) CT in the evaluation of emergent thoracic aortic syndromes. Traumatic aortic rupture, aortic aneurysm, aortic dissection, intramural hematoma, and penetrating atherosclerotic ulcer. Radiol Clin North Am 1999; 37:575–89.

21. Sebastia C, Pallisa E, Quiroga S, Alvarez-Castells A, Dominguez R, Evangelista A. Aortic dissection: diagnosis and follow-up with helical CT. Radiographics 1999; 19:45–60.

22. Rubin GD, Shiau MC, Schmidt AJ, et al. Computed tomographic angiography: historical perspective and new state-of-the-art using multi detector-row helical computed tomography. J Comput Assist Tomogr 1999; 23(Suppl. 1):S83–90.

23. Elefteriades JA, Hammond GL, Gusberg RJ, Kopf GS, Baldwin JC. Fenestration revisited. A safe and effective procedure for descending aortic dissection. Arch Surg 1990; 125:786–90.

24. Slonim SM, Miller DC, Mitchell RS, Semba CP, Razavi MK, Dake MD. Percutaneous balloon fenestration and stenting for life-threatening ischemic complications in patients with acute aortic dissection. J Thorac Cardiovasc Surg 1999; 117:1118–26.

25. Chavan A, Hausmann D, Dresler C, et al. Intravascular ultrasound-guided percutaneous fenestration of the intimal flap in the dissected aorta. Circulation 1997; 96:2124–7.

26. Beregi JP, Prat A, Gaxotte V, Delomez M, McFadden EP. Endovascular treatment for dissection of the descending aorta. Lancet 2000; 356:482–3.

27. Lookstein RA, Mitty H, Falk A, Guller J, Nowakowski FS. Aortic intimal dehiscence: a complication of percutaneous balloon fenestration for aortic dissection. J Vasc Interv Radiol 2001; 12:1347–50.

29 | Traumatic Aortic Injury (Indication for Endovascular Repair, Troubleshooting and Current Results, Comparison with Conventional Surgery)

Rossella Fattori
Cardiovascular Department, University Hospital S. Orsola, University of Bologna, Bologna, Italy

INTRODUCTION

Traumatic aortic injury (TAI) is a lesion extending from the intima to the adventitia, occurring as a result of trauma. The first annotation of TAI was in 1557 by Vesalius, who described a patient with an aortic rupture after a fall from a horse. In 1923 Dshanelidze in Russia reported the first successful repair of TAI in a penetrating lesion of ascending aorta, followed in the 1950s by the surgical reports of Gerbode et al., Klassen et al., Passaro and Pace (1). The era of high-speed motor vehicles has brought with it an increased incidence of TAI. The more sophisticated prehospital care and the proliferation of rapid transport for patients have resulted in an average increase in the number of patients treated. Several recent investigations have shown that TAI occurs in 10% to 30% of adults sustaining fatal blunt trauma. TAI therefore represents one of the most common causes of death at the scene of vehicular accidents, accounting for 8000 victims/yr in the United States. (2–8).

The lesion may be generated by many different types of sudden deceleration injury, including car and motorcycle collisions, falls from a height or blast injuries, airplane and train crashes, skiing and equestrian accidents. The region subjected to the greatest strain is the isthmus, where the relatively mobile thoracic aorta joins the fixed arch and the insertion of the ligamentum arteriosus. Aortic ruptures occur at this site in 80% of the pathological series and in 90% to 95% of the clinical series (2, 4, 5, 7, and 8). The mandatory use of a seat belt, first introduced in the 1970s in Finland, and progressively throughout the world, has partially modified the characteristics of the trauma impact that leads to aortic injury. However, air bags and seat belts do not protect against this type of impact. Such injuries can be expected to gain prominence in road traffic injury statistics (2), since the frequency of lethal injuries in head-on collisions is lowered by the mandatory use of restraints, which protect the victim from thoracic and head lesions but not from the mechanism producing aortic injury.

PATHOLOGY

According to the Parmley study (9) on 296 aortic injuries, the lesion may be classified as follows:

1. intimal hemorrhage
2. intimal hemorrhage with laceration
3. medial laceration
4. complete laceration of the aorta
5. false aneurysm formation
6. periaortic hemorrhage

Areas of intimal hemorrhage were noted at autopsy in patients who died of other fatal lesions. The endothelial layer may be intact or the hemorrhage may be associated with circumscribed laceration of the endothelial and internal elastic lamina of the intima. The tear is transverse in 80% to 90% of patients and involves all or part of the aortic circumference. When the lesion involves intimal and medial layers, a false aneurysm is formed.

The aneurysm is fusiform in the case of a circumferential lesion involving the entire wall on the transversal plane, while in a partial lesion in which only a portion of the wall is lacerated, it appears as localized diverticulum. Periaortic hemorrhage is frequently associated with the aortic injury independently of the type of lesion. Complete rupture of the aorta including the adventitia and the periadventitial connective tissue will often lead to immediate death. However, mediastinal hematoma may permit temporary survival. In the Parmley report, 9 of 38 patients who survived temporarily had complete transection, their survival being dependent on the hematoma contained in periaortic and mediastinal tissues.

MEDICAL AND SURGICAL MANAGEMENT

It is conventional to consider traumatic aortic injury to be a highly lethal injury. This concept is primarily based on the historical study by Parmley and associates in 1958 (9) who reported autopsy findings in 296 nonpenetrating TAI. Remarkably, Parmley's analysis estimated that 85% of the victims died on the scene from free aortic rupture; of those who survived at least for one hour, 30% died within six hours, 49% within 24 hours and 90% within four months. This article has been referenced in every subsequent report on this topic and has influenced the general opinion over the next 50 years, leading to the concept that immediate surgery should be advocated in traumatic aortic injury. However, as reported in several clinical series (10), the risk of a complete rupture of the aorta is not very high after four to six hours, especially if patients, once admitted to the hospital, are immediately submitted to pharmacological treatment with controlled hypotension.

The best time to intervene in the aortic lesion and whether surgery should be preceded or followed by the treatment of associated traumatic lesions remains a matter of debate (10–20). Immediate surgery has been characterized by a high mortality and morbidity rate (20–40%). In a report of 144 patients undergoing surgery within an average of six hours after arrival in hospital, there was an intraoperative mortality of 10.2% and postoperative mortality of 18.4% with major postoperative morbidity such as paraplegia reaching 10.5% (4). In a recent prospective multicenter trial (11) among 274 patients collected over 2.5 years, the overall mortality was 31%, with 14% operative mortality in stable patients undergoing planned thoracotomy.

This first phase after the trauma is life threatening and accident victims should be taken to hospital as quickly as possible. A prompt diagnosis of aortic wall injury is mandatory and an aggressive intravenous therapy with vasodilators and beta-blocking drugs must be started to reduce the aortic wall stress and the risk of lethal aortic rupture. According to Pate (10), the risk of rupture of a periaortic hematoma contained in the mediastinum can be avoided if the systolic blood pressure is constantly maintained below 120 mmHg. On the subsequent days a process of organization of the hematoma usually develops and with time it will turn into a strong fibrous tissue, with the formation of a pseudoaneurysm (21), that has the same risk of rupture as a true aneurysm of similar size. Patients must be admitted to an intensive care unit with continuous monitoring of electrocardiogram, arterial and central venous pressure, renal function and peripheral metabolism. An arterial systolic pressure exceeding 90 mmHg should be an indication to limit fluid replacement and any hemodynamic support in hypotensive patients. Monitoring of respiratory function and eventual intubation and mechanical ventilation is fundamental in polytraumatized patients with respiratory insufficiency due to central nervous system injury, pulmonary contusion and pleural effusion with measurement of chest tube outputs.

The overall mortality and the incidence of major complications are lower when it is possible to delay surgery (Table 1). It is important to remember that 90% of patients with aortic injury have associated other open and closed traumatic lesions of different areas (orthopedic, abdominal, closed-head injury) which may cause a rapid evolution into shock and coma, thus influencing the patient's outcome. Therefore, the treatment of associated lesions is fundamental

TABLE 1 Overall Mortality in Patients Treated with Delayed Surgery

Author	Year	Patients (*N*)	Overall mortality *N* (%)	Mortality related to aortic rupture (%)
Akins	1981	19	2 (10.5)	–
Kipfer	1994	10	0 (0)	0 (0)
Maggisano	1995	44	2 (4.5)	–
Pate	1995	112	21 (18.8)	6 (5.4)
Fabian	1997	21	11 (52.4)	0 (0)
Holmes	2002	30	8 (26.7)	1 (3.3)
Kwon	2002	10	1 (10)	0 (0)
Langanay	2002	19	3 (15.8)	0 (0)
Pacini	2005	48	2 (4.2)	1 (2.1)

in these patients and it is another incentive to delay surgical intervention in the aorta. Computed tomography scan and magnetic resonance imaging offer noninvasive assessment of the anatomical characteristics of the aortic lesions and can be used to monitor their evolution (18,22–25). Signs indicative of imminent free rupture, such as an increase in size of the periaortic hematoma or pseudoaneurysm, recurrent hemothorax, associated with a poorly controlled arterial pressure, can be promptly identified and therefore provide an indication for emergency surgery.

ENDOVASCULAR TREATMENT

Early Results and Comparison with Open Surgery

From 1996 the introduction of endovascular techniques for the thoracic aorta offered less invasive options, especially for patients in which emergency treatment is necessary. After initial limited series and case reports, endovascular treatment has become the method of choice in the management of TAI (26–30). At present, several reports in literature provide data on comparative results of endovascular therapy with respect to open surgery, supporting the use of stent graft in traumatic injuries, both in acute and chronic cases (31–34). Because of the lower invasiveness, avoiding thoracotomy and the use of heparin, endovascular repair can be applied in acute patients without the risk of destabilizing pulmonary, head or abdominal traumatic lesions. In early clinical series, endovascular treatment demonstrated lower morbidity and mortality in comparison with open surgical repair even in high-risk patients. The Talent Thoracic Retrospective Registry (35), which collected data on 457 patients treated for thoracic aortic lesions in seven major European centers, reported excellent results of endovascular repair in traumatic lesions: among 85 acute and chronic aortic injuries, this type of aortic lesions resulted in the lowest morbidity and mortality and represented the best long-term outcome. Significantly a very low rate of primary and secondary endoleaks is reported in case series, probably due to the good wall conditions (no atherosclerotic alteration of the aortic wall, no mural thrombus) at the neck sites.

Endovascular Management of Acute and Chronic Cases

At present, several standard sizes of thoracic stent grafts are promptly available, allowing their use in the emergency setting. In the past few years, initial medical management and delayed surgery of the aortic traumatic injury represent an important advance in the difficult management of polytrauma, substantially reducing operative and overall mortality. However, there are some patients in whom delayed surgery cannot be applied. Even if the majority of traumatic aortic injuries are stable lesions, in approximately 5% of them the risk of rupture may be high in the acute phase. Signs of impending rupture such as periaortic hematoma, repeated hemothorax, and uncontrolled blood pressure are considered signs of instability. Sometimes the aortic tear, acting with a valve mechanism, may cause a pseudocoarctation syndrome producing a reduction of flow in the descending aorta with lower extremity ischemia. This complication, which represents a surgical emergency, is observed in 10% of victims (36).

In these unstable patients endovascular techniques offer a suitable alternative to emergency open repair.

There is no requirement for full heparinization and the blood loss is minimal during the procedure. The risk of paraplegia seems to be very low even in extensive atherosclerotic aneurysms in which the aortic coverage extends from the left subclavian artery to the celiac axis. Therefore, due to the limited longitudinal extension of a traumatic lesion, only one segment of stent graft is used with very low risk of intercostal artery occlusion (Fig. 1A–E).

In the chronic posttraumatic aneurysm, endovascular treatment represents a favorable alternative treatment of an asymptomatic disease that is frequently recognized several years after the trauma. Death from rupture may occur many years after injury sometimes without any signs and symptoms of onset (21). Because it is impossible to predict which aneurysm still remains quiescent, elective repair is always recommended for both symptomatic and asymptomatic lesions. Advances in surgical techniques and spinal cord protection over the years have significantly reduced operative mortality and paraplegia rates in elective surgical repair of the thoracic aorta. In the largest surgical series, operative mortality for chronic posttraumatic aneurysms ranges from 0% to 10% and paraplegia accounts for 5% of cases. The risk of paraplegia in surgery of chronic posttraumatic aneurysm is very low as compared to atherosclerotic ones, because of the limited extension of the pseudoaneurysm that usually does not extend beyond the first pair of intercostal arteries. Endovascular treatment may play an important role in the management of chronic posttraumatic aneurysms, allowing a low invasive option with limited risk of complications (Fig. 2A–D).

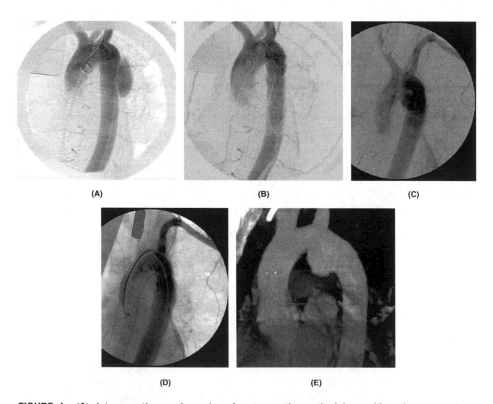

(A)   (B)   (C)

(D)   (E)

FIGURE 1 (**A**) Intraoperative angiography of a traumatic aortic injury with a large pseudoaneurysm in the posterior aortic wall, 15 mm below left subclavian artery. (**B**) After stent deployment there is a good aneurysm sealing. (**C**) Intraoperative angiography of a traumatic aortic injury involving the anterior aortic wall, very close to the left subclavian artery (proximal neck 4 mm). (**D**) The stent graft is deployed adjacent to the left subclavian artery, without occlusion: a good aneurysm sealing is achieved. (**E**) Computed tomography image (maximum intensity projection reconstruction) of a traumatic injury above the left subclavian artery (no proximal aortic neck). Revascularization of the left subclavian artery is necessary before stent-graft treatment.

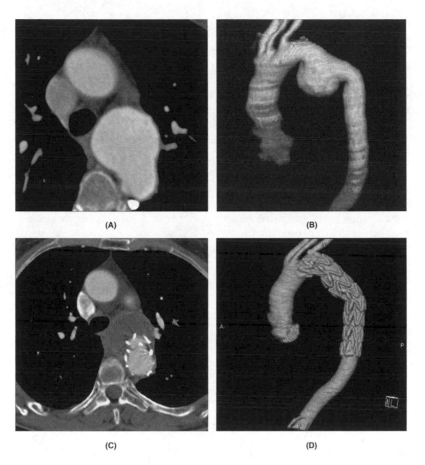

(A)   (B)

(C)   (D)

FIGURE 2   (**A**) Axial Multi Detector Computer Tomography (MDCT) image of a chronic posttraumatic aneurysm involving 2/3 of aortic circumference. (**B**) MDCT image [volume rendering (VR) reconstruction] of the same case: a proximal aortic neck of at least 10 mm is visible. (**C**) Axial MDCT image after stent-graft treatment: thrombosis of the aneurysm sac is complete. (**D**) MDCT image (VR reconstruction) of the same case after stent-graft treatment.

Assessment of Morphology for Stent-Graft Deployment

Endovascular treatment of TAI requires a favorable aortic morphology. Adequate vascular access (7–8 mm of diameter of femoral or iliac artery) is necessary, but is not always available especially in young patients. The most important anatomical characteristic of any lesion allowing endovascular treatment is the presence of an adequate proximal neck. The aortic isthmus is usually very close to the left subclavian artery and sometimes the lesion is in contiguity or a limited distance from the vessel. Several studies have reported the artificial creation of an aortic neck, covering the left subclavian artery with the stent graft, with or without previous subclavian to carotid transposition or bypass grafting.

However subclavian-to-carotid transposition and bypass grafting are adjunctive procedures which in some centers carries the risk of mortality and stroke (4.2%), while the abrupt closure of the left subclavian artery may evolve into chronic or acute subclavian steal syndrome. The risk of vertebral ischemia and cerebellar infarction is reported up to 5% for interventional treatment of intracranial aneurysm treated by vertebral ligation, therefore one may expect the same rate of complication for endovascular coverage of the left subclavian and vertebral artery without previous revascularization (37, 38). Moreover, the long life adjacency of the uncovered part of the stent graft to the left carotid artery is a potential source of emboli.

It is important to consider that the absence of atherosclerotic wall involvement of the aorta in posttraumatic aneurysms impacts on endovascular treatment, with successful aneurysm sealing even with short aortic neck (4–5 mm), without the need of left subclavian artery coverage. Preoperative imaging studies are fundamental in order to define the precise measurement of aortic morphology. If left subclavian artery coverage is necessary with previous bypass grafting, it may be questionable if endovascular treatment is preferable to elective open surgery.

Accurate measurements are also necessary to verify the efficacy of the procedure during follow-up. Usually, the aneurysm sac in both acute and chronic cases demonstrates a high rate of shrinkage (28).

CONCLUSIONS

For many years traumatic aortic injury has been considered a highly lethal lesion and a potential cause of death in blunt chest trauma. Despite evidence in the literature of lower morbidity and mortality, initial medical management of uncomplicated aortic injury and subsequent delayed surgery has not been easily accepted in the clinical practice. The development of endovascular techniques represents a viable alternative with very low risk and limited impact on trauma destabilization.

REFERENCES

1. Passaro E, Pace WG. Traumatic rupture of the aorta. Surgery 1959; 46:787–91.
2. Richens D, Kotidis K, Neale M, Oakley C, Fails A. Rupture of the aorta following road traffic accidents in the United Kingdom 1992–1999. The results of the co-operative crash injury study. Eur J Cardiothorac Surg 2003; 23:143–8.
3. Eddy CA, Rush VW, Marchioro T, Ashbaugh D, Verrier ED, Dillard D. Treatment of traumatic rupture of the thoracic aorta. Arch Surg 1990; 125:1351–5.
4. Hunt JP, Baker CC, Lentz CW, et al. Thoracic aorta injuries: management and outcome of 144 patients. J Trauma 1996; 40:547–56.
5. Greendyke RM. Traumatic rupture of the aorta. Special reference to automobile accidents. JAMA 1966; 195:527–30.
6. Arajarvi E, Santarvirta S, Tolonen J. Aortic ruptures in seat belt wearers. J Thorac Cardiovasc Surg 1989; 98:355–61.
7. Ben-Menachem Y. Rupture of the thoracic aorta by broadside impacts in road traffic and other collisions: further angiographic observations and preliminary autopsy findings. J Trauma 1993; 35:363–7.
8. Shorr RM, Crittenden M, Indeck M, Hartunian SL, Rodriguez A. Blunt thoracic trauma. Analysis of 515 patients. Ann Surg 1987; 206:200–5.
9. Parmley LF, Mattingly TW, Manion WC, Jahnke EJ, Jr. Nonpenetrating traumatic injury of the aorta. Circulation 1958; 17:1086–101.
10. Pate JW, Fabian TC, Walker W. Traumatic rupture of the aortic isthmus: an emergency? World J Surg 1995; 19:119–26.
11. Fabian TC, Richardson JD, Croce MA, Smith JS, Rodman GJ, Kearney PA, Flynn W, Ney AL, Cane JB, Luchette FA, et al. Prospective study of blunt aortic injury: multicenter trial of the American Association for the Surgery of Trauma. J Trauma Inj Infect Crit Care 1997; 42(3):374–83.
12. Fattori R, Celletti F, Bertaccini P, et al. Delayed surgery of traumatic aortic rupture: role of magnetic resonance imaging. Circulation 1996; 94:2865–70.
13. Maggisano R, Nathens A, Alexandrova NA, et al. Ruptures traumatiques de l'aorte thoracique: l'intervention d'urgence est-elle toujours indiquee? Ann Chir Vasc 1995; 9:44–52.
14. Jahromi AS, Kazemi K, Safar HA, Doobay B, Cinà C. Traumatic rupture of the thoracic aorta: cohort study and systematic review. J Vasc Surg 2001; 34:1029–34.
15. Kipfer B, Leupi F, Schuepbach P, Friedli D, Althaus U. Acute traumatic rupture of the thoracic aorta: immediate or delayed surgical repair? Eur J Cardiothorac Surg 1994; 8:30–3.
16. Blegvad S, Lippert H, Lund O, Hansen OK, Christensen T. Acute or delayed surgical treatment of traumatic rupture of the descending aorta. J Cardiovasc Surg 1989; 30:559–64.
17. Pacini D, Angeli E, Fattori R, et al. Traumatic rupture of the thoracic aorta: 10 years of delayed management. J Thorac Cardiovasc Surg 2005; 129(4):880–4.
18. Fattori R, Celletti F, Descovich B, et al. Evolution of post traumatic aneurysm in the subacute phase: magnetic resonance imaging follow-up as a support of the surgical timing. Eur J Cardiothorac Surg 1998; 13:582–7.
19. Hess PJ, Howe HR, Robicsek F, et al. Traumatic tears of the thoracic aorta: improved results using the Bio-Medicus Pump. Ann Thorac Surg 1989; 48:6–9.

20. Safi HJ, Bartoli S, Hess KR, et al. Neurologic deficit in patients at high risk with thoracoabdominal aortic aneurysms: the role of cerebral spinal fluid drainage and distal aortic perfusion. J Vasc Surg 1994; 20:434–43.
21. Finkelmeyer BA, Mentzer RM, Kaiser DL, Tegtmeyer CJ, Nolan SP. Chronic traumatic thoracic aneurysm. Influence of operative treatment on natural history: an analysis of reported cases, 1950–1980. J Thorac Cardiovasc Surg 1982; 84:257–66.
22. Mirvis SE, Shanmuganathan K, Miller BH, White CS, Turney SZ. Traumatic aortic injury: diagnosis with contrast-enhanced thoracic CT- five-year experience at a major trauma center. Radiology 1996; 200:413–22.
23. Gavant ML. Helical CT grading of traumatic aortic injuries. Impact on clinical guidelines for medical and surgical management. Rad Clin North Am 1999; 37:553–74.
24. Downing SW, Sperling JS, Mirvis SE, et al. Experience with spiral computed tomography as the sole diagnostic method for traumatic aortic rupture. Ann Thorac Surg 2001; 72:495–501.
25. Patel NH, Hahn D, Comess KA. Blunt chest trauma victims: role of intravascular ultrasound and transesophageal echocardiography in cases of abnormal thoracic aortogram. J Trauma 2003; 55(2):330–7.
26. Rousseau H, Soula P, Perreault P, et al. Delayed treatment of traumatic rupture of the thoracic aorta with endoluminal covered stent. Circulation 1999; 99(4):498–504.
27. Lachat M, Pfammatter T, Witzke H, et al. Acute traumatic aortic rupture: early stent-graft repair. Eur J Cardiothorac Surg 2002; 21:959–63.
28. Fattori R, Napoli G, Lovato L, et al. Indications for, timing of and results after treatment of catheter based treatment of the injury of aorta. AJR 2002; 178(6):125–32.
29. Waldenberger P, Fraedrich G, Mallouhi A, et al. Emergency endovascular treatment of traumatic aortic arch rupture with multiple arch vessel involvement. J Endovasc Ther 2003; 10(4):728–32.
30. Melnitchouk S, Pfammatter T, Kadner A, et al. Emergency stent-graft placement for hemorrhage control in acute thoracic aortic rupture. Eur J Cardiothorac Surg 2004; 25:1032–8.
31. Doss M, Balzer J, Martens S, et al. Surgical versus endovascular treatment of acute thoracic aortic rupture: a single-center experience. Ann Thorac Surg 2003; 76:1465–9.
32. Andrassy J, Weidenhagen R, Meimarakis G, Lauterjung L, Jauch KW, Kopp R. Stent versus open surgery for acute and chronic traumatic injury of the thoracic aorta: a single-center experience. J Trauma 2006; 60(4):765–71.
33. Rousseau H, Dambrin C, Marcheix B, Richeux L, Mazerolles M, Cron C, Watkinson A, Mugniot A, Soula P, Chabbert V, et al. Acute traumatic aortic rupture: a comparison of surgical and stent-graft repair. J Thorac Cardiovasc Surg 2005; 129(5):1050–5.
34. Schumacher H, Bockler D, von Tengg-Kobligk H, Allenberg JR. Acute traumatic aortic tear: open versus stent-graft repair. Semin Vasc Surg 2006; 19(1):48–59.
35. Fattori R, Nienaber CA, Rousseau H, Beregi JP, Heijmen R, Grabenwoger M, et al. Results of endovascular repair of the thoracic aorta with the Talent Thoracic Stent-Graft: the TTR registry. J Thorac Cardiovasc Surg 2006; 132(2):332–9.
36. Malm JR, Deterling RH. Traumatic aneurysm of the thoracic aorta simulating coarctation. J Thorac Cardiovasc Surg 1960; 40:271–8.
37. Cina CS, Safar HA, Lagana A, Arena G, Clase CM. Subclavian carotid transposition and bypass grafting: consecutive cohort study and systematic review. J Vasc Surg 2002; 35(3):422–9 (Review).
38. Steinberg GK, Drake CG, Peerless SJ. Deliberate basilar or vertebral artery occlusion in the treatment of intracranial aneurysms. Immediate results and long-term outcome in 201 patients. J Neurosurg 1993; 79(2):161–73.

30 | Embolization in Thoracic Hemorrhage

Tony Nicholson
Leeds Teaching Hospitals NHS Trust, Leeds, U.K.

INTRODUCTION

Thoracic hemorrhage may be traumatic or nontraumatic in origin. It is invariably life threatening and formerlly surgery was the only means of controlling such bleeding. Since 1970 embolization has become a widely used alternative treatment for bleeding from the lungs, and stent-grafting increasingly effective for bleeding from the aorta and great vessels. This chapter will deal with those causes of thoracic hemorrhage where embolization is most appropriate. These include bronchial artery hemorrhage and pulmonary hemorrhage related to penetrating trauma.

HEMOPTYSIS CAUSED BY BRONCHIAL ARTERY HEMORRHAGE

The bronchial circulation is the source of 90% of causes of massive hemoptysis, one of the most dreaded of all respiratory emergencies. Chest X ray and bronchoscopy have been important in the early diagnosis as both can indicate the side and the lobe that the bleeding is coming from and bronchoscopy can occasionally be useful in hemorrhage control. However multi-slice computed tomography (CT) is becoming increasingly important for the same reasons but in addition it is capable of giving information about bronchial artery anatomy which saves time during later angiography.

Knowledge of bronchial artery anatomy and the underlying pathophysiology of hemoptysis are essential if minimally invasive treatment by embolization is to succeed.

Conservative management of massive hemoptysis carries a mortality of 50% to 100% (1). It is important to note the cause of death is usually asphyxiation not exsanguination. It is therefore vital that in all these cases the airway is checked and secured prior to any further definitive treatment. Emergency surgery for massive hemoptysis has a mortality rate of up to 40% (2).

The first report of bronchial artery embolization for massive hemoptysis was in 1973 (3). However, this technique had been used successfully prior to this in Hanoi during the Vietnam War in 1970 as treatment for bleeding from contused lung. Subsequently much has been written about the safety and efficacy of bronchial artery embolization (4–10). It is important to remember that embolization, though extremely effective, is often not a long-term solution to the underlying pathophysiological process. Active tuberculosis and aspergilloma that is resistant to conventional drug therapy and other active processes such as hydatid disease and benign and malignant tumors will require surgery once the initial acute episode has been controlled.

Causes of Massive Bronchial Hemoptysis

It is generally accepted that massive hemoptysis has occurred when a patient coughs up between 300 and 600 mL of blood in 24 hours (1). However, smaller amounts may be life threatening if they threaten the patient's airway and in this regard the definition might apply to any hemoptysis that threatens a patient's life.

The causes of massive hemoptysis differ around the world: in developing countries tuberculosis in the commonest underlying cause. In the West, bronchogenic carcinoma, bronchiectasis, cystic fibrosis, and aspergillosis are the most common causes. Bronchial artery aneurysms are rare but are seen as a result of chronic inflammatory disease and in hereditary hemorrhagic telangiectasia. These are either juxta-aortic or intrapulmonary and are also amenable to embolization.

Diagnosis

Massive hemoptysis should initially be treated by an assessment of the airway, the breathing and the circulation. Following this it is important to find the cause of bleeding and to localize the lobe from which the bleeding is originating.

Chest X ray is useful but is normal or unhelpful in localization in 17% to 81% of patients (11–13). Fibro-optic bronchoscopy is often used as it is occasionally good at localizing the lobe where the bleeding is coming from, can diagnose a central bronchial lesion and can also be used to control bleeding by the injection of vasoactive drugs. However there is still controversy over this issue. Where the chest X ray is normal or nonlocalizing, bronchoscopy is said to be helpful in between 10% and 43% of patients (12,13). Where bleeding is massive and active, bronchoscopy often cannot localize the site or lobe because blood obscures the view.

Some believe that fibro-optic bronchoscopy prior to bronchial artery embolization is unnecessary where a chest X ray has indicated the site and size of bleeding (11). There are also some risks associated with fibro-optic bronchoscopy including airway compromise, delays in definitive treatment, hypoxemia and relatively high cost.

Where there is time, CT is becoming increasingly useful as it diagnoses bronchiectasis, bronchogenic carcinoma and aspergilloma accurately (13,14). CT can suggest a specific diagnosis in between 39% and 88% of patients where a chest X ray is non-diagnostic (14). The site of bleeding can also be localized by CT in between 63% and 100% of patients (11,15). Multi-slice CT evaluation can also produce exquisite images of bronchial artery anatomy assisting the interventionist hugely.

Bronchial Artery Anatomy

The bronchial arteries usually originate directly from the thoracic aorta, between the T5 and T6 vertebrae. They may arise directly from the aorta's ventral or ventrolateral surface or, if arising from an intercostobronchial trunk (ICBT), dorsolaterally or lateral on the right side. Four classic patterns are described (16):

- In 40% of cases there are two bronchial arteries on the left and one on the right arising from an ICBT in 70%.
- In 21%, one on the left and an ICBT on the right.
- In 20% there are two on the left and two on the right, one of which arises usually from an ICBT.
- In 10% one on the left and two on the right, one of which arises from an ICBT.

Occasionally both right and left bronchial arteries have a common trunk from the aorta (Fig.1). The prevalence of bronchial arteries with anomalous origins is quite high, ranging from 8.3% to 35% (17,18). Such arteries may arise from the aortic arch (the commonest anomalous site), the internal mammary artery, the thyrocervical trunk, the costocervical trunk, the brachiocephalic artery, the subclavian artery, the pericardiophrenic artery, the inferior phrenic artery or the abdominal aorta. The way to tell that these are bronchial rather than systemic arteries is that they always extend along the course of the major bronchi whereas systemic collateral vessels enter the pulmonary parenchyma through the pulmonary ligament or the pleura and their course is not parallel to the major bronchi. Rather than carrying out a complete search of all these potential aberrant sites the interventionist should simply be aware of the possible presence of aberrant bronchial arteries and search for them when bronchial arteries do not arise from the usual sites between T5 and T6 to supply areas of abnormal lung. It is also worth searching for aberrant bronchial arteries when no abnormality is demonstrated from more usual sites or where successful embolization fails to arrest hemoptysis.

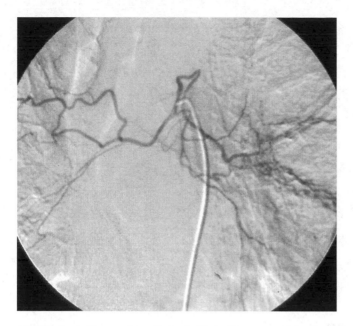

FIGURE 1 A 21-year-old patient admitted with pneumonia and massive hemoptysis. Using a Cobra catheter, a common trunk which occurs in about 4% of patients has been found. Bronchial angiography demonstrates abnormal left bronchial arteries, later embolized with 300 to 500 U polyvinyl alcohol via a microcatheter with resolution of symptoms.

Having understood bronchial artery origin anatomy it is important to realize that bronchial arteries and ICBTs can also supply other arteries as collaterals. These include anterior medullary spinal arteries which are recognized by their characteristic hairpin configuration (Fig. 2) as they arise close to the origin of the bronchial artery or ICBT. Very rarely, bronchial arteries can anastamose with coronary arteries (especially when these are stenosed and subclavian arteries). Clearly in all these cases extra care has to be taken to avoid reflux of embolization materials.

Bronchial Artery Embolization

Descending thoracic aortography is recommended initially using a pigtailed catheter in order to determine the number and sites of origin of the bronchial arteries (Figs. 3 and 4B). A decision can then be made as to which catheter is most suitable for selective studies and these are usually the Cobra, Simmons 1 or occasionally Headhunter or Lefjudkins catheters. Superselective catheterization using microcatheters permits safe positioning beyond the origin of any spinal cord and other branches and minimizes reflux of particles.

Bronchial arteries larger than 2 mm on a CT are considered to be abnormal (19).

Certainly adult bronchial arteries should not measure more than 1.5 mm diameter at their origin and 0.5 mm in the broncho-pulmonary segment. If they are larger than this they are considered to be hypertrophic. Other signs that may be seen in massive hemoptysis include severe tortuosity, neovascularity, hypervascularity, and extravasation of contrast medium and shunting into the pulmonary artery or vein. Very rarely bronchial artery aneurysms can be seen.

Although gelatine sponge is inexpensive and often used as an embolic material in bronchial artery embolization, recannalization is common and it is thought to be responsible for cases of recurrent bleeding (20). Polyvinyl alcohol particles are the embolization materials of choice. They are nonabsorbable and extremely effective. A size range of 300 to 500 U in diameter is usually used but it must be understood that because of clumping they are actually larger than this. It is very important to avoid the use of any embolic material that can pass

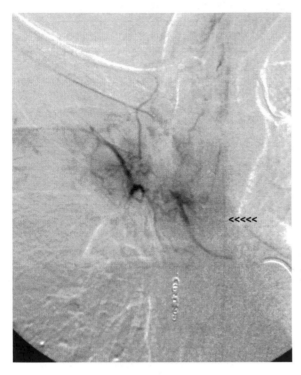

FIGURE 2   Left bronchial angiography for recurrent hemoptysis in a patient who had previous emboliza-tion of an aberrant internal mammary artery bronchial circulation. An anterior spinal artery with its characteristic hairpin bend is seen ($\lll$) arising from the proximal left intercostobronchial trunk.

through broncho-pulmonary anastomoses. In a human lung the largest of these anastomoses appears to be around 325 U (21).

If particles smaller than this are used or if any of the newer spherical or trisacryl particles are used at this size they will pass through and cause pulmonary and systemic infarction. Even where broncho-pulmonary fistulae are seen, 350 to 500 U polyvinyl alcohol (PVA) is considered safe (Fig. 4A–D). It is best not to use coils or liquid embolic agents such as glue or onyx, as these occlude the proximal artery and prevent repeat embolization if recurrent hemoptysis occurs.

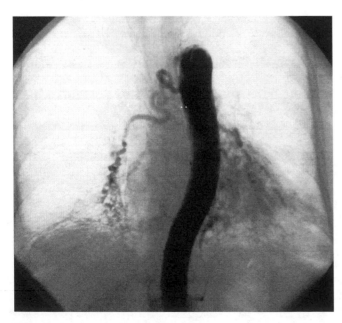

FIGURE 3   Thoracic aortography with the pigtail catheter just proximal to the left sub-clavian artery immediately reveals the bronchial arterial anatomy. In this case the most common pattern of one right and two left. This patient has bilateral basal bronch-iectasis and the enlarged, tortuous bronchial arteries with parenchymal staining are very visible.

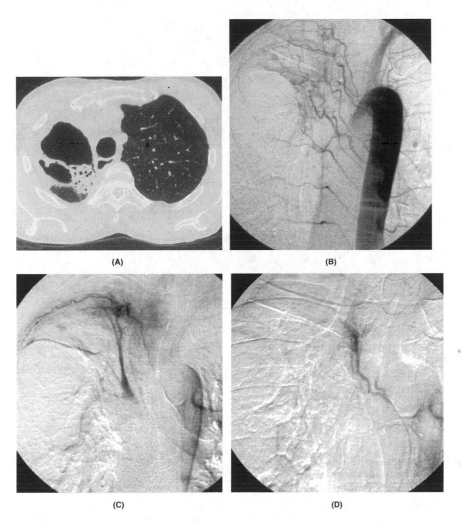

FIGURE 4 (**A**) Computed tomography scan reveals a large cavity at the right apex with a solid mobile area diagnosed as an aspergilloma in this 56-year-old with massive hemoptysis. (**B**) Aortography and (**C**) right bronchial angiography reveal the abnormal bronchial and intercostal circulation with fistula into the pulmonary veins. (**D**) Embolization using 300 to 500 U polyvinyl alcohol resulted in a good clinical result and the patient later had amphotericin instillation into the cavity with resolution of the aspergilloma.

They can however be used to occlude internal mammary arteries, to prevent embolization of normal tissue and the development of collateral arteries (Fig. 5A,B).

Results

Bronchial artery embolization is very affective at controlling acute massive hemoptysis. Nonrecurrence rates are between 73% and 98% (10). However where ongoing inflammation is present, up to 52% of patients will develop recurrent hemoptysis (22). Therefore in those patients who have active inflammatory processes causing their abnormal bronchial arteries, embolization is a palliative procedure.

Complications

Chest pain is the most common complaint after embolization occurring in up to 90% of patients (18). Such chest pain is usually transient. Dysphagia due to embolization of esophageal branches occurs rarely and usually regresses spontaneously. The most disastrous complication

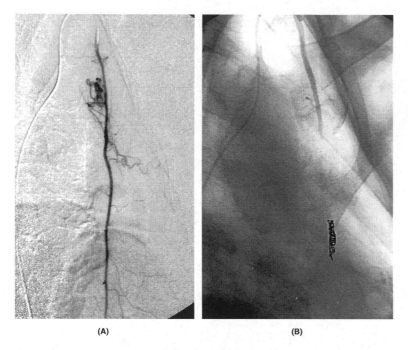

(A)   (B)

FIGURE 5 (**A** and **B**) Massive hemoptysis caused by bleeding from bronchial arteries arising from the left internal mammary artery. The distal inferior mesenteric artery has been coil embolized to prevent nontarget embolization and then 300 to 500 U polyvinyl alcohol used to affect treatment.

is spinal cord ischemia. This can occur in up to 6.5% of patients (20). This complication can be avoided if careful embolization is performed distal to any, carefully searched for, spinal artery. If there is any doubt at all whether embolization can be performed safely then either the attempt should be abandoned or distal coils should be inserted rather than particles.

Other complications that have been sporadically reported in the literature include transient cortical blindness, nontarget embolization, bronchial necrosis and dissection of the aorta and iliac arteries. These are all excessively rare and many are due to inadvertent embolization via broncho-systemic collaterals.

HEMOPTYSIS CAUSED BY NON-BRONCHIAL SYSTEMIC ARTERIES

Intervention is useful if systemic arteries cause massive hemoptysis. This occurs in less than 5% of all cases. Sometimes these are due to inflammatory processes in the pleura and bleeding can be from intercostal arteries, subclavian and axillary branches, internal mammary arteries or inferior phrenic arteries, all of which may become enlarged and rupture due to local inflammatory processes.

In addition penetrating trauma, iatrogenic trauma particularly from SwanGantz catheters and infection can cause bleeding from aneurysms and pseudoaneurysms of the main pulmonary arteries. Such pseudoaneurysms can usually be controlled by either packing the pseudoaneurysm with coils, glue or onyx or by embolizing the "front door/back door" pulmonary arteries (Fig. 6).

SUMMARY

Embolization has replaced surgery as the procedure of choice for acute hemoptysis, though surgery is often the definitive treatment for the underlying pathology. Experience and training in airway maintenance, a thorough knowledge of bronchial and systemic anatomy and

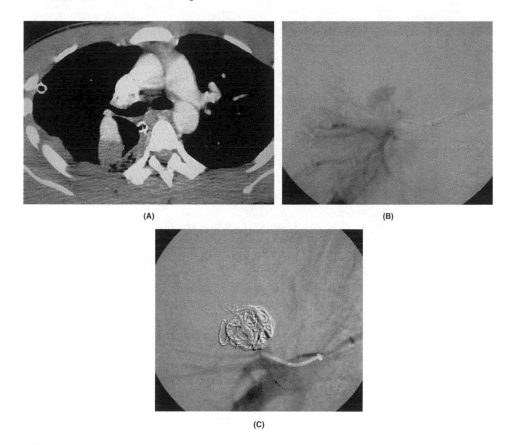

(A)

(B)

(C)

FIGURE 6   A 24-year-old man stabbed in the back developed chest pain and low volume hemoptysis several days after the incident. (**A**) A computed tomography scan revealed a large pulmonary artery pseudoaneurysm which was (**B**) confirmed by pulmonary angiography and (**C**) treated by packing the pseudoaneurysm with coils. No pulmonary infarction was caused and the patient made a full recovery.

embolization techniques, a team approach with surgeons and respiratory physicians and, in the future, access to CT are essential if lives are to be saved and complications avoided.

ACKNOWLEDGMENTS

My thanks go to Mrs. Lin Thomas for typing this manuscript and Dr. Simon McPherson for providing images.

REFERENCES

1. Najarian KE, Morris CS. Arterial embolization in the chest. JTORAC Imaging 1998; 13:93–104.
2. Fernando HC, Stein M, Benfield JR, et al. Role of bronchial artery embolization in the management of haemoptysis. Arch Surg 1998; 133:862–6.
3. Remy J, Foisin C, Ribet M, et al. Treatment by embolization of severe or repeated haemoptysis associated with systemic hypervascularisation. Nouv Presse Med 1973; 2:2060–8.
4. Wholey MH, Chamorro HA, Rao G, et al. Bronchial artery embolization for massive haemoptysis. JAMA 1976; 236:2501–4.
5. Remy J, Anraud A, Fardou H, et al. Treatment of haemoptysis by embolization of bronchial arteries. Radiology 1977; 122:33–7.
6. Uflacker R, Kaemmerer A, Neves C, et al. Management of massive haemoptysis by bronchial artery embolization. Radiolody 1983; 146:627–34.

7. Uflacker R, Kaemmerer A, Picon PD, et al. Bronchial artery embolization in the management of haemoptysis: technical aspects and long term results. Radiology 1985; 157:637–44.
8. Keller FS, Rosch J, Loflin TG, et al. Non-bronchial systemic collateral arteries: significance in percutaneous embelotherapy from haemoptysis. Radiology 1987; 164:687–92.
9. Hayakawa K, Tanaka F, Torizuka T, et al. Bronchial artery embolization for haemoptysis: immediate and long term results. Cardiovasc Intervent Radiol 1992; 15:154–9.
10. Kato A, Kudo S, Matsumoto K, et al. Bronchial artery embolization of haemoptysis due to benign disease: immediate and long term results. Cardiovasc Intervent Radiol 2000; 23:351–7.
11. Hsiao EI, Kirsch CM, Kagawa FT, et al. Utility of fibro optic bronchoscopy before bronchial artery embolization for massive haemoptysis. Am J Roentgenol 2001; 177:861–7.
12. Naidich DP, Funt S, Ettengern A, et al. Haemoptysis: CT-Bronchoscopic correlation in 58 cases. Radiology 1990; 177:357–62.
13. Hirschberg B, Biran I, Glazer M, et al. Haemoptysis: aetiology evaluation and outcome in a tertiary referral hospital. Chest 1997; 112:440–4.
14. Millar AB, Boothroyd AE, Edwards D, et al. The role of computer tomography (CT) in the investigation of unexplained haemoptysis. Respir Med 1992; 86:39–44.
15. Abala T, Nair PC, Cherian J. Haemoptysis: aetiology evaluation outcome—a prospective study in a third world country. Respir Med 2001; 95:548–52.
16. Cauldwell EW, Siekert RG, Lininger RE, et al. The bronchial arteries: an anatomic study of 105 human cadavers. Surg Gynecol Obstet 1948; 86:395–412.
17. Sancho C, Escilante E, Dominguez J, et al. Embolization of bronchial arteries of anomalous origin. Cardiovasc Intervent Radiol 1998; 21:300–4.
18. Cohan AM, Doershuk CF, Stern RC. Bronchial artery embolization to control haemoptysis in cystic fibrosis. Radiology 1990; 175:401–5.
19. Furuse M, Saito K, Kunieda E, et al. Bronchial arteries: CT demonstration with arteriographic correlation. Radiology 1987; 162:393–8.
20. Tanaka N, Yamakado K, Murashima S, et al. Super-selective bronchial artery embolizations for haemoptysis with a co-axial micro catheter system. J Vasc Intervent Radiol 1997; 8:55–70.
21. Pump K. Distribution of bronchial arteries in human lungs. Chest 1972; 62:447–51.
22. Katoh O, Kishikawa T, Ymada H, et al. Recurrent bleeding after arterial embolization in patients with haemoptysis. Chest 1990; 97:541–6.

31 | Assessment and Imaging of Abdominal Aneurysms (Comparison of Modalities and Selection of Patients for Endovascular Repair)

M. Truijers
Department of Surgery, Division of Vascular Surgery, Radboud University Nijmegen Medical Centre, Nijmegen, The Netherlands
L. J. Schultze-Kool
Department of Radiology, Radboud University Nijmegen Medical Centre, Nijmegen, The Netherlands
J. D. Blankensteijn
Department of Surgery, Division of Vascular Surgery, Radboud University Nijmegen Medical Centre, Nijmegen, The Netherlands

INTRODUCTION

The success of endovascular aneurysm repair (EVR) largely depends on an accurate preoperative assessment of aneurysm morphology. The use of EVR in patients considered anatomically unsuitable increases the risk for adverse outcome, including endoleak, stent migration and aneurysm rupture (1). Several imaging modalities have been proposed to facilitate the preoperative assessment of aortic morphology. The ideal modality should be noninvasive and still provide all information needed for EVR. This includes information on the dimensions and quality of the arterial access site, aneurysm and proximal and distal seal zones (2).

IMAGING MODALITIES

The imaging modalities discussed in this chapter are trans-abdominal ultrasound (US), intravascular ultrasound (IVUS), digital subtraction angiography (DSA), computed tomography angiography (CTA) and magnetic resonance angiography (MRA). All these modalities have been proposed for the preoperative assessment of aneurysm morphology and have their distinct advantages and pitfalls.

Trans-abdominal Ultrasound

US is the method of choice to detect aortic aneurysms; it is noninvasive, generally available and allows accurate diameter measurements. US, however, fails to visualize comprehensively the orifices of aortic side branches, tortuous vessels and infrarenal dimensions. Because of these disadvantages US is insufficient for the preoperative planning of EVR.

Intravascular Ultrasound

IVUS is a catheter-based invasive imaging modality. IVUS catheters are advanced through the femoral and iliac arteries into the aneurysm and infrarenal neck. This produces real-time information on vascular anatomy and vessel wall morphology. Because of this real-time imaging some authors advocate the use of IVUS intraoperatively during endograft deployment (3,4). Preoperatively, IVUS produces detailed axial images. An automated vessel analysis protocol is used to generate longitudinal reconstructions. These reconstructions facilitate the anatomical characterization of the proximal seal zone and provide comprehensive insight in the relation of side branches to the aorta (5).

IVUS, however, has limitations as the measurement of vessel diameter and length depend on the position of the catheter. Unfortunately, the catheter does not always follow the true vessel centerline. This tendency results in less accurate length measurements and elliptical-shaped artifacts, compromising diameter assessment (6). Although IVUS provides quantitative and qualitative information on the extent and composition of atherosclerotic plaques, heavily calcified plaques produce severe shadowing, complicating image interpretation.

In conclusion, IVUS potentially delivers valuable information during endograft deployment. However due to the invasive character, inaccurate diameter and length measurements, additional costs and procedure time, the use of IVUS as sole imaging modality for aneurysm morphology assessment is limited.

Digital Subtraction Angiography

The introduction of DSA significantly reduced examination time, contrast material load and patient discomfort compared to conventional angiography (7). Magnification artifacts caused by divergence of the X ray beam are reduced by using calibrated catheters. Although this improves aortic length and angulation measurements super stiff guidewires are needed to reduce length underestimation in tortuous vessels and length overestimation in saccular aneurysms (Fig. 1). DSA allows the accurate assessment of aortic side-branch patency, which is particularly important for the construction of tailor-made branched or fenestrated endografts for complex aneurysms (Fig. 2) (8). DSA also facilitates adjunctive endovascular procedures in patients with adverse aneurysm or access artery morphology. Arterial access is improved by balloon angioplasty of focal iliac artery narrowing and aorto-iliac aneurysms often require fluoroscopy-controlled coil embolization of the internal iliac artery to allow safe endograft coverage of the internal iliac artery orifice.

The main limitations of DSA are its invasive nature and that it fails to visualize mural thrombus, compromising diameter measurement and landing zone assessment. To overcome this shortcoming DSA has to be combined with axial computed tomography (CT) or magnetic resonance imaging (MRI) for preoperative EVR planning (9). With the ongoing development of noninvasive imaging modalities like CT and MRI and their image post-processing tools, the preoperative use of DSA is limited, especially since DSA is still associated with a small but definite risk of complications (10).

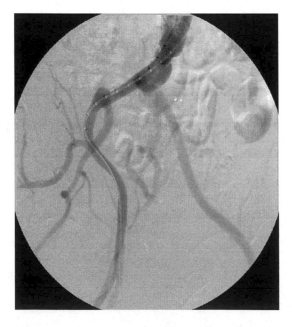

FIGURE 1 Digital subtraction angiography using a calibrated catheter. Note that the calibrated catheter does not follow true vessel centerline.

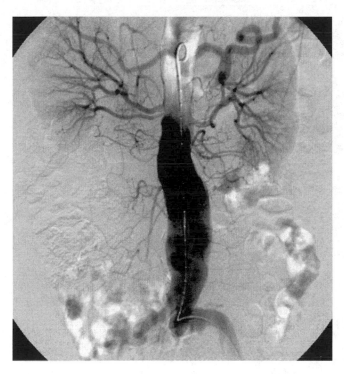

FIGURE 2 Digital subtraction angiography with measuring pigtail. Note double renal artery on the right.

Computed Tomography Angiography

In helical or spiral CT the X ray tube and detector (gantry) rotate continuously as the patient moves through the scanner. The result is a raw dataset, representing the helical path of the X ray beam through the scanned volume. From this primary raw data, images can be reconstructed (post-processed) in several planes and even into three-dimensional models (Fig. 3). By the additional infusion of intravenous contrast, spiral CTA potentially combines the advantages of conventional slices-by-slice CT and angiography. The diagnostic performance of spiral CTA however depends on the appropriate choice of acquisition parameters (11). The most important acquisition parameters are table feed (TF) per gantry rotation and slice thickness or collimation (SC). Both TF and SC are determined by overall scan range and data acquisition time. CTA of the abdominal aorta starts above the celiac artery and includes the external iliac artery and preferably the femoral bifurcation, resulting in a large scan range. In an attempt to keep scanning time, subsequent tube heating and motion artifacts limited the patient has to be moved through the scanner at high table speeds, leading to an increase in slice collimation and suboptimal spatial resolution.

This inverse relation between scan range and slice collimation has been overcome by the introduction of multi-slice spiral computed tomography (MSCT) (12). MSCT allows the simultaneous acquisition of multiple slices during one gantry rotation.

Besides an improvement in acquisition parameters, MSCT also allows an improvement in reconstruction parameters (12). MSCT acquires large amounts of data. A special interpolation scheme (z-filtering) uses of all these data for the final reconstruction. The final slice thickness or spatial resolution is therefore only determined by scanner configuration (number of slices and effective detector size) and the selected reconstruction increment (RI). RI determines the degree of overlap between subsequent slices. The most useful post-processing tools for the assessment of aortic morphology include, multiplanar reconstruction (MPR), maximum intensity projection (MIP), volume rendering (VR) and shaded surface display (SSD).

Multiplanar reconstructions are generated to visualize the aorta in axial, coronal, sagittal and orthogonal orientation. A commercially available workstation is used to scroll through the two-dimensional stack of images (cine mode). Orthogonal images, reconstructed around

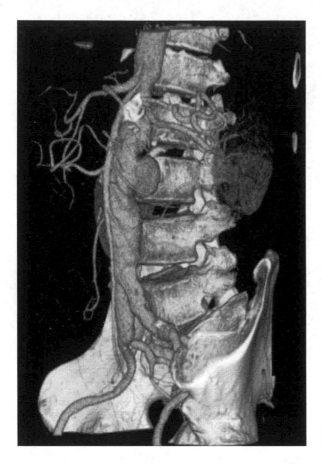

FIGURE 3 Computed tomography angiography, three-dimensional reconstruction.

the central axis (centerline) of the vessel, allow the visualization of the aorta and iliac arteries in a plane perpendicular to blood flow. The perpendicular images and centerlines are used for diameter and length measurements (Fig. 4) (13). Early diameter assessment using axial CT images was often inaccurate as tortuous vessels appeared elliptical, leading to an overestimation of vessel diameter. To compensate for this elliptical appearance, it has been proposed that true diameter corresponded with the smallest diameter on axial images. This however resulted in diameter underestimation for truly elliptical vessels. The use of orthogonal images has overcome this problem and renders true aneurysm diameter (14). Centerlines are used in length measurements. Unlike IVUS or DSA catheters the virtual centerline follows the vessel lumen without bulging into an aneurysm sac or following the shorter route through tortuous vessels. Furthermore the final graft length and diameter can be calculated by manually adjusting the centerline and planar reformats to the expected endograft path. Some software applications even allow the placement of a Virtual Graft® (Medical Metrx Solutions, West Lebanon, New Hampshire, U.S.A.) within the vessel lumen.

The second useful image post-processing tool is MIP. This tool visualizes the densest voxels for the identification of luminal contrast and wall calcifications. The result is an angiographic-like two-dimensional image. This image can be visualized from every desired angle which is useful for the preoperative assessment of iliac artery calcification or occlusion.

The final image post-processing tools, VR and SSD provide three-dimensional virtual images of the aorta and relevant side branches (Fig. 5). Both techniques rely on the difference in voxel attenuation factor for different anatomical structures, a process called segmentation. In SSD only pixels above a certain threshold are retained for the identification of surfaces. An illusion of depth is created by displaying virtual gray scale reflections on these created surfaces. VR allows the segmentation of the entire dataset by applying color codes to preset attenuation

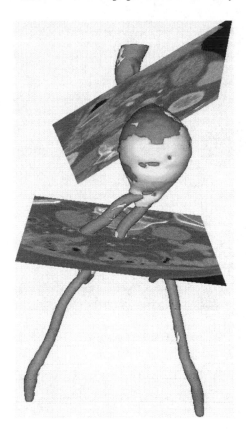

FIGURE 4 Computed tomography angiography, centerline and perpendicular reconstruction.

factors. This results in the identification of lumen, thrombus and calcification. VR produces reliable three-dimensional images of tortuous vessels. By rotating the model, accurate measurements of aortic neck and iliac artery angulations can be made.

CTA has two main disadvantages. The use of ionizing radiation and the necessity for nephrotoxic contrast. With the use of MSCT, radiation exposure initially increased. In order to resolve this problem effective milliampere was introduced. This allows adjustment of radiation dose in function of slice collimation and table speed. The use of thin collimation however still requires fair amounts of ionizing radiation. The second disadvantage of CTA is the use of nephrotoxic contrast. MSCT reduces the need for nephrotoxic contrast by allowing shorter data acquisition and by optimizing the delay between contrast admission and data acquisition (bolus triggering). In bolus triggering a region of interest is selected (e.g., aorta) after which the contrast is injected. When the contrast attenuation in the region of interest exceeds the preset trigger threshold (120 Houndsfeld Units) the scanner starts acquiring data reducing the need for contrast. In spite of this reduction in contrast dose prehydration is often necessary for patients with renal impairment. Furthermore even in limited dose intravenous contrast has the inherent risk for idiosyncratic reactions.

In conclusion, CTA with the use of MSCT and image post-processing, combines the advantages of conventional CT and DSA. CTA is the only single imaging modality that allows a thorough assessment of aortic morphology and provides all the information needed for EVR (15–17).

Magnetic Resonance Angiography

Since the introduction of MRA several imaging protocols have been proposed. All these protocols have their distinct advantages and disadvantages.

Spin-echo MRA depends upon a signal void (black-blood) created inside the vessel lumen by flowing blood. This allows the identification of the vessel wall and intraluminal thrombus.

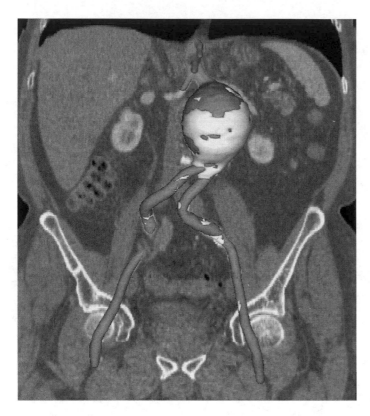

FIGURE 5 Computed tomography angiography, volume rendering.

Both spin-echo MRA and bright-blood techniques, like time-of-flight MRA, rely on the visualization of blood flow to distinguish between vessel lumen and arterial wall. Due to this flow dependency the visualization of aortic aneurysms is often limited as flow through the aneurysm is usually slow. In addition, both black- and bright-blood techniques require fairly long acquisition times which can result in motion artifacts (18).

The introduction of contrast-enhanced MRA resolved the problem of flow dependency by the application of gadolinium. Gadolinium induces a T1 shortening effect, limiting saturation problems due to slow blood flow and allowing faster data acquisition (19). By lowering the required acquisition time new applications of MRA became feasible. In cine-MRA, images are obtained during different phases of the cardiac cycle resulting in a dynamic view of the vessel wall. The potential of this technique to visualize actual vessel translation and endograft motion after EVR has been demonstrated (20). Besides the continuous development of MRA, the main advantages of MRA remain the lack of ionizing radiation, and the ability of image post-processing. Like CTA, image post-processing of MRA includes MPR, maximum intensity projection (MIP), VR and SSD (Fig. 6).

MRA however, has practical limitations due to poor equipment availability, associated high costs and relatively long acquisition times (up to one hour). Furthermore not all patients are eligible for MRA because of metallic implants (prosthesis, pacemaker or endograft) or claustrophobia. The main limitation of MRA is the low sensitivity for iliac artery and seal zone calcification which could lead to complicated arterial access and inappropriate endograft fixation. Like ionizing contrast, gadolinium is nephrotoxic. MRA however still plays an important role in patients with renal impairment as the dose of gadolinium used during MRA is limited.

MORPHOLOGICAL CRITERIA

The technical success of EVR, uncomplicated and complete exclusion of the aneurysm, depends on arterial access, safe and accurate device deployment and adequate fixation of

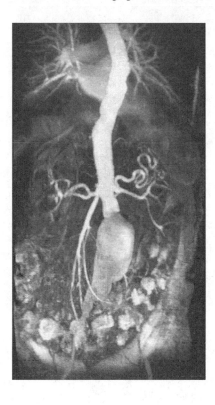

FIGURE 6   Magnetic resonance angiography, maximum intensity projection.

the graft above and below the aneurysm (2). Arterial access is needed for device delivery. If the iliac or femoral arteries are too small, tortuous or calcified, access is impaired possibly precluding EVR. Safe device deployment is possible if the deployed device does not cover essential branch vessels or cause distal embolization. The main anatomical criteria that could exclude patients for EVR however concern the dimensions and morphology of the proximal and distal aneurysm neck. Mismatch of graft-aneurysm dimensions at one of the seal zones could result in type I endoleak, graft migration and increase the risk for aneurysm rupture. Several criteria have been proposed to standardize and stratify the morphological risk factors associated with adverse outcome after EVR. These criteria are summarized in Table 1 and Figure 7 (2,21). Table 1 also contains the recommendations for access site and seal zone dimensions made by three manufacturers of commercially available endografts.

Arterial Access

Iliac and femoral artery anatomy is an important factor for EVR. High vessel tortuosity, heavy calcification and small arterial dimensions could complicate EVR and preclude percutaneous access artery closure, requiring femoral artery cutdown. Unfavorable access artery dimensions are associated with an increased risk of arterial dissection, failure to deliver the endograft and distal embolization (22). Although focal narrowing and near iliac artery occlusions can be treated by balloon angioplasty and iliac or femoral artery tortuosity can be overcome by straightening the vessels using traction, adverse access artery anatomy could lead to iliac artery damage and subsequent conversion to open or combined endovascular and open (hybrid) aneurysm repair.

Device Deployment

Safe device deployment is possible if the device does not cover essential side branches or cause distal embolization. Consequently, the anatomy of the aneurysm and potentially related side branches should be assessed before deployment. The assessment of aneurysm morphology includes aneurysm diameter and length measurement, estimation of tortuosity and calculation

TABLE 1 Stratification of Morphological Criteria

Morphology	None	Mild	Moderate	Severe	Aneurx® (Medtronic, Santa Rosa, California, U.S.A.)	Zenith® (Cook Inc., Bloomington, Indiana, U.S.A.)	Excluder® (W.L. Gore & Associates, Inc., Flagstaff, Arizona, U.S.A.)
Access site (iliac)							
Diameter (mm)	>10	8–10	7–8	<7	>7	>7.5	>6
Stenosis	Absent	Diameter >7 mm Length <3 cm	Diameter <7 mm Length <3 cm	Diameter <7 mm Length >3 cm (or multifocal)			
Calcification	Absent	<25% vessel length	25–50% vessel length	>50% vessel length			
Tortuosity[a]	<1.25	1.25–1.5	1.5–1.6	>1.6			
Angulation[b] (°)	160–180	120–160	90–120	<90			
Deployment							
Aneurysm							
Angulation[c] (°)	160–180	140–160	120–140	<120			
Tortuosity[a]	<1.05	1.05–1.15	1.15–1.2	>1.2			
Thrombus	Absent	25% CSA	25–50% CSA	>50% CSA			
Side branches							
Aortic side branches	None	One vessel	Two vessels	Two vessels with paired IA or LA; IMA >4 mm			
Hypogastric artery	Patent	Unilateral occlusion	Unilateral occlusion Contralateral >50% stenosis	Bilateral occlusion			
Seal zone							
Proximal neck							
Length (mm)	>25	15–25	10–15	<10	>10	>15	>15
Diameter (mm)	<24	24–26	26–28	>28	18–26	18–28	19–26
Angulation[d] (°)	>150	135–150	120–135	>120	>135	>120	>120
Calcification/thrombus	<25% Circumference	25–50% Circumference	50–75% Circumference	>75% Circumference			<2 mm thick <25% Circumference
Distal neck							
Length (mm)	>30	20–30	10–20	<10	>10	>10	>10
Diameter (mm)	<12.5	12.5–14.5	14.5–17	>17	11–15	7.5–20	8–13.5

[a] Tortuosity = centerline distance/straight lumen distance.
[b] Access site angulation = angle between common femoral artery and aortic bifurcation.
[c] Aortic angulation = most acute angle in the pathway between the lowest renal artery and the aortic bifurcation.
[d] Proximal neck angulation = angle between the axis of the proximal neck and the axis of the aneurysm.
Abbreviations: CSA, cross-sectional area; IA, intercostal artery; IMA, inferior mesenteric artery; LA, lumbar artery.
Source: Adapted from Refs. 2, 21.

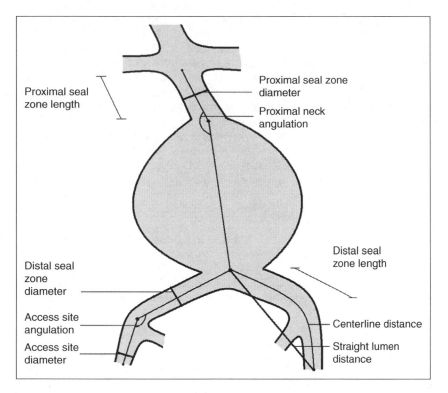

FIGURE 7 Main definitions regarding the morphological criteria for endovascular aneurysm repair. *Source:* Adapted from Ref. 2.

of luminal thrombus load. Although no absolute contraindication for EVR, large aneurysms (>6 cm) often have more complex anatomical characteristics and are associated with a significantly longer operation time and more proximal endograft migration (23). Length assessment of the infrarenal aorta (lowest renal artery to aortic bifurcation) is important before deployment of modular bifurcated endografts. These endografts are comprised of two or more components, the main body with ipsilateral iliac limb and the contralateral iliac limb. Fixation and deployment of the contralateral limb within the main body requires catheterization of the main body from the contralateral access artery. This is only possible when the bifurcation of the selected main body is located above the aortic bifurcation. Aneurysm thrombus load and tortuosity should be assessed as the risk of embolization during EVR is determined by the amount of intraluminal thrombus and the severity of tortuosity of the entire deployment pathway (2).

The identification of patent aortic side branches is essential before deployment of the endograft. Accessory renal arteries are present in 15% to 30%, failure to identify these aberrant vessels, could lead to coverage and subsequent renal impairment or type II endoleak. The inferior mesenteric arteries are generally excluded from the circulation after deployment. Although this rarely causes complications, patients with (near) occlusions of both the superior mesenteric artery and celiac artery could suffer from bowel ischemia.

Proximal and Distal Seal Zone

Complete and durable aneurysm exclusion demands an adequate seal between the endograft and the arterial wall. Failure to achieve an adequate seal results in type I endoleak, graft migration and persistent risk of rupture. Seal quality is largely determined by the morphology of the proximal and distal landing zone or "aneurysm neck." The proximal neck is defined as the distance between the most caudal renal artery and the beginning of the aneurysm.

Most commercially available endografts require a minimal proximal neck length of 15 mm and a maximum neck diameter of 30 mm. Other morphological factors related to proximal endograft fixation include the amount of thrombus and calcium within the proximal neck, the angle between the axis of the infrarenal neck and aneurysm and the shape of the proximal neck (e.g., tapered, reverse tapered, straight or bell shaped) (24,25). In the absence of a suitable infrarenal landing zone, several commercially available endografts allow suprarenal fixation with bare wire struts. Whether suprarenal fixation protects against proximal migration and is safe in regard to renal artery patency, remains to be investigated (26).

The distal seal zone or neck determines the type of endograft used. Since the introduction of EVR several different endograft designs have been proposed. The first straight or tube endografts were used in patients with aneurysms confined to the aorta. These grafts required a distal seal zone, between the aneurysm and the aortic bifurcation, with a length of at least 20 mm and a diameter no larger than 25 mm. Because only few patients met these anatomical criteria the need for endografts passing the aorta bifurcation was established. This has lead to the development of modular bifurcated endografts and aorto-uni-iliac devices with contralateral iliac occlusion and femoral crossover bypass. These devices are anchored distally in the common or external iliac artery. Fixation in the external iliac artery however, requires adjunctive coil embolization of the internal iliac artery to prevent type II endoleak (chap. 37). The morphological criteria for the distal seal zone vary for the different commercially available endografts. Generally the distal seal zone should be at least 10 mm long and maximum 20 mm wide.

Although the number of patients eligible for EVR is often limited by adverse proximal and distal seal zone anatomy, new developments in endograft design and operative procedures render more patients suitable for EVR. Scalloped, fenestrated, and even branched endografts have been developed (chap. 38). These endografts allow suprarenal fixation while visceral side branches like the renal, mesenteric and even celiac artery remain patent (27). Furthermore complex aneurysm and vascular anatomy can be modified by adjunctive endovascular or surgical (hybrid) procedures (28).

CONCLUSION

Since the introduction of modular bifurcated endografts more patients are considered suitable for EVR. These devices allow the distal seal zone to be chosen between the common iliac and femoral artery. Although the development of new endovascular devices allows more flexibility, the dimensions and quality of the proximal and distal seal zone, access site and aneurysm side branches still determine the success of EVR. The selection of patients based on morphological criteria requires accurate preoperative and preferably noninvasive imaging.

Multi-slice CTA is the only single source imaging modality that provides all necessary information for the preoperative assessment of aortic morphology. Raw scan data are acquired in a single breath hold and transferred to an image post-processing workstation for MPR, MIP, three-dimensional SSD and VR. MPR and MIP allow the accurate assessment of thrombus, calcium, diameter and length, while iliac artery and infra renal neck tortuosity and angulation are assessed with VR and SSD reconstructions. Although CTA has disadvantages (nephrotoxic contrast and ionizing radiation), CTA is the method of choice for patient selection based upon morphological criteria.

MRA has been introduced as a possible replacement for CTA. However, in spite of recent developments in image post-processing and contrast enhanced scanning protocols, CTA remains the primary single source imaging modality for EVR planning. This is mainly due to practical considerations and the low sensitivity of MRA for intravascular calcium.

REFERENCES

1. Brewster DC, Cronenwett JL, Hallett JW, Jr., et al. Guidelines for the treatment of abdominal aortic aneurysms. Report of a subcommittee of the Joint Council of the American Association for Vascular Surgery and Society for Vascular Surgery. J Vasc Surg 2003; 37:1106–17.

2. Chaikof EL, Fillinger MF, Matsumura JS, et al. Identifying and grading factors that modify the outcome of endovascular aortic aneurysm repair. J Vasc Surg 2002; 35:1061–6.
3. White RA, Donayre C, Kopchok G, et al. Intravascular ultrasound: the ultimate tool for abdominal aortic aneurysm assessment and endovascular graft delivery. J Endovasc Surg 1997; 4:45–55.
4. Slovut DP, Ofstein LC, Bacharach JM. Endoluminal AAA repair using intravascular ultrasound for graft planning and deployment: a 2-year community-based experience. J Endovasc Ther 2003; 10:463–75.
5. van Essen JA, Gussenhoven EJ, Blankensteijn JD, et al. Three-dimensional intravascular ultrasound assessment of abdominal aortic aneurysm necks. J Endovasc Ther 2000; 7:380–8.
6. Beebe HG, Kritpracha B. Imaging of abdominal aortic aneurysm: current status. Ann Vasc Surg 2003; 17:111–8.
7. Katzen BT. Peripheral, abdominal, and interventional applications of DSA. Radiol Clin North Am 1985; 23:227–41.
8. Anderson JL, Berce M, Hartley DE. Endoluminal aortic grafting with renal and superior mesenteric artery incorporation by graft fenestration. J Endovasc Ther 2001; 8:3–15.
9. Fillinger MF. New imaging techniques in endovascular surgery. Surg Clin North Am 1999; 79:451–75.
10. Singh H, Cardella JF, Cole PE, et al. Quality improvement guidelines for diagnostic arteriography. J Vasc Interv Radiol 2003; 14:S283–8.
11. Prokop M, Schaefer-Prokop C, Galanski M. Spiral CT angiography of the abdomen. Abdom Imaging 1997; 22:143–53.
12. Prokop M. General principles of MDCT. Eur J Radiol 2003; 45(Suppl. 1):S4–10.
13. Broeders IA, Blankensteijn JD, Olree M, et al. Preoperative sizing of grafts for transfemoral endovascular aneurysm management: a prospective comparative study of spiral CT angiography, arteriography, and conventional CT imaging. J Endovasc Surg 1997; 4:252–61.
14. Kritpracha B, Wolfe J, Beebe HG. CT artifacts of the proximal aortic neck: an important problem in endograft planning. J Endovasc Ther 2002; 9:103–10.
15. Broeders IA, Blankensteijn JD. Preoperative imaging of the aortoiliac anatomy in endovascular aneurysm surgery. Semin Vasc Surg 1999; 12:306–14.
16. Sprouse LR, Meier GH, III, Parent FN, et al. Is three-dimensional computed tomography reconstruction justified before endovascular aortic aneurysm repair? J Vasc Surg 2004; 40:443–7.
17. Qanadli SD, Mesurolle B, Coggia M, et al. Abdominal aortic aneurysm: pretherapy assessment with dual-slice helical CT angiography. AJR Am J Roentgenol 2000; 174:181–7.
18. Ludman CN, Yusuf SW, Whitaker SC, et al. Feasibility of using dynamic contrast-enhanced magnetic resonance angiography as the sole imaging modality prior to endovascular repair of abdominal aortic aneurysms. Eur J Vasc Endovasc Surg 2000; 19:524–30.
19. Nienaber CA, Fattori R. Aortic diseases—do we need MR techniques? Herz 2000; 25:331–41.
20. Vos AW, Wisselink W, Marcus JT, et al. Cine MRI assessment of aortic aneurysm dynamics before and after endovascular repair. J Endovasc Ther 2003; 10:433–9.
21. Hellinger JC. Endovascular repair of thoracic and abdominal aortic aneurysms: pre- and post-procedural imaging. Tech Vasc Interv Radiol 2005; 8:2–15.
22. Tillich M, Bell RE, Paik DS, et al. Iliac arterial injuries after endovascular repair of abdominal aortic aneurysms: correlation with iliac curvature and diameter. Radiology 2001; 219:129–36.
23. Waasdorp EJ, de Vries JP, Hobo R, et al. Aneurysm diameter and proximal aortic neck diameter influence clinical outcome of endovascular abdominal aortic repair: a 4-year EUROSTAR experience. Ann Vasc Surg 2005; 19:755–61.
24. Albertini J, Kalliafas S, Travis S, et al. Anatomical risk factors for proximal perigraft endoleak and graft migration following endovascular repair of abdominal aortic aneurysms. Eur J Vasc Endovasc Surg 2000; 19:308–12.
25. Balm R, Stokking R, Kaatee R, et al. Computed tomographic angiographic imaging of abdominal aortic aneurysms: implications for transfemoral endovascular aneurysm management. J Vasc Surg 1997; 26:231–7.
26. Parmer SS, Carpenter JP. Endovascular aneurysm repair with suprarenal vs. infrarenal fixation: a study of renal effects. J Vasc Surg 2006; 43:19–25.
27. Verhoeven EL, Zeebregts CJ, Kapma MR, et al. Fenestrated and branched endovascular techniques for thoraco-abdominal aneurysm repair. J Cardiovasc Surg (Torino) 2005; 46:131–40.
28. Carroccio A, Spielvogel D. Combined open and endovascular techniques for the treatment of complex vascular disease. Mt Sinai J Med 2004; 71:12–6.

32 | Techniques of Endovascular Graft Placement for Abdominal Aortic Aneurysm

J. P. Becquemin and J. Marzelle
Henri Mondor Hospital, University Paris XII, Creteil, France

INTRODUCTION

Since Parodi demonstrated the feasibility of endovascular repair, endovascular aneurysm repair (EVAR) has emerged as the gold standard for aneurysm repair. In North America, more patients undergo EVAR than open surgery. Although the results of the Dutch Randomized Endovascular Aneurysm Management trial and EVAR I and II trials have raised controversy regarding longer term results when compared to conventional repair, most advocates of stent-grafting have continued to expand the indications for the use of endovascular technology. This chapter describes the technical aspects of EVAR, including tips and tricks for trouble shooting problems. Recent advances regarding fenestrated and branched stent grafts are described elsewhere.

Pre-Operative Aneurysm Evaluation

Three-dimensional computed tomography (CT) reconstructions and computerized measurements facilitate pre-operative planning (Fig. 1). With the current generation of stent grafts, it is recommended to oversize the stent diameter by 10% to 20% compared to the diameter of the proximal landing zone. When embarking on a programme of endovascular stent-grafting, it is desirable to have a large range of stent grafts, devices and endovascular equipment "on the shelf" to deal with a spectrum of unexpected findings or events. Though the list of anatomical constraints has shifted over recent years, there remain certain criteria which deem aneurysms unsuitable or unfavourable for EVAR.

Pre-Operative Patient Evaluation

The EVAR-I trial demonstrated that, compared to open surgery, early mortality from stent-grafting is reduced threefold. Conversely, the EVAR II trial demonstrated that, in patients not fit for open surgery, EVAR produced no survival benefit. While it may be concluded that EVAR should only be offered to patients who are considered between mild to moderate risk from open surgery, there remains controversy regarding the EVAR-II results and the suitability of unfit patients for stent-grafting. The role and extent of pre-operative cardiac evaluation is also controversial, but it should be noted that beta-blockers and statins seem to have an effect in reducing postoperative cardiac complications. Severe pulmonary dysfunction is less relevant for EVAR than open repair, since EVAR can be performed under local anaesthesia without laparotomy. Renal function is of paramount importance since EVAR requires iodine-based contrast injection, which can provoke acute renal failure. However, the volume of contrast agent can be reduced dramatically (<50 cc) and it is possible to perform EVAR with carbon dioxide injection.

Setting for EVAR

EVAR can be performed in the operating room (OR) or endovascular suite. In the OR, modern mobile C-arms are adequate for the required quality of imaging for EVAR. The operating table must be radio-translucent. In the endovascular suite, imaging is usually superior but great

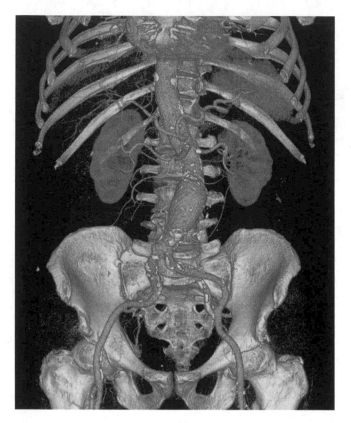

FIGURE 1   Three-dimensional reconstruction of a abdominal aortic aneurysm amenable to stent graft.

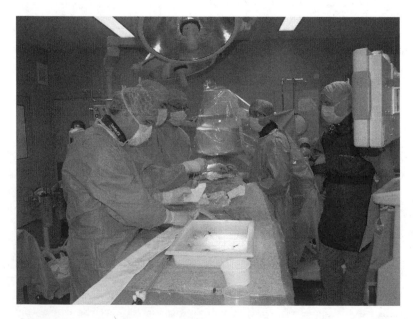

FIGURE 2   Modern combined operative room and angio-suite for endovascular procedures.

care must be taken to ensure a sterile environment which matches that provided in the OR. Many institutions now have specialized endovascular rooms designed with fixed imaging and operating theatres conditions (Fig. 2).

Positioning the Patient

Figure 3 shows our recommended position of the patient, staff and equipment for performing EVAR. Anaesthesiologists remain at the head of the patient. The operators and scrub nurse are on the right side of the patient. Before starting the procedure, it is essential to ensure unrestricted movement of the C-arm around the patient. It is important that adequate imaging is possible from thoracic aortic arch to below the groins. To set landmarks, we still place a ruler below the operating table, to the left of the lumbar spine.

Anaesthesia

General, regional and local anaesthesia can be used. Local anaesthesia is possible in frail patients, though ischemic leg pain during deployment can be problematic. When an aortoiliac repair is required in combination with a femorofemoral cross over graft, general anaesthesia is preferable.

Approach

We routinely use a percutaneous approach, though others prefer surgical cut-downs. We start the procedure by puncturing both groins. A standard guidewire is positioned in the iliac artery. Then, a Perclose® arterial closure system (Abbott Vascular Systems, Abbott Park, Illinois, U.S.A.) is placed. According to the introducer sheath diameter, we used two Perclose devices on the side of the main body of the graft introduction and one on the contralateral side (Fig. 4). The needles are removed and the suture threads left in place.

Groins are surgically exposed when additional surgical repair is required, such as cross-over graft, femoral endarterectomy or an iliac conduit to bypass a severely diseased external

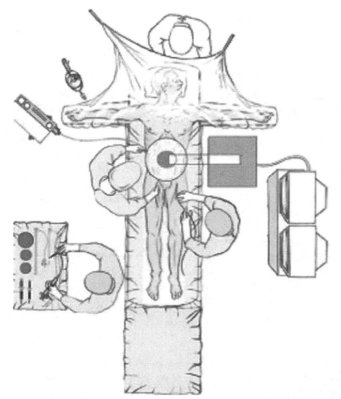

FIGURE 3 Drawing of the operative setting for endovascular aneurysm repair.

iliac artery. We usually perform a short horizontal incision above the inguinal ligament. The main advantage of this approach is to avoid the lymph's nodes of the triangle of Scarpa.

Catheterization Techniques

Nine-French introducer sheaths are placed in the common femoral arteries through which $0.035'' \times 1.50$ m hydrophilic wires, such as the Terumo wire, are introduced through the iliac arteries to the supra-renal aorta. On the side chosen for the long limb extension, contralateral to the graft main body, a marked pig-tail catheter is positioned over the wire to the L1/L2 level, the expected level of the renal arteries. On the opposite side, the Terumo wire is exchanged for a stiff wire, such as the Lunderquist wire (0.035 in., 2.80 m long), using an angled catheter such as the Vanschie (Cook). The upper tip of the wire is positioned carefully with radiological imaging, to ensure that it remains in the aortic arch and does not enter the arch vessels, most dangerously the left common carotid artery.

Stent-Graft Introduction

The sheath containing the main body of the graft is flushed with saline. The position of the markers identifying the short limb of the graft is identified by X-ray screening and the stent positioned in the correct orientation. Systemic heparin is given intravenously (0.5 mg/kg body weight) prior to insertion of the delivery device. With the current introducer systems formal arteriotomy is not required, so the artery is punctured directly. The sheath is advanced under fluoroscopic guidance. When the markers identifying the upper level of the graft material are at the approximate level of the renal arteries, or slightly above, digital subtraction angiography is performed with a contrast run through the pigtail catheter. The origin of the renal arteries should be identified precisely. With road-mapping, the relative positions of the graft and renal arteries are assessed and the markers placed precisely at the level, or just below, the renal arteries.

Main Body and Long Leg Graft Deployment

Depending upon the grafts used the deployment differs somewhat. The deployment of the three commonest grafts utilized in Europe are described. Further details of available grafts are described in Chapter 33.

The Cook Zenith Device
The Cook Zenith stent graft (Fig. 5) includes a row of bare stents with hooks at the proximal part of the graft. The deployment of the body starts from the second row of the stent which is covered by the Dacron fabric. The proximal uncovered stent is held within the hollow nose cone of the delivery sheath at this stage. By holding the pusher firmly with the right hand and pulling the outer sheath with the left hand, the second and third rows of the graft can be deployed. A second angiogram is performed to check the positioning of the graft in relation to the renal arteries. At this stage, it is still possible to modify the position of the graft either by pushing the system proximally or by pulling it distally. Once the positioning is optimal, the bare stent is released by unscrewing the safety locker, removing the metallic thread of the safety locker and advancing the hollow nose cone. The bare stent opens and the hooks engage with the aortic wall above the renal arteries. At this stage the graft can no longer be moved (Fig. 6A,B).

   The remainder of the stent graft is now deployed by continued backward pressure on the outer sheath while holding the introducer stationary. The correct opening of the contralateral short limb is apparent due to the radio-opaque markers and metallic stent.

The Gore Excluder Device
The Gore Excluder graft (Fig. 7) comprises a nitinol stent and polytetrafluorethylene graft with no bare suprarenal fixation stent. The stent graft is released by pulling a wire which maintains the device on the delivery system. Once the wire is removed the device deploys in an "all-or-nothing" fashion, with no way of repositioning the graft. It is of paramount importance that positioning is extremely accurate prior to deployment.

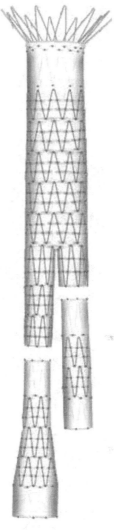

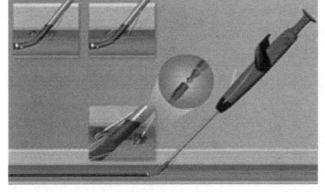

FIGURE 4 Drawing of a preclosing system used for endovascular aneurysm repair: the Perclose system (Abbott).

FIGURE 5 Cook Zenith stent graft.

The Medtronic Talent Device

The latest generation of the Talent device (Fig. 8) comprises a dacron graft supported by a self-expanding nitinol stent. There is a bare proximal stent with no hooks or barbs, and fixation relies upon the radial force exerted by the device. The delivery catheter has an integrated handle to aid controlled deployment. Rotating or releasing and retracting the integrated handle deploys the device by retracting the outer sheath cover. Deployment can commence slightly high as it is still possible to draw the device more distally as deployment continues. It is not possible to advance the device any further proximally once the first row opens.

Contra Lateral Limb Catheterization

Cathetarization of the contralateral limb can be challenging in difficult anatomy. The graduated catheter is removed and replaced by an angled catheter such as the Vanschie (Cook), which is available with three different angles. The catheter is positioned in the aneurysm, close to the opening of the short limb. An angulated Terumo wire is introduced through the catheter and by

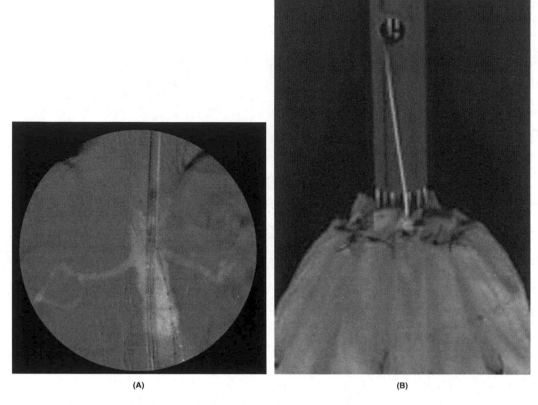

(A)   (B)

FIGURE 6   (**A,B**) Proximal deployment of a Cook stent graft.

exercising different rotations of the catheter and wire, the short limb of the graft is catheterized (Fig. 9). Once in place, the catheter is advanced to the level of the upper neck of the aneurysm. It is essential at this stage to ensure that the limb has been cannulated and the catheter is not within the aneurysm sac. The wire is removed in order for the catheter to regain its nominal curve and a rotation is exercised on the proximal tip. If the radio opaque extremity turns freely, the catheter is within the graft. If not, the catheter is outside the graft and should be withdrawn. If there is any doubt, a small amount of contrast can be injected. A stiff wire such as the Linderquist wire is then advanced through the catheter into the thoracic aorta and the catheter withdrawn so that the contralateral limb can be deployed.

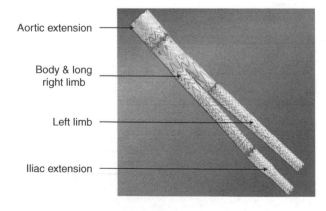

Aortic extension

Body & long right limb

Left limb

Iliac extension

FIGURE 7   W.L. Gore Excluder stent graft.

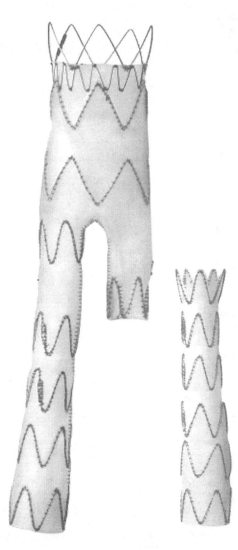

FIGURE 8   The talent Medtronic stent graft.

Distal Limbs Placement

The technique for both limbs is similar, with marking of the internal iliac arteries essential if these are to be preserved. Ideally, if the limbs are to be placed in the common iliac arteries, the full length of these should be engaged with the endograft limb. The C-arm is adjusted to an oblique position (Fig. 10 and contrast medium (10 mL) is injected through the sheath. The length and distal diameter of the limb are checked (occasionally by placing the graduated catheter on the wire). The appropriate limb is then passed over the stiff wire to the desired location. An overlap of at least one full stent length is recommended to avoid disconnection.

Ballooning and Completion

An extra large compliant balloon is inflated at the level of the landing zones to firmly apply the device to the arterial wall. However, the native arteries above and below the fabric of the graft must not be dilated due to the risk of arterial rupture.

The final angiogram is performed with a pigtail catheter positioned at the level of the renal arteries, to identify endoleaks, graft compression or kinking and to ensure preservation of the renal and internal iliac arteries. Occasionally it is necessary to aspirate blood from sheaths in both groins to encourage passage of contrast through the stent, particularly if the internal iliac arteries have been intentionally covered.

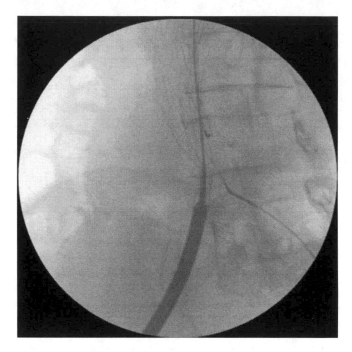

FIGURE 9 Short limb catheterizm with a Vanschie catheter during endovascular aneurysm repair.

Delayed pictures may be required to detect type II endoleaks, which require no immediate intervention as 60% thrombose in the early postoperative period. Contrast may be identified entering the aneurysm sac from the ostia of the inferior mesenteric or lumbar arteries. If a type I endoleak is identified, additional measures must be taken to ensure a seal is achieved Initially, re-ballooning of the landings zones should be considered. If this is insufficient to achieve a seal, extension cuffs can be placed either proximally or distally depending upon the location of the endoleak. Palmaz stents may also be deployed in the proximal neck to ensure good apposition of the stent to the vessel wall.

In case of severe kinking, particularly of the stent limbs, balloon or self expandable stents must be placed to prevent acute limb thrombosis (Fig. 11).

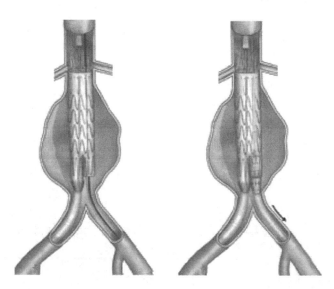

FIGURE 10 Distal limb placement during endovascular aneurysm repair.

Aortouniiliac Graft

We preferentially use bifurcated grafts which avoid routine groin incisions and the risk of infection and occlusion associated with cross over grafts. However, if one iliac artery is occluded, severely diseased or excessively tortuous, or when the aorta around the level of the bifurcation is less than 20 mm diameter (preventing full expansion of the two limbs of a bifurcated graft), we place an aortouniiliac graft. Horizontal groin incisions are performed bilaterally. The control angio catheter is placed on the side contralateral to that chosen for graft deployment. The renal arteries are located and the graft is deployed in the usual manner. An occluder is placed in the contralateral common iliac artery unless already occluded. Once the endovascular part is complete, a cross over femorofemoral graft is performed. The anastomosis on the receiving side is performed end-to-end if no occluder is required or end to side. For the graft, we generally choose a subcutaneous route which should be tunnelled prior to the administration of heparin (Fig. 12).

Puncture Site Closure

If performed percutaneously with arterial closure devices, the sutures threads are tied, extremities cut and steri-strips are placed on the wound. If performed with open groin cut-downs, the arteries are repaired with a fine non-absorbable suture and wounds closed with running absorbable sutures. The patient is prescribed aspirin 75 mg/day.

Efficacy Control

Within one month, a Duplex scan and/or a CT scan are performed to check the position of the graft and to exclude late endoleaks (Fig. 13).

Tips and Tricks for Trouble Shooting Problems

Access

Small caliber and/or severely diseased iliac arteries may prevent the introduction of the sheath. Gentle dilatation with a balloon or preferably with dilatators may overcome the problem. If these manoeuvres fail, the external or common iliac artery should be exposed through a short retroperitoneal incision. An 8 mm dacron tube graft conduit is anastomosed end to side to the artery. The delivery device can then usually be delivered through the conduit. Once the

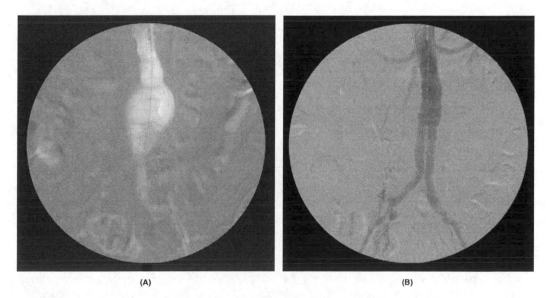

(A)   (B)

FIGURE 11   (**A,B**) Pre and final angio for abdominal aortic aneurysm treated by endovascular aneurysm repair.

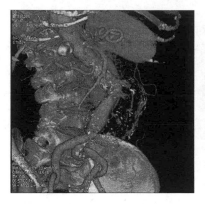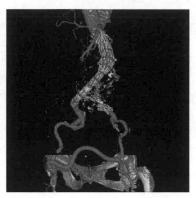

FIGURE 12 Postoperative computed tomography scan of abdominal aortic aneurysm treated with an aortouniiliac stent graft.

stent graft has been deployed, the graft is removed or sutured to the common femoral artery (Fig. 14).

Severe angulation of the iliac artery may prevent stent-graft delivery. A groin incision can be made to expose the common femoral artery. Tributaries are ligated and the external iliac artery exposed beneath the inguinal ligament. It is often then possible to straighten the external iliac artery with the second finger of the left hand, while with the right hand advances the delivery sheath (Fig. 15).

Internal Iliac Artery Involvement

In 15% to 30% of cases, the graft limbs are extended into the external iliac artery which poses two potential problems (see chap. 41). The first is retrograde flow from the internal iliac tributaries into the aneurysm causing endoleak, and the second is internal iliac occlusion causing buttock colonic or pelvic ischemia. When the internal iliac is likely to be covered, back bleeding can be prevented by coil embolization of the origin of the artery. This can be performed at the time of surgery, from an ipsilateral or contralateral approach (Fig. 16). If both internal iliacs are to be occluded it is advisable to perform embolizations as a staged procedure.

Conversely if preservation of the internal iliac artery is deemed critical, a side branch graft or combined technique should be considered. This latter comprises an internal iliac translocation to the distal external iliac, or a bypass graft from the common iliac to the internal iliac (Fig. 17).

Angulated Proximal Necks

Severe neck angulation may preclude endovascular repair. However, if the neck is long enough it is possible to straighten an angulated neck with a large (25 mm) Palmaz stent (Cordis) either before or after stent-graft deployment (Fig. 18). Excessive angulation or tortuosity can also be straightened by the use of two stiff wires prior to stent deployment.

Short Limb Catheterization

Although usually straightforward, catheterization of the contralateral limb can occasionally be technically challenging, particularly if the short limb is not fully open and compressed by aneurysm thrombus, or when the axis of the common iliac is not in line with the graft. If proving difficult, snaring a wire from the opposite side should be considered. The wire is caught below the orifice of the contralateral limb with a snare-goose neck catheter and withdrawn from the introducer (Fig. 19). This is exchanged for a stiff wire and the limb of the graft deployed as before. Alternatively the wire can be inserted from the left arm. When these techniques fail, the only solution is to place a aortouniiliac converter into the stent graft, occlude the contralateral limb and perform a femorofemoral graft.

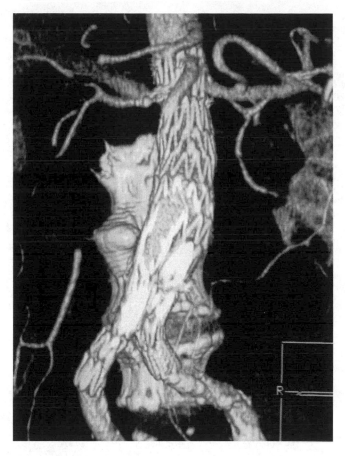

FIGURE 13   Postoperative computed tomography scan of abdominal aortic aneurysm treated with a bifurcated stent graft.

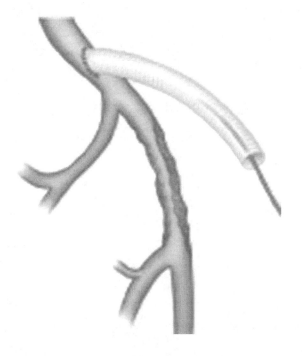

FIGURE 14   Ilio-femoral graft prior to endovascular aneurysm repair to facilitate access.

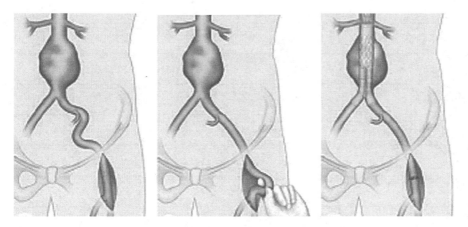

FIGURE 15   The Parodi manoeuvre to straighten angulated external iliac artery before endovascular aneurysm repair.

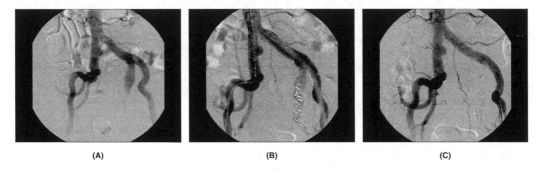

(A)   (B)   (C)

FIGURE 16   (**A,B,C**) Ipsilateral approach for coils embolization of the internal iliac artery before endovascular aneurysm repair.

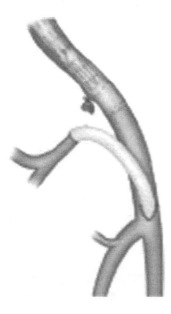

FIGURE 17   Common femoral to internal iliac artery bypass to preserve pelvic flow before endovascular aneurysm repair.

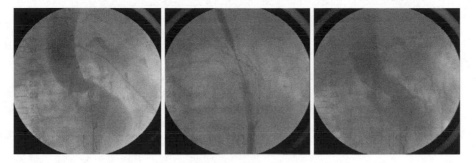

FIGURE 18   Extra large Palmaz stent placement to deal with severely angulated neck.

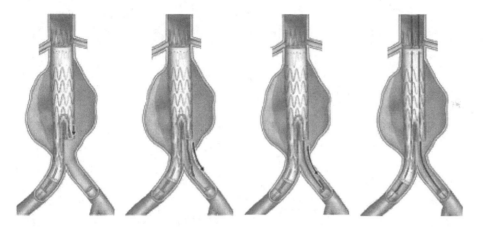

FIGURE 19   Snare technique to deal with difficult short limb catheterization during endovascular aneurysm repair.

Limb or Graft Occlusion

In cases where EVAR is particularly long and complex, or where there is a kinked stent graft or severely diseased outflow, stent limbs or the entire graft may occlude in the early peri-operative period. Fresh clot can be cleared by thrombolysis but this is usually contra-indicated. Open conversion with a femorofemoral or axillo bifemoral graft may be performed, though open graft thrombectomy and correction of any recognized technical defect should be considered (see chap. 52).

Rupture

In difficult anatomy, the aneurysm or the iliac arteries may rupture. Depending upon the time of occurrence there are several endovascular options. When rupture occurs before stent deployment, prompt placement of the stent graft should stop the bleeding. When the iliac ruptures, if the wire is still in place a covered graft is placed across the arterial injury. To gain immediate control a balloon can be inflated to isolate the arterial injury. If the wire has been removed direct surgical repair may be the most appropriate action.

ACKNOWLEDGMENT

Drawings by Virginie Ratel.

33 | Current Endografts for Abdominal Aortic Stenting

Vincent Riambau and Ivan Murillo
Vascular Surgery, Thorax Institute, Hospital Clínic, University of Barcelona, Barcelona, Spain

INTRODUCTION

The widespread application of endovascular aneurysm repair (EVAR) has been affected by limitations to the technology. The percentage of aneurysms considered suitable for endovascular repair has been increasing over the past decade, with improvements in graft design. However, long term durability, endoleaks and graft related complications still limit the efficacy of EVAR.

HISTORICAL PERSPECTIVE

Pioneering work on the endovascular treatment of abdominal aortic aneurysms (AAA) was initially reported in 1968 and continued in an experimental setting with major contributions from Palmaz and Gianturco (1,2). In 1988 Volodos (3) reported the first clinical experience in a descending thoracic pseudoaneurysm using a home-made endograft. In 1991 Juan Parodi (4) reported the first five human cases of abdominal aneurysm exclusion, which heralded the modern era of EVAR. In the past two decades up to 20 types of aortic endografts have been developed and more than 100,000 endografts have been implanted worldwide. At the present time many endografts are available for clinical use, and many more have been withdrawn from the market following adverse clinical incidents. As present, the ideal endograft and delivery system has yet to be defined. The remainder of this chapter focuses on current endografts and their differing design parameters.

IDEAL AORTIC ENDOGRAFT DESIGN

An ideal aortic endograft may be defined as an endovascular prosthesis that excludes the aneurysm from the circulation, protects indefinitely from aortic rupture and allows normal blood flow through the aorta and its branches. An ideal endograft needs to demonstrate permanent fixation, long durability and hemodynamic function over time. The endograft should be easy and accurate to deploy and applicable to difficult and challenging anatomy.

Other endograft parameters to be considered in choosing an endograft for a particular case might include:

- Global design: modular, uni-body, bifurcated, aortouniiliac (AUI).
- Stent configuration: endo or external skeleton; full or partially supported.
- Fabric composition: thin-polyester, surgical polyester, polytetrafluoroethylene (PTFE), thin-PTFE, ultra thin material.
- Fixation mechanism: friction, bare stent, barbs, spikes, hooks.
- Sizes: diameters and lengths.
- Delivery system: diameter, hemostatic behavior, flexibility, tracktability, pushability, accuracy on deployment.
- Company with research and development data on product design and behavior or only with commercial purposes.
- Price.

CURRENT ENDOGRAFTS

Many endografts have been introduced into clinical practice around the world. Some (Stentor™, Vanguard™, Ancure™, Lifepath™) have already disappeared from the market for different reasons, most of them related to poor clinical outcomes and issues with durability. This chapter will review the current commercially available endografts with attention directed to their advantages and disadvantages.

Anaconda™

The Anaconda AAA stent-graft system is manufactured by Vascutek (Inchinnan, Scotland, U.K.) (5). The concept for the Anaconda originated with Prof. Lutz Lauterjung from Munich. The first vascutek Anaconda system was the subject of a clinical study from 1999–2000. The device, which had no active fixation mechanism, but which relied on a high radial force for both sealing and anchoring, led to infrarenal neck dilatation and migration in some patients. The study was discontinued and the device was re-engineered to include four pairs of hooks for positive fixation and a modified top ring stent to address the neck dilatation. A second 60 patients study was carried out from 2002–2004. After successful results at 12 months follow up (zero migration, zero neck dilatation and zero Type I or Type III endoleaks), the Conformité Européenne (CE) mark was awarded in April 2005. The device is currently under clinical investigation in Food and Drug Administration (FDA) study in the U.S.A.

The Anaconda is a modular system, comprising of a body and two limbs. Limb extensions and aortic cuffs are available. Vascutek made use of its extensive textile technology to create an ultra thin woven polyester graft with similar physical properties (burst and porosity) to conventional surgical prostheses. The ring stents at the top of the body and the ring stents which provide support in the limbs are nitinol (Fig. 1).

The system is designed to be placed infrarenally and is anchored in place by four pairs of nitinol hooks. The body of the device can be fully repositioned after it is unsheathed, to ensure optimal placement. Cannulation of the contralateral limb is achieved with the use of a unique magnet system.

The Anaconda system can be used in infrarenal aortic necks up to 31.5 mm diameter (max graft diameter is 34 mm) and in iliac arteries up to 17 mm diameter (flared legs up

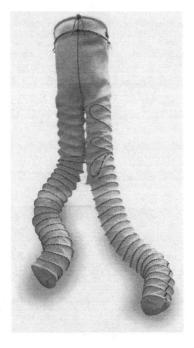

FIGURE 1   Anaconda™ stent graft.

to 21 mm in diameter). Neck angulations up to 60° can be treated and a study to evaluate the device in severely angled necks is planned. Delivery system uses 18 F internal diameter (ID) for bodies up to 24 mm diameter and 20 F ID for bigger bodies. Leg introducer system uses 18 F ID sheaths.

Potential advantages of the Anaconda system are the flexibility and ability to be repositioned, while a disadvantage is that not all legs fit all bodies. Additionally, very short clinical experience constitutes another current limitation, and no data regarding widespread use and long term durability are available. There are no published studies regarding this graft at the time of writing.

AneuRx™

The AneuRx stent-graft was initially designed by Dr. Thomas Fogarty and introduced in Europe in 1996 by Medtronic AVE, Santa Rosa, California, U.S.A (6). This graft received FDA approval in 1999. More than 40,000 implants worldwide have been performed.

AneuRx is a modular bifurcated endograft with two main self-expandable pieces, designed with a thin-walled noncrimped woven polyester fabric, fully supported by a nickel–titanium (nitinol) exoskeleton with diamond-shaped stent rings (Fig. 2).

There is no proximal bare stent, nor any hooks or barbs. Proximal fixation relies on the radial force provided by the self-expandable nitinol stent. Initially, the bifurcated endograft was too stiff. This was changed to a more flexible, segmented bifurcation graft after some aneurysm ruptures were reported in the U.S. FDA trial. AneuRx is available with aortic diameters from 20 to 28 mm and iliac leg diameters of 12 to 16 mm. The length of the primary access side is 16.5 cm and contralateral legs are available in lengths of 8.5 up to 11.5 cm. Aortic and iliac extenders are available in different diameters as well as an AUI convertor.

In November 2004 Medtronic introduced the Xcelerant delivery system. This new delivery system is more intuitive, and contributes to precise placement of the stent graft. The Xcelerant delivery system also employs kink-resistant catheter material, which serves to facilitate tractability of the stent graft through tortuous access vessels.

The most important advantage for AneuRx was the ease and simplicity to deploy. The stiffness is one of its major limitations as well as the lack of conformability in angulated necks. Migration has been described in the AneuRx (7) graft, but this endograft has a substantial literature base to support its clinical use.

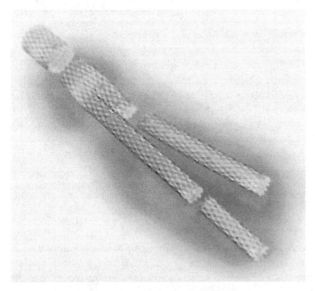

FIGURE 2 AneuRx™ device with some ancillary elements.

Aorfix™

Aorfix is the brand for two endograft products: bifurcated and uniiliac. Aorfix is manufactured by Lombard Medical, Oxfordshire, U.K. (8). Aorfix was conceived, specified and reviewed by Prof. Brian Hopkinson and was designed and developed by Dr. Peter Phillips and his team at Anson Medical.

Aorfix was first launched as an AUI device with a CE mark in 2001. The success of the design led directly to the Aorfix bifurcated device which was initially utilized in cases with very angulated aortic necks in situations where open surgery was not appropriate and where the clinicians concluded that no other implant would be effective.

Aorfix bifurcated device received its CE mark in November 2004 and conditional approval to start its U.S. Investigational Device Exemption (IDE) trial in November 2005.

Aorfix is designed as a modular bifurcated endograft with microfiber polyester graft fabric stitched under computer control to a nitinol interconnected hoop structure as exoskeleton (Fig. 3). Four pairs of hooks contribute to a fixation. Endograft aortic sizes range from 24 to 31 mm in steps of 1 mm with a recommended over sizing is 10%. Iliac sizes start in 10 mm up to 20 mm in steps of 2 mm. Distal ends are flared from a nominal diameter of 12 mm to the selected final diameter which extends for the last 20 mm of the device.

The major advantages are represented by the capability to treat angulated aortic necks and highly tortuous iliac arteries, and to treat a wider range of anatomy than any other single stent graft. In contrast, some disadvantages should be noted. The implantation technique may be difficult with respect to orientation of the graft and precise placement. Another major disadvantage is the lack of clinical data regarding short, mid or long term outcomes.

Apolo™

Apolo is manufactured by Nano Endomulinal, Brazil (9). This endograft is available in Brazil and in a few South American countries. CE mark and FDA approval remain pending. Apolo is a modular stent graft with an endoskeleton of nitinol and ultra thin wall-expanded polytetra-fluoroethylene (ePTFE) fabric (Fig. 4). Fixation is achieved by a transrenal bare stent and radial force. The attractive feature of this graft is the small caliber of its introducer system. Two-step delivery systems appear to be more accurate than other single staged systems.

Braile Stent-Graft

Braile Biomedica (10) is located in Sao Jose do Rio Preto in Sao Paulo, Brazil. This endograft has a modular design with z-stents of stainless steel covered with thin polyester (Fig. 5). Main body with two stumps is preloaded in an introducer sheath of 20 F outer diameter (OD). Iliac legs use a 17 F delivery system. The deployment is following a simple pullback movement. Fixation is allowed by a proximal bare stent and friction forces.

Ella Stent-Graft®

The Ella stent-graft is manufactured by Dr. Karel Volenec—ELLA—CS, Hradec Kralove, Czech Republic (11). Ella stent-graft is modular endograft, with Fer-X design in two types: Compact and Segmented. Fer-X Compact design has high longitudinal stability—especially for cases requiring a long stent graft, and Fer-X Segmented design has high flexibility—especially focused in cases with tortuous iliac arteries. Different shapes are available: tubular, conical, bifurcated, AUI, with aortic and iliac extenders (Fig. 6). A recent publication (12) demonstrates an acceptable six-year experience with this endograft.

EndoFit™

EndoFit stent graft system is a product of LeMaitre Vascular (Burlington, Massachusetts, U.S.A.). This graft was co-designed by Dr. Edward B. Diethrich and William Colone. At present time EndoFit is only available as AUI design with an occluder. The stent graft is built following an encapsulated nitinol z-stent frames between two ePTFE layers. A proximal bare stent is part of the fixation mechanism (Fig. 7). The delivery system uses an 18 to 20 F (OD) sheaths for 20 mm up

FIGURE 3 Aorfix™ stent graft.

FIGURE 4 Apolo™ endograft: (*left*) main body and ipsilateral leg and (*right*) contralateral leg.

FIGURE 5 Braile stent graft.

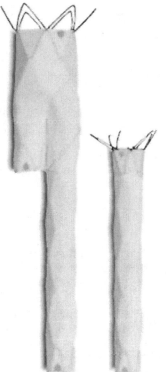

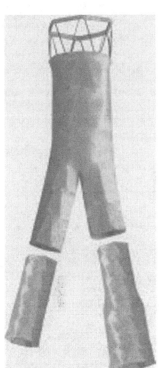

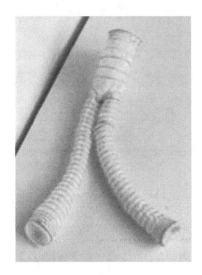

FIGURE 3

FIGURE 4

FIGURE 5

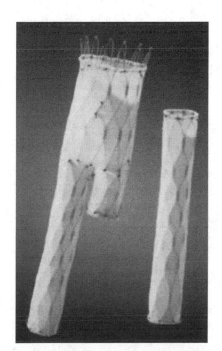

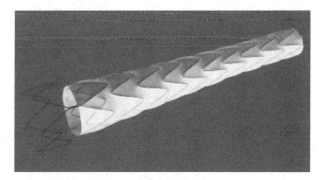

FIGURE 7

FIGURE 6

FIGURE 6 Ella stent graft®.

FIGURE 7 Endofit™ stent graft.

to 36 mm proximal diameter. Iliac diameters range from 20 mm down 12 mm. This device can be deployed in 90° angulated necks. Custom made diameters and lengths are part of its catalogue. The deployment system is a simple pullback movement. The system is limited by its uni-iliac design and little clinical information is available (13).

Fortron™

Fortron AAA stent-graft system is a product of Cordis Corporation (Warren, New Jersey, U.S.A.) (14). This endograft was originally designed by Dr. Michael L. Marin. CE-mark was obtained in August 2001. At present time this endograft is not available due to product withdrawal.

Fortron is a modular stent graft with three basic pieces. An endoskeleton with nitinol z-stent and low porosity seamless woven Dacron™ graft with multiple polyester point and blanket sutures. Multiple infrarenal barbs act as part of fixation system in addition to a proximal transrenal bare stent and friction (Fig. 8).

Gore Excluder®

Gore Excluder® endoprosthesis is a product of W.L. Gore & Associates, Inc. (Newark, Delaware, U.S.A.) (15). In 2002, this graft obtained the FDA approval. In 2004, a new low permeability material into the device design was integrated.

Gore Excluder is a modular stent graft configurated with an exoskeleton of nitinol and multilayer ePTFE graft material (Fig. 9). This device uses an active fixation mechanism with infrarenal anchors in addition to radial force and friction. The delivery system uses separate introducer sheaths. For aortic trunk up to 28 mm proximal diameter 18 F (ID) introducer system is recommended. For trunk with 31 mm proximal diameter a 20 F (ID) introducer is applied.

The maximum proximal diameter is 31 mm for the aorta and 20 mm for iliac limbs. Not more than 60° of aortic neck angulation is acceptable for this particular device. No AUI or convertor configurations are available.

The clearest advantages for Gore Excluder are the low profile of the delivery system, when considered without the sheath and its flexible design for tortuous anatomy. Also, the easy delivery system, just removing a suture line, is one of the most appreciable advantages, although there are some concerns as to how accurate deployment may be in angulated necks. In contrast, the lack of AUI design and bigger proximal diameters represent the major limitations of the current Gore Excluder endograft.

Many published papers are present in the medical literature in the last five years concerning the overall clinical outcomes and applications of Gore Excluder stent-graft (16–18).

PowerLink™

Powerlink system for AAA is a product of Endologix®, Irvine, California. This device was utilized in the first all Japanese patients AAA clinical study, and in Phase 1 FDA feasibility trials. Those early designs evolved into the current PowerLink™ System. The company conducted several studies in Europe and received CE Mark in March 2000. The company completed a FDA pivotal trial and obtained FDA marketing approval in October 2004.

Powerlink endograft has a bifurcated and unibody stent-graft using ePTFE. Cobalt chromium alloy stents are arranged as an endoskeleton. Powerlink endograft uses radial force to provide a proximal seal combined with column strength of the long main body to inhibit late migration by sitting near the anatomic bifurcation. Infrarenal and suprarenal configurations are available (Fig. 10).

Endograft diameters for aorta are 25, 28 and 34 mm (34 mm is in clinical trials in the U.S.). For iliac arteries, 16 and 20 mm endograft designs are available.

Two theoretical advantages should be mentioned: Powerlink represents a unique design of unibody device (long main body) allowing the stent graft to be deployed on the aortic bifurcation to reduce the possibility of late migration. The single wire stent construction and attachment of graft only at proximal and distal ends of stent cage allow graft material to "balloon" off of stent cage during cardiac cycle in order to reduce wear and fatigue on stent providing a very durable stent graft. To date there have been no reported stent fractures or graft failures. But at the same time some disadvantages are associated with this particular endograft. "Bottom-up" deployment from the bifurcation involves re-training versus typical stent graft planning and placement. In consequence, a longer learning curve is necessary. Proximal stent-graft extension is necessary with this deployment method so reducing the advantage of having a single body. Finally, the endoskeleton provides durability, but requires more caution when re-wiring through the endograft. From the literature it appears that mid-term results are acceptable (19).

SETA®

The System for Endovascular Treatment of Arteries (SETA) is a graft produced by Latecba, SA, Buenos Aires, Argentina. SETA has different models and designs (Fig. 11). The stents are balloon expandable and made of stainless steel, except both iliac stumps that are supported by nitinol self expandable stents. The graft is made of knitted polyester and the porosity ranges from 2000 to 4000 mL/cm^2/min. The fixation is transrenal due to plastic deformation of the stent and friction.

There are few morphological limitations to use as it can be use to treat aneurysms with short necks (close to 0 mm), angulations up to 90°, and 35 mm in diameter. No late leaks due to the balloon expandable proximal stent and the non stented body of the aortic trunk have been observed. However, the deployment method for the bifurcated model requires an additional access from the left subclavian artery. There are very little clinical data reported in the literature.

Talent™

Talent is a product manufactured by Medtronic Vascular (Santa Rosa, California, U.S.A.) (20). In 1998 Talent obtained the CE mark approval for AAA and AUI Flex-Tip™ delivery system. In 1999 Talent AAA and AUI CoilTract™ delivery system got the CE mark. Finally, AAA/AUI Xcelerant™ delivery system obtained its CE mark in 2004. Talent is a proven platform with more than 25,000 implants throughout the world.

Talent is a modular endograft with nitinol exoskeleton z-stents and low profile polyester graft material (Fig. 12). Fixation is ensured by a combination of actions from suprarenal bare springs, radial force and columnar strength provided by a longitudinal nitinol connecting bar. The endograft is preloaded in its delivery system using a 22 F (OD) introducer sheath for proximal graft diameter from 24 up to 28 mm and 24 F for proximal diameters between 30 and 36 mm. Contralateral limbs use 18 F (OD) for distal diameters between 8 and 20 mm and 20 F for 22 and 24 mm distal diameters.

The current platform has several advantages. The first is the possibility to treat a wide spectrum of AAA due to a large range of available sizes, different models and a high conformability (nitinol+spring design). Secondly, the high-performance of the Xcelerant delivery system with improved tracktability, smoother deployment, exceptional control, accuracy has widened indications. The large numbers of grafts implanted and the literature surrounding clinical practice appears (21) to indicate that this is a safe and durable graft when implanted for the correct indications.

Future directions are ongoing in Medtronic™ in order to improve the Talent platform. Greater flexibility in the device, smaller device profile, greater durability in device material and designs to treat short necks (<10 mm) are some of these goals.

VI AUF Stent Graft™

VI AUF stent graft and the VI EXTENDER CUFF™ are products of Vascular Innovation Co., Binzen, Germany, and are similar to many of the first "home-made" devices. The VI AUF stent graft is an unibody aorto-uni-femoral endograft with a balloon expandable Palmaz stent attached to a Vascutek ePTFE graft (Vascutek-Terumo, Inchinnan, Scotland, U.K.) with zero porosity (Fig. 13). Proximal fixation is provided by radial force and a suprarenal bare stent segment. Delivery system uses a 19.5 F (OD) introducer sheath. Endograft proximal diameter is 25 to 26 mm. Distal diameter of the graft is 8 mm and it is sewn to the femoral artery.

FIGURE 8   Fortron™ stent graft.

FIGURE 9   Gore Excluder™ and its ancillary components.

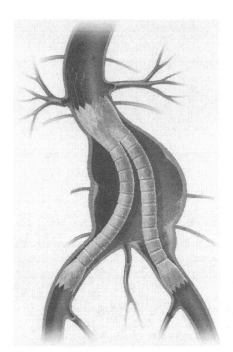

FIGURE 8

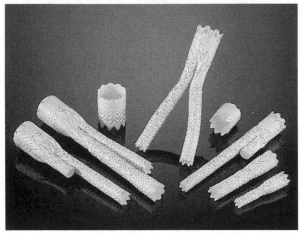

FIGURE 9

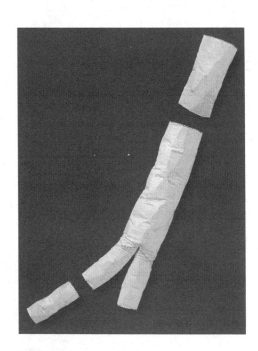

FIGURE 10

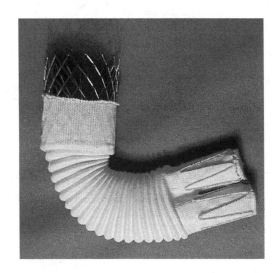

FIGURE 11

FIGURE 10   PowerLink™ endograft without proximal bare stent and with some ancillary elements.

FIGURE 11   SETA® graft from Argentina.

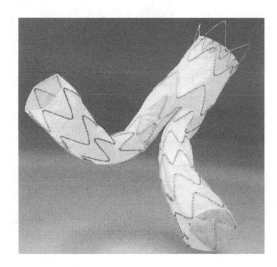

FIGURE 12 Talent™ stent graft.

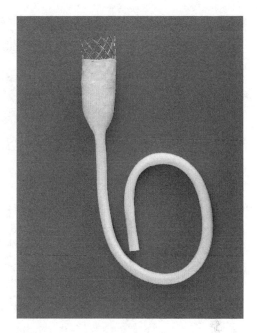

FIGURE 13 VI AUF™ stent graft.

This particular endograft can be useful for ruptured aneurysms, difficult anatomies and as a repair for some migrated endografts. Nevertheless, its major limitation is to have only a aorto-uni-femoral design with a proximal diameter up to 26 mm. Its use represents always a coverage of the ipsilateral internal iliac artery (22).

Zenith®

The Zenith endovascular graft with the H&L-B (Hartley and Lawrence-Brown) One-Shot® introduction system are products of Cook (Bloomington, Indiana, U.S.A.) (23). Today over 10,000 Zenith AAA Endovascular Graft have been implanted worldwide with promising results. CE-mark was accepted in September 1999 and FDA clearance was obtained in May 2003.

Zenith AAA endovascular graft is a bifurcated, modular system consisting of fully supported, self-expandable stainless steel z-stents (exoskeleton except for the proximal stent in the main body and proximal and distal stents for iliac legs) and standard thickness woven polyester graft material. The endovascular graft is a three-component device (an aortic main body and two iliac legs), the sizes of with can be selected to match a variety of patient anatomy and specific treatment goals. Proximal fixation is provided by transrenal bare stent with spikes and radial force in the infrarenal sealing stent (Fig. 14).

Zenith AAA endovascular graft is preloaded in the One-Shot introduction system with two sizes: 18 F (ID) for main bodies of 22, 24 and 26 mm and 20 F (ID) for 28, 30, 32, 34 and 36 mm. Iliac legs use 14 F (ID) for 8 up to 16 mm and 16 F (ID) from 18 up to 24 mm in diameter. The deployment system uses a staged method providing a very precise positioning and attachment.

Similar to the Talent graft the principle advantages are the ability to treat a wide spectrum of aneurysms and the extensive documentation of graft performance (24). One disadvantage is that the z-stent configuration some times does not conform well in tortuous iliac arteries and can lead to a kinking in the iliac graft.

DEVICE SPECIFIC OUTCOMES

In the absence of randomized trial data it is difficult to compare between devices. The problem is compounded by clinicians choosing different grafts for differing indications. Often, grafts

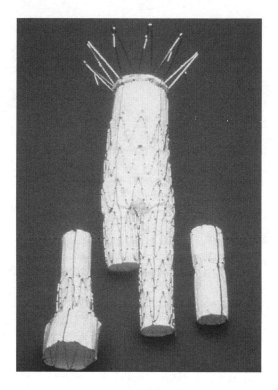

FIGURE 14 Zenith® endovascular graft and its components.

with suprarenal fixation are utilized for patients with challenging anatomy and grafts with infrarenal fixation are used for patients with easier proximal necks. Clearly, a comparison between supra and infrarenal fixation in these circumstances may be difficult (25).

Several publications have attempted to compare outcomes. Ouriel et al. presented data from a single center experience of 703 patients (26). Importantly, these authors demonstrated that aneurysm related death and freedom from rupture was similar for all devices analyzed. They reported that limb occlusion rates were higher in the ancure group and that the endoleak and sac expansion rate was highest in the excluder group.

A more recent publication for several centers has suggested that endoleak rate, principally related to Type II endoleaks, may be different at differing time points between devices. In this study, however, the rate of reintervention was similar for all groups (27).

The Eurostar registry recently published an analysis of 6787 patients with varying devices. The authors suggested that the first generation devices compared unfavorably with later designs in terms of aneurysm rupture and all cause mortality (16). The EVAR trial has collected data on device outcome and these are awaited.

ACKNOWLEDGMENTS

To all companies that contributed their information (Vascutek, Medtronic, Lombard Medical, Ella-CS, LeMaitre, Cordis, W.L. Gore & Associates, Endologix, Latecba, Vascular Innovations, and Cook).

REFERENCES

1. Balko A, Piasecki GJ, Shah DM, Carney WI, Hopkins RW, Jackson BT. Transfemoral placement of intraluminal polyurethane prosthesis for abdominal aortic aneurysm. J Surg Res 1986; 40(4):305–9.
2. Palmaz JC, Sibbitt RR, Reuter SR, Tio FO, Rice WJ. Expandable intraluminal graft: a preliminary study. Work in progress. Radiology 1985; 156(1):73–7.

3. Volodos' NL, Karpovich IP, Shekhanin VE, Troian VI, Iakovenko LF. A case of distant transfemoral endoprosthesis of the thoracic artery using a self-fixing synthetic prosthesis in traumatic aneurysm. Grudn Khir 1988; 6:84–6.
4. Parodi JC, Palmaz JC, Barone HD. Transfemoral intraluminal graft implantation for abdominal aortic aneurysms. Ann Vasc Surg 1991; 5(6):491–9.
5. www.vascutek.com
6. www.medtronic.com
7. Conners MS, III, Sternbergh WC, III, Carter G, Tonnessen BH, Yoselevitz M, Money SR. Endograft migration one to four years after endovascular abdominal aortic aneurysm repair with the AneuRx device: a cautionary note. J Vasc Surg 2002; 36(3):476–84.
8. www.lombardmedical.com
9. www.nano.com.br
10. www.braile.com.br
11. www.ellacs.cz
12. Kocher M, Utikal P, Koutna J, et al. Endovascular treatment of abdominal aortic aneurysms—6 years of experience with Ella stent-graft system. Eur J Radiol 2004; 51(2):181–8.
13. Saratzis N, Melas N, Lazaridis J, et al. Endovascular AAA repair with the aortomonoiliac EndoFit stent-graft: two years' experience. J Endovasc Ther 2005; 12(3):280–7.
14. www.cordis.com
15. www.goremedical.com
16. van Marrewijk CJ, Leurs LJ, Vallabhaneni SR, Harris PL, Buth J, Laheij RJ. Risk-adjusted outcome analysis of endovascular abdominal aortic aneurysm repair in a large population: how do stent-grafts compare? J Endovasc Ther 2005; 12(4):417–29.
17. Kibbe MR, Matsumura JS. The Gore Excluder U.S. multi-center trial: analysis of adverse events at 2 years. Semin Vasc Surg 2003; 16(2):144–50.
18. Kong LS, MacMillan D, Kasirajan K, et al. Secondary conversion of the Gore Excluder to operative abdominal aortic aneurysm repair. J Vasc Surg 2005; 42(4):631–8.
19. Albertini JN, Lahlou Z, Magnan PE, Branchereau A. Endovascular repair of abdominal aortic aneurysms with a unibody stent-graft: 3-year results of the French Powerlink Multicenter Trial. J Endovasc Ther 2005; 12(6):629–37.
20. www.medtronic.com
21. Espinosa G, Ribeiro M, Riguetti C, Caramalho MF, Mendes WD, Santos SR. Six-year experience with talent stent-graft repair of abdominal aortic aneurysms. J Endovasc Ther 2005; 12(1):35–45.
22. Malas MB, Ohki T, Veith FJ, et al. Absence of proximal neck dilatation and graft migration after endovascular aneurysm repair with balloon-expandable stent-based endografts. J Vasc Surg 2005; 42(4):639–44.
23. www.zenithstentgraft.com
24. Greenberg RK, Chuter TA, Sternbergh WC, III, Fearnot NE. Zenith AAA endovascular graft: intermediate-term results of the U.S. multicenter trial. J Vasc Surg 2004; 39(6):1209–18.
25. Nevelsteen A, Maleux G. Endovascular abdominal aortic aneurysm treatment: device-specific outcomes. J Cardiovasc Surg (Torino) 2004; 45(4):307–19.
26. Ouriel K, Clair DG, Greenberg RK, et al. Endovascular repair of abdominal aortic aneurysms: device-specific outcome. J Vasc Surg 2003; 37(5):991–8.
27. Sheehan MK, Ouriel K, Greenberg R, et al. Are type II endoleaks after endovascular aneurysm repair endograft dependent? J Vasc Surg 2006; 43(4):657–61.

34 | Endovascular Aneurysm Repair (EVAR) Lessons from the Registries

Peter Harris
University of Liverpool, Liverpool, U.K.

INTRODUCTION

In order to gain acceptance in clinical practice today all new technologies, therapeutic devices, drugs, operations and interventional procedures must pass through a number of phases of evaluation to establish their safety and efficacy. Although cumbersome, this process makes sense not only in the interests of patient safety but also to ensure proper use of limited heathcare resources. The different phases of evaluation generate standards of proof that correspond approximately to the well-known and accepted Levels of Scientific Evidence (1). This is a hierarchical system with anecdotal case reports at the bottom of the scale and meta-analysis of randomized trials at the top. While clinical scientists naturally aspire to the highest standards of proof, it is self-evident that this cannot often be achieved in one step from the inception of a new therapeutic concept. Progression from one phase to the next, starting at the bottom is the logical way to proceed.

Randomized controlled trials (RCTs) represent the final, most definitive and most expensive phase in the process of clinical evaluation. Increasingly RCTs seem to be regarded as an absolute prerequisite for acceptance of a new therapy, drug or device as a valid clinical tool. But, launching into randomized trials without having determined beforehand that the performance of the new treatment is similar to that of the established treatment would be illogical and irresponsibly wasteful. Furthermore, there is an ethical requirement that clinicians who involve their patients in an RCT must be in equipoise in respect of the efficacy of the treatments being compared.

A properly organized registry is a powerful tool for the evaluation of a new clinical technology, and an essential stepping-stone towards the attainment of an appropriate standard of proof of efficacy. Whilst RCTs, provide no more than a "snapshot" of the comparative value of two or more treatment options at one point in time, registries are able to track the benefits and disadvantages of new iterations of an evolving technology over a long period.

The progressive and ongoing modification of the design of aortic endografts is an excellent example of this type of evolution. Stringent, independent monitoring of this process is essential, primarily in the interests of patient safety. This chapter will describe how these diverse functions of registries have been applied specifically in the case of endovascular aneurysm repair (EVAR) and the lessons that have been learned. There are a number of national registries including the Registry for Endovascular treatment of Aneurysms in the U.K. In this chapter data will be drawn exclusively from the pan-European European Collaborators on Stent-graft Techniques for Aortic Aneurysm Repair (EUROSTAR) registry.

THE EUROSTAR REGISTRY

The EUROSTAR Registry was established in 1996, shortly after the first commercial stent/graft for abdominal aortic aneurysm (AAA) repair became available. All commercial endografts introduced subsequently have been included in the registry. In 2003, data relating to early generations of device, with demonstrably flawed designs or engineering, were excluded from the aggregated database. The database was continually updated on-line and

TABLE 1 The Make and Number of Commercial Endografts
Included in the Aggregated EUROSTAR Abdominal Aortic
Aneurysm Registry in January 2006

Endograft	Number of patients
Anaconda	53
AneuRx	983
Endologix	156
Ancure	73
Excluder	1105
Fortron	91
Lifepath	134
Talent	2220
Zenith	3114

published in a paper report twice yearly. Reports on the aggregated database were freely available to anyone while contributors and commercial companies had privileged access to center and device-specific data, respectively. In December 2005, 10 years after its inception the EUROSTAR project was discontinued. Data are no longer available on-line, but the database continues to be the source of papers in peer-reviewed journals and other publications.

EUROSTAR was a voluntary registry and was therefore subject to the potential disadvantage of selective case reporting. To counter this risk there is now a requirement for patients to be registered in advance of the intervention. Submission of data to the registry is open to all vascular units throughout greater Europe, not just the European Union. However, continued membership of the project is subject to compliance with minimal standards of performance in terms of data submission. In order to preserve the quality and credibility of the database, it has been necessary to enforce this condition from time to time by deleting all data from centers that have consistently failed to submit follow-up data.

Between January 1996 and December 2005 more than 10,000 patients in total were registered but, with the exclusion in 2003 of data on early generations of stent/grafts a total of 7968 patients treated in 177 centers were included in the aggregated AAA database. Table 1 shows the number of each make of commercial endograft included in the current abdominal registry.

LESSONS LEARNED FROM THE EUROSTAR REGISTRY

EVAR Is a Safe Procedure

This was apparent from analyses of the earliest data, which showed 30-day mortality rates consistently less than 4% overall and less than 2% for American Society of Anesthesiologists (ASA) one and two categories of patients. The definitive analysis included a 30-day mortality rate for all patients of 2.4% and an early conversion rate of 0.9%. Nonfatal systemic complications were encountered in 11% of patients, renal and pulmonary being most common. Device-related complications including graft migration and thrombosis and secondary interventions were reported in 2.6% and access-site complications in 6%. Thirty-percent of the procedures were carried out under either regional or local anesthesia. Eighty eight operations were carried as day-case procedures but the mean duration of hospital stay was 5.9 days.

Type 2 Endoleaks Are Benign

Type 2 endoleaks were detected on completion angiography in 10% of the patients registered with EUROSTAR. This compares to 4% of patients with Type 1 endoleaks and 2% with Type 3 endoleaks. Invariably steps are taken to resolve Types 1 and 3 endoleaks at the primary

TABLE 2 Statistically Significant Risk Factors for Late Rupture Following Endovascular Aneurysm Repair Identified in a Univariate Analysis Model (EUROSTAR Data)

Risk factor	Hazard ratio	P value
Age	1.11	0.009
Preop diam AAA	1.056	0.0001
Last diam AAA	1.056	0.001
↑ diam AAA	1.099	0.0004
Any endoleak	3.435	0.0056
Prox Type 1 endoleak	3.998	0.0266
Midgraft Type 3 endoleak	5.999	0.0001
Migration	7.49	0.0001

Abbreviation: AAA, abdominal aortic aneurysm.

procedure but Type 2 endoleaks are very rarely treated. Justification for this policy is supported by EUROSTAR data, which demonstrate that Types 1 and 3 endoleaks are associated with a significant risk of postoperative rupture and aneurysm-related death, whereas Type 2 endoleaks are not (Table 2) (2). More than half of Type 2 endoleaks detected on completion angiography resolve spontaneously within three years. Generally those that do not connect relatively wide inflow and outflow channels with high volume and velocity flow. The majority of EUROSTAR clinicians intervene secondarily to treat Type 2 endoleak only if there is continued expansion of the aneurysm—"endotension." This policy seems reasonable although there is no clear evidence in support of it from the EUROSTAR registry or any other source. Reports of isolated Type 2 endoleak being responsible for late rupture of the aneurysm are rare anecdotes.

Migration Is the Principal Cause of Late Failure

The first generations of commercial endografts were associated with an unacceptably high rate of late failure. In 2000, EUROSTAR reported a cumulative rupture rate of 12.44% six years after treatment. The devices included in this study were mainly Stentor (Mintec) and Vanguard (Boston Scientific) endografts (3). These devices were withdrawn from the market long ago but the data acquired by EUROSTAR provided an invaluable insight into the failure modes of aortic endografts and enabled a detailed analysis of the critical risk factors associated with late rupture (3). Although Type 1 endoleak was associated with rupture in a univariate analysis model (Table 2) it did not feature when the data were subjected to multivariate analysis (Table 3). Three factors only were found to be independently associated with rupture, large aneurysm diameter, Type 3 endoleak and migration (Table 3). Of these only Type 3 endoleak and migration were clinically important, the risk ratios being 7.5 and 5.3, respectively. These data provide a clear indication that Type 1 endoleaks invariably occur secondarily to migration. Some Type 3 endoleaks were also secondary to migration in the form of separation of component parts of modular devices, while others were due to breaches of structural integrity due to fabric wear or metal fatigue. These findings have played an important role in informing the continued evolution of endograft design and construction. More recent evidence from EUROSTAR has confirmed that the performance of modern endografts is significantly superior to that of earlier iterations (4).

TABLE 3 Statistically Significant Risk Factors for Late Rupture Following Endovascular Aneurysm Repair Identified in a Multivariate Analysis Model (EUROSTAR Data)

Risk factor	Hazard ratio	P value
Last diam AAA	1.057	0.0028
Midgraft Type 3 endoleak	7.474	0.0024
Migration	5.335	0.0156

Abbreviation: AAA, abdominal aortic aneurysm.

Early Detection of Migration and Structural Deformity of the Endograft Are the Main Priorities for Postprocedural Surveillance

In the early days, postoperative surveillance was directed mainly toward the identification of endoleaks. However, the EUROSTAR data described above show that the only endoleaks that matter, Types 1 and 3, are late precursors of impending rupture. Anecdotal experience suggests that the onset of a new endoleak, especially proximal Type 1 endoleak, may be followed very rapidly by rupture of the aneurysm. For this reason, reliance upon endoleak to indicate the need for secondary intervention is unsafe. It follows that postprocedural surveillance should be focused mainly upon detection of migration and evidence of impending or actual structural failure of the device in order to identify the patient at risk. Changes in aneurysm morphology may be relevant also; an aneurysm that continues to expand being cause for concern while reassurance may be derived from evidence of the sac shrinking. Although intuitive there is little or no objective evidence to support a policy of secondary intervention for continued expansion of the aneurysm sac as an isolated finding. Analysis of EUROSTAR data shows a weak but statistically significant association between the risk of rupture and both the original and last measured size of the aneurysm but no association with continued expansion.

Revision of the priorities for postoperative surveillance has led to changes in the modalities used and the frequency of examination. Although computed tomography (CT) scanning probably remains the "gold standard," a standardized procedure for plain X ray provides excellent information about migration and stent deformation. Changes in the size of the aneurysm can be monitored with ultrasound scans. Therefore, CT scans are unnecessary for routine surveillance and should be reserved for further detailed investigation of patients in whom there is a suspicion of adverse change. In this way the radiation dose to the patient and the cost to the health-care system of EVAR can be reduced significantly without detriment in terms of quality of care. Unfortunately, currently there is no adequate alternative to CT for follow up of patients after thoracic EVAR.

The Rate of Secondary Interventions After EVAR Is Reducing

The rate of secondary intervention after endovascular the AAA repair is falling (Fig. 1) (4). There are two reasons for this. First, modern endografts are constructed from more durable materials than earlier iterations of these devices and they are better engineered to resist migration. Most secondary interventions today are transfemoral endovascular procedures. Kinking, stenosis or thrombosis of a limb of the endograft are the most common indications, complications of this type being observed in approximately 2% of EUROSTAR patients each year. Conversions still occur but at a low rate of approximately 0.5% per year. The second

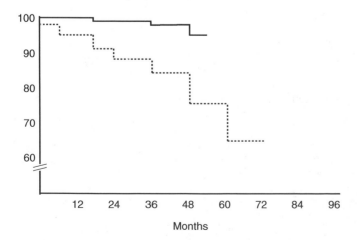

FIGURE 1 Kaplan-Meier plots comparing the risks of secondary intervention associated with early (*dotted line*) and later (*solid line*) generations of abdominal aortic endografts (EUROSTAR data).

reason for the falling rate of secondary intervention is better understanding of what constitute appropriate indications. Recognition of the benign nature of Type 2 endoleaks means that they are rarely considered to be an indication for secondary treatment. The accepted exception to the policy of watchful waiting is progressive expansion of the aneurysm sac and Type 2 endoleak as the only identifiable cause. But, even here evidence to support secondary intervention is lacking.

A significant obstacle to the wider dissemination of EVAR is its cost relative to the established alternatives. Progressive reduction in the rate of secondary intervention will impact significantly upon cost-efficiency and the acceptability of this treatment to cash-limited health-care systems around the world.

All Currently Available Stent Grafts Have Strengths and Weaknesses and None Are Superior in All Clinical Performance Indicators

In 2005, EUROSTAR published a comparison of the performance of different commercial makes of stent grafts for endovascular repair of AAAs (5). The data were risk adjusted to account for differences in aneurysm morphology, patient characteristics and postoperative events. Although statistically significant differences between stent grafts were identified no single device was found to be superior to the others in respect of all of the events analyzed. Each device was found to have strengths and weaknesses. For example, Zenith (Cook) stent grafts are highly resistant to migration but more prone to kinking and occlusion of the limbs of the device compared to other makes. Statistically significant differences between the devices are listed in Table 4.

TABLE 4 Stastically Different Unadjusted Hazard Ratios of Outcome Events among Current Makes of Aortic Endografts

	AneuRx		**Excluder**		**Talent**	
AneuRx						
Excluder	T2-endo	0.61 (0.5–0.8)				
	Migration	3.59 (1.9–6.9)				
	Occlusion	2.23 (1.1–4.5)				
	Conversion	2.62 (1.2–5.6)				
	Secondary intervention	2.10 (1.4–3.1)				
	Death	1.64 (1.2–2.3)				
Talent	Growth	0.68 (0.5–1.0)	T2-endo	1.98 (1.5–2.6)		
	Shrinkage	0.75 (0.6–0.9)	Shrinkage	0.68 (0.6–0.8)		
	Migration	1.71 (1.2–2.4)	Migration	0.48 (0.2–0.9)		
			Occlusion	0.44 (0.2–0.9)		
			Conversion	0.39 (0.2–0.8)		
			Secondary intervention	0.51 (0.3–0.7)		
			Death	0.64 (0.5–0.9)		
Zenith	T1/3-endo	1.44 (1.1–1.9)	T2-endo	1.37 (1.1–1.8)	T1/3-endo	1.64 (1.3–2.1)
	Shrinkage	0.66 (0.6–0.8)	Shrinkage	0.60 (0.5–0.7)	T2-endo	0.70 (0.5–0.9)
	Migration	6.18 (3.6–10.6)	Occlusion	0.29 (0.2–0.6)	Shrinkage	0.88 (0.8–1.0)
	Occlusion	0.65 (0.4–1.0)	Secondary intervention	0.65 (0.4–1.0)	Migration	3.61 (2.1–6.4)
	Conversion secondary intervention	3.60 (2.0–6.6)	Death	0.62 (0.4–0.9)	Occlusion	0.67 (0.5–1.0)
	Death	1.37 (1.1–1.8)			Conversion secondary intervention	3.50 (1.9–6.3)
					Death	1.29 (1.0–1.6)

Example: patients with an AneuRx stent graft have a 39% ($= 1 - 0.61$) decreased risk of Type 2 endoleak, and a 3.59 times increased risk of migration compared to patients with an Excluder.

The Future of EVAR Registries

Following publication of the results of randomized trials, which have confirmed the clinical efficacy of EVAR, at least in relatively "good risk" patients (6,7), enthusiasm for registries in this area has declined. EUROSTAR experienced a dramatic reduction in the number of new patients being registered following publication of the results of these trials. Is this appropriate? We do seem to have reached a plateau as far as the evolution in the design of endografts is concerned and there is perhaps little value in adding more of the same data to an already very large database. However, the present apparent stalling of the basic technology is likely to be temporary. New concepts and materials may be just around the next corner and we need to have the tools available to assess them. More immediate is the need to continue to monitor new and evolving applications of the established technologies, fenestrated and branched endografts for treatment of juxta-renal and thoraco-AAAs and the challenges of aortic arch disease are good examples. EUROSTAR was conceived as a 10-year project and was discontinued as planned after this period of time had elapsed having achieved all of its primary objectives. The clear and obvious need for continuing data collection for the purposes of audit and quality control is a matter primarily for locally-based initiatives supported by national registries rather than for an international study group.

ACKNOWLEDGMENTS

The author acknowledges gratefully the vascular surgeons and radiologists throughout Europe who have contributed data to the EUROSTAR registry, members of the EUROSTAR International Advisory Board, the EUROSTAR Data Managers and the Executive Director of the EUROSTAR Data Registry Centre in Eindhoven, The Netherlands, Dr Jacob Buth.

REFERENCES

1. Sackett DL. Rules of evidence and clinical recommendations on use of thrombotic agents. Chest 1986; 89(Suppl. 2):2S–3.
2. van Marrewijk C, Buth J, Harris PL, Norgren L, Nevelsteen A, Wyatt MG. Significance of endoleaks after endovascular repair of abdominal aortic aneurysms: the EUROSTAR experience. J Vasc Surg 2002; 35:461–73.
3. Harris PL, Vallabhaneni SR, Desgranges P, Becquemin JP, van Marrewijk CJ, Laheijh RJ. Incidence and risk factors of late rupture, conversion and death after endovascular repairof infrarenal aortic aneurysms: the EUROSTAR experience. J Vasc Surg 2000; 32:739–49.
4. Torrela F for the EUROSTAR collaborators. Effect of improved endograft design on outcome of endovascular aneurysm repair. J Vasc Surg 2004; 40:216–21.
5. van Marrewijk CJ, Leurs LJ, Vallabhaneni SR, et al. Risk-adjusted outcome analysis of endovascular abdominal aortic aneurysm repair in a large population: how do stent-grafts compare? J Endovasc Ther 2005; 12:417–29.
6. EVAR trial participants. Endovascular aneurysm repair versus open repair in patients with abdominal aortic aneurysm (EVAR 1 trial): randomised controlled trial. Lancet 2005; 365:2179–86.
7. Blankensteijn JD, de Jong SE, Prinssen M, et al. Two-year outcomes after conventional or endovascular repair of abdominal aortic aneurysms. N Engl J Med 2005; 352:2398–405.

35 | Trials Comparing Endovascular Abdominal Aortic Aneurysm Repair with Open Surgical Repair or Conservative Management (Design, Results, and Future Work)

Janet T. Powell
Department of Vascular Surgery, Imperial College at Charing Cross, London, U.K.

INTRODUCTION

Vascular surgery is becoming dominated by and changing through the introduction of new technologies. What evidence is needed before a new technology can be recommended for routine clinical practice? The best level of evidence (level 1) is obtained from randomized clinical trials. These may take several years to establish the trial, recruit the patients and then follow them up for several years to establish whether the new technologies can provide durable results, equivalent to, or better than, the previous gold standard. Since the time from idea of the trial to results can be five years or more, such trials are best conducted early when the technology is satisfactory, but before the technology has stabilized.

RANDOMIZED TRIALS

For abdominal aortic aneurysm (AAA), the gold standard treatment has been open surgical repair which is associated with significant operative (30 days) mortality. Despite improvements in anesthetic technique and postoperative care, the operative mortality remains high, up to 8% in population series (1). Endovascular aneurysm repair (EVAR) was first reported over 15 years ago (2,3). However, it took 10 years for the first randomized trials to start, the EVAR trials, which started recruiting in 1999 (4). These trials were rapidly followed by the Dutch Randomised Endovascular Aneurysm Management (DREAM) trial in the Netherlands and Belgium (5), the anticoagulation in cardioversion using enoxaparin (ACE) trial in France and the open versus endovascular repair (OVER) trial in the Veterans Administration hospitals of the U.S.A. (6,7). The outline characteristics of these trials are shown in Table 1.

DESIGN

The basic design of the EVAR-1 and the other three trials outside of the U.K. was to randomize patients after their infrarenal aneurysm had been deemed to have morphology suitable for EVAR and the patients were considered fit enough to undergo open surgery (Fig. 1). None of the trials had the resources to carefully document the outcome of all the patients who were unsuitable for endovascular repair. Although some of the trials will provide an indication of the proportion of patients with large AAA considered suitable for endovascular repair, such figures are only rough indicators. Therefore the generalizability of the findings is uncertain, although as endograft technology continues to develop a greater proportion of patients are likely to be suitable for endovascular repair. Similarly, only a single trial (EVAR-1) documented the patients considered unfit for open repair. Fitness criteria are likely to be different across the four trials and some patients considered fit for open surgery in one country might not be considered fit for open surgery in another country. None of the trials are prescriptive in respect of fitness indicators, although some trials provided guidelines.

TABLE 1   The Four Randomized Trials for Comparison of Endovascular Aneurysm Repair Versus the Gold Standard of Open Repair in Patients with Large Aneurysms, Fit for Either Procedure

Trial	Abdominal aortic aneurysm diameter for entry (cm)	Recruitment target (actual)	Primary endpoint	Reporting
EVAR-1, U.K.	5.5	900 (1082) closed	Mortality	30-day 2004 4-year 2005
DREAM, The Netherlands and Belgium	5	400 (351) closed	30-day mortality	2004 2-year 2005
ACE, France	5	600 (~300)	Mortality and complications	2007 ?
OVER, U.S.A.	5.5	900 (~700)	Mortality	2008–2009

Abbreviations: ACE, Anticoagulation in Cardioversion Using Enoxaparin; DREAM, Dutch Randomised Endovascular Aneurysm Management; EVAR-1, Endovascular Aneurysm Repair-1; OVER, Open Versus Endovascular Repair.

The fit patients suitable for endovascular repair were randomized to receive either traditional open surgical repair or endovascular repair, using the endograft of choice at the participating center. All the trials focused on large AAA, although the entry diameter criterion varied across the trials (Table 1). The primary outcome measure also varied across the four trials and accounts for the very different sample sizes planned in the different trials (Table 1). Nevertheless it is likely that data from the separate trials can be pooled for meta-analyses of postoperative and long-term mortality. Each trial also has several secondary endpoints, including quality of life, costs, and cost-effectiveness. There has been no attempt used to standardize the quality of life assessments used in the different trials and it is likely to be impossible to synthesize such data in a meta-analysis. Already the DREAM trial has suggested that quality of life short-form (SF-36) at one year is better in patients randomized to open repair, whereas this was not evident from EuroQuol evaluations in the EVAR-1 trial (8,9).

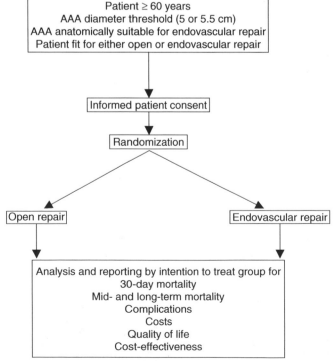

FIGURE 1   Basic design of all the trials listed in Table 1.

Although endovascular repair initially was mooted for patients considered unfit for open surgical repair of AAA, only the EVAR-2 trial has put this possibility to the rigorous test of a randomized controlled trial. Patients considered unfit for open surgery with aneurysm morphology suitable for endovascular repair were randomized to either early endovascular repair or no intervention (Fig. 1). It is important to stress that patients entered into the EVAR-2 trial were considered unfit for open surgery at the time of randomization and as such were very different from the high risk patient series published from the United States, where patients are fit for open repair (10,11). Being unfit at the time of randomization does not necessarily mean that fitness cannot be improved and this could lead, at a much later date, to patients crossing over from the no intervention allocated to endovascular repair. Application of a risk scoring system to the patients in the EVAR-1 and EVAR-2 trials showed that the mean "unfitness" score [Customized Probability Index (12)] was three times higher in EVAR-2 patients than EVAR-1 patients, confirming the appropriate allocation of patients between these two trials.

RESULTS

For patients considered fit for open surgery, both the EVAR-1 and DREAM trials have reported 30-day operative mortality, with analysis by intention to treat (13,14). In the EVAR-1 trial there was a threefold reduction in 30-day mortality, from 4.6% for open repair to 1.6% for endovascular repair, $p < 0.001$. The smaller DREAM trial was underpowered and showed similar 30-day mortalities of 4.8% for open repair and 1.5% for endovascular repair, $p = 0.09$. Even before the OVER and ACE trials report, there appears to be a clear early advantage to endovascular repair.

Longer-term follow up has been reported, to four years for the EVAR-1 trial and to two years for DREAM (9,15). Both trials show that after two years, there was no difference in all-cause mortality between patients randomized to endovascular repair and those to open repair. In the DREAM trial the two-year survival was 89.6% and 89.7% for open and endovascular repair groups, respectively. In the EVAR-1 trial the two-year survival was similar and the four-year survival was approximately 72% in both open and endovascular groups.

Longer-term aneurysm-related mortality was assessed in both trials. At the midterm there continued to be an approximately twofold reduction in aneurysm-related mortality in the endovascular repair groups, but this difference was attributable principally to the difference in 30-day mortality. For the patient and his or her family, the actual cause of death may be less important than good quality of life gained. The early advantage of endovascular repair cannot be disputed.

The reasons why the early advantage of endovascular repair is not sustained are not entirely clear. Although both trials reported a significant number of reinterventions in the endovascular groups over this time period, this was rarely associated with mortality. There appear to be an increased number of deaths from cardiovascular causes in the endovascular groups compared to the open repair groups in the time period between 30 days and two years. It has been hypothesized that there is considerable occult cardiac disease in the AAA patients and whereas the greater stress of open versus endovascular surgery causes mortality within 30 days for open repair, these deaths occur later in the endovascular groups. In other words, the stress of open surgery precipitates a death waiting to happen and there is a rapid "catch up" in the endovascular group. However, the absolute number of deaths involved is small and there may be other explanations for the catch up mortality in the endovascular group.

The results of the EVAR-1 and DREAM trials have allowed the calculation of cost-effectiveness. The Belgian authorities have already decided that endovascular repair is not cost-effective (16). Modeling studies conducted by both EVAR-1 and DREAM trialists also are likely to show that, with current pricing of endografts, current complication rates and the require-ment for long-term surveillance, endovascular repair is unlikely to be cost-effective. In this context, the results of the OVER trial with more recent graft technology will be important. If reinterventions and surveillance after endovascular repair can be minimized, endovascular repair may become cost-effective in the future.

Despite the differences between these trials of EVAR in patients fit for either procedure, there is consensus in the results to date. With vascular interventionists the results are not controversial: the controversies will arise if more funding agencies adopt the Belgian attitude, reserving endovascular repair for research funded studies only.

The results of the EVAR-2 trial are controversial. The trial was established to show the benefit of endovascular repair versus no intervention in this group of patients with numerous and severe comorbidities: their four-year survival was only 36% (17). However the 30-day mortality rate in the endovascular repair group was 9%, similar to the rupture rate in the no intervention group. Therefore, there at four years there was no difference in either all-cause mortality or aneurysm-related mortality between the randomized groups. Neither was there any significant difference in quality of life between the two randomized groups at one year (17). On the basis of these results, the only level of (level 1) evidence available, endovascular repair cannot be recommended in such patients.

It is true that some 20% of the no intervention group eventually underwent aneurysm repair, with relatively good results. There is circumstantial evidence that many of this group who breached protocol had been treated to reduce cardiac morbidities before aneurysm repair, for instance time elapsed since myocardial infarction, arrhythmias controlled and blocked coronary arteries stented or bypassed. Anesthetists had reassessed these patients as fit for open repair and some of them actually had open repair. To assess the impact of these crossovers, per protocol analysis was conducted, but this too failed to show any advantage for early endovascular repair. These findings have been very unpopular in the U.S.A. and other quarters. Although others have attempted to show the good results of endovascular repair in high risk patients, patients unfit for repair and those who die from aneurysm rupture before being treated are ignored (10,11). The index for these series is aneurysm repair (treatment received) versus the index of randomization (intention to treat) in the trials. Further, the high risk patients evaluated in the U.S.A. have four-year survival of 60% or more, very different from the 36% four-year survival in the EVAR-2 trial.

FUTURE WORK

The issue of greatest concern to most practicing clinicians and future patients is whether the regulatory authorities, in Europe and beyond, will approve endovascular grafts for routine clinical practice; in many cases this means proving the cost-effectiveness of endovascular repair. Both the EVAR-1 and DREAM trials are continuing to follow up the randomized patients, so that actual long-term data will supplant modeling for cost-effectiveness evaluations in about five years.

The second major issue relates to patient fitness. In editorial comment which accompanied the midterm results of the EVAR-1 and EVAR-2 trials, Cronenwett published a format for when to choose open or endovascular repair based on patient fitness and morphological suitability for endovascular repair (18). The latter criterion is being extended all the time, through fenestrated and branched grafts that can be used in patients without a clearly defined and suitable aneurysm neck. In the guidelines proposed by Cronenwett, open repair would remain the treatment of choice for younger, fitter patients. Evidence, based on the EVAR-1 trial, was presented first at the Society of Vascular Surgery meeting (June 2006, Philadelphia, U.S.A.), to suggest the converse, the fittest patients benefit most by endovascular repair (19). These issues remain to be teased out, by development of a robust fitness scoring system that can be applied to both trial and single series center patient data. Several fitness scoring systems have been published. Currently only the Glasgow Aneurysm Score has been evaluated for EVAR (20). Other scoring systems, such as the revised Goldman index focus on cardiac events and do not perform well for open aneurysm repair (21). The Customized Probability Index has been developed for vascular surgery and takes account of recent knowledge about the perioperative benefits of statins and beta-blockers in high risk patients (12). The development of a robust scoring system to predict both short and long-term mortality is likely to require collaboration between the different trials, so that a scoring system developed from one trial can be validated in a second trial, before being applied to single center data sets.

Robust scoring systems for fitness also would help settle the debate as to when a high risk patient becomes too unfit, or has too high a comorbidity burden, to consider endovascular repair. It is interesting that even in the context of large AAAs, there appears to be time to improve patient fitness because the risk of aneurysm rupture appears to be reduced in patients with clearly defined aneurysm necks. The annual risk of rupture in the EVAR-2 trial was only 9%, whereas we had expected rates much closer to 20% based on previously published series (17,22). Therefore, within the EVAR-2 trial there is important work to be done identifying risk factors for aneurysm rupture as well as using the computed tomography data to evaluate detailed stress/strain relationships in large aneurysms.

In his editorial, Cronenwett also identified a middle ground, where patient preference would dominate the decision for either open or endovascular repair (18). We know nothing of patient preference and how the weight of continued surveillance and high risk of further interventions after endovascular repair impacts on their lives. Generic quality of life questionnaires would not be sufficiently sensitive to identify such issues. For these reasons research into patient preference has commenced and results should be available to feed into final decisions concerning cost-effectiveness in about five years time. Other areas of future work from the existing trials include the comparison of different grafts, for instance Zenith versus Talent in EVAR-1, with outcomes that include mortality, endoleaks, and reinterventions (23).

Others are revisiting the scenario of small AAAs, questioning whether early endovascular repair would be better than surveillance. Two such trials have started, both company sponsored, one in Europe (24) and one in the U.S.A. Both trials are scheduled to be smaller than the previous small aneurysm trials, which is one of the reasons why they may not provide convincing results. Another important reason is the still unrecognized burden of cardiovascular disease in these patients, leading to a heightened risk of cardiovascular death. In the small aneurysm trials about one-fourth of patients never required surgery, either because their aneurysm diameter did not increase or they died of another cause before the aneurysm reached the threshold diameter of 5.5 cm. With endovascular repair costing at least 25% more than open repair, the decision to sanction surgery on all small AAAs from publicly funded health care economies would be in serious doubt.

There also are unanswered questions that the trials will not be able to address. These include questions about generalizability, maintaining competence and training in open repair, the role of endovascular repair at the time of rupture and issues of gender and ethnicity. The rapid pace of technology in the medical device arena will impact upon these unknowns. The introduction of fenestrated and branched grafts may improve generalizability (proportion of patients suitable for endovascular repair), training and assessments of competence may place increasing reliance on simulators. Above all, the unanswered question of durability of endografts may not be answered by long-term follow up for any of the trials, since at the time of such analyses, much newer generation devices will be on the market place and the results from earlier versions of endografts may not be applicable.

REFERENCES

1. Blankensteijn JD. Mortality and morbidity rates after conventional abdominal aortic aneurysm repair. Semin Interv Cardiol 2000; 5:7–13.
2. Volodos NL, Shekhanin VE, Karpovich IP, Troian VI, Gur'ev IuA. A self-fixing synthetic blood vessel endoprosthesis. Vestn Khir Im I I Grek 1986; 137:123–5.
3. Parodi JC, Palma JC, Barone HD. Transfermoral intraluminal graft implantation for abdominal aortic aneurysm. Ann Vasc Surg 1991; 5:491–7.
4. Brown LC, Epstein D, Manca A, Beard JD, Powell JT, Greenhalgh RM. The U.K. EndoVascular Aneurysm Repair (EVAR) trials: design, methodology and progress. Eur J Vasc Endovasc Surg 2004; 27:372–81.
5. Prinssen M, Buskens E, Blankensteijn JD. The Dutch Randomised Endovascular Aneurysm Management (DREAM) trial. Background, design, methods. J Cardiovasc Surg 2002; 43:379–84.
6. Becquemin J. ACE trial: elective abdominal aortic aneurysm—open versus endovascular repair. NCT 00224718. Creteil, France: Hopital Henri Mondor, 2005 (http://clinicaltrials.gov).
7. Lederle F. CSP#498: Open versus endovascular repair (OVER) trial for abdominal aortic aneurysms. Minneapolis: West Haven Cooperative Studies Program Coordinating Center, 2005. (http://clinicaltrials.gov)

8. Prinssen M, Buskens E, Blankensteijn JD, DREAM Trial Participants. Quality of life after endovascular and open AAA repair. Results of a randomised trial. Eur J Vasc Endovasc Surg 2002; 27:121–7.
9. EVAR Trial Participants. Endovascular aneurysm repair versus open repair in patients with abdominal aortic aneurysm (EVAR trial 1): randomised controlled trial. Lancet 2005; 365:2179–86.
10. Sicard GA, Zwolak RM, Sidawy AN, White RA, Siami FS. Endovascular abdominal aortic aneurysm repair: long-term outcome measures in patients at high-risk for open surgery. J Vasc Surg 2006; 44:229–36 (E-pub April 27).
11. Bush RL, Hedayati N, Johnson ML, et al. Performance of endovascular aortic aneurysm repair in high-risk patients: results from the VA National Surgical Quality Improvement Program. J Vasc Surg 2007; 45:227–33.
12. Kertai MD, Boersma E, Klein J, van Urk H, Poldermans D. Optimizing the prediction of perioperative mortality in vascular surgery by using a customized probability model. Arch Int Med 2005; 165:898–904.
13. EVAR Trial Participants. Comparison of endovascular aneurysm repair with open repair in patients with abdominal aortic aneurysm (EVAR trial 1), 30-day operative mortality results: randomised controlled trial. Lancet 2004; 364:843–8.
14. Prinssen M, Verhoeven EL, Buth J, et al. A randomised trial comparing conventional and endovascular repair of abdominal aortic aneurysms. New Engl J Med 2004; 351:1607–18.
15. Blankensteijn JD, de Jong S, Prinssen M, van der Ham A. Two year outcomes after conventional or endovascular repair of abdominal aortic aneurysms. New Engl J Med 2005; 352:2398–405.
16. Bonneux L, Cleemput I, Vrijeng F. HTA endovasculaire behandeling van het AAA: KCE reports Volume 23A. Brussel: Federaal Kenniscentrum vor Gezondheidszorg, 2005.
17. EVAR Trial Participants. Endovascular aneurysm repair and outcome in patients unfit for open repair of abdominal aortic aneurysm (EVAR trial 2): randomised controlled trial. Lancet 2005; 365:2187–92.
18. Cronenwett JL. Endovascular aneurysm repair: important mid-term results. Lancet 2005; 365:2156–8.
19. EVAR Trial Participants. Patient fitness and survival after abdominal aortic aneurysm repair in patients from the UK EVAR trials. Br J Surg 2007; 94:709–16.
20. Biancari F, Hobo R, Juvonen T. Glasgow aneurysm score predicts survival after endovascular stenting of abdominal aortic aneurysm in patients from the EUROSTAR registry. Br J Surg 2006; 93:191–4.
21. Lee TH, Marcantonio ER, Mangione CM, et al. Derivation and prospective validation of a simple index for prediction of cardiac risk of major noncardiac surgery. Circulation 1999; 100:1043–9.
22. Lederle FA, Johnson GR, Wilson SE, et al. Rupture rate of large abdominal aortic aneurysms in patients refusing or unfit for elective repair. JAMA 2002; 287:2968–72.
23. EVAR Trial Participants. Secondary interventions and mortality following endovascular aortic aneurysm repair: device-specific results from the UK EVAR trials. Eur J Vasc Endovasc Surg 2007; (September; accessed online June 2007).
24. Cao P, CAESAR Trial Collaborators. Comparison of surveillance vs Aortic Endografting for Small Aneurysm Repair (CAESAR) trial: study design and progress. Eur J Vasc Endovasc Surg 2005; 30:245–51.

36 | Outcomes After Endovascular Abdominal Aortic Aneurysm Repair

Harjeet S. Rayt, Robert D. Sayers, and Matthew J. Bown
Department of Cardiovascular Sciences, University of Leicester, Vascular Surgery Research Group, Leicester Royal Infirmary, Leicester, U.K.

INTRODUCTION

Since the introduction of endovascular abdominal aortic aneurysm ($\Lambda\Lambda\Lambda$) repair endovascular aneurysm repair (EVAR) by Parodi (1) in 1991, this technique has continued to gain popularity and widespread acceptance by the vascular surgical community. This has mainly been due to the accepted perioperative benefits of elective EVAR on morbidity and mortality. This chapter presents the results of elective EVAR in terms of perioperative mortality and longer-term mortality and morbidity rates.

PERIOPERATIVE MORTALITY

Perioperative mortality has been assessed principally by two large randomized trials comparing EVAR and open AAA repair, the EVAR (2) and Dutch Randomized Endovascular Aneurysm Management (DREAM) (3) trials, several data registries and a single meta-analysis of observational studies (4).

EVAR-1 and EVAR-2 Trials

The EVAR-1 and EVAR-2 trials were setup in 1999 to assess the safety and efficacy of EVAR against best current treatment for large (≥ 5.5-cm diameter) AAA. Both were multicenterd randomized controlled trials across 41 suitable U.K. centers. Suitability of centers was assessed after they had performed at least 20 EVAR procedures and data had been sent to the Registry of Endovascular Treatment of Aneurysms (5). The EVAR-1 trial compared EVAR and open AAA repair in patients considered fit for open repair of their AAA. EVAR-2 compared EVAR with best medical therapy against best medical therapy alone in patients considered unfit for open repair (6). Patient recruitment occurred between 1999 and 2003. Male and female patients aged 60 and over with a documented AAA of at least 5.5-cm diameter on computed tomography scan were assessed for anatomical suitability for EVAR. Such patients were offered entry into EVAR-1 if considered fit for an open repair or EVAR-2 if considered unfit.

The EVAR-1 trial initial results showed significantly lower 30-day mortality in the EVAR group compared to the open group (1.7% vs. 4.7%; $p=0.009$) (2). The in-hospital mortality rate followed a similar trend, with deaths from EVAR being almost a third lower (2.1% vs. 6.2%; $p=0.001$). Other early results from the trial showed a lower median length of hospital stay with EVAR (7 vs. 12 days; $p<0.001$); and lower median length of operation (180 vs. 200 minutes; $p<0.001$). The trial also reported secondary interventions either during the 30-day postoperative period or during the primary admission, whichever was longer. EVAR had a significantly higher rate of reintervention when compared to open repair (9.8% vs. 5.8%; $p=0.025$).

The EVAR-2 trial was much smaller than EVAR-1. EVAR-1 recruited a total of 1082 patients prior to randomization whilst EVAR-2 consisted of a total of only 338 patients. From this; 166 were randomized to EVAR and 172 were offered best medical therapy. The main differences between patients in EVAR-2 and EVAR-1 were a high rate of symptomatic cardiac disease (~70%), a lower mean forced expiratory volume at one second (1.7 L), higher rates of diabetes mellitus (14% of patients) and a higher mean creatinine concentration of 110 µmol/L (7). The 30-day operative mortality from elective EVAR in EVAR-2 was 7%, considerably higher than that seen in the EVAR-1 trial (1.7%), however many participants crossed from the best medical therapy to surgery arms of the trial and many deaths occurred in those patients awaiting surgery.

DREAM Trial

The DREAM trial recruited patients from 28 centers in The Netherlands and Belgium who had at least a 5-cm diameter AAA and were suitable for elective repair via open or endovascular techniques (3,8). Three hundred and forty-five patients between November 2000 and December 2003 were randomly assigned to either repair by endovascular (171 patients) or open (174 patients) methods.

The operative mortality from open repair was 4.6% and 1.2% in the endovascular group. The rates of mortality and severe complications combined were 9.8% in the open group and 4.7% in the EVAR group. However, neither finding was statistically significant ($p=0.1$). When considering complications alone, it was found that there were less systemic and local complications in the endovascular group. Moderate and severe systemic complications were seen in 26.4% of open repairs but only for 11.7% in the endovascular group ($p<0.001$). In the open group the majority of these were pulmonary complications and in the endovascular group cardiac problems were more prevalent. The DREAM trial also demonstrated a significant ($p=0.001$) reduction in mean duration of surgery (151 vs. 135 minutes), mean estimated blood loss (1654 vs. 394 mL), hospital stay and intensive care utilization.

The authors of the DREAM trial concluded that endovascular repair was preferable to open repair in patients with an AAA that was at least 5-cm diameter. Unfortunately, the data presented in their results does not support these claims. Firstly, the authors state that due to time restrictions, their study was 12% underpowered, which automatically has implications on any results obtained. Secondly, results given for operative mortality do not show any statistically significant difference.

Registry Data

The EUROSTAR (European Collaborators on Stent/Graft Techniques for Aortic Aneurysm Repair) Registry was setup in 1996 with a view to collate data on results of endovascular AAA repair. One hundred and thirty-five centers in 18 different European countries contributed data to the EUROSTAR Registry. By July 2003, 5466 patients had been registered into the trial although since then 1224 of these patients have been excluded from analysis as they were fitted with early generation grafts that are now no longer in production (Ancure, Stentor, Vanguard) (9). Results from the EUROSTAR Registry published in 2000 considered 2464 patients. The 30-day mortality rate quoted was 3.2% with death rates from all cause mortality occurring in 5.5% in the first four years (10).

The Lifeline Registry of EVAR was established in the United States of America in 1998 with the purpose of evaluating long term outcomes of infrarenal EVAR (11). Data was collected from five endodovascular stent-graft manufacturers in the U.S.A. that had been approved by the Food and Drug Administration (FDA) since 1999. A total of 2998 patients were considered in the study, of which only 334 had open repair of their AAA. Patients undergoing EVAR had more comorbidities than those having open repair. EVAR patients were on average three years older, and had more coronary heart disease and congestive heart failure (all p values <0.01). The open repair cohort also had significantly more women (21% vs. 13%; $p<0.01$) (12). The results showed no significant 30-day operative mortality between EVAR and open repair (1.7% vs. 1.4%; $p=0.72$). Furthermore, they concluded that 80% of AAA related deaths occurred within the initial 30-day period in EVAR patients. There were a further 11 deaths up to six years. The open repair group was only followed up for one year, but only four deaths were seen within the first 30 days of the operation.

Although the authors of the reports from the Lifeline Registry conclude that EVAR is a safe and effective treatment for selected patients with infrarenal AAA, it must be remembered that this is not a randomized control trial. Data has been collated retrospectively from manufacturers' records. The authors touch upon the problems of combining data which has not been recorded uniformly in the first instance. For example, definitions of endpoints vary among all manufacturers. The authors use it to their advantage in that the two cohorts were different, stating that this enhances the argument for EVAR, as the mortality rates between the two groups are not significant. It must also be noted that while the results are encouraging, the mortality rates from open repair (1.4%) are much lower than the mortality rates for open repair seen in other large trials (5.8% U.K. small aneurysm trial, 4.7% Canadian Aneurysm Study (13,14) and 4.7% EVAR-1).

The Lifeline Registry included data regarding patients who had been implanted with the Ancure, AneuRx, Excluder, Powerlink and Zenith grafts. Of these five, the Ancure and AneuRx grafts have already come under criticism (15,16).

Meta-Analysis

Aside from the studies discussed above there are in excess of 800 electronically identifiable studies that pertain to EVAR. The most recent meta-analysis of the outcome of EVAR by Franks et al. (4) has compiled all of the relevant data from the world literature on EVAR. A similar meta-analysis was performed by Drury et al. (17) previously but since the study by Franks et al. draws data from all of the papers assimilated in the earlier study and also includes more recent literature only the results of the most recent study (4) are presented below. This systematic review found 161 articles pertaining to 28,862 patients that were suitable for a meta-analysis. Articles were included in the analysis if they gave details of the outcome of patients undergoing elective EVAR. All reports of patients with ruptured or symptomatic AAA were excluded. There was an overall operative mortality of 3.3% (95% confidence interval 2.9–3.6%). This figure is higher than those found in other studies (3,18,19) but the reports included in the meta-analysis included those from the early development of EVAR when both techniques and grafts were new and clinicians were inexperienced.

One of the most interesting techniques used in this meta-analysis was the application of meta-regression. This enables factors that are associated with changes in the outcome measures of a meta-analysis to be determined. On a simplified basis this involves comparing an outcome measure against other variables (such as time or average age of patients in the study), then fitting a linear regression model to the data but weighting studies to have a larger influence in the regression depending on their size (actually the inverse of the variance of the outcome variable being examined for each individual study). When operative mortality was examined in this fashion it was found that the most significant factor that affected outcome was the date when the study was performed ($p < 0.001$) This demonstrated there had been a steady decrease in operative mortality over time (Fig. 1) and was the first study to show an improvement in the results of EVAR since the procedure had been introduced in 1991.

LONG-TERM OUTCOME

Data regarding the short-term results of EVAR are relatively abundant in the literature, however because of the relatively recent introduction of the procedure and ongoing developments of techniques and devices, assessment of longer-term outcome is more difficult. The majority of reliable data is drawn from the same studies that detail accurate short-term outcomes.

Mortality

In the EVAR-1 trial four-year results show little difference in all cause mortality (28%) between the EVAR and open groups, but do demonstrate a lower rate of aneurysm related mortality in the EVAR group (4% vs. 7%; $p = 0.04$) (19). In the EVAR-2 trial at four years projected mortality

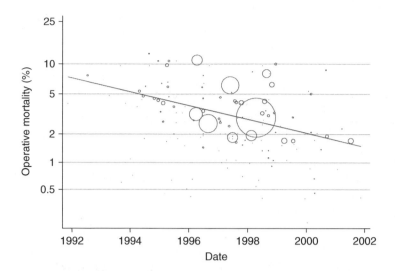

FIGURE 1   Meta-regression analysis of reported EVAR mortality rate over time. Circles represent individual studies; the size of the circle is proportional to the influence of each study in the meta-analysis. *Source*: From Ref. 4.

was 64% of the total participants, with no difference in all cause mortality or aneurysm related mortality between the two groups (7).

The Lifeline study did not show any significant difference in all cause survival between the two groups up to four years.

Morbidity

In the EVAR-1 trial at four years post randomization, 41% of patients in the EVAR group had postoperative complications, of which Type 2 endoleak was the most common (79%). This compares poorly with the 9% rate of postoperative complications at four years in the open repair group. The number of patients with at least one reintervention at four years was 20% in the EVAR group and only 6% in the open repair group although many of the secondary interventions in the EVAR were trans-femoral catheter related procedures. Interestingly, of the 81 patients that required a reintervention, almost a quarter of these (23%) were during the primary hospital admission.

Long-term analysis of the EVAR-2 trial found that 43% of EVAR patients had suffered at least one postoperative complication at the end of four years, with more than a quarter (26%) needing reintervention. This compares with only 18% of the no intervention group having postoperative complications (because of the crossover of those randomized to best medical therapy eventually undergoing EVAR and the use of intention to treat analysis) of which 4% required further treatment. In the EVAR group, endoleaks constituted the majority of post-operative problems (55%), with Type 2 endoleaks predominating (53%).

In the reports from the registries, the Eurostar collaborators published in 2006 a secondary intervention rate of 8.7% at a mean time of 12 ±13 months post surgery. This was higher amongst patients treated for larger aneurysms (≥5.5-cm diameter) at the two-year time point (9.9% vs. 7.1%) (20). In the Lifeline registry of the 487 patients in the EVAR group 18.2% required secondary intervention, of which only a small minority (15%) occurred after the immediate postoperative period. Unfortunately no further data was recorded regarding the interventions.

Systemic Complications

Major concerns after open AAA repair focus on cardiorespiratory complications and major organ dysfunction/failure. In this respect, EVAR offers many potential benefits such as avoidance of laparotomy and aortic cross clamping, absence of bowel manipulation and cooling, reduced postoperative pain, ileus, blood and fluid loss. Elkouri et al. (21) reported cardiac complications in 11% of EVAR patients compared to 22% in open repair. Similarly there was a lower rate of respiratory complication with EVAR compared to open repair (3% vs. 16%).

Despite these advantages, many people develop an unexplained pyrexia and leucocytosis after successful EVAR (22). This is thought to be due to thrombosis of the contents of the excluded aneurysm sac which causes release of inflammatory mediators into the systemic circulation. However, it is known that less inflammatory mediators are produced after EVAR than after open repair, especially Interleukin-6 (IL-6) (23–26). Other factors such as C-reactive protein, endotoxin and IL-1 receptor antagonist levels have all been shown to be less post EVAR repair (27–30). EVAR has also been associated with other beneficial physiological responses such as reduced complement activation (29,31), reduced adrenaline and cortisol production (32) and reduced intestinal ischemia (26,30).

Local Complications

Endoleaks

Endoleaks (33) refer to the persistent perfusion of the aneurysm sac after EVAR and affects 15% to 21% of patients (34–41). Endoleak rates range from 7% to 22% at one month postprocedure depending on the type of graft used. This figure stays constant when looking at midterm data with leak rates in the proportion of 7% to 20% at one to two years (42). Although it is useful to have a generalized view of endoleaks, the clinical outcome can vary immensely amongst the different types.

Types 1 and 3 endoleaks are usually grouped together when considering clinical outcomes and management because they both lead to persistent blood flow into the aneurysm sac at high pressure, leading to rapid aneurysm expansion and potential rupture. Type 1 or Type 3 endoleaks occur in 7% to 16% of patients at one year post EVAR. The EUROSTAR collaborators have identified several predictors of Type 1/3 endoleak including large preoperative aneurysms, large diameter aneurysm neck, severe angulation of the proximal neck and less intra-sac thrombus. Different stents also appear to be associated with different leak rates. The Stentor (27%), Endovascular Technologies (EVT)/Ancure (24%), and Vanguard (15%) stents have higher rates of Type 1/3 endoleaks when compared to the Talent (10%), AneuRx (7%), Excluder (6%) and Zenith (6%) devices (43).

Although there have been cases of rupture following Type 2 endoleaks post EVAR, they are not classed with the same severity as their Type 1/3 counterparts. This is mainly because Type 2 endoleaks are low pressure leaks caused by retrograde flow into the aneurysm sac from branching vessels. Zarins et al. estimated the incidence of Type 2 endoleaks following EVAR to be 10% to 20% (42). whilst the meta-analysis by Drury et al. found a rate of 10.3% at one year after surgery (17).

In the meta-analysis performed by Franks et al. (4) the overall endoleak rate was 22.8% (95% confidence interval 20.6–25.2%), with 10.5% of these being Type 1. Meta regression analysis demonstrated that endoleak rates have also been reducing in frequency over time (Fig. 2). This represents a fall in endoleak rates from 43% in 1992 to 13.5% in 2002.

Migration

Distal movement of the graft within the aortic sac due to continuous downward displacement forces from pulsatile blood flow is another complication seen with EVAR. Migration of the stent can lead to a Type 1 endoleak, therefore predisposing the patient to aneurysm rupture. There have been similar rates of migration with all FDA approved endovascular devices of 2% at one year. The AneuRx clinical trial has reported stent graft migration rates of 8.4% at a mean time post EVAR of 30 ± 11 months. Furthermore, Kaplan–Meier analysis for freedom from migration was 99% at one year, 93% at two years and 81% at three years.

Stent-Graft Fatigue

Stent graft fatigue is defined as "an actual change in the mechanical nature of the device, such as suture disruption, metal fracture or fabric erosion," and can lead to a wide range of problems

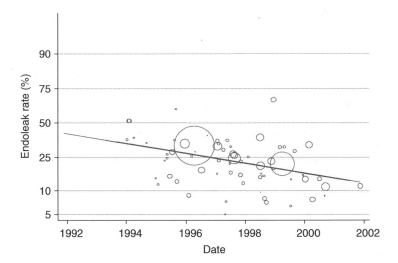

FIGURE 2 Meta-regression analysis of reported post EVAR annual endoleak rates over time. Circles represent individual studies; the size of the circle is proportional to the influence of each study in the meta-analysis. *Source*: From Ref. 4.

including endoleaks, migration, aneurysm sac expansion and rupture (44). Much of the literature in this area is device specific. Zarins et al. studied 120 explanted AneuRx stents and concluded that migration was associated with more stent strut fractures and that suture breaks were seen in most of the devices. Despite this, there was no relationship between device failures and clinical outcomes (45).

Jacobs et al. reviewed EVAR data from 686 patients over a 10-year period and found that 60 patients (15%) had stent graft fatigue with an average time to fatigue of 19 months. Of these 60, 43 had metallic stent fractures (72%); 14 had suture-stent disruptions (23%); and three had graft holes (5%). Stress fatigue and metallic corrosion have been postulated as causes for metallic stent fractures. Breakdown of the fabric is thought to be due to the micromotion of the bare metal stent against the fabric (44).

Graft Limb Occlusion

The incidence of graft limb occlusion following an open repair is approximately 2% (46). A recent study by Cochennec et al. found that 7.2% of patients suffered from occluded endovascular grafts between 0 and 71 months (one or both limbs); with an average time to occlusion of 9.5 months. This accounted for occlusion in 4.3% of all the limbs (36 occlusions in 829 limbs) (47). Although this figure seems very high, it is not representative of other studies. Erzurum et al. identified a patient incidence of endograft limb occlusion of 2.67%, with a median time of 34.9 days to occlusion, after considering 823 EVAR procedures over a seven-year period (48).

In a review of the ANCURE stent, Parent et al. found an occlusion rate of 10.4% (7 patients of 67) (49). Although it is easy to say that the rates of endograft limb occlusion are higher than open repair, one must also bear in mind that much of the data available on this topic is limited to smaller studies.

Graft Infection

As with open repair, infection of endovascular stent grafts can be devastating. Since Chalmers et al. (50) reported the first case of stent graft infection in 1993; there have been a multitude of case reports on the topic (51,52). A review conducted by Ducasse et al., demonstrated a mean frequency of infection of 0.43% (53). This value compares well with the accepted rates of infection for prosthetic grafts used in open repair (0.5–3%) (54) and contradicts experimental data showing that endovascular devices present lower bacterial resistance and greater infectivity. However, the low rates at present could be due to the lack of long term follow-up data for EVAR patients. Interestingly, the authors also commented on the fact that 62.5% of the stent graft infections occurred in patients treated in interventional radiology suites, compared to 37.5% of infections occurring after EVAR in an operating theater.

Wound Infection

Access to the aorta is usually achieved via the transfemoral route using a groin incision. Although actual wound infection is low (2%), seroma formation occurs in approximately 15% of patients. Fortunately, no further treatment is required and these seromas resolve within the first six months of surgery. The large sheaths used in EVAR when compared to angiography also predispose to false aneurysm formation (55).

Hip and Buttock Claudication

This is commonly seen after EVAR and is due to occlusion of one or both internal iliac arteries. On deploying the stent, these may unintentionally be covered or alternatively coil embolization of the internal iliac artery is also carried out preoperatively in patients with an AAA and unilateral or bilateral aneurysms of common iliac arteries to allow the stent to be landed in the external iliac without a Type 2 endoleak from the internal iliac artery. Hip and buttock claudication after this procedure occurs in 26% to 41% of patients (56–61).

SUMMARY

EVAR remains a new technology that is under constant development. There are clear advantages in perioperative outcome that are partially offset by the relatively high long-term complications of the procedure. More recently evidence has come to light that outcomes are improving with time (4) and if this continues into the future it could be expected that better patient selection, device design and clinician experience should reduce the long-term complications of EVAR that prevent its widespread application.

REFERENCES

1. Parodi JC, Palmaz JC, Barone HD. Transfemoral intraluminal graft implantation for abdominal aortic aneurysms. Ann Vasc Surg 1991; 5(6):491–9.
2. The EVAR Trial Participants. Comparison of endovascular aneurysm repair with open repair in patients with abdominal aortic aneurysm (EVAR trial 1), 30-day operative mortality results: randomised controlled trial. Lancet 2004; 364:843–8.
3. Prinssen M, Verhoeven EL, Buth J, et al. A randomized trial comparing conventional and endovascular repair of abdominal aortic aneurysms. N Engl J Med 2004; 351(16):1607–18.
4. Franks SC, Sutton AJ, Bown MJ, Sayers RD. Systematic review and meta-analysis of 12 years of endovascular abdominal aortic aneurysm repair. Eur J Vasc Endovasc Surg 2007; 33(2):154–71.
5. Thomas SM, Gaines PA, Beard JD, Vascular Surgical Society of Great Britain and Ireland, British Society of Interventional Radiology. Short-term (30-day) outcome of endovascular treatment of abdominal aortic aneurism: results from the prospective Registry of Endovascular Treatment of Abdominal Aortic Aneurism (RETA). Eur J Vasc Endovasc Surg 2001; 21(1):57–64 (see comment).
6. Brown LC, Epstein D, Manca A, Beard JD, Powell JT, Greenhalgh RM. Endovascular Aneurysm Repair (EVAR) trials: design, methodology and progress. Eur J Vasc Endovasc Surg 2004; 27(4):372–81.
7. The EVAR Trial Participants. Endovascular aneurysm repair and outcome in patients unfit for open repair of abdominal aortic aneurysm (EVAR trial 2): randomised controlled trial. Lancet 2005; 365(9478):2187–92.
8. Prinssen M, Buskens E, Blankensteijn JD. The Dutch Randomised Endovascular Aneurysm Management (DREAM) trial. Background, design and methods. J Cardiovasc Surg 2002; 43(3):379–84.
9. EUROSTAR Registry. (Accessed April 6, 2007 at https://nancy.kikamedical.com/eurostar/kika/eventa/eurostar/pdf/aaa_2004.pdf)
10. Harris PL, Vallabhaneni SR, Desgranges P, Becquemin JP, van Marrewijk C, Laheij RJ. Incidence and risk factors of late rupture, conversion, and death after endovascular repair of infrarenal aortic aneurysms: the EUROSTAR experience. European Collaborators on Stent/graft techniques for aortic aneurysm repair. J Vasc Surg 2000; 32(4):739–49.
11. Lifeline Registry of Endovascular Aneurysm Repair Steering Committee. Lifeline registry: collaborative evaluation of endovascular aneurysm repair. J Vasc Surg 2001; 34(6):1139–46.

12. Registry TL. Lifeline registry of endovascular aneurysm repair: long-term primary outcome measures. J Vasc Surg 2005; 42(1):1–10.
13. Johnston KW. Nonruptured abdominal aortic aneurysm: six-year follow-up results from the multi-center prospective Canadian aneurysm study. Canadian Society for Vascular Surgery Aneurysm Study Group. J Vasc Surg 1994; 20(2):163–70.
14. Johnston KW, Scobie TK. Multicenter prospective study of nonruptured abdominal aortic aneurysms. I. Population and operative management. J Vasc Surg 1988; 7(1):69–81.
15. May J, White GH, Yu W, Sieunarine K. Importance of plain x-ray in endoluminal aortic graft surveillance. Eur J Vasc Endovasc Surg 1997; 13(2):202–6.
16. Guidant. (Accessed April 7, 2007 at http://www.ashcraftandgerel.com/ancure.html)
17. Drury D, Michaels JA, Jones L, Ayiku L. Systematic review of recent evidence for the safety and efficacy of elective endovascular repair in the management of infrarenal abdominal aortic aneurysm. Br J Surg 2005; 92(8):937–46.
18. White GH, Yu W, May J, Chaufour X, Stephen MS. Endoleak as a complication of endoluminal grafting of abdominal aortic aneurysms: classification, incidence, diagnosis, and management. J Endovasc Surg 1997; 4(2):152–68.
19. The EVAR Trial Participants. Endovascular aneurysm repair versus open repair in patients with abdominal aortic aneurysm (EVAR trial 1): randomised controlled trial. Lancet 2005; 365(9478):2179–86.
20. Hobo R, Buth J. Secondary interventions following endovascular abdominal aortic aneurysm repair using current endografts. A EUROSTAR report. J Vasc Surg 2006; 43(5):896–902.
21. Elkouri S, Gloviczki P, McKusick MA, et al. Perioperative complications and early outcome after endovascular and open surgical repair of abdominal aortic aneurysms. J Vasc Surg 2004; 39(3):497–505.
22. Velazquez OC, Carpenter JP, Baum RA, et al. Perigraft air, fever, and leukocytosis after endovascular repair of abdominal aortic aneurysms. Am J Surg 1999; 178(3):185–9.
23. Bolke E, Jehle PM, Storck M, et al. Endovascular stent-graft placement versus conventional open surgery in infrarenal aortic aneurysm: a prospective study on acute phase response and clinical outcome. Clinica Chimica Acta 2001; 314(1–2):203–7.
24. Rowlands TE, Homer-Vanniasinkam S. Pro- and anti-inflammatory cytokine release in open versus endovascular repair of abdominal aortic aneurysm. Br J Surg 2001; 88(10):1335–40.
25. Burger T, Heucke A, Halloul Z, et al. Interleukin pattern, procalcitonin level and cellular immune status after endovascular aneurysm surgery. Zentralblatt fur Chirurgie 2000; 125(1):15–21.
26. Syk I, Andreasson A, Truedsson L, Risberg B. Postoperative downregulation of MHC class II antigen on monocytes does not differ between open and endovascular repair of aortic aneurysms. Eur J Surg 1999; 165(11):1035–42.
27. Odegard A, Lundbom J, Myhre HO, et al. The inflammatory response following treatment of abdominal aortic aneurysms: a comparison between open surgery and endovascular repair. Eur J Vasc Endovasc Surg 2000; 19(5):536–44.
28. Boyle JR, Goodall S, Thompson JP, Bell PR, Thompson MM. Endovascular AAA repair attenuates the inflammatory and renal responses associated with conventional surgery. J Endovasc Ther 2000; 7(5):359–71 (see comment).
29. Swartbol P, Norgren L, Albrechtsson U, et al. Biological responses differ considerably between endovascular and conventional aortic aneurysm surgery. Eur J Vasc Endovasc Surg 1996; 12(1):18–25.
30. Elmarasy NM, Soong CV, Walker SR, et al. Sigmoid ischemia and the inflammatory response following endovascular abdominal aortic aneurysm repair. J Endovasc Ther 2000; 7(1):21–30.
31. Galle C, De Maertelaer V, Motte S, et al. Early inflammatory response after elective abdominal aortic aneurysm repair: a comparison between endovascular procedure and conventional surgery. J Vasc Surg 2000; 32(2):234–46.
32. Salartash K, Sternbergh WC, III, York JW, Money SR. Comparison of open transabdominal AAA repair with endovascular AAA repair in reduction of postoperative stress response. Ann Vasc Surg 2001; 15(1):53–9.
33. White GH, Yu W, May J. Endoleak—a proposed new terminology to describe incomplete aneurysm exclusion by an endoluminal graft. J Endovasc Surg 1996; 3(1):124–5.
34. Zarins CK, White RA, Moll FL, et al. The AneuRx stent graft: four-year results and worldwide experience 2000. J Vasc Surg 2001; 33(2 Suppl.):S135–45 (erratum appears in J Vasc Surg 2001; 33(6):1318).
35. Faries PL, Brener BJ, Connelly TL, et al. A multicenter experience with the talent endovascular graft for the treatment of abdominal aortic aneurysms. J Vasc Surg 2002; 35(6):1123–8.
36. Makaroun MS, Deaton DH. Is proximal aortic neck dilatation after endovascular aneurysm exclusion a cause for concern? J Vasc Surg 2001; 33(2 Suppl.):S39–45.
37. Zarins CK, White RA, Schwarten D, et al. AneuRx stent graft versus open surgical repair of abdominal aortic aneurysms: multicenter prospective clinical trial. J Vasc Surg 1999; 29(2):292–305 (see comment; discussion 306–8).

38. Greenberg RK, Lawrence-Brown M, Bhandari G, et al. An update of the Zenith endovascular graft for abdominal aortic aneurysms: initial implantation and mid-term follow-up data. J Vasc Surg 2001; 33(2):S157–64.
39. Bush RL, Najibi S, Lin PH, et al. Early experience with the bifurcated Excluder endoprosthesis for treatment of the abdominal aortic aneurysm. J Vasc Surg 2001; 34(3):497–502.
40. Criado FJ, Wilson EP, Fairman RM, Abul-Khoudoud O, Wellons E. Update on the Talent aortic stent-graft: a preliminary report from United States phase I and II trials. J Vasc Surg 2001; 33(2):S146–9.
41. Matsumura JS, Katzen BT, Hollier LH, Dake MD. Update on the bifurcated EXCLUDER endoprosthesis: phase I results. J Vasc Surg 2001; 33(2):S150–3.
42. Zarins CK, Heikkinen MA, Lee ES, Alsac JM, Arko FR. Short- and long-term outcome following endovascular aneurysm repair. How does it compare to open surgery? J Cardiovasc Surg (Torino) 2004; 45(4):321–33.
43. Bown MJ, Fishwick G, Sayers RD. The post-operative complications of endovascular aortic aneurysm repair. J Cardiovasc Surg 2004; 45(4):335–47.
44. Jacobs TS, Won J, Gravereaux EC, et al. Mechanical failure of prosthetic human implants: a 10-year experience with aortic stent graft devices. J Vasc Surg 2003; 37(1):16–26.
45. Zarins CK, Arko FR, Crabtree T, et al. Explant analysis of AneuRx stent grafts: relationship between structural findings and clinical outcome. J Vasc Surg 2004; 40(1):1–11.
46. Hallett JW, Jr., Marshall DM, Petterson TM, et al. Graft-related complications after abdominal aortic aneurysm repair: reassurance from a 36-year population-based experience. J Vasc Surg 1997; 25(2):277–84 (discussion 285–6).
47. Cochennec F, Becquemin JP, Desgranges P, Allaire E, Kobeiter H, Roudot-Thoraval F. Limb graft occlusion following EVAR: clinical pattern, outcomes and predictive factors of occurrence. Eur J Vasc Endovasc Surg 2007; 34(1):59–65.
48. Erzurum VZ, Sampram ES, Sarac TP, et al. Initial management and outcome of aortic endograft limb occlusion. J Vasc Surg 2004; 40(3):419–23.
49. Parent FN, III, Godziachvili V, Meier GH, III, et al. Endograft limb occlusion and stenosis after ANCURE endovascular abdominal aneurysm repair. J Vasc Surg 2002; 35(4):686–90 (see comment).
50. Chalmers N, Eadington DW, Gandanhamo D, Gillespie IN, Ruckley CV. Case report: infected false aneurysm at the site of an iliac stent. Br J Radiol 1993; 66(790):946–8.
51. Flora HS, Chaloner EJ, Sweeney A, Brookes J, Raphael MJ, Adiseshiah M. Secondary intervention following endovascular repair of abdominal aortic aneurysm: a single centre experience. Eur J Vasc Endovasc Surg 2003; 26(3):287–92.
52. Clouse WD, Brewster DC, Marone LK, et al. Durability of aortouniiliac endografting with femor-ofemoral crossover: 4-year experience in the Evt/Guidant trials. J Vasc Surg 2003; 37(6):1142–9.
53. Ducasse E, Calisti A, Speziale F, Rizzo L, Misuraca M, Fiorani P. Aortoiliac stent graft infection: current problems and management. Ann Vasc Surg 2004; 18(5):521–6.
54. Jackson MR, Clagett GP. Aortic graft infection. In: Cronenwett JL, Rutherford RB, eds. Decision Making in Vascular Surgery. Philadelphia: WB Saunders, 2001:186–91.
55. Slappy AL, Hakaim AG, Oldenburg WA, Paz-Fumagalli R, McKinney JM. Femoral incision morbidity following endovascular aortic aneurysm repair. Vasc Endovasc Surg 2003; 37(2):105–9.
56. Criado FJ, Wilson EP, Velazquez OC, et al. Safety of coil embolization of the internal iliac artery in endovascular grafting of abdominal aortic aneurysms. J Vasc Surg 2000; 32(4):684–8.
57. Lee CW, Kaufman JA, Fan CM, et al. Clinical outcome of internal iliac artery occlusions during endovascular treatment of aortoiliac aneurysmal diseases. J Vasc Interv Radiol 2000; 11(5):567–71 (see comment).
58. Lee WA, O'Dorisio J, Wolf YG, Hill BB, Fogarty TJ, Zarins CK. Outcome after unilateral hypogastric artery occlusion during endovascular aneurysm repair. J Vasc Surg 2001; 33(5):921–6.
59. Cynamon J, Lerer D, Veith FJ, et al. Hypogastric artery coil embolization prior to endoluminal repair of aneurysms and fistulas: buttock claudication, a recognized but possibly preventable complication. J Vasc Interv Radiol 2000; 11(5):573–7 (see comment).
60. Razavi MK, DeGroot M, Olcott C, III, et al. Internal iliac artery embolization in the stent-graft treatment of aortoiliac aneurysms: analysis of outcomes and complications. J Vasc Interv Radiol 2000; 11(5):561–6 (see comment).
61. Sanchez LA, Patel AV, Ohki T, et al. Midterm experience with the endovascular treatment of isolated iliac aneurysms. J Vasc Surg 1999; 30(5):907–13.

37 | Management of Endoleaks and Graft Failure Following Endovascular Aneurysm Repair

G. D. Treharne and J. A. Brennan
Royal Liverpool University Hospital, Liverpool, U.K.

INTRODUCTION

The widespread introduction of endovascular aneurysm repair (EVR) has introduced a new spectrum of potential complications. While some, such as groin access complications, were predictable; others, including endoleak and stent migration were unique to EVR. Most worrying was the potential for continued aneurysm expansion and rupture despite apparent successful aneurysm exclusion. Uncertainty about the significance of these complications tempered the appeal of EVR to many, and initial optimism was replaced by considerable scepticism regarding the durability of EVR, compared with the proven track record for open repair.

It became clear that careful appraisal of EVR-specific complications was essential to quantify their significance, and identify what, if any, intervention was required. Enthusiasts remained convinced that the concept of EVR was not inherently flawed, and that technique-specific complications could be overcome. Indeed it became apparent that many of the early problems related to design flaws of the first-generation devices, poor patient selection and inadequate stent oversizing. Improvements in these areas have vastly improved the performance of stent grafts, leading to widespread acceptance of EVR for the management of abdominal aortic aneurysms (AAAs).

EVR was more closely scrutinized than many preceding new surgical techniques. Subsequently, some "complications" were treated prior to recognition that they were natural consequences of the new approach that could be safely managed conservatively. It has also been necessary to identify which complications pose a significant risk to the patient.

Complications following EVR have been categorized by the Ad Hoc Committee of the Joint Societies of Vascular Surgery and American Association for Vascular Surgery (1). This chapter will concentrate on the specific issues of endoleaks (including endotension) and graft failure.

ENDOLEAKS

Endoleak is defined as "persistence of blood flow outside the lumen of the endoluminal graft but within an aneurysm sac or adjacent vascular segment being treated by the graft" (2). They are classified by their site of origin (Table 1) (1).

Endoleaks are one of the most common phenomena observed following EVR, and indicate a failure to isolate the aneurysm from the circulation. Depending on type and severity, endoleaks may convey a risk of continued aneurysm expansion and rupture. Not all endoleaks require intervention and growing experience gained by careful patient follow-up has indicated that a significant proportion may be managed conservatively.

Furthermore, the incidence of significant endoleaks can be minimized by meticulous attention to detail during preoperative planning to select appropriately (over)sized grafts, to anticipate possible intraoperative difficulties (iliac tortuosity) and to reject patients with unfavorable morphology.

TABLE 1   Classification of Endoleak by Site of Origin

Type I: Graft attachment site endoleak
  Type Ia: Proximal
  Type Ib: Distal
  Type Ic: Iliac occluder
Type II: Retrograde endoleak from aortic side branches
  Lumbar
  Mesenteric
  Iliac
Type III: Endoleak due to a breach of integrity of the device
  Type IIIa: Modular disconnection
  Type IIIb: Incomplete seal
  Type IIIc: Fabric tear
Type IV: Graft porosity
  Only applicable up to 1 mo after the procedure. After this, the endoleak should be reclassified as Type III
Type V: Site undefined/"endotension"

DETECTION OF ENDOLEAK

A significant proportion of endoleaks are detectable intraoperatively with completion angio-graphy following graft deployment. Demonstration of a Type I or Type III endoleak requires immediate remedial intervention. Conversely, Type II endoleaks (which are more common) are generally of little concern at this stage, but should be noted and observed during follow-up. Type IV endoleaks are of little consequence.

    Duplex ultrasonography can be used effectively for endoleak detection postoperatively (3), though computed tomographic angiography (CTA) is used most frequently (Fig. 1) (4,5). Magnetic resonance imaging (MRI) has been compared favorably to CTA and offers advantages in terms of reduced contrast nephrotoxicity and radiation dose (6).

    Endoleaks are defined as "primary" if they are identified at the time of operation, or "secondary" if they are discovered during postoperative surveillance.

MANAGEMENT OPTIONS FOR ENDOLEAK

Secondary endovascular or open intervention for endoleak is required when there is a perceived risk of aneurysm rupture (7). Unfortunately, it has been difficult to quantify rupture risk in practice. Previously, many institutions adopted an aggressive approach on the basis that any endoleak was a potential risk, but experience has shown that both endovascular and open solutions confer significant risks themselves. Furthermore, certain

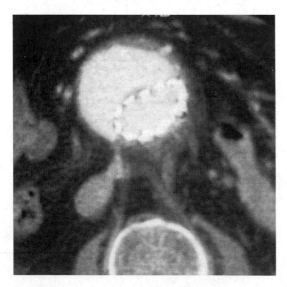

FIGURE 1 Computed tomography with contrast demonstrating a large Type I endoleak.

endoleaks are now generally regarded to be benign, leading to a shift toward conservative strategies.

Proximal Type I Endoleak

Proximal Type I endoleaks are more common with short (less than 10 mm) infrarenal aortic necks, or where the neck demonstrates an irregular contour with atherosclerotic "shelves" and/or significant angulation (Fig. 2). When self-expanding devices are used, it is necessary to oversize by 10% to 20% at the neck to obtain an adequate seal. Where there is a short infrarenal neck, the use of a device with a suprarenal uncovered stent is advisable to extend the fixation zone.

There is evidence that the infrarenal neck of AAA following endovascular repair undergoes progressive enlargement (8,9). This may lead to stent-graft migration, development of a secondary Type I endoleak and the potential for aneurysm rupture (7,10). Careful post-stent surveillance is required.

The main concern with proximal Type I endoleaks is the associated risk of aneurysm rupture. It has been postulated that large primary type I endoleaks with significant flow into the aneurysm sac confer a higher risk of rupture to the patient than the untreated aneurysm, due to the fact that arterial blood is flowing into a closed system. Similarly secondary Type I endoleaks should be treated as they have been associated with a significant aneurysm rupture rate (11).

Management Options

Proximal endoleak secondary to an irregular or angulated neck may be seen on completion angiography. This can often be sealed using a moulding balloon to affect an hemostatic seal. Alternative strategies include the use of a Palmaz® (Cordis, Miami Lakes, Florida, U.S.A.) stent to aid conformity within an irregular neck (Fig. 3), or a proximal extension cuff. Stent-graft systems that comprise a short aortic body can be disadvantageous in this situation, as there may not be enough space to deploy a cuff extension without compromising patency of the renal arteries and

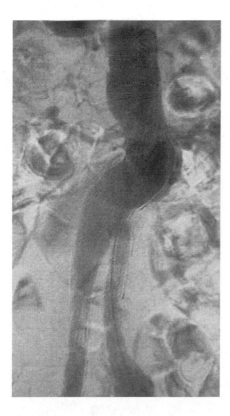

FIGURE 2 Completion angiography following endovascular aneurysm repair with an angulated neck demonstrating a proximal Type I endoleak.

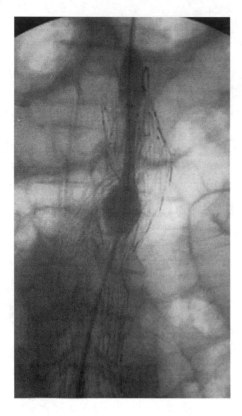

FIGURE 3   A Palmaz stent being deployed to seal a proximal Type I endoleak.

stent-graft limbs. A recent option is the use of a proximal fenestrated cuff which enables extension of the seal zone into the suprarenal aorta whilst maintaining visceral artery patency.

If attempts to resolve a proximal Type I endoleak are unsuccessful, very small low-flow Type I endoleaks may initially be managed conservatively in preference to open conversion. A proportion may resolve spontaneously within three months. Coiling of the perigraft channel has been described for proximal Type I endoleaks (12), but the long-term efficacy of such treatment is questionable and it has not gained widespread acceptance. There are concerns that, while flow may be abolished, there may still be pressure transmission through the induced thrombus leaving the aneurysm at risk of continued expansion.

If endovascular techniques fail, open banding of the aortic neck may be performed. The aorta is encircled with one or more nylon tapes, tied down onto the proximal portion of the stent graft to create an artificial neck and closing the endoleak channel. A balloon should be inflated within the stent graft when securing the tapes. Theoretical concerns of inducing aortic wall necrosis have not been reported.

If all of the maneuvres described prove ineffective, open conversion should be considered. This is a major undertaking, especially if the presence of a suprarenal stent. Immediate conversion after EVR is associated with a high mortality and a staged procedure is advisable.

Distal (iliac) Type I Endoleak

Distal type I endoleaks are usually secondary to graft sizing error and therefore largely preventable, but are easier to treat than proximal leaks. If the iliac limb is positioned correctly, balloon angioplasty is recommended initially. If the stent has been deployed too proximally, the limb should be extended with a further device. If it is not possible to seal within the distal common iliac it may be necessary to extend into the external iliac after coil embolization of the internal iliac. Small persistent distal type I endoleaks may be managed conservatively, as many will resolve spontaneously and are thought to confer a low risk for aneurysm rupture. We would advocate careful surveillance for up to six months before considering further intervention. Persistence of the endoleak with evidence of aneurysm sac enlargement warrants further treatment, and open conversion should be considered.

Secondary distal Type I endoleaks can occur as a result of proximal migration of the iliac limbs due to the "fire-hose" effect whereby pulsatile flow within a capacious aneurysm sac causes distortion of the endograft and tugs the iliac components from the native arteries. One way to minimize such an effect is to ensure maximal use or "engagement" of the common iliac arteries with the stent-graft limbs at the time of initial device deployment. This is difficult to achieve in patients with short common iliac arteries. Proximal iliac limb migration should be detectable with careful postoperative surveillance to allow further extension before limb disengagement occurs.

Type II Endoleak

Type II endoleaks identified intraoperatively are managed conservatively. They are the most common type of endoleak following EVR. Usually arising from patent lumbar arteries or the inferior mesenteric artery (IMA, Fig. 4), most Type II leaks thrombose spontaneously, usually within six months (13). A recent review of contemporary EVR trial data suggests that intervention for Type II endoleak is only indicated where there is demonstrated aneurysm sac enlargement after six months, persistence of the endoleak for more than 12 months without sac enlargement, or an aneurysm sac pressure more than 20% of mean arterial blood pressure (14).

Coil embolization of the responsible aortic side branches is the favored approach if conservative treatment fails (15). This is usually performed transarterially but may also be carried out via translumbar approach (Fig. 5) (16). Lumbar endoleaks are usually accessible via one of the internal iliac arteries into the iliolumbar arcade. The IMA is generally accessed through the superior mesenteric artery (SMA), accessing the marginal artery with a microcatheter system.

Alternative approaches to side branch perfusion include laparoscopic clipping of the patent side branch(es), direct ligation via retroperitoneal exposure and open aortic aneurysmotomy with under-running of the responsible vessel origins.

Prevention of Type II endoleak by prophylactic embolization of the aneurysm sac has been described with coils or fibrin glue (17), but this is generally unnecessary due to the benign and usually self-limiting nature of these endoleaks.

Type III Endoleaks

Type III endoleaks can occur intraoperatively, or are more commonly identified during follow-up, secondary to iliac limb dislocation or material fatigue.

Intraoperatively they most commonly occur at the junctions of modular devices. Separation of the components is unusual, the leak usually occurring as a result of failure of the self-expanding components to conform effectively. This is usually easily corrected with a

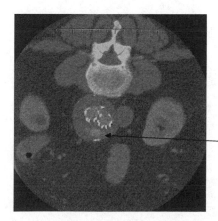

Type 2 endoleak from patent IMA

FIGURE 4 Peristent Type II endoleak following endovascular aneurysm repair from patent inferior mesenteric artery.

moulding balloon. If the endoleak persists, it may be necessary to deploy a further covered stent-graft limb across the junction.

In the intermediate and longer term limb dislocation is occasionally seen either due to disconnection of the modular overlap within the aneurysm (stump limb disconnection) or to dislocation of the stent-graft limb from the common iliac artery back into the aneurysm sac (Fig. 6). Though uncommon, Type III leaks are potentially serious and easily rectified by deployment of a further covered stent-graft. If the native common iliac is short it may be necessary to embolize the internal iliac and extend into the external iliac artery.

Type IV Endoleaks

It is generally accepted that Type IV or "porosity" endoleaks are insignificant and resolve spontaneously—usually within 48 hours. The incidence varies depending on the weave, suture holes, and thickness of the material used in each graft system. It is important to exclude other types of endoleak before confirming a diagnosis of Type IV, although the characteristic late "blush" on angiography is characteristic.

Type V Endoleaks

The management of Type V endoleaks is usually conservative, but they are not all benign in nature. The concept of "endotension" refers to the continued transmission of pressure into the aortic sac, through a channel occluded by thrombus or secondary to intermittent endoleak (18). Close monitoring of the aneurysm sac is vital since continued sac expansion requires reintervention. Options include re-lining of the original device with a further stent graft. This may not be technically possible if a device with a short body has been used, and conversion with an aortouni-iliac device with contralateral iliac artery occlusion and femoro-femoral crossover graft may be necessary. Consideration of conversion to open repair should be made if endovascular options are unavailable.

Intrasac Pressure Measurements

Over recent years, interest has been expressed as to whether intrasac pressure measurements can predict aneurysms at risk of rupture after EVR. Catheters attached to a suitable pressure

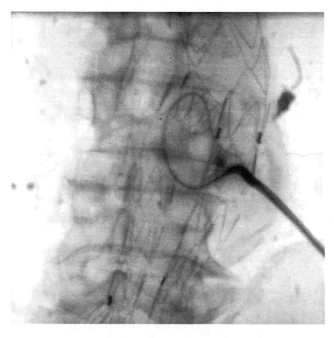

FIGURE 5 Direct puncture of an aneurysm sac after endovascular aneurysm repair to enable embolization of a persistent Type II endoleak.

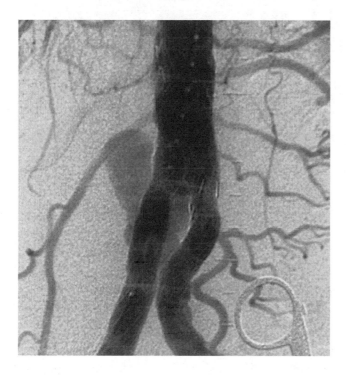

FIGURE 6 Large type III endoleak due to dislocation of the iliac stent limb from the main body of the endovascular aneurysm repair device.

transducer can be placed within the aneurysm sac outside the device at the time of surgery, and usually withdrawn 48 to 72 hours postoperatively. Permanent implantable devices with radiotelemetry monitoring are now under trial (19) and one such device, the EndoSure™ (CardioMEMS, Atlanta, GA, U.S.A.) device, is being marketed.

A continuous arterial waveform within the aortic sac correlates with the presence of Type I endoleaks, but is less reliable for other types (20). Direct measurement of pressure transmission within thrombus lining aortic aneurysms during open surgery has demonstrated wide variations, presumably related to the thrombus microstructure (21). This casts some doubt as to whether intrasac pressure measurements can be reliably used to predict endoleaks. Computed tomography (CT)-guided trans-lumbar puncture of the aortic sac and may confirm significant endoleaks if doubt exists.

GRAFT FAILURE

Structural Failure

A variety of structural failures have been reported for a variety of commercially available devices. Depending on severity, this has prompted either revision or voluntary withdrawal of devices from the market. Failures have included fabric defects, seam failure, tie breaks, hook fractures, spring fractures, disintegration of the frame, and separation of the modular components. Knowledge of the prevalence of device failures has been hampered by sporadic reporting, and often the clinical consequences have been ill defined. The value of continued long-term follow-up for EVR patients is supported by reports of structural failures two years or more after surgery, often related to component fatigue.

Management of structural failure is dependent on the individual type and its perceived consequences.

Fabric Defects

Fabric tears, seam failure, and microleaks have been reported in the Stentor (MinTec, Freeport, Grand Bahama), Vanguard™ (Boston Scientific, Natick, Massachusetts, U.S.A.), and AneuRx® (Medtronic, Sunnyvale, California, U.S.A.) devices (2). If the resulting endoleak is detected perioperatively and is small, it may be managed conservatively with regular duplex and/or CT follow-up—a proportion will seal spontaneously with thrombosis of the aneurysm sac.

Late presentation of an endoleak related to a fabric defect usually requires intervention, particularly if it is accompanied by evidence of aneurysm expansion. Therapeutic strategies include the deployment of a covered stent or a further bifurcated device to seal the defect. Ultimately, open conversion may be required.

Device Degradation

Conformational changes secondary to metal and fabric fatigue cause loss of device integrity. Mintec's Stentor device and the Vanguard II endograft were both withdrawn from the market after design defects were demonstrated. Suture breaks occurred in up to 60% of devices, often resulting in segmental separation and dislocation. Late aneurysm ruptures subsequent to the inevitable endoleaks prompted the withdrawal.

Other devices have benefited from redesign and strengthening of components as defects were demonstrated, but separation of modular components can occur with current endografts, and without any apparent structural defects. This can conceivably result from continued lengthening of the native aneurysmal artery, or by component diameter mismatch.

When device separation occurs, intervention is almost always required as the resultant endoleak is usually significant and there is perceived to be a high risk of late aneurysm rupture. Endovascular deployment of a covered stent to bridge the separated components may be performed, but if this is not possible, open conversion should be considered.

With all endografts, frequent surveillance is required to identify component degradation. Plain radiological films are adequate to reveal failure of the metallic frame. Fabric degradation may be identified by duplex sonography, but more accurately by CTA or magnetic resonance angiography.

Iliac Limb Occlusion

Iliac limb occlusion is related to adverse anatomy of the iliac artery (tortuosity, calcification and stenosis) and the conformability of the stent-graft limb. This can prevent satisfactory limb deployment, despite use of a moulding balloon, risking early limb thrombosis. It is advisable to remove any stiff wires during completion angiography to reveal any excessive tortuosity, or abutting of the stent against the vessel wall. Oblique projections may also be useful to ensure favorable deployment. Significant kinking of a limb at this stage indicates a strong likelihood of subsequent iliac limb occlusion and should be addressed by deployment of a rigid uncovered stent to maintain patency.

When iliac limb occlusion occurs as a late event, it usually manifests as limb claudication or as critical limb ischemia. When intervention is indicated, femoro-femoral bypass is recommended. Graft thrombectomy can be hazardous—re-thrombosis is common and there is a theoretical risk of displacing the endograft or causing separation of its components.

INFECTION OF ENDOGRAFT

Endovascular graft infections are rare, with a reported incidence iof 0.37% to 1.1% (22). Information regarding the causes and therapeutic strategies for stent infection are scarce.

Approximately one-third of endovascular aortic graft infections occur within four months of deployment, presumably from bacterial contamination during surgery. The pathogenesis of late infection is unclear. The most common organism isolated from infected aortic prostheses is *Staphylococcus aureus*. Less common opportunistic pathogens have been identified in patients with immune suppression (24).

Diagnosis of graft infection requires a high level of clinical suspicion, as symptoms are often nonspecific. Low-grade pyrexia, and raised inflammatory markers are not uncommon following endograft placement and may be related to post-implantation syndrome. Laboratory results may therefore be unhelpful. The demonstration of gas within the aneurysm sac has high diagnostic significance and is most commonly identified with a CT scan. Other imaging options that may assist in the diagnosis include ultrasound, MRI, and radio-labeled leucocyte scanning.

CT-guided aspiration of perigraft fluid may yield positive cultures to aid diagnosis and guide appropriate antibiotic therapy.

Once an infected endovascular prosthesis has been diagnosed, treatment requires excision of the graft with either in situ replacement or extra-anatomical bypass. Published mortality rates are high (16.3–20%) (22).

REFERENCES

1. Chaikof EL, Blankensteijn JD, Harris PL, et al. Reporting standards for endovascular aortic aneurysm repair. J Vasc Surg 2002; 35:1048–60.
2. White GH, Yu W, May J, Chaufour X, Stephen MS. Endoleak as a complication of endoluminal grafting of abdominal aortic aneurysms: classification, incidence, diagnosis and management. J Endovasc Surg 1997; 4:152–68.
3. McLafferty RB, McCrary BS, Mattos MA, et al. The use of color-flow duplex scan for the detection of endoleaks. J Vasc Surg 2002; 36(1):100–4.
4. Rozenblit AM, Patlas M, Rosenbaum AT, et al. Detection of endoleaks after endovascular repair of abdominal aortic aneurysm: value of unenhanced and delayed helical CT acquisitions. Radiology 2003; 227:426–33.
5. Stavropoulos SW, Baum RA. Imaging modalities for the detection and management of endoleaks. Semin Vasc Surg 2004; 17:154–60.
6. Pitton MB, Schweitzer H, Herber S, et al. MRI versus helical CT for endoleak detection after endovascular aneurysm repair. AJR Am J Roentgenol 2005; 185(5):1275–81.
7. Harris PL, Vallabhaneni SR, Desgranges P, Becquemin JP, Van Marrewijk C, Laheij RJ. Incidence and risk factors of late rupture, conversion, and death after endovascular repair of infrarenal aortic aneurysms: the EUROSTAR experience. J Vasc Surg 2000; 32:739–49.
8. Palombo D, Valenti D, Ferri M, et al. Changes in the proximal neck of abdominal aortic aneurysms early after endovascular treatment. Ann Vasc Surg 2003; 17(4):408–10.
9. Liapis C, Kakisis J, Kaperonis E, et al. Changes of the infrarenal aortic segment after conventional abdominal aortic aneurysm repair. Eur J Vasc Endovasc Surg 2000; 19(6):643–7.
10. England A, Butterfield JS, Jones N, et al. Device migration after endovascular abdominal aortic aneurysm rupture: experience with a talent stent-graft. J Vasc Interv Radiol 2004; 15(12):1399–405.
11. Veith FJ, Baum RA, Ohki T, et al. Nature and significance of endoleaks and endotension: summary of opinions expressed at an international conference. J Vasc Surg 2002; 35:1029–35.
12. Amesur NB, Zajko AB, Orons PD, Makaroun MS. Embolotherapy of persistent endoleaks after endovascular repair of abdominal aortic aneurysm with the ancure-endovascular technologies endograft system. J Vasc Interv Radiol 1999; 10:1175–82.
13. Van Marrewijk C, Buth J, Harris PL, Norgren L, Nevelsteen A, Wyatt MG. Significance of endoleaks after endovascular repair of abdominal aortic aneurysms: the EUROSTAR experience. J Vasc Surg 2002; 35:461–73.
14. Gelfand DV, White GH, Wilson SE. Clinical significance of type II endoleak after endovascular repair of abdominal aortic aneurysm. Ann Vasc Surg 2006; 20:69–74.
15. Baum RA, Cope C, Fairman RM, Carpenter JP. Translumbar embolization of type II endoleaks after endovascular repair of abdominal aortic aneurysms. J Vasc Interv Radiol 2001; 12:111–6.
16. Baum RA, Carpenter JP, Golden MA, et al. Treatment of type II endoleaks after endovascular repir of abdominal aortic aneurysms: comparison of transarterial and translumbar techniques. J Vasc Surg 2002; 35:23–9.
17. Zanchetta M, Faresin F, Pedon L, Riggi M, Ronsivalle S. Fibrin glue aneurysm sac embolization at the time of endografting. J Endovasc Ther 2005; 12(5):579–82.
18. Gilling-Smith GL, Brennan J, Harris P, et al. Endotension after endovascular aneurysm repair: definition, classification, and strategies for surveillance and intervention. J Endovasc Surg 1999; 6:305–7.
19. Ellozy SH, Carroccio A, Lookstein RA, et al. First experience in human beings with a permanently implantable intrasac pressure transducer for monitoring endovascular repair of abdominal aortic aneurysms. J Vasc Surg 2004; 40(3):405–12.
20. Chaudhuri A, Ansdell LE, Grass AJ, Adiseshiah M. Intrasac pressure waveforms after endovascular aneurysm repair (EVR) are a reliable marker of type I endoleaks, but not type II or combined types: an experimental study. Eur J Vasc Endovasc Surg 2004; 28(4):373–8.
21. Vallabhaneni SR, Gilling-Smith GL, Brennan JA, et al. Can intrasac pressure monitoring reliably predict failure of endovascular aneurysm repair? J Endovasc Ther 2003; 10(3):524–30.
22. Fiorani P, Speziale F, Calisti A, et al. Endovascular graft infection: preliminary results of an international enquiry. J Endovasc Ther 2003; 10:919–27.

38 | Fenestrated and Branched Endografts for the Management of Juxta-Renal Aneurysms

Eric E. Roselli
Department of Thoracic and Cardiovascular Surgery, Cleveland Clinic, Cleveland, Ohio, U.S.A.
Roy K. Greenberg
Department of Vascular Surgery, Cleveland Clinic, Cleveland, Ohio, U.S.A.

CLINICAL RELEVANCE

Endovascular repair of aortic aneurysms has been limited to patients whose anatomy provides a favorable fit for the available endografts. Until recently patients with short (less than 15 mm) or conical infrarenal aortic necks, aneurysms encroaching on the visceral segment from above or below, or involving the distal aortic arch have been deemed not amenable to endovascular repair because the seal zone could not provide adequate substrate for a durable repair. Although some of these patients can be treated with an open surgical procedure at an acceptable risk using an infrarenal clamp, many require suprarenal clamping, circulatory arrest or a staged procedure with the inherent increased risks (1–3). Furthermore, patients deemed high risk for open surgery and with unfavorable anatomy for endovascular surgery are often relegated to medical management (4,5). Fenestrated and branched stent grafts designed to accommodate tributary arteries allow for placement of the sealing stent into a greater extent of the aorta (Fig. 1A,B) (6–8). The development of these devices has expanded the indications for endovascular repair of aneurysmal disease (Fig. 2) (9,10).

PATIENT SELECTION

This chapter will specifically address the use of fenestrated or branched grafts for the treatment of aneurysmal disease abutting the distal visceral segment, i.e., juxtarenal aneurysms. For endovascular therapy of these patients, several conditions must be met:

1. Presence of an aortic aneurysm at higher risk for rupture than the risk of repairing it using a fenestrated graft (greater than 5.5 cm).
2. Relatively high risk for open surgical repair based on a thorough assessment of comorbidities and an understanding that the durability of these endovascular devices is yet unknown.
3. Infrarenal anatomy deemed unfavorable to endovascular repair (Fig. 3A,B) with commercially available stent grafts because of one of the following:
   a. Proximal aortic neck length less than 15 mm
   b. Funnel-shaped aortic neck
   c. Extensive thrombus-lined aortic neck
   d. Severe angulation
4. Anatomy conducive to fenestrated or branched stent grafting including all of the following:
   a. Normal caliber visceral aortic segment
   b. Parallel visceral aortic segment

The choice of graft design is governed by the proximal neck anatomy. If the proximal infrarenal aortic neck length is greater than or equal to 3 mm then a fenestrated device

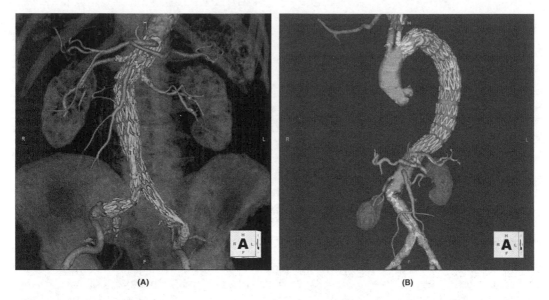

(A)   (B)

FIGURE 1 Volume rendered 3D reconstruction images following the completion of fenestrated stent-graft repair of (**A**) a juxtarenal aneurysm with stents deployed within both renal and the superior mesenteric arteries and (**B**) a distal arch and descending aneurysm with a stent deployed across a fenestration to accommodate the left common carotid artery.

is appropriate; if the neck is less than 3 mm or nonexistent, then the patient requires the use of a branched device.

Patients whose comorbidities predict a life expectancy not warranting aneurysmal repair and who otherwise do not meet the indications above are contraindicated to undergo endovascular repair. Furthermore, patients with iliac lesions not amenable to angioplasty or recanalizable to allow passage of the delivery system are contraindicated. Other contra-indications include allergies to device materials such as stainless steel or polyester graft material, and systemic infection. All patients should be able to undergo the required follow-up imaging.

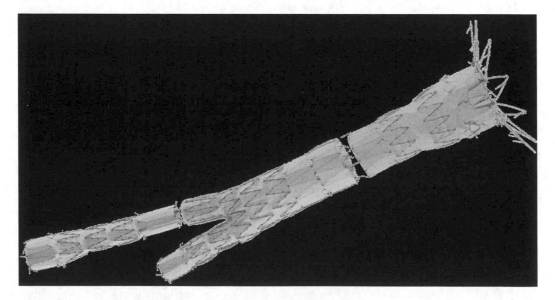

FIGURE 2 The Zenith modular fenestrated stent-graft system.

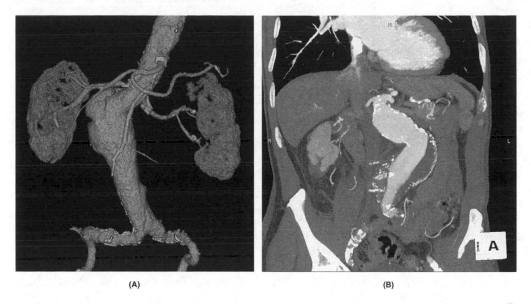

(A)   (B)

FIGURE 3   3D reconstructions of computed tomography images demonstrating infrarenal aneurysms not amenable to endovascular repair with commercially available devices because of (**A**) severe angulation and (**B**) short length of the neck.

PROCEDURE

Planning

A clear understanding of the aortic, iliac, and femoral anatomy based on preoperative imaging is critical to proper patient selection, device design, and accurate delivery. Other important landmarks are the lowest renal artery, the aortic bifurcation and the origins of the internal iliac arteries. A site of delivery of the main body must be selected based on the size, extent of calcification and tortuosity of the access vessels (Fig. 4A–C).

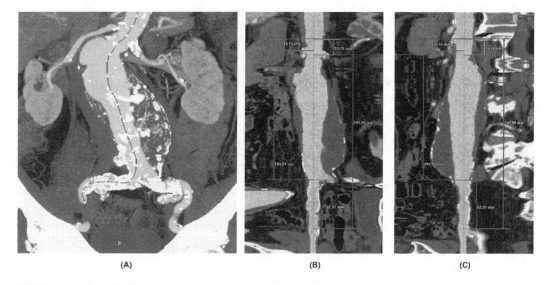

(A)   (B)   (C)

FIGURE 4   Various 3D techniques are critical to accurate design of these devices including (**A**) center line of flow analysis which can be further evaluated in the stretched mode. (**B,C**) By rotating the stretched views about the center line axis, the various landmarks can be identified. Maximum intensity projections are helpful to evaluate the tortuosity of access vessels and aorta to determine best side of delivery.

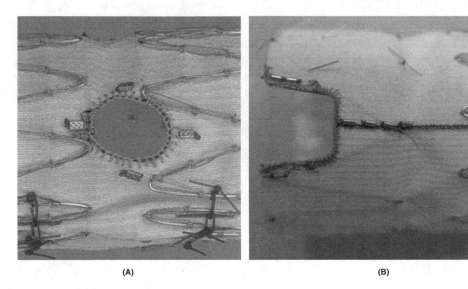

FIGURE 5   (**A**) Small reinforced fenestration and (**B**) proximal scallop.

Accurate preoperative planning is required, ideally with high-resolution imaging and three-dimensional reconstructions. The design of devices must follow particular guidelines as described below:

- Grafts may include no more than two of any one type fenestration (small, large, or scallop) within a single sealing stent (Fig. 5A,B).
- The distance between fenestrations must be more than 5 mm in a longitudinal axis (generally approximately two hours of clock position, depending on graft diameter).
- It is not possible to place a fenestration distal to the lowest sealing stent.
- The outside diameter of the graft is typically chosen to be 10% to 25% larger than the proximal implantation site.
- The attachment sites for distal implantation are oversized by approximately 10% to 20%. In vessels with diameters greater than 16 mm, oversizing can be increased.
- The proximal body length should place the distal end of the graft between 20 and 30 mm above the aortic bifurcation when the fenestrations are aligned.
- The distal body length should place the distal end of the contralateral limb between 5 and 10 mm above the aortic bifurcation, and provide maximum overlap between body components without covering the tapered or fenestrated area of the proximal body. *Note*: A 2-stent overlap is the absolute minimum, with a 3 to 4-stent overlap being preferable.
- The lengths of the integral ipsilateral leg and the modular contralateral leg are chosen to land the distal end just above the common iliac bifurcation.
- The contralateral leg length must provide for at least a 1-stent overlap with the distal body contralateral limb, with an upper limit of approximately a 2-stent overlap. An overlap of about 1-$\frac{1}{2}$ stents is optimal.

Practical Points

The following explains the sequence of tasks necessary for proper device design and planning and are delineated on a standardized sizing sheet:

1. Plan the seal/fenestration zone
2. Select side for graft body introduction
3. Choose fenestration configuration

4. Choose proximal body diameter
5. Determine inner aortic vessel diameter
6. Choose proximal graft length
7. Choose distal body length
8. Choose distal body ipsilateral leg diameter
9. Choose distal body ipsilateral leg length
10. Choose contralateral leg diameter
11. Choose contralateral leg length

Imaging

Preoperatively, high-resolution helical computed tomography (CT) scan of the chest, abdomen, and pelvis is required, utilizing a narrow collimation set between 0.5 and 1 mm intervals, gantry rotation of 0.5 seconds, and table feed of 12 mm to allow for the acquisition of the appropriate data. The CT scan should be performed without oral contrast and with the intravenous contrast (low osmolar, nonionic) bolus timed for the arterial phase. Non-contrast and venous phase images are also obtained. Reconstructions with 1 to 1.5 mm slices are helpful to accurately select patients, design the device and plan the operation. A three-dimensional work station should be accessible to the surgeon designing the device (see Techniques below).

An endovascular suite with a fixed imaging system with 12 to 16 in. image intensifier is best for the multiple views and occasionally prolonged imaging necessary for this procedure. Handheld ultrasound can be helpful for difficult to obtain percutaneous access.

DEPLOYMENT

Deployment is described for the Cook fenestrated graft as this is the most commonly used iteration. The operator needs to re-familiarize himself with the specific device design prior to beginning the procedure. Particular attention should be directed at understanding the location of the fenestrations in relation to the edge of the graft material and to one another and also the predetermined sites of delivery and access to branch vessels.

Bilateral common femoral arteries are exposed in the standard fashion with oblique incisions unless the patient requires placement of an iliac conduit via a retroperitoneal approach, which has been described elsewhere (11).

Femoral artery puncture on the side of delivery is performed in the usual fashion and access is established with a 0.035-in. wire. The catheter is then directed to the aortic arch and exchanged for a stiff guidewire (0.035 Amplatz or Lunderquist).

Contralateral access can be accomplished using one of two techniques: either multiple punctures to provide access to the branch vessels or single puncture with a large-bore (20–24-F Check Flow) sheath which is subsequently multiply punctured.

Once bilateral wire access has been obtained, the patient is heparinized. A straight angiography catheter is then placed via the contralateral side and positioned at the level of the renal arteries. Angiography is then performed to delineate the visceral segment.

The device is then oriented so that the vertical markers are anterior, horizontal markers are posterior, and the right-handed check mark is midline by imaging it outside of the patient's body under fluoroscopy. The device is then advanced through the femoral artery to the level of the visceral segment until the markers for the scallop and/or fenestrations are aligned with the appropriate arteries. Doing so may require multiple low-dose contrast injections.

It is important to verify that the distal aspect of the device is above the aortic bifurcation. Once orientation of the proximal body has been confirmed, the top two stents are partially deployed. The device position is then adjusted as necessary in both the longitudinal and rotational planes. The sheath is then completely withdrawn to expand the stent graft throughout its length. The next step entails cannulation of the fenestrations. The contralaterally placed wire and angiocath should be withdrawn at this point and the main body of the device recannulated. Using an appropriately angled catheter and flexible angled guidewire, at least two fenestrations and their corresponding arteries should be cannulated. With catheter access to the artery, the wire should be exchanged for a stiffer access wire (Rosen). An access sheath (Ansel) or guiding catheter (Multi-Purpose B style) should then be advanced through the fenestration into the artery (Fig. 6). This step should be repeated for both renal arteries if the stent graft is designed with two small fenestrations.

Once secure access to the fenestrations and their corresponding arteries has been obtained, complete deployment of the main device may proceed in a standard fashion by removing the trigger wires and deploying the proximal uncovered stent.

Stenting the branch vessels can now be performed via the previously placed access sheaths. Balloon expandable stents measuring 15 to 24 mm in length and 6 to 8 mm in diameter are deployed. The stents should be placed mostly into the target vessel with approximately 3 mm extending proximally into the aorta (Fig. 7). The aortic portion of the stents should then be flared with a 10 mm×2 cm balloon to rivet them in place within the main device (Fig. 8). Further flaring with a larger compliant balloon is selectively employed. Each stent should be completely deployed including the flaring process before proceeding to the subsequent one (Fig. 9).

The completion of the device deployment is similar to that previously described for the Zenith system (12). The second component is delivered through the ipsilateral side, oriented, and deployed until the contralateral limb expands at the level above the aortic bifurcation. The contralateral limb is then cannulated and the limb extensions deployed.

Immediately postoperatively, the decision to transfer patients to an intensive care unit is based on comorbidities and the course of the operation. Patients are to be hydrated to maintain euvolemia. Patients are closely monitored for signs of embolization, especially with regard to renal function. Blood urea nitrogen and serum creatinine are followed daily and once shown to be normal or stabilized, the patient undergoes completion CT with the protocol as described above prior to discharge.

All patients are imaged again in 1 month, 6 months, and 12 months and annually thereafter with CT and plain radiographs. The CT is performed using a high kernal protocol both with and without IV contrast and a delayed venous phase. Attention is directed at the aneurysm sac to determine size and look for endoleaks, and at the device for migration and stent integrity (13). Furthermore, patients have plain radiographs performed from the anterior, lateral and oblique views to assist in the detection of stent fractures.

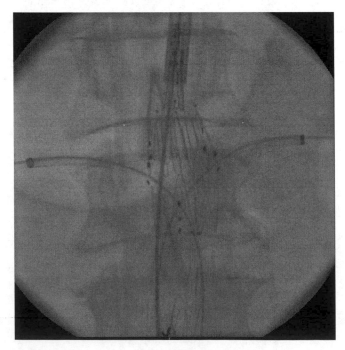

FIGURE 6 Fluoroscopic image demonstrating bilateral renal artery access with two 7-F sheaths within the partially deployed main body device. Note the markers depicting the proximal edge of the graft, the fenestrations, and the orienting markers below.

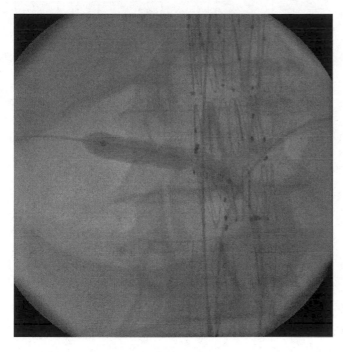

FIGURE 7 Fluoroscopic image depicted delivery of right renal stent with proximal-most portion within the body of the main device.

OUTCOMES

The results of the first 119 patients undergoing fenestrated stent grafting at the Cleveland Clinic are available. Technical success was achieved in 100% of patients who had a mean aneurysm size of 6.5 cm with a single acute mortality. Mean follow-up was 19 months and Kaplan–Meier estimates of survival at 1, 12, 24, and 36 months are 0.99, 0.92, 0.83 and 0.79, respectively (Fig. 10). There were no late aneurysm related deaths and no conversions to open procedures (14).

Endoleak and migration are inherent to all endovascular devices and the rate of occurrence in our experience with these devices is described in Figure 11 (14). Furthermore, clinical complications may include any issues typically seen following aortic surgery (15,16).

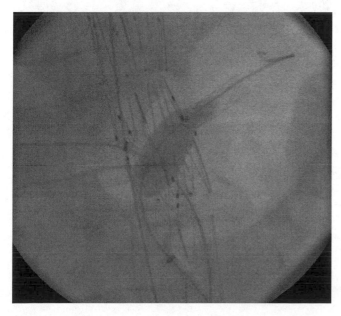

FIGURE 8 Fluoroscopic image demonstrated flairing of the proximal portion of the stent within the main device with a 10 mm×2 cm balloon to rivet the components together.

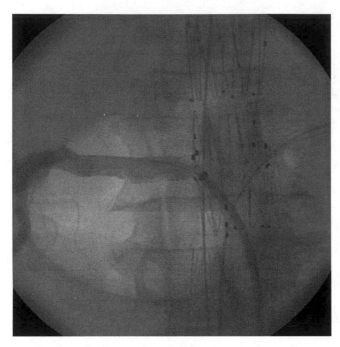

FIGURE 9 Selective angiographic image after completed stenting and flairing of the right renal artery. Notice the sheath within the left renal artery. Each branch vessel is completed before moving on to the next.

Intraoperatively persistent type I endoleaks around the proximal graft material are treated with inflation of a compliant balloon, and occasionally with placement of a large Palmaz™ stent (Cordis, Miami, Florida, U.S.A.) to ensure circumferential apposition within the sealing segment of the graft material to the aortic wall. If the Type I leak is from a fenestration then direct ballooning into the stent or stent graft with the compliant balloon should resolve it. Alternatively, deployment of an additional balloon expandable stent graft can address this problem. Type III endoleaks between the main device components are

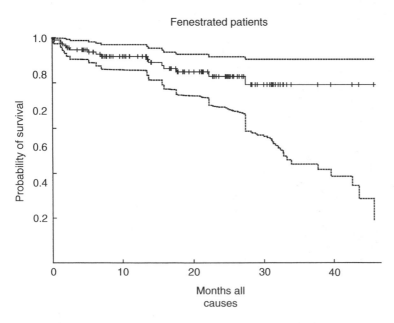

FIGURE 10 Kaplan–Meier estimates of survival from all causes of mortality after fenestrated stent grafting. *Source*: From Ref. 14.

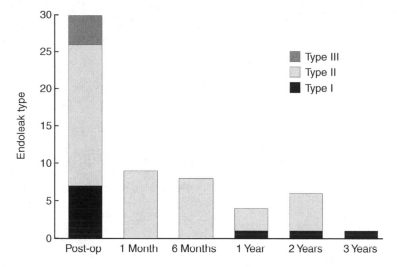

FIGURE 11 Endoleaks by type at various follow-up intervals. *Source*: From Ref. 14.

easily treated with dilation using the compliant balloon (Coda, Cook, Indianapolis, Indiana) or if delayed, with the addition of an extension cuff or balloon expandable stent. Most Type II endoleaks will resolve. If they persist and are associated with enlargement of the aneurysm sac, the source vessel must be embolized. We prefer a trans-arterial approach with glue embolization.

CONCLUSION

In conclusion, the development of fenestrated and branched devices has expanded the use of endovascular techniques to treat patients with juxtarenal aneurysms. This approach is safe and reproducible with excellent outcomes but several factors are key to achieving success. Accurate preoperative planning is required, ideally with high-resolution imaging and three-dimensional reconstructions. Durability of repair is dependent upon adequate seal and fixation in a normal and parallel segment of aorta. A broad understanding of arterial access and the use of angiographic wires and catheters is required for consistent technical success.

REFERENCES

1. Bicknell CD, Cowan AR, Kerle MI, Mansfield AO, Cheshire NJ, Wolfe JH. Renal dysfunction and prolonged visceral ischaemia increase mortality rate after suprarenal aneurysm repair. Br J Surg 2003; 90(9):1142–6.
2. Shortell CK, Johansson M, Green RM, Illig KA. Optimal operative strategies in repair of juxtarenal abdominal aortic aneurysms. Ann Vasc Surg 2003; 17(1):60–5 (Epub 2003 January 15).
3. Sarac TP, Clair DG, Hertzer NR, et al. Contemporary results of juxtarenal aneurysm repair. J Vasc Surg 2002; 36(6):1104–11.
4. Greenberg RK, Clair D, Srivastava S, et al. Should patients with challenging anatomy be offered endovascular aneurysm repair? J Vasc Surg 2003; 38:990–6.
5. Linsen MA, Vos AW, Diks J, Rauwerda JA, Wisselink W. Fenestrated and branched endografts: assessment of proximal aortic neck fixation. J Endovasc Ther 2005; 12(6):647–53.
6. Verhoeven EL, Prins TR, Tielliu IF, et al. Treatment of short-necked infrarenal aortic aneurysms with fenestrated stent-grafts: short-term results. Eur J Vasc Endovasc Surg 2004; 27(5):477–83.
7. Kruger AJ, Holden AH, Hill AA. Endoluminal repair of a thoracic arch aneurysm using a scallop-edged stent-graft. J Endovasc Ther 2003; 10(5):936–9.
8. Park JH, Chung JW, Choo IW, Kim SJ, Lee JY, Han MC. Fenestrated stent-grafts for preserving visceral arterial branches in the treatment of abdominal aortic aneurysms: preliminary experience. J Vasc Interv Radiol 1996; 7(6):819–23.

9. Roselli EE, Greenberg RK, Pfaff K, Francis C, Svensson LG, Lytle BW. Endovascular treatment of thoracoabdominal aortic aneurysms. J Thorac Cardiovasc Surg. 2007; 133(6):1474–82. Epub 2007 May 2.
10. Greenberg RK, Haulon S, Lyden SP, et al. Endovascular management of juxtarenal aneurysms with fenestrated endovascular grafting. J Vasc Surg 2004; 39(2):279–87.
11. Abu-Ghaida A, Clair D, Greenberg R, Srivastava S, O'Hara P, Ouriel K. Broadening the applicability of endovascular aortic aneurysm repair: the use of iliac conduits. J Vasc Surg 2002; 36:111–7.
12. Greenberg RK, Lawrence-Brown M, Bhandari G, et al. An update of the Zenith endovascular graft for abdominal aortic aneurysms: initial implantation and mid-term follow-up data. J Vasc Surg 2001; 33(Suppl. 2):S157–64.
13. Greenberg RK, Turc A, Haulon S, et al. Stent-graft migration: a reappraisal of analysis methods and proposed revised definition. J Endovasc Ther 2004; 11(4):353–63.
14. O'Neill S, Greenberg RK, Haddad F, Resch T, Sereika J, Katz E. A prospective analysis of fenestrated endovascular grafting: intermediate-term outcomes. Eur J Vasc Endovasc Surg 2006; 32:115–23 (Epub ahead of print).
15. Haddad F, Greenberg RK, Walker E, et al. Fenestrated endovascular grafting: the renal side of the story. J Vasc Surg 2005; 41(2):181–90.
16. Sampram ES, Karafa MT, Mascha EJ, et al. Nature, frequency, and predictors of secondary procedures after endovascular repair of abdominal aortic aneurysm. J Vasc Surg 2003; 37(5):930–7.

39 Therapeutic Options for Thoracoabdominal and Pararenal Aortic Aneurysms

Timothy A. M. Chuter
Division of Vascular Surgery, University of California San Francisco, San Francisco, California, U.S.A.

INTRODUCTION

Thoracoabdominal aortic aneurysms (TAAA) occupy an inaccessible location high in the retroperitoneum, and they have branches to organs, such as the liver, kidneys and small intestine, with little tolerance for ischemia. Consequently, traditional surgical repair of these aneurysms has produced high rates of mortality and morbidity (1). Endovascular techniques employ a transarterial route of access to the aneurysm and do not interrupt flow for more than a few seconds, and therefore have the potential to greatly reduce mortality, morbidity, hospital stay, pain, and debility. Given these advantages, endovascular repair would have replaced surgical repair a long time ago were it not for one challenge; how to exclude the aneurysm from the circulation without also excluding flow to its branches.

Implantation of a simple tubular stent graft is not an option, unless vital arterial branches to the intra-abdominal organs have already been provided with an alternative source of blood through extra-anatomic bypass (2). Any completely endovascular method of TAAA repair requires the creation of internal visceral and renal artery bypasses, using branched stent grafts, of which there are two types, unibody and modular. Unibody stent grafts are inserted whole and held in a partially expanded state while their branches are manipulated into position using a system of catheters. Modular stent grafts are assembled in situ from a collection of separately inserted components.

UNIBODY BRANCHED STENT GRAFTS

Only one group has ever reported successful insertion of a multibranched unibody stent graft (3). Their device was, and still is (4), custom made to match the findings of three-dimensional reconstructions of contrast-enhanced computed tomography. The trunk and limbs of the graft are constructed from woven polyester fabric, sutured to a series of transaxial nitinol hoops. These hoops are folded and maintained in a compressed state, even after withdrawal of the delivery sheath, so that the branches can be inserted into the renal, superior mesenteric and celiac arteries. As if the simultaneous insertion of multiple branches were not enough, the necessary catheter-based mechanisms have to function in the absence of downstream access to the branches of the thoracoabdominal aorta. The hoop-like attachment wires endow the stent graft with great flexibility, and the ability to seal within short, angulated, irregular segments of aorta. Although this feature is a great advantage in the proximal thoracic aorta (where other versions of this unibody device have been used successfully), it is of less value in the thoraco-abdominal aorta. Indeed, endoleak has been a persistent problem with this type of device, regardless of location.

The inherent complexities of unibody construction increase exponentially with every additional branch. The first challenge is stent-graft design and manufacture. Each branch of the stent graft has to be of the right length, diameter, position and orientation on the stent graft. Stent-graft delivery is also complicated by the presence of multiple branches, all preattached to the same prosthesis. There is no opportunity for staging the procedure and no such thing as partial success. The whole thing fails or succeeds as a unit.

MODULAR BRANCHED STENT GRAFTS

The modular branched stent graft consists of multiple single-lumen stent grafts, joined where the lines of insertion intersect and the stent grafts overlap. All the current systems of modular branched stent-graft construction are members of the Zenith family of devices, manufactured by Cook (Bloomington, Indiana, U.S.A.), for a variety of reasons. The characteristic features of Zenith technology allow the addition of holes or cuffs at various locations for patient-specific design; partial deployment and bridging catheter insertion for precise positioning; and secure aortic attachment for migration prevention.

The technology of branched stent-graft insertion has evolved over the past five years to include: constraining wires to hold the stent graft in a state of partial deployment; markers to aid in orientation; indwelling catheters and wires to aide in transgraft catheterization; and a wide variety of attachment sites on the primary aortic stent graft to create secure, hemostatic intercomponent connections. These attachment sites fall into two main groups, fenestrations and cuffs. A fenestration is, at its simplest, just a hole in the wall of the primary stent graft. Nitinol rings may be added to reinforce the fenestration, but there is no zone of contact between the rim of the fenestration and the branch, just a discrete ring no deeper than the graft is thick. A cuff, on the other hand, has a margin of fabric, which creates and overlap zone between the primary stent graft and the branch stent graft (covered stent). In that regard, a cuff resembles the attachment site for the contralateral limb of a typical modular bifurcated stent graft. Cuffs can extend outward or inward, upward or downward, from the wall of the primary stent graft. They can be short or long, straight or curved, depending on the location and orientation of the corresponding target artery.

Fenestrations and Balloon-Expanded Covered Stents

The substitution of a covered stent for the usual open stent of standard fenestrated stent-graft technique moves the site of sealing from the branch artery orifice to the branch artery lumen, turns the fenestration into a branch, and extends the range of treatable anatomy (5). An open stent helps to keep the margin of the fenestration in close apposition to the margin of the renal artery, but it cannot bridge any gap between the two. In cases of juxtarenal aneurysm, the aorta is not dilated at the level of the renal arteries and there is no space between the wall of the stent graft and the wall of the aorta.

If the aneurysm extends proximally to involve the pararenal aorta, there is a gap between the wall of the stent graft and the wall of the aneurysm. A covered stent can bridge this gap and prevent type I endoleak, but only if there is a permanent hemostatic seal at the junction between the covered stent (branch) and the primary stent graft. Since the fenestration provides no overlap zone at this site, the intercomponent connection depends on the creation of a waist in the covered stent where the fenestration resists expansion of a slightly oversized balloon. This form of balloon driven flaring is only possible using *balloon-expanded* covered stents (Fig. 1). No degree of oversizing will induce the necessary attachment or seal between the margin of the fenestration and a *self-expanding* covered stent.

In cases of pararenal aneurysm, the technique of fenestrated stent-graft implantation is largely unaffected by the substitution of a covered stent for an uncovered stent. However, the treatment of TAAA adds several levels of complexity.

Firstly, there are more branches. It is relatively easy to line up one fenestration with one renal artery, and secure the position using a covered stent. The partial deployment mechanisms allow adjustments of stent-graft position. Accurate deployment of two branches depends on the relative positions of the two fenestrations and the two target arteries (usually renal arteries). Adjustments in stent-graft position and orientation may help line up one fenestration, but not necessarily both of them. With every additional branch, the opportunities for failure expand exponentially.

Secondly, the target artery often passes in a caudal direction, and its orifice may be far from the fenestration. Under these circumstances, the path of catheterization passes around an acute bend through a large space. It can be difficult to provide covered stent delivery systems with enough support to follow this path.

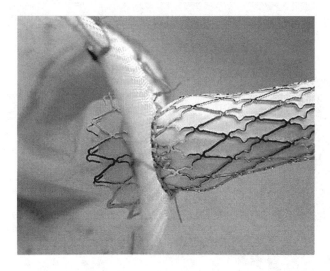

FIGURE 1 The junction between a fenestrated stent graft and a JoMed (JoMed International AB, Helsingborg, Sweden) balloon-expanded covered stent.

Thirdly, traditional fenestrated technique calls for all bridging catheters to be in place before the constraining wires are removed. When there are four fenestrations and four bridging catheters, the insertion route from the contralateral femoral artery becomes a little crowded.

All these complexities notwithstanding, this form of repair is clearly feasible, especially with modifications in stent-graft and delivery system design. For example, the covered stents can be inserted through the transbrachial route, especially if the proximal end of the stent graft has accessory fenestrations or scallops to allow access to the partially deployed stent graft.

Cuffs and Self-Expanding Covered Stents

The presence of a cuff on the primary stent graft changes the line of covered stent insertion (6). If the inside of the cuff is oriented toward the head, it can only be entered from a brachial access point. The catheter will tend to continue in a caudal direction once it exits the stent graft and enters the aneurysm sac. Its path to the orifice of the target artery then curves outward toward the target arterial orifice. The goal in cuffed stent-graft design is to manipulate the shape, position and orientation of the cuff to keep this path as straight as possible, thereby facilitating target artery catheterization. For example, upgoing renal arteries are best reached through upgoing cuffs, while downgoing visceral arteries almost always call for downgoing cuffs.

In most cases, the cuffed portion of the primary stent graft has a dog bone shape, with a wide top, a narrow middle, and a wide bottom. The narrow central segment provides additional space for catheter manipulation and ensures continuing sac (and visceral) perfusion right up to the point at which the last covered stent is inserted. Partial constraining wires can be used, in combination with a cap over an uncovered proximal stent, to keep the stent graft partially deployed, provide additional space, and allow adjustments in stent-graft position. They are not as useful with cuffed designs as they are with fenestrations, because they have to be removed to allow free access through the proximal end of the stent graft.

Some of the more exotic options, such as spiral cuffs, and combinations of fenestrated and cuffed stent grafts have a role in complex cases. Nevertheless, the author tends toward a standard stent graft with multiple barrel-shaped cuffs, a standard delivery system without additional indwelling catheters or a top cap, and a standard insertion technique with two distinct stages, transfemoral and transbrachial. Our preferred cuff consists of a short, wire-supported cylinder, measuring 15 to 18 mm in length and 6 to 8 mm in diameter (Fig. 2A). The cuff has one end on the inside (Fig. 2B) and one end on the outside of the wall of the stent graft, depending on the orientation of the corresponding target artery. Our preferred covered stent (Fluency®; CR Bard Inc., Murray Hill, New Jersey) measures 60 mm in length and 7 to 9 mm in diameter (Fig. 2C). We routinely line each covered stent with a slightly larger (8–10 mm) and longer Wallstent®. We usually insert the large aortic stent graft, or grafts, and any

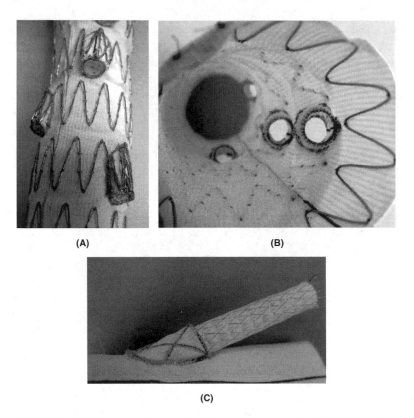

(A)   (B)

(C)

FIGURE 2 (**A**) The external appearance of a cuffed stent graft. (**B**) The internal appearance of a cuffed stent graft. (**C**) A Fluency® self-expanding stent within a cuff.

upgoing covered stents through the femoral arteries, then remove all the transfemoral catheters, sheaths and wires, close the groins, and re-prep for covered stent insertion via brachial access. Access for covered stent insertion is through a series of coaxial sheaths, with French sizes of 6, 8, 10 and possibly 12. All are kink resistant (Flexor®, Cook Medical Inc., Bloomington, Indiana, U.S.A.), except the 8, which, for size compatibility with the 10, has to be of standard wall construction. The longest of these sheaths is 90 cm in length, so all the selective catheters and covered stent delivery systems for this phase of the operation have to be 100 cm, or longer.

We have found the renal arteries to be the most difficult of the target arteries. They often arise far from the stent graft, project outward or upward (not downward), and branch early. Under these circumstances, the Fluency delivery system requires the support of a stiff guidewire. Even with a stiff wire in place, the catheters, sheaths, and delivery systems may hang up on the orifice of the cuff, the orifice of the artery, or any acute angulation along the way. When this happens, the wire pushes back, only to advance again as soon the catheter is withdrawn. The moving tip of a stiff guidewire is a dangerous object. Fortunately, modular technique allows one to stop the procedure at any point and return another day, should inadvertent renal artery injury necessitate reversal of heparinization. The safest technique involves frequent selective angiograms, and the safest wire has a short floppy segment and a curved tip (Rosen®, Cook Medical Inc., Bloomington, Indiana, U.S.A.). When the renal arteries are truly upgoing (Fig. 3A), the cuffs should be similarly oriented for ease of covered stent insertion (Fig. 3B).

COMPARISONS

The author believes that multibranched stent grafts of cuffed modular design will ultimately become the primary treatment for TAAA. The main determinant of this technology's role will

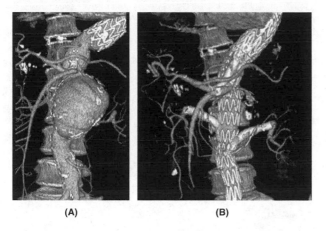

(A)   **(B)**

FIGURE 3 (**A**) Preoperative computed tomograph showing upgoing renal arteries and downgoing visceral arteries. (**B**) Postoperative computed tomograph showing upgoing cuffs and covered stents to the renal arteries, and downgoing cuffs and covered stents to the visceral arteries.

be the rate of paraplegia, but there are other factors to consider, and some of the alternative techniques may have particular advantages under certain circumstances.

Open Surgery Alone

The traditional surgical approach has one potential advantage over all the endovascular alternatives: the opportunity for intercostal reimplantation. Every vascular surgeon has seen cases in which intraoperative changes in evoked potentials normalized after intercostal reimplantation, yet wide variations in this part of open surgical technique persist. Many other factors, such as cerebrospinal fluid pressure, spinal temperature, blood pressure, and reperfusion, contribute to the risk of paraplegia, and many other interventions have been incorporated into prophylactic measures. If reperfusion injury and hemodynamic instability are more important than the restoration of intercostal flow, the rate of paraplegia following endovascular will be less than open surgery. Experience with endovascular repair of the descending thoracic aorta suggests that this is the case.

Visceral Bypass and Endovascular Aneurysm Exclusion

The combined approach has several advantages over surgery alone. The exposure is less, especially in the more extensive aneurysms, which might otherwise have required thoracotomy, and division of the diaphragm. Since the bypasses originate on the iliac arteries, there is no need to clamp the aorta and no need to institute partial left heart bypass or manipulate afterload pharmacologically. Some interruption of visceral perfusion is unavoidable during the creation of the distal anastomoses to the celiac and superior mesenteric arteries, but this may be minimal if collaterals, such as the pancreaticoduodenal artery and middle colic artery, are well developed.

    The combined approach may even have advantages over the implantation of a branched stent graft in the following circumstances:

1. Short, stenotic visceral arteries complicate the insertion of a stent-graft branch. Stenosis limits access, while early branching limits the length of the implantation site.
2. In cases of distal Type IV TAAA the space required for downgoing stent-graft branches is sometimes obtained by lengthening the amount of supraceliac aorta that must be covered which may increase the risk of paraplegia. The endovascular portion of the combined operation, on the other hand, has no such requirement; the proximal end of the stent graft goes only as high as it needs to obtain secure, hemostatic implantation.

3. Impending rupture or contained rupture mandate immediate repair, which is currently impossible using branched stent grafts. Some forms of modular branched stent graft might one day permit generic components to be held in stock. However, at this point in their development these devices are custom made, a process that takes weeks. Most centers have various unbranched stent grafts on the shelf, and are able to obtain the less commonly used sizes from industry stock within a day or two.

Multibranched Stent Grafts of Unibody Design

The potential advantage of the unibody design is freedom from risk of component separation. The limitations of this approach stem from the irreducible complexity of stent-graft design, manufacture and delivery, all of which represent barriers to widespread application.

Multibranched Stent Grafts of Modular Design

Although the fenestrated and cuffed versions of this approach may appear similar, they have different methods of insertion, employ different types of covered stent, and have different methods of stent-graft connection.

In theory, fenestrated technique may have lower risk of paraplegia in cases of pararenal aneurysm and Type IV TAAA. Because the fenestrated graft can obtain a seal at the level of the celiac and superior mesenteric arteries, while the presence of cuffs inevitably prevents the apposition of stent graft to aorta.

Cuffed stent grafts, on the other hand, are less susceptible to misalignment, and probably more stable. In comparison with a fenestration, a cuff usually provides a straighter path to the target artery, and a more secure attachment site for a covered stent attachment. Moreover, the self-expanding covered stents, used in conjunction with cuffs, are more robust than the balloon-expanded covered stents used in conjunction with fenestrations. They have a capacity for recovery, which balloon-expanded stents lack.

CONCLUSION

While there remain many unknowns, such as the risk of paraplegia, it appears likely that each of these methods will have a role to play in the treatment of aortic aneurysms. Fenestrated stent grafts will be used in combination with flared (uncovered) stents to treat juxtarenal aortic aneurysms. Fenestrated stent grafts will be used in combination with balloon-expanded covered stents to treat pararenal aortic aneurysms. Cuffed multibranched stent grafts will be used in conjunction with self-expanding covered stents to treat thoracoabdominal aortic aneurysms. Simple stent grafts will be used in conjunction with extra-anatomic visceral bypass to treat symptomatic thoracoabdominal aortic aneurysms. Open surgery will be reserved for thoracoabdominal aneurysms in young patients, especially those whose complex luminal pathology precludes stent-graft insertion.

REFERENCES

1. Svensson LG, Crawford ES, Hess KR, Coselli JS, Safi H. Experience with 1509 patients undergoing thoracoabdominal aortic operations. J Vasc Surg 1993; 17:357–70.
2. Castelli P, Caronno R, Piffaretti G, et al. Hybrid treatment for thoracic and thoracoabdominal aortic aneurysms in patients unfit for open conventional repair. Acta Chir Belg 2005; 105:602–9.
3. Hosokawa H, Iwase T, Sato M, et al. Successful endovascular repair of juxtarenal and suprarenal aortic aneurysms with a branched stent graft. J Vasc Surg 2001; 33:1087–92.
4. Saito N, Kimura T, Toma M, et al. Endovascular repair of a thoracoabdominal aortic aneurysm involving the celiac artery and the superior mesenteric artery. Ann Vasc Surg 2006; 20:659–63.
5. Anderson JL, Adam DJ, Berce M, Hartley DE. Repair of thoracoabdominal aortic aneurysms with fenestrated and branched endovascular stent grafts. J Vasc Surg 2005; 42:600–7.
6. Chuter TAM, Gordon RL, Reilly LM, Goodman JD, Messina LM. An endovascular system for thoracoabdominal aortic aneurysm repair. J Endovasc Ther 2001; 8:25–33.

40 | Endovascular Treatment of Ruptured Abdominal Aortic Aneurysm (Indications, Technical Aspects, Troubleshooting and Current Results)

Chee V. Soong, William Loan, and Bernard Lee
Vascular and Endovascular Surgery Unit, Belfast City Hospital, Belfast, Northern Ireland

INTRODUCTION

Abdominal aortic aneurysm (AAA) is considered a chronic degenerative disease with a predisposition to gradual enlargement and eventual rupture. The mortality of conventional open repair (OR) of ruptured abdominal aortic aneurysm (rAAA) remains around 41% despite a constant, albeit slow, improvement in mortality of around 3.5% per decade (1). Although it has been speculated that patient selection may account for some of this steady improvement, Bown et al. (1) were unable to demonstrate any clear association with preoperative selection, intraoperative or postoperative factors. In addition to this persistent high mortality, recovery amongst the survivors may be protracted with prolonged stay in the intensive therapy unit (ITU) and in hospital.

During the last decade, the use of endovascular repair (EVR) has become increasingly popular in the management of elective AAA. The debate as to whether EVR has an advantage in elective cases remains unresolved, despite the two multicenter trials in The Netherlands and the U.K. demonstrating that EVR was associated with a lower aneurysm-related postoperative mortality up to two years and three years, respectively (2,3). Given the high mortality of rAAA, there has been a reasonable expectation that the option of EVR may lead to a significant improvement in perioperative death. Since the first published report by Yusuf et al. (4) in 1994 on the use of emergency EVR (eEVR) on rAAA, there have been a small number of case series reporting both feasibility and putative benefit in reducing morbidity and mortality compared to OR (4–8).

At present, the undoubted theoretical attractions of eEVR for ruptured aneurysms have still to be confirmed in practice: there may be a possible reduction in mortality rates and in ITU/hospital stay, but it appears likely that the postoperative recovery following eEVR may be attended by just as many complications as following OR (7). Unfortunately, at this stage, even if the results were to demonstrate a clear advantage of eEVR over OR, many vascular units would not currently be in a position to provide a round-the-clock emergency endovascular service. The establishment of an eEVR service is logistically challenging, wholly dependent on enthusiastic and committed personnel, requiring specific equipment and a rigorous attention to protocols and technique. More importantly, even well-established endovascular units have found the provision of an eEVR service difficult and have failed to offer this option of treating rAAA to all their patients (5,9).

INDICATIONS FOR ENDOVASCULAR MANAGEMENT

The option to offer an eEVR service for rAAA depends on a number of factors, most notably the imaging modality, the availability of suitable stent grafts, and the availability of trained and experienced personnel. The decision to seek further imaging to assess stent-graft suitability is a critical first step in the process, and needs careful consideration.

Preoperative Imaging and Patient Selection

Conventional vascular teaching has always been to operate on rAAA as soon as the diagnosis is made, based on clinical findings of abdominal pain, with or without back pain, hypotension, and collapse. eEVR potentially defies this traditional practice by delaying surgery in order to allow further investigations to assess for endovascular suitability, and to arrange for the endovascular option. Resch et al. (9) found a preoperative delay of 11 hours with eEVR compared to one hour with OR, from time of presentation. In the stable patient this delay may be inconsequential, but in the unstable patient any delay in treatment may be difficult to accept and justify, especially when there is the possibility that the patient may in the end be morphologically unsuitable for stent graft. However, the delay with eEVR should improve with experience and the entire process expedited by good teamwork.

If the patient is sufficiently stable, spiral computed tomography (CT) scanning is the current imaging modality of choice, providing information which can allow detailed planning and also confirm the diagnosis. The use of angiography alone has been shown to be feasible by some workers, while others are skeptical of its accuracy in sizing for stent grafts (Fig. 1) (10). Measurements by angiography are intraluminal while CT measurements are made from "adventitia-to-adventitia." The presence of thrombus within the lumen may further compromise the accuracy of angiography. It can be argued that accuracy may not be as important in a life-and-death situation and if angiography were to be used, then slightly more oversizing may be all that is required, and a thin concentric lining of thrombus does not always signify unsuitability (11). A reasonable approach that is adopted by some is to proceed directly to angiography for those patients who are deemed too unstable for CT scan (6,7,9). However, Lloyd et al. (12) have demonstrated that patients with rAAA who do not undergo surgery have a median survival time from admission of about 10 hours, with nearly 90% surviving more than two hours after admission. Based on these data, preoperative CT should be feasible for most patients with rAAA, if this can be performed expeditiously and does not lead to the delay in surgery observed by Resch et al. (9) Therefore, good teamworking, planning, and adherence to a stringent protocol are vital in dealing with patients considered for eEVR. Intravascular ultrasound has been used by some practitioners, but is not a technique with which many are familiar (7).

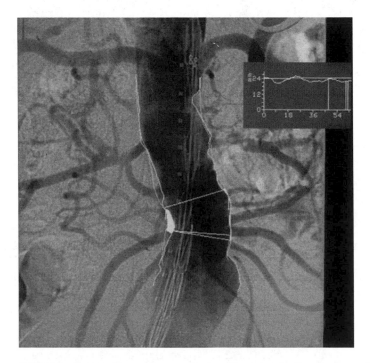

FIGURE 1 Angiography measurements at aortic neck may allow assessment without computed tomography.

TABLE 1 Anatomic Criteria for Endovascular Repair Suitability Based on Computed Tomography Scan (as Recommended by Stent-Graft Manufacturers)

Neck length	>15 mm
Neck diameter	<30 mm
Neck angle	<60°
Iliac diameter	<23 mm
Iliac length	>35 mm
External iliac diameter	>7 mm

Anatomic Suitability

CT scan criteria for elective EVR suitability are generally similar for most of the commercially available graft systems (Table 1). If these criteria were to be applied to the emergency situation, only about 20% of rAAA patients will be suitable for EVR, the largest limiting factor being adverse proximal neck morphology (11). However, the proportion of patients reported to be suitable appears to be higher, as most practitioners are more tolerant of adverse anatomical features that would normally prejudice against EVR in the elective setting (Figs. 2 and 3). Neck diameter of up to 32 mm and iliac diameter of 22 mm are probably still acceptable, as there are commercially available off-the-shelf devices of 36 and 24 mm, allowing for an oversize of approximately 10%, respectively. Although some workers have treated neck lengths <1 cm and achieved hemostatic seal, necks this short should only be attempted in the absence of other unfavorable features such as calcification or angulation (5,10).

While the neck of the aneurysm is the most critical area, at least one iliac system needs to be suitable for delivery of the stent graft. Likewise, the presence of one unfavorable factor in the iliac artery alone may not rule out EVR, but any combination of wall calcification, diameter of ≤7 mm and tortuousity should deter any attempts at stenting (Fig. 4). Short segments of stenosis may be angioplastied and rendered endosuitable. The presence of a unilateral iliac artery aneurysm does not preclude eEVR if the contralateral iliac is suitable, but if the aneurysm involves both iliac systems to their bifurcation, exclusion of the aneurysm complex will be arduous. Coiling of the internal iliac arteries and extending the stent graft beyond the aneurysmal segments to the external iliac artery can be performed, except that this can lead to long delays in excluding the aneurysm and can increase the risk of colonic ischemia (13). Gluteal claudication and impotence may also prove disabling to some patients.

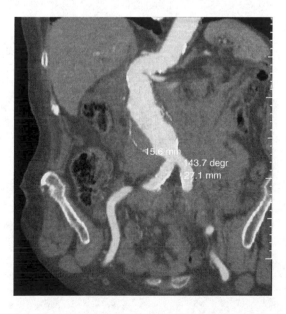

FIGURE 2 Adverse neck anatomy may be tolerated in emergency endovascular repair.

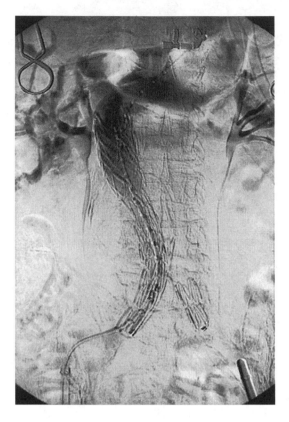

FIGURE 3 Same adverse neck as in Figure 2 but with stent graft in place.

Patient Resuscitation and Anesthesia

Unless the patient is grossly unstable, any attempts at aggressive fluid resuscitation of patients with rAAA must be resisted. The blood pressure should be allowed to stabilize rather than raised above the level at initial presentation, unless the patient's level of consciousness is affected. The exact criteria for "stability" remain to be defined, with the level of what constitutes

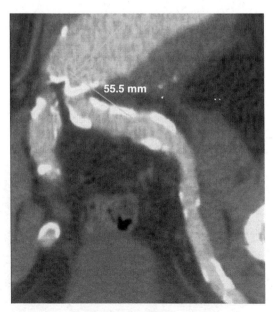

FIGURE 4 Calcified and tortuous iliac unsuitable emergency endovascular repair.

"hypotensive" varying among practitioners, and ranges from 50 to 100 mmHg (5,6,14,15). The level of consciousness and the development of cardiac dysrhythmia are useful guides (11). There is compelling evidence in animal studies and in trauma patients that the use of "hypotensive resuscitation" or "permissive hypotension" leads to improved survival compared to normotensive or immediate resuscitation (16–18). Permissive hypotension is believed to allow clot formation and avoid coagulopathy which are vital determinants in the outcome of patients with rAAA. Some workers, in fact, recommend the active reduction of systolic pressure to <100 mmHg using nitroprusside infusion although this practice may mask the effect of further blood loss (19).

Patients with rAAA are in a state of compensated shock with maximal vasoconstriction. Induction of general anesthesia is associated with a loss of arterial sympathetic tone and relaxation of the abdominal wall musculature. This causes loss of tamponade, frequently causing complete circulatory collapse and a significant increase in mortality. The type of anesthesia used for eEVR differs from center to center, although the majority of practitioners would attempt the procedure under local anesthesia, at least until the aneurysm is excluded (5,6,9,13,14). In a series by Peppelenbosch et al. (5), 58% of patients had local or regional anesthesia.

The entire eEVR procedure including femorofemoral crossover may be performed under local anesthesia and appropriate level of sedation, avoiding the precipitous hypotension associated with general anesthesia (20). Sedation should be just adequate to enable the patient to be comfortable and serene but still compliant. Unfortunately, some patients can become so agitated and restless that they require general anesthesia. In most of these cases, induction of general anesthesia may be deferred until the stent graft has been deployed and aneurysm excluded (8,18).

Regardless of the type of anesthesia, the patient should always be prepared and draped as for OR, with access to both groins, allowing rapid conversion to OR if required. With experience it is feasible to perform percutaneous access even in hypotensive patients with the aide of an ultrasound machine and closure devices (21). However, at present the closure devices available require placement prior to introduction of any large device, introducing a delay. In any event, surgical exposure of the common femoral arteries is necessary for femorofemoral crossover anastomoses if an aortic uniiliac (AUI) system is used.

TECHNICAL ASPECTS

Operating Room Equipment and Venue

Whether eEVR is performed in a purpose-built endovascular suite or in theater with a mobile c-arm is probably irrelevant, providing the procedure can be carried out safely and effectively, the imaging is optimal, and conversion to open surgery can rapidly be facilitated. Accurate positioning of the graft and the ability to identify and characterize any endoleak precisely and rapidly requires high quality imaging systems and good angiographic techniques.

Adequate operative illumination is mandatory, usually because of the need to perform a femorofemoral bypass when an AUI device is used. Furthermore, with the more adverse anatomy associated with emergency AAA, the potential for adjuvant surgical intervention is quite high during eEVR. There is an increased risk of iliac dissection and distal embolization due to adverse iliac morphology (6,13,14). Conversion to OR will be required if the aneurysm cannot be excluded and the patient fails to stabilize (6). Some patients will develop a profoundly tense abdomen and necessitate prophylactic decompression to prevent abdominal compartment syndrome (ACS) (10).

Type of Stent Graft

There is still much controversy as to whether the bifurcated or AUI stent-graft system is superior for rAAA and the preference again varies from center to center. The overwhelming requirements for any graft system must be simplicity of usage and rapid exclusion of the aneurysm. The AUI system satisfies these conditions, and has the added advantage of requiring

TABLE 2 Emergency Endovascular Repair Stent-Graft Preference of Individual Institutions

Author	AUI	Bifurcated system	Tube grafts
Peppelenbosch et al.	19	5	2
Hinchliffe et al.	20	—	—
Scharrer-Pamler et al.	1	19	4
Resch et al.	12	9	—
Lachat et al.	—	20	1

Abbreviation: AUI, aortic uniiliac.

a smaller "shelf stock" of endovascular devices to allow management of an adequate range of aneurysm morphology. Thus, it is currently the preferred option in many centers (Table 2). There are some commercially available AUI devices which come in two components with a universal joint that will allow the length to be adjusted by "tromboning" the distal iliac extension into the proximal main body as required. Although these attractive features should make the AUI an obvious choice for rAAA, opponents of this system would argue that it necessitates a femorofemoral crossover bypass to revascularize the contralateral leg. This leads to prolongation of the procedure and has the added risk of graft infection and graft thrombosis. However, the extra-anatomical bypass is only performed when the aneurysm is already excluded and the latter two complications are uncommon (13).

Some workers prefer the bifurcated system and certainly, in stable patients, this is unlikely to pose difficulties (20). It will certainly give a more anatomic graft system. Unfortunately, with the unpredictable nature of rAAA, any delay in cannulating the contralateral limb will risk the loss of hemostasis and further blood loss. There is evidence to suggest that delays in cannulating the contralateral limb are associated with an increased risk of ACS (22). Inability to cannulate the contralateral limb may inevitably require conversion with its associated dire consequences (23). To minimize these risks, Jongkind et al. (24) have described a bifurcated graft with a hemostatic valve in the contralateral limb stump. The presence of the hemostatic valve will allow rapid exclusion of the aneurysm and at the same time avoid the need for an extra-anatomical bypass, and its accompanying catalog of problems.

Aortic Occlusion Procedures

These are only necessary when the patient becomes unstable (6,13). An occlusion balloon may be passed into the descending aorta via a transbrachial or transfemoral approach and many different techniques have been proposed (10,25,26). Unfortunately, maintaining the position of the occluding balloon which has been passed via the femoral approach remains a problem due to its tendency to be expelled by the pulsatile force of blood within the abdominal aorta. Passing the balloon over a stiff wire may help but this alone is usually ineffective. Suprarenal occlusion should be avoided as much as possible because of the bulk of visceral tissue that this renders ischemic. In Belfast, infrarenal occlusion is preferred and this may be quickly achieved through a femoral approach without detailed angiography by firstly, passing a balloon over a guidewire through a long 14- or 16-F introducer sheath into the aneurysm sac. The balloon can then be inflated within the aneurysm and advanced with the sheath so that it wedges in the aneurysm neck from below. With the balloon in this position, if a second guidewire has previously been passed, the stent graft can still be delivered into position without having to deflate the balloon. Unfortunately, the balloon requires deflation during deployment of the graft but if catastrophic hypotension ensues, the balloon may be repositioned more proximally.

Some workers, prefer the brachial approach (10,25). Matsuda et al. (23) described a technique of passing the occlusion balloon via the brachial artery down into the aneurysm sack and then pulling back until the balloon is lodged in the aneurysm neck from below. This approach has advantages in that it does not interfere with the passage of devices from the groin, but there is a risk of arterial embolism during manipulation around the aortic arch. The brachial artery may be difficult to access in hypotensive patients and the artery itself can be too small to accommodate a large bore introducer sheath, which is necessary for a balloon catheter.

TROUBLESHOOTING

The presence of an endoleak is a more immediate concern in eEVR than in elective patients. The checklist for endoleaks should be methodical, starting at the proximal neck with anteroposterior and lateral views. It is worth emphasizing again that many rAAA patients have less favorable necks than their elective counterparts and Type I endoleaks will be more common than in elective patients (6,15,22,26). As a result, the use of a balloon expandable Palmaz^{TM} stent (Cordis Corp., Miami, Florida, U.S.A.) as an adjunctive measure is a reasonable proposition to resolve any proximal endoleaks (Figs. 5 and 6). These giant stents are crimped onto large balloons (Cristal Valvoplasty, Balt, Montmorency, France) but can easily be dislodged during its passage through artery and graft unless it is passed through a long, large bore (16 F) sheath to its deployment position.

If there is difficulty identifying the site of a potential proximal endoleak, it is advisable to perform a low-injection rate run within the stent graft. If contrast reflux back to the top of the graft is avoided, a proximal Type I endoleak can be excluded or confirmed, depending on whether the leak persists (Fig. 7). A Type II and IV endoleak may be treated expectantly if the patient remains stable, and some would suggest intervention at one month if such an endoleak persists (5). Type III leaks are unusual, unless the overlap between the two components of the stent graft is inadequate. However, Type I and Type III endoleaks will require immediate intervention.

After the above checklist has been exhausted, and Type I and III leaks excluded, if a small endoleak is still visible it is acceptable to speculate a degree of Type IV endoleak. The latter is probably more commonly seen in rAAA than in elective cases because of hemodilution and coagulopathy, which are consequent on the large volumes of blood loss and the fluid given for resuscitation. In these circumstances, if the patient remains stable it is reasonable to complete the procedure and reimage a couple of days postoperatively using a duplex ultrasound or CT scan. If the patient becomes unstable at any stage, reintervention including conversion to OR may be necessary.

In the presence of continuing instability, it is possible to reinflate an occlusion balloon in the proximal neck of the graft, preserving renal and mesenteric perfusion. However, beware the

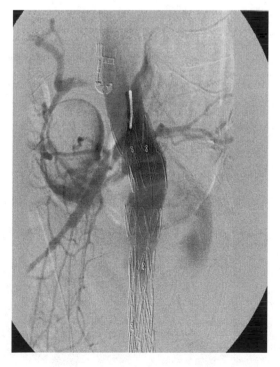

FIGURE 5 Type I endoleak in emergency endovascular repair.

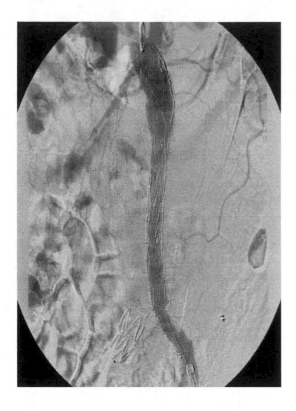

FIGURE 6 Type I endoleak (as seen in Fig. 5) successfully treated by Palmaz stent.

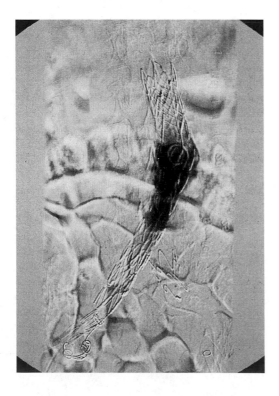

FIGURE 7 Contrast injected inside stent graft identifies Type IV endoleak.

water-hammer effect of this procedure, which may dislodge the stent graft from the aneurysm neck. A systematic approach to investigating continuing blood loss should be adopted, including a check of the rest of the aortic segments. Nevertheless, it is important to bear in mind that ruptured aneurysm in any circumstances will carry significant mortality, that the risk of EVR failure will be greater than in elective cases, especially when patients with less than ideal anatomy are to be offered eEVR. In these situations, it might be best to convert to OR earlier rather than later (6).

CURRENT RESULTS

Postoperative Recovery and Complications

The image of a patient able to eat and mobilize the day after surgery, has been used to champion eEVR as a better technique of repairing rAAA than OR (4). Although there are many anecdotal reports of patients recovering rapidly following eEVR without the need to stay in intensive care unit, the physiological stress suffered by these patients must not be taken lightly. The amount of blood lost by patients undergoing eEVR is often underestimated by the immeasurable volume concealed within abdomen. The hypotension during induction of general anesthesia for OR, which indicates significant hypovolemia, may not occur during eEVR if this is performed under local anesthesia. Nevertheless, the physiological stress that accompanies rAAA, even if repaired endovascularly, may still lead to the same spectrum of complications that is often associated with OR. In addition, there are also potential problems that are unique to eEVR that must be recognized.

One obvious potential drawback of eEVR is failure to successfully exclude the aneurysm sac resulting in continued blood loss. If this is subtle it can be difficult to detect at the time of surgery and only manifest as an inability to maintain a stable blood pressure during the recovery phase. Blood loss may be exacerbated by the presence of coagulopathy, which can also perpetuate the endoleak (5). The prophylactic use of clotting factors and fresh frozen plasma should always be considered in patients who require large volumes of fluid and blood replacement. In fact, some workers administer these blood factors in the majority of their patients, recognizing the problems associated with established coagulopathy (15). There is also evidence that presence of coagulation defect may also predispose to the development of ACS (22).

Most patients presenting with rAAA are elderly and often have other comorbidities that may be unknown even to the patient. The presence of these comorbid conditions will serve to delay recovery and lead to a poorer outcome, and could well have accounted for the 45% mortality observed by Hinchliffe et al. (6). Many of their patients were unfit for OR and this is reflected by the number of patients who died from failure of various organs.

Cardiovascular events, pulmonary complications and renal impairment account for the majority of the morbidity seen postoperatively. In the series by Scharrer-Pamler et al. (23), myocardial infarction was responsible for 75% of deaths and Peppelenbosch et al. (5) found in their series, cardiac events contributed to one-fourth of all complications. Renal impairment may affect up to 33% of patients following eEVR (6,14). It is likely that the hypotensive insult, large doses of contrast and inadvertent coverage of the renal arteries may aggravate latent renal impairment (9). Fortunately, the majority of patients escape without requiring long-term renal dialysis although there is a small proportion who will subsequently suffer a fatal outcome (14). In addition, the combination of hypotension, occlusion of the internal iliac arteries in some patients and increased abdominal compartment pressure can compromise mesenteric blood flow with the subsequent development of bowel ischemia (5,6).

Another underdiagnosed complication that may occur following eEVR is ACS (10,14,22). This occurs because of an increase in intraabdominal pressure due to blood within the abdominal cavity and intestinal distension, which may be precipitated by the large volume of fluid infused and ischemia-reperfusion injury. Factors found to increase the risk of ACS following eEVR (22) are: (*i*) the need for aortic occlusion balloon, (*ii*) an increase in activated partial thromboplastin time, (*iii*) large volume of blood transfusion, and (*iv*) delay in cannulating the contralateral limb. Failure to recognize and treat ACS will result in increased risk of renal impairment, visceral and intestinal ischemia, respiratory failure and death. There is a likelihood that some of the multiple organ dysfunction syndromes observed following eEVR may have resulted from unrecognized ACS. The possibility of acute ACS should be assumed if intraabdominal pressure is ≥ 20 mmHg, associated with diminishing urinary output and increasing airways pressure. If this is suspected an abdominal decompression must be considered (10,22,27). It is however, plausible to treat ACS nonsurgically by intubation, relaxation of abdominal muscles and hemofiltration (14).

Wound complications are not uncommon following eEVR, ranging from hematoma to deep graft infection. The development of perigraft collection has been observed in the tract of the femorofemoral crossover bypass. The majority of perigraft collections are sterile but infection of the femorofemoral crossover graft can develop and the prophylactic use of antibiotics should be considred (5).

The more unfavorable anatomy of rAAA will predispose to stent graft complications (5,28). In addition, the aneurysm neck of rAAA has been found to dilate at a greater rate than elective AAA (29). As a result, the cumulative risk of secondary procedures, was found to be around 35% at two years with a late conversion rate to OR of 9% due to migration. Consequently, there is a temptation to counter these potential complications by increasing the percentage oversize of the stent graft (29). However, greater oversizing may cause more dilatation as the radial force of self-expanding stents is proportional to the percentage of oversize.

In view of the adverse anatomy and high incidence of complications, it has been proposed that eEVR should be considered a temporizing procedure, used to convert an acute unstable situation to a controlled stable one, to allow the patient to be optimized for late open conversion if necessary (26). Although this contentious practice may be a logical proposal in fit patients who have evidence of irredeemable stent graft complication and adverse anatomy, it may be difficult in those who have multiple comorbidities. Nevertheless, in patients who are unfit, it is possible to limit the extent of open conversion by using the stent graft as the conduit and suturing the graft to the neck of the aneurysm and securing the junction of the different components. This will avoid the need to cross-clamp the aorta and replace the stent graft even though it is advisable to control the aneurysm neck in case the graft were to be displaced accidentally.

Mortality

Reflecting the pattern for OR of rAAA, mortality rates for eEVR differ widely amongst reporting institutions (Table 3). There is no doubt that the approach is different between EVR and OR, even though there are common factors that may determine good or poor outcomes. OR necessitates a long incision followed by cross-clamping of the infrarenal aorta. Identifying the neck of the aneurysm may be made difficult by blood obscuring view and as a result, injury to neighboring structures is common. Proponents of supraceliac clamping of the aorta would argue that identifying and exposing the aorta at this level is easier and safer, but if the blood continues to flood the abdomen, the view would similarly be impeded. The ease of identifying and clamping the infrarenal aorta also depends on aortic morphology. A "reasonable" neck length will be much easier to clamp than if the neck were wide, short, and angulated. Unfortunately, in centers which are championing eEVR, only unstable patients who are actively bleeding and patients who have adverse anatomy of the aneurysm neck and iliac vessels are offered OR. Therefore, these centers reporting their series comparing OR with eEVR are not necessarily comparing like with like. A meta-analysis of the world experience from 48 centers involving 442 patients demonstrated an average mortality of 18% (30). There was however, selective usage of eEVR, and the proportion of stented patients ranged between 18% and 76%. This again illustrates the role of reporting bias and patient selection, especially when most reports were based on patients who were hemodynamically stable and who may otherwise have done just as well with OR.

The one prospective nonrandomized study evaluating the efficacy of the two techniques was an international multicenter trial evaluating the use of eEVR in rAAA, which was an uncontrolled and nonrandomized study (7). However, despite selecting only patients who were hemodynamically and morphologically suitable, it failed to demonstrate any difference in mortality rates between EVR and OR and this has fuelled the controversy further (7).

TABLE 3 Mortality Rate Following Emergency Endovascular Repair

Author	Year of publication	Number of patients	Mortality rate (%)
Ohki et al.	2000	20	10
Hinchliffe et al.	2001	20	45
Yilmaz et al.	2002	24	17
Scharrer-Pamler et al.	2003	24	20
Resch et al.	2003	21	19
Hechelhammer et al.	2005	37	10.8
Peppelenbosch et al.	2005	49	35
Veith World Series	2005	442	18

An intention-to-treat study by the same principal team of investigators demonstrated that overall mortality is reduced as a result of stenting patients who are endosuitable. However, there are a few discrepancies in this report. In the historical control group only 28 patients were diagnosed with rAAA over a two-year period, whereas during the one-year study period 40 patients were diagnosed with rAAA. This is three times the numbers presenting per year before the study was commenced. Not all patients who underwent eEVR had CT angiogram nor open confirmation of rAAA. In addition, only patients who were stable or responded to resuscitation and had favorable anatomy were offered eEVR. In view of these disparities the results of this study should be treated with caution. At best, the study showed that eEVR is feasible in various hospital settings for ruptured aneurysm patients, with at least equivalent short-term outcomes to OR.

CONCLUSION

eEVR has been shown to be a feasible alternative of repairing rAAA although most case series are reported by enthusiasts with a wealth of elective and emergency endovascular experience. Unfortunately, there is no strong evidence yet to support the view that eEVR is better than OR in managing rAAA, especially in unstable patients. It is particularly in this unstable group of patients that eEVR needs to show better outcome before it can supersede the conventional approach. There is currently a multicenter randomized study underway in the Netherlands and its results will be awaited with anticipation. At this stage, more evidence is necessary before any health authority will find the strategic challenge of setting up an emergency endovascular service a worthwhile proposition.

REFERENCES

1. Bown MJ, Sutton AJ, Bell PRF, et al. A meta-analysis of 50 years of ruptured abdominal aortic aneurysm repair. Br J Surg 2002; 89(6):714–30.
2. Blankensteijn JD, de Jong SECA, Prinssen M, et al. Two-year outcomes after conventional or endovascular repair of abdominal aortic aneurysms. N Engl J Med 2005; 352(23):2398–405.
3. EVR Trial Participants. Endovascular aneurysm repair versus open repair in patients with abdominal aortic aneurysm (EVR trial 1): randomized controlled trial. Lancet 2005; 365(9478):2179–86.
4. Yusuf SW, Whitaker SC, Chuter TAM, et al. Emergency endovascular repair of leaking aortic aneurysm. Lancet 1994; 344(8937):1645.
5. Peppelenbosch N, Yilamz N, van Marrewijk M, et al. Emergency treatment of acute symptomatic or ruptured abdominal aortic aneurysm. Outcome of a prospective intent-to-treat by EVR protocol. Eur J Vasc Endovasc Surg 2003; 26(3):303–10.
6. Hinchliffe RJ, Yusuf SW, Macierewicz JA, et al. Endovascular repair of ruptured abdominal aortic aneurysm—a challenge to open repair? Results of a single centre experience in 20 patients Eur J Vasc Endovasc Surg 2001; 22(6):528–34.
7. Peppelenbosch N, Geelkerkeen RH, Soong C, et al. Endograft treatment of ruptured abdominal aortic aneurysm using the Talent AUI system. International multicenter study. Abstract Book. In: Annual Meeting of the American Society for Vascular Surgery, 2005.
8. Hinchliffe RJ, Braithwaite BD, Hopkinson BR. The endovacular management of ruptured abdominal aortic aneurysms. Eur J Vasc Endovasc Surg 2003; 25(3):191–201.
9. Resch T, Malina M, Linbald B, et al. Endovascular repair of ruptured abdominal aortic aneurysms: logistics and short term results. J Endovasc Ther 2003; 10(3):440–6.

10. Ohki T, Veith FJ. Endovascular grafts and other image-guided catheter based adjuncts to improve the treatment of ruptured aortoiliac aneurysms. Ann Surg 2000; 232(4):466–79.
11. Rose DF, Davidson JR, Hinchcliffe RJ, et al. Anatomical suitability of ruptured abdominal aortic aneurysms for endovascular repair. J Endovasc Ther 2003; 10(3):453–7.
12. Lloyd GM, Brown MJ, Norwood MG, et al. Feasibility of preoperative computer tomography in patients with ruptured abdominal aortic aneurysm: a time-to-death study in patients without operation. J Vasc Surg 2004; 39(4):788–91.
13. Yilmaz N, Peppelenbosch N, Cuyper PWM, et al. Emergency treatment of symptomatic or ruptured abdominal aortic aneurysm. The role of endovascular repair. J Endovasc Ther 2002; 9(4):449–57.
14. Lachat ML, Pfammatter Th, Witzke HJ, et al. Endovascular repair with bifurcated stent-grafts under local anaesthesia to improve outcome of ruptured aortiliac aneurysms. Eur J Vasc Endovasc Surg 2002; 23(6):528–36.
15. Veith FJ, Ohki T. Endovascular approaches to ruptured infrarenal aorto-iliac aneurysms. J Cardiovasc Surg (Torino) 2002; 43(3):369–78.
16. Owens T, Watson WT, Prough MD, et al. Limiting initial resuscitation of uncontrolled haemorrhage reduces internal bleeding and subsequent volume requirements. J Trauma 1995; 39(2):200–9.
17. Bickell WH, Wall MJ, Jr., Pepe PE, et al. Immediate versus delayed fluid resuscitation for hypotensive patients with penetrating torso injuries. N Engl J Med 1994; 331(17):1105–9.
18. Roberts K, Revell M, Youssef H et al. Hypotensive rescucitation in patients with ruptured abdominal aortic aneurysm. Eur J Vasc Endovasc Surg 2006; 31:339–44.
19. Peppelenbosch N, Zannetti S, Barbieri B, et al. Endograft treatment in ruptured abdominal aortic aneurysm using the Talent AUI stentgraft system. Design of a feasibility study. Eur J Vasc Endovasc Surg 2004; 27(4):366–71.
20. Verhoeven EL, Prins TR, van den Dungen JJ, et al. Endovascular repair of acute AAAs under local anesthesia with bifurcated endografts: a feasibility study. J Endovasc Ther 2002; 9(2):158–64.
21. Howell M, Villarel R, Krajcer Z. Percutaneous access and closure of femoral artery access sites associated with endoluminal repair of abdominal aortic aneurysms. J Endovasc Ther 2001; 8(1):68–74.
22. Mehta M, Darling RC, III, Roddy SP, et al. Factors associated with abdominal compartment syndrome complicating endovascular repair of ruptured abdominal aortic aneurysm. J Vasc Surg 2005; 42(6):1047–51.
23. Scharrer-Pamler R, Kotsis T, Kapper X, et al. Endovacular stent-graft repair of ruptured aortic aneurysms. J Endovasc Ther 2003; 10(3):447–52.
24. Jongkind V, Diks J, Linsen MA, et al. A temporary hemostatic valve in the short limb of a bifurcated stent-graft to facilitate endovascular repair of ruptured aortic aneurysm: experimental findings. J Endovasc Ther 2005; 12(1):66–9.
25. Matsuda H, Tanaka Y, Hino Y, et al. Transbrachial arterial insertion of aortic occlusion balloon in patients with shock from ruptured abdominal aortic aneurysm. J Vasc Surg 2003; 38(6):1293–6.
26. Malina M, Veith F, Ivancev K, Sonesson B. Balloon occlusion of the aorta during endovascular repair of ruptured abdominal aortic aneurysm. J Endovasc Ther 2005; 12(5):556–9.
27. Meldrum DR, Moore FA, Moore EE, et al. Prospective characterization and selective management of the abdominal compartment syndrome. Am J Surg 1997; 174(6):667–72.
28. Hechelhammer L, Lachat ML, Wildermuth S, et al. Midterm outcome of endovascular repair of ruptured abdominal aortic aneurysms. J Vasc Surg 2005; 41(5):752–7.
29. Badger SA, O'Donnell ME, Makar R, et al. Aortic necks of ruptured abdominal aneurysms dilate more than asymptomatic aneurysms following endovascular repair. J Vasc Surg 2006; 44:244–9.
30. Veith FJ. Update on endovascular repair of ruptured abdominal aortic and thoracic aneurysms: the collected world experience. Vascular 2005; 13:S38–9.

41 | Iliac Artery Aneurysms (Indications for Endovascular Repair, Technical Aspects, Troubleshooting, Current Results, and Comparison with Open Surgery)

T. J. Parkinson, J. D. G. Rose, and M. G. Wyatt
Northern Vascular Centre, Freeman Hospital, Newcastle, U.K.

INTRODUCTION

Iliac artery aneurysms (IAAs) can occur in the presence of abdominal aortic aneurysms (AAAs), but it is uncommon for them to occur in isolation (1). Due to their pelvic anatomy, detection can be difficult, and presentation varied. If treated conservatively IAAs are likely to expand, and ultimately rupture (2). With increasing use of detailed imaging, and less invasive treatment options, the high mortality associated with IAAs (3) may be rectified.

EPIDEMIOLOGY

IAAs occur in 10% to 20% of patients with AAAs, with an overall reported incidence of 0.3% to 2.2% for all intra-abdominal aneurysms (1). Brunkwall et al. (4) studied the autopsy reports and theater records of Malmo for a 15-year period up to 1985. Within a cohort of 26,251 hospital autopsies, 1267 (4.8%) had aortoiliac aneurysms, and only 7 (0.03%) had solitary iliac artery aneurysms (SIAAs). The distribution of these SIAAs included five confined to the common iliac artery, one to the internal and another to the external iliac. The frequency of IAA association with AAAs was 19.7%.

With the advent of better imaging, it has become easier to diagnose IAAs, and follow them on a prospective basis. Vammen et al. (5) reported two studies. In the first one, 5470 men were invited to screening for AAA using ultrasonography. Of the 5470 invited, 4176 (76.1%) attended, with 171 aneurysms detected. Twenty-one (0.5%) of these were referred for surgery, due to an aneurysm diameter exceeding 5 cm. Five (25%) of the 21 also had a common iliac aneurysm, and a further two were referred for surgery due to isolated common iliac aneurysms measuring greater than 3.5 cm in diameter. For common iliac aneurysms requiring surgery, the total prevalence was 0.17%, and for isolated IAAs this was lower at 0.05%.

In the second part of the report, retrospective data from the 350 patients having undergone aneurysm repair between 1989 and 1997 were analyzed. There were 75 patients with IAA, representing an incidence of 18.4 per million per year. Sixty-three of the cases had coexisting aortic and iliac aneurysm, producing an incidence of 15.5 per million per year. The final 12 patients had isolated IAA, producing an incidence of 2.9 per million per year.

ANATOMICAL SITE OF IAAs

The most common site for IAAs is the common iliac artery, with the external iliac the most rarely affected (1). In their series of patients, Greenfield and Richardson (1) reported 55 patients with a total of 72 aneurysms of the iliac arteries. For the common, internal and external arteries, the number of isolated aneurysms were 6, 12 and 0 respectively, while for multiple aneurysms they were 42, 10 and 2 respectively. These results were compared to those of Norman et al. (6), who analyzed the data from an endoluminal stent-graft database of 223 patients and reported 15 cases of internal IAA.

NATURAL HISTORY OF IAAs

The natural history of IAAs is unclear, but is believed to follow that of aortic aneurysms, with increasing diameter being associated with an increased risk of rupture (7). The reported rupture rate varies wildly between studies, with numbers ranging from 14% to 75% of patients (1). Large series (1) have reported rupture rates between 14% and 70%, with an average IAA size at a rupture of 5.6 cm. A recent review revealed that the rupture rate varied between 0% and 82%, with an adjusted total of 31% (97 patients), for a total of 311 patients with 473 IAAs (8).

A recent study has also reported the outcomes of IAAs, with a specific consideration regarding expansion. Santilli et al. (2) reported 189 patients with a total of 323 IAAs that varied from 1.5 to 10 cm. No patients died of ruptured aneurysm (AAA or IAA) during follow-up. Survival rates ranged from 96.3% at one year to 78.2% at three and four years. IAAs were found at multiple sites in 84% of the patients, and 321 of the 323 aneurysms involved the common iliac artery, with one involving the internal iliac and the other the external iliac. All IAAs measuring between 4.0 and 4.9 cm in diameter increased in size during the follow-up period. The expansion rates for aneurysms measuring 3 cm or less at diagnosis were between 0.05 and 0.15 cm/yr, whereas aneurysms 3 cm or larger expanded at between 0.25 to 0.28 cm/ yr ($p < 0.003$). All IAAs had similar expansion rates regardless of their anatomical position.

In this study only 3.1% of IAAs were symptomatic, all being greater than 4 cm in diameter, and only 24 (13%) of the 189 patients had a palpable mass, 72% of those aneurysms being greater than 4 cm in diameter. Based on the above findings, any IAA over 3 cm should be closely monitored with ultrasonography or computed tomography on a six-monthly basis. Due to the high risk of rupture, and increased expansion rates, it is currently recommended that elective repair should be undertaken in good risk patients with an IAA size greater than 3.5 cm (8).

CLINICAL FEATURES

IAAs may be asymptomatic, rupture, or cause symptoms due to their presence in the pelvis. Chronic pain associated with nerve root (sciatica) or visceral compression, iliac-enteric fistulas, claudication, heart failure due to arteriovenous fistulas, urologic obstruction with frequency and urgency have all been reported (1,3). In addition, patients may present with hydrone-phrosis (9), lower limb edema and cellulitis (10) and bleeding hemorrhoids secondary to IAA rupture (11).

CLASSIFICATION OF IAAs AND SUITABILITY FOR REPAIR

The classification for IAAs described by Sandhu et al. (8) is useful when considering the options for open or endovascular repair. These categories are listed below, together with the potential implications for open or endovascular repair.

Category A

These are classified as common iliac aneurysms with a proximal and distal neck length of at least 1 cm, with minimal mural thrombus or calcification in the neck. These patients can receive either open aneurysmorraphy with inlay interposition graft, or endovascular repair with the endograft placed within the common iliac artery. Large variations in diameter between the proximal and distal neck may occasionally dictate the use of a tapered endograft.

Category B

Common iliac aneurysms with an adequate proximal neck, but extending distally to the bifurcation (Fig. 1). Open repair involves proximal anastomosis to the common iliac artery with the distal anastomosis to the iliac bifurcation or external iliac with ligation of the common iliac just proximal to the bifurcation.

Endovascular repair entails endograft placement across the internal iliac, with proximal fixation in the common iliac and distal fixation in the external iliac (Fig. 2). Transcatheter coil embolization of the internal iliac is required, preferably using coils made of nonferromagnetic

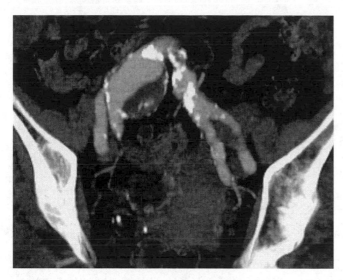

FIGURE 1 A reconstructed computed tomography scan showing a 4.4-cm common iliac artery aneurysm.

metals (such as platinum) that are magnetic resonance compatible. If the ostium of the internal iliac is aneurysmal, then the more distal main stem is coiled, taking care that no more than the proximal portions of any patent outflow branches are blocked.

Modern embolic devices, such as the Amplatzer Vascular Plug® (AGA Medical Corporation, Plymouth, Minnesota, U.S.A.), are now available in small sizes, and these can abolish the need for multiple embolization coils. Assuming the outflow of the internal iliac is blocked and the ostium is to be covered with stent graft, then it is not necessary to pack the aneurysm with coil.

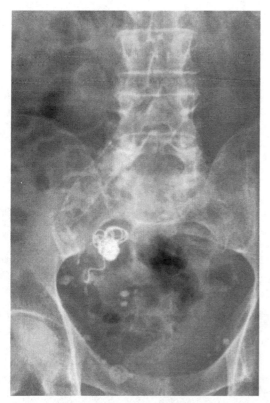

FIGURE 2 Plain abdominal film showing a straight interposition graft used for the treatment of a common iliac artery aneurysm (IAA). Note coiling of the internal IAA.

Category C

Common iliac aneurysms with an adequate proximal neck, but extending distally beyond the bifurcation to involve both external and internal iliac vessels. Open repair is similar to above. If the proximal internal iliac is aneurysmal, then a jump graft can be performed to the distal internal iliac. If this is not the case, the IAA should be excluded by opening the sac, and oversewing the branches from inside the aneurysm.

Endovascular repair would follow the same pattern as for category B.

In addition, a combination of open and endovascular repair can be considered, with coil embolization of the internal iliac artery and open aneurysm repair.

Category D

The common iliac artery is normal, but the internal iliac artery is aneurysmal. Open repair involves exclusion and oversewing of the internal iliac branches from within. If the internal iliac origin is aneurysmal, then an inlay graft bridging the common and external iliac can be used.

Endovascular repair may require the placement of an endograft across the internal iliac, following coil occlusion of the aneurysm (Fig. 3). Alternatively, where there is sufficient proximal and distal "neck" in the internal iliac main stem, the aneurysm may be excluded by placing embolization coils at either end, or by packing the sac with embolic material. The current preference to pack the aneurysm sac would be to use multiple (30 cm) platinum coils, in the largest sizes initially, and then gradually reduced in diameter to allow tight packing. Liquid embolic material is not advisable in these circumstances.

Category E

Common iliac aneurysms with an inadequate proximal neck, those which are bilateral, and those associated with AAA are placed within this category. Open repair involves a bifurcated aortoiliac graft with a variable distal configuration. Endovascular repair follows much the same route with either a bifurcated endograft (Fig. 4), or aortouniiliac graft placement, contralateral iliac occlusion followed by femoral–femoral crossover.

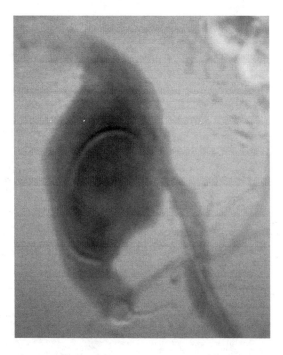

FIGURE 3 Digital subtraction angiogram showing the early stages of coil embolization of an internal iliac artery aneurysm.

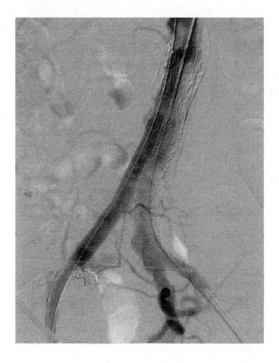

FIGURE 4 Operative angiogram showing a bifurcated aortic graft used for the treatment of an abdominal aortic aneurysm and 4-cm right common iliac artery aneurysm.

In patients suitable for repair, the type of procedure is dependent on the patients' health status, the number and anatomy of aneurysms, the accessibility of the aneurysm, and any involvement of the aorta (8).

OPEN SURGICAL REPAIR

Mortality remains variable for open repairs, with figures ranging from 0% to 42% for elective operations, and 0% to 80% for emergencies (3). An overall analysis including 367 patients, with 500 IAAs revealed an emergency mortality of 40%, an elective mortality of 7%.

ENDOVASCULAR REPAIR

With the emergence of endovascular technology in the 1980s, it soon became possible to treat IAAs with less invasive techniques than open surgery. In 1983, Perdue et al. (12) reported the transcatheter embolization of an internal IAA with Gianturco Embolization Coils® (Cook Medical, Bloomington, Indiana, U.S.A.) and gelfoam. It has long been clear that such minimally invasive treatments may be of great value in those patients with significant medical comorbidities. However, the level of evidence regarding the routine use of such techniques is poor.

Parsons et al. (13) reported a series of patients treated over a period of four years. There were 25 patients, with 24 common and 4 internal iliac aneurysms. Combined aneurysms were noted in three of the patients. The mean preoperative aneurysm size was 4.4 cm (range 3.1–7.8 cm). Postoperatively, 90% of the patients showed a decrease in aneurysm size (mean 5%), and no aneurysm was shown to expand.

Cumulative survival rates following operation were 100% up to nine months, falling to 86% at 45 months. One patient was shown to have rupture of a successfully excluded 8-cm isolated common iliac aneurysm at 17 months, but recovered following open repair. In total there were four (12%) procedure-related complications and no procedure-related deaths.

Cardon et al. (14) presented similar results. For 27 patients undergoing endovascular repair, one death was documented, but there was an immediate failure rate of 18.5%, including two open conversions and two postoperative endoleaks. In the follow-up period (mean 11.8

months, range 6–19 months), 22 of the 24 grafts remained patent, but with one thrombosis and one stenosis, treated by operation and angioplasty respectively.

Cormier et al. (15) reported on 32 patients, with 34 IAAs. Stent deployment was successful in 33. The internal iliac artery, originally patent in 28 cases, could be preserved in only four either because preoperative Gianturco coil treatment was required, or because stent occlusion of the internal iliac artery ostium was undertaken. Postoperatively, there was an endoleak in two patients (one requiring placement of a second stent), late reperfusion of an unembolized internal iliac artery in one case (requiring surgical ligation), and two cases of iliac artery stenosis >70% (both requiring balloon dilation). Buttock claudication occurred in six patients and was disabling in four, but all cases eventually resolved within 13 months. Out of the 34 IAAs, there were five late complications.

A recent review of the available published series has shown the perioperative mortality to range between 0% and 4%, with only one death among a total of 106 patients (117 IAAs, 111 operations) (8,15).

RECOMMENDATIONS FOR TREATMENT

From the literature, the endovascular option seems to convey a smaller mortality risk than open surgical repair of IAAs. However, there is concern regarding the development of long-term complications such as kinking and endoleak formation, as was seen with the early aortic endografts. These grafts require close and lifelong follow-up, and to date there are no data with respect to their relative cost effectiveness when compared to open repair.

The complications of impotence and gastrointestinal ischemia are well known following both internal iliac embolization and open surgery for iliac aneurysms. A recent case (16) has also highlighted the rare, but catastrophic complication of unilateral lower limb paralysis (due to ischemia of the lumbosacral plexus) following unilateral coil embolization of an internal iliac artery.

Due to the rarity of the condition, all of the published data have been derived from small prospective or retrospective case series. While a large multicenter randomized trial of open versus endovascular repair would be ideal for an accurate comparison of the two treatments, it is unlikely that enough patients could be recruited, even in a multicenter setting.

There may be a further role for endovascular repair in the selective treatment of medically unfit patients with contained iliac ruptures (17). This could lead to a significant reduction in the mortality rate from ruptures, when compared to open repair. Nevertheless, the rarity and severity of such cases again prevents accurate comparison to more traditional methods.

Despite a lack of long-term evidence, the development of endovascular techniques continues. Vascular plugs have been used in place of coils to occlude the iliac segments (18,19), with the potential benefit of a reduction in the risk of complications such as internal iliac ischemia, as well as reduced cost.

Nevertheless, with the continuing development of endografts and analysis of operative results, it seems likely that endovascular repair will eventually prove itself a safe and reliable method of IAA treatment.

REFERENCES

1. Richardson JW, Greenfield LJ. Natural history and management of iliac aneurysms. J Vasc Surg 1988; 8(2):165–71.
2. Santilli SM, Wernsing SE, Lee ES. Expansion rates and outcomes for iliac artery aneurysms. J Vasc Surg 2000; 31(1 Pt 1):114–21.
3. Krupski WC, Selzman CH, Floridia R, et al. Contemporary management of isolated iliac aneurysms. J Vasc Surg 1998; 28(1):1–11 (Discussion 11–13).
4. Brunkwall J, Hauksson H, Bengtsson H, et al. Solitary aneurysms of the iliac arterial system: an estimate of their frequency of occurrence. J Vasc Surg 1989; 10(4):381–4.
5. Vammen S, Lindholt J, Henneberg EW, et al. A comparative study of iliac and abdominal aortic aneurysms. Int Angiol 2000; 19(2):152–7.
6. Norman PE, Lawrence-Brown M, Semmens J, et al. The anatomical distribution of iliac aneurysms: is there an embryological basis? Eur J Vasc Endovasc Surg 2003; 25(1):82–4.

7. Dix FP, Titi M, Al-Khaffaf H. The isolated internal iliac artery aneurysm—a review. Eur J Vasc Endovasc Surg 2005; 30(2):119–29.
8. Sandhu RS, Pipinos II. Isolated iliac artery aneurysms. Semin Vasc Surg 2005; 18(4):209–15.
9. O'Driscoll D, Fitzgerald E. Isolated iliac artery aneurysms with associated hydronephrosis. J R Coll Surg Edinb 1999; 44(3):197–9.
10. Bhasin N, Jones SM, Patel J, et al. Internal iliac artery aneurysm—a cause of leg swelling and cellulitis. J R Soc Med 2004; 97(10):483–4.
11. Singh A, Amin A, Riaz AA, et al. Bleeding prolapsed hemorrhoids as a presentation of ruptured internal iliac artery aneurysm: report of a case. Surg Today 2005; 35(10):893–5.
12. Perdue GD, Mittenthal MJ, Smith RB, III, et al. Aneurysms of the internal iliac artery. Surgery 1983; 93(2):243–6.
13. Parsons RE, Marin ML, Veith FJ, et al. Midterm results of endovascular stented grafts for the treatment of isolated iliac artery aneurysms. J Vasc Surg 1999; 30(5):915–21.
14. Cardon JM, Cardon A, Joyeux A, et al. Endovascular repair of iliac artery aneurysm with endoprosystem I: a multicentric French study. J Cardiovasc Surg (Torino) 1996; 37(3 Suppl. 1):45–50.
15. Cormier F, Al Ayoubi A, Laridon D, et al. Endovascular treatment of iliac aneurysms with covered stents. Ann Vasc Surg 2000; 14(6):561–6.
16. Kritpracha B, Comerota AJ. Unilateral lower extremity paralysis after coil embolization of an internal iliac artery aneurysm. J Vasc Surg 2004; 40(4):819–21.
17. Ricci MA, Najarian K, Healey CT. Successful endovascular treatment of a ruptured internal iliac aneurysm. J Vasc Surg 2002; 35(6):1274–6.
18. Ha CD, Calcagno D. Amplatzer vascular plug to occlude the internal iliac arteries in patients undergoing aortoiliac aneurysm repair. J Vasc Surg 2005; 42(6):1058–62.
19. Diehm N, Kickuth R, Silvestro A, et al. Endovascular treatment of an internal iliac artery aneurysm using a nitinol vascular occlusion plug. J Endovasc Ther 2005; 12(5):616–9.

42 | Aneurysms of the Lower Limb

Ignace Tielliu, Eric Verhoeven, Clark Zeebregts, and Jan van den Dungen
Department of Surgery, Division of Vascular Surgery, University Medical Center Groningen, Groningen, The Netherlands

INTRODUCTION

Aneurysms of the lower limb arteries are uncommon. They usually involve the popliteal artery (PA) and the common femoral artery (CFA). Aneurysms involving the superficial femoral (SFA) and deep femoral arteries are rare. The main treatment of CFA aneurysms is conventional surgery. As the main role of endovascular therapy is in the treatment of popliteal artery aneurysms (PAAs), the majority of the following account is devoted to a description of the management of PAAs.

COMMON FEMORAL ARTERY

CFA aneurysms may be true aneurysms arising de novo or they may be pseudoaneurysms related to surgical anastomoses or a previous arterial puncture. Saccular aneurysms with a narrow neck, which are the usual type related to arterial puncture, can usually be treated percutaneously by the injection of thrombin into the aneurysm sac (chap. 48). The majority of true and anastomotic aneurysms are fusiform and are not amenable to thrombin embolization. Unlike peripheral aneurysms in other locations, CFA aneurysms cannot be treated by endovascular placement of a stent graft because the device would likely occlude or fracture because of repetitive movement at the hip joint. Moreover, placement of a covered stent would probably result in occlusion of the deep or superficial femoral artery. Therefore, the vast majority of CFA aneurysms are treated by open repair and placement of an interposition graft.

POPLITEAL ARTERY

PAAs occur predominantly in men older than 60 years. Cohort series of conservative management indicate that symptoms occur in up to 70% of patients (1). Symptomatic aneurysms may present with ischemia resulting from peripheral embolization, acute thrombosis of the aneurysm, or local compression of nerves and deep veins. Rupture of a PAA is very uncommon.

The occurrence of peripheral embolization into the calf vessels is related to aneurysm size, distortion of the PA, and the presence of thrombus lining the wall of the aneurysm (2). Acute embolization is a potentially devastating complication, which may lead to acute critical limb ischemia with the risk of subsequent amputation if prompt treatment is not instituted. Chronic embolization results in progressive obstruction of the crural vessels and patients usually present with progressive intermittent claudication. The presence of occlusion of most or all of the runoff vessels makes treatment by surgical bypass problematic because of the lack of distal vessels to anastomose a graft to. Clearly, the best way to deal with these complications is to prevent them by treating the aneurysms before they cause symptoms.

Patients who present with symptoms of acute critical limb ischemia should be assessed for the presence of a PAA. If a PAA is diagnosed by a duplex ultrasound, consideration should be given to transarterial thrombolysis to see if any of the occluded tibial vessels can be reperfused prior to definitive treatment of the aneurysm itself. Most interventionalists prefer to thrombolyze the occluded runoff vessels rather than the thrombosed popliteal aneurysm itself because of a risk of further distal embolization. After improvement of the runoff, endovascular or surgical bypass of the aneurysm can be performed (3–5).

Indications for Intervention

While it is generally accepted that a PAA should be treated to prevent limb-threatening complications such as thrombosis and distal embolization, the ideal timing for elective treatment is not defined. Many vascular specialists believe that PAAs larger than 2 cm should be treated (6–9). However, others believe that any intervention should be delayed until they attain a diameter of 3 cm, unless there is a large amount of thrombus or significant distortion of the PA (2,10).

Surgical Repair of PAA

For decades, open repair has been the golden standard of treatment for PAAs. The most common surgical procedures involve either medial or posterior approaches to the aneurysm. Until recently, the majority of surgeons preferred the medial approach with proximal and distal ligation of the aneurysm. However, due to evidence that the medial approach procedure can lead to further aneurysm growth and rupture due to retrograde filling of the aneurysm through genicular side branches, the posterior approach with exclusion of the aneurysm and an interposition graft is preferred by many surgeons.

Endovascular Repair of PAA

This involves the exclusion of the aneurysm by placement of a stent graft starting from the normal caliber artery proximally onto a normal artery distal to the aneurysm. The normal caliber arteries above and below the aneurysm are known as the proximal and distal landing zones.

Contraindications for endovascular repair are the lack of proximal or distal landing zones (Fig. 1), or compromised inflow or outflow arteries. In our practice, we have treated several cases with only one good outflow artery, but we consider that the quality of the inflow vessels is very important and we always optimize the inflow vessels by angioplasty, stenting or conventional surgery if they are significantly diseased. If the inflow cannot be improved, an endovascular graft is unlikely to remain patent for long and these patients are not treated by endovascular repair. A large discrepancy in the diameter between the proximal and distal landing zones is a technical contraindication. If the difference in diameter between the landing zones is only a few millimeters, this can be managed by placement of more than one contiguous overlapping stent graft of slightly different diameters. If there is a much larger discrepancy (greater than 3 mm), placement of overlapping grafts of significantly different diameters may result in a fold in one of the grafts which may cause an endoleak between the adjacent endografts. Graft infolding may obstruct the lumen and lead to occlusion of the endograft.

Preoperative Work-Up

The PA can be imaged by several modalities including conventional angiography, computed tomography (CT) angiography, magnetic resonance (MR) angiography and ultrasound. At the present time, duplex ultrasound is the main imaging method used by most departments to confirm the clinical diagnosis of a PAA.

When the patient is admitted for elective treatment, the duplex examination should be repeated to confirm that the aneurysm remained patent. During this second duplex examination, the diameters of the proximal and distal landing zones of the PA are measured from the intima

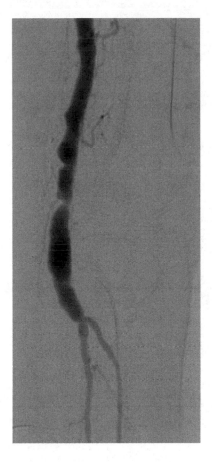

FIGURE 1 Angiogram of a popliteal artery showing inadequate landing zone for endovascular repair due to extension of the aneurysm up to the popliteal bifurcation.

of one wall to the intima of the opposite wall. The choice of the stent-graft diameter is based on these measurements, together with data from the preoperative and intraoperative angiogram.

In addition, marks are drawn on the patient's leg to indicate the proximal and distal extent of the aneurysm. This is because mural thrombus in the aneurysm sac may obscure the differentiation between the normal vessel and aneurysmal vessel during intraoperative angiography.

Although it is possible to plan the procedure in terms of device selection on the basis of the duplex imaging alone, conventional angiography with a calibrated pigtail provides the optimal information for this purpose. In addition to information on the length of the aneurysm to be stented, and the caliber of the proximal and distal landing zones, important information on the quality of the iliac and femoral inflow, and the crural outflow vessels is provided by this procedure. CT and MR angiography can also provide this information, although conventional calibrated angiography is preferable.

Using the imaging information, stent grafts are selected to adequately bridge the distance between the proximal and distal landing zones, so that the aneurysm is excluded. If more than one endograft is required, allowance should be made for the overlap distance required between adjacent devices. The diameter of the stent grafts should be oversized by 10% to 20% in relation to the diameters of the landing zones. A similar degree of oversizing should be applied between adjacent endografts to ensure an adequate seal.

Stent Grafts

Clearly, a stent graft which has to cross the knee joint must have specific properties. The stent has to withstand the repetitive flexion-extension movements associated with daily life.

In addition, it must be resistant to kinking in response to knee flexion of up to at least 90°. Finally, it should be available in a range of appropriate diameters and lengths. The largest experience so far for this indication has been gained with nitinol-expanded polytetrafluoroethylene (ePTFE) stent grafts (Hemobahn® and Viabahn®, W.L. Gore, Flagstaff, Arizona, U.S.A.) (11,12). These are self-expanding stent grafts, which have an ePTFE lining on the inside of the nitinol stent.

Endovascular Procedure

Access to the femoral artery through a small cutdown under local anesthesia is our preferred method, although the procedure can be performed percutaneously using arterial closure devices. The CFA is punctured and a 30-cm long sheath is introduced into the SFA. Five thousand units of heparin are injected. A calibrated straight tip angiocatheter is introduced over the guidewire and is positioned with the tip at the level of the tibioperoneal trunk. The pencil markings on the leg of the patient are supported by radiopaque needles in order to visualize them by fluoroscopy. A final length estimation of the required length of endograft coverage is obtained by angiography performed through the sheath in conjunction with the radiopaque markers on the catheter and skin.

Endografts are placed from the distal to the proximal landing zones. A road map may be useful during endograft deployment, although the skin markers defining the landing zones are usually adequate. Several stent grafts are often required because the maximal available length of one stent graft is usually insufficient to cover the distance (Fig. 2). In our unpublished series of 66 aneurysms, the mean total stented length was 20.2 cm (range 10–34) and a mean of two stent grafts (range, 1–4) were used. Stent grafts of different diameters can be deployed to overcome discrepancies in landing zone diameter as described previously. The length of

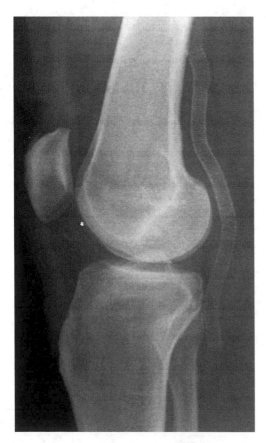

FIGURE 2 X-ray of the knee in lateral view showing two overlapping stent grafts in the popliteal artery.

overlap between adjacent endografts should be at least 3 cm to avoid disconnection. In respect to the overlap between two stent grafts, the smallest diameter endograft should be deployed first followed by the wider diameter endografts to enable a seal. This is usually the most distal endograft. If the smaller caliber endograft is deployed into a wider endograft, there will obviously be a leak.

Accurate positioning of the stent graft in the distal PA can be difficult with the Hemobahn because deployment commences at the proximal end of the endograft. When the release thread is pulled, both the catheter and the distal stent graft are placed under tension which can result in deployment of the endograft a little more proximal than is desired. In some patients, this effect can result in the device being totally deployed within the aneurysm sac, especially in cases when the aneurysm is large and without thrombus. (Fig. 3) This phenomenon occurred twice in our series. To prevent this problem, it is advisable to use a stiff guidewire (e.g., Amplatz Super Stiff, Boston Scientific Corp, Galway, Ireland) to provide added support. Finally, the Viabahn may be better than the Hemobahn for deployment at the distal landing zone because deployment commences distally first which reduces the effect described above.

After deployment, the endografts are dilated with percutaneous transluminal angioplasty (PTA) balloons of the same size, in order to ensure that the endografts are closely applied to the wall of the artery and to eliminate possible folds within the endografts. It is important to examine the stent grafts meticulously with fluoroscopy only, to detect any folding of the endografts (Fig. 4). Balloon dilatation of the stent grafts usually solves this problem and limits any future risk of thrombosis. Finally, a completion angiogram is performed and should demonstrate complete exclusion of the aneurysm and intact outflow.

Postoperative Treatment and Follow-Up

Antiplatelet therapy is be commenced on the day of the intervention. Patients are administered a daily dose of 100 mg acetyl salicylic acid. We also recommend that patients take clopidogrel

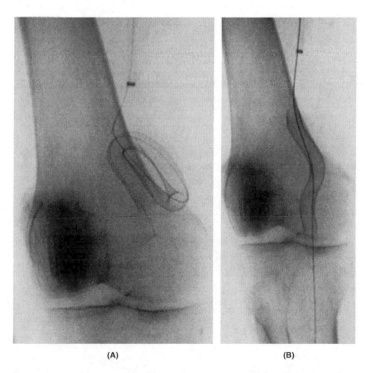

(A) (B)

FIGURE 3 **(A)** Stent graft curled up in large aneurysm sac which could be stretched with a catheter over the guidewire **(B)**.

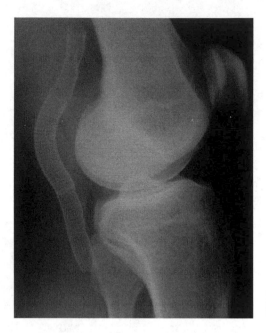

FIGURE 4   Fold in proximal part of Hemobahn® (W.L. Gore, Flagstaff, Arizona) stent graft.

75 mg daily for about six weeks after the procedure as this proved to be a significant factor for maintaining patency of the stent graft in our prospective series (11). However there are no data to indicate the optimal dose or length of treatment required (12).

Follow-up is essential to confirm continued exclusion of the aneurysm, and any complications that might arise. Patients are followed up by duplex ultrasound and plain radiography of the knee every six months for the first two years and annually thereafter. The role of duplex is the detection of endoleaks and the assessment of the PAA sac diameter. The radiographs are performed with the knee in extension (anteroposterior and lateral views) and in 90° flexion (lateral view) to detect migration, kinking, and fractures of the stent graft. The radiograph performed immediately after implantation of the endografts is used as a reference for later comparison. Bony landmarks are helpful for the assessment of migration.

Complications

Occlusion

The most feared complication is occlusion. In our current series of 66 aneurysms treated with stent grafts, 9 of the 16 occlusions (56%) resulted in limb ischemia. The reasons for occlusion are not always clear: stenosis due to intimal hyperplasia, inadequate anticoagulation, mechanical problems due to knee movement, and insufficient outflow, can all play a role. If a patient with occluded endografts presents with only mild or moderate claudication, treatment is not mandatory. Patients presenting with more severe ischemia should be treated immediately. Transarterial thrombolysis may be effective at clearing acute thrombus and restoring patency to the graft and runoff vessels. After patency has been restored, the underlying cause should be treated. In our series, none of the occlusions resulted in amputation.

To avoid mechanical obstruction, patients are advised not to bend their knee more than 90° for a prolonged period of time. The impact of this measure on the prevention of occlusions is unclear.

Migration

Migration of stent grafts may occur at the landing zones and at the overlap zones. Migration is usually easily diagnosed on the lateral radiographs of the knee with the use of bony landmarks.

Treatment involves placement of additional endografts to either extend graft coverage at the landing zones or to bridge disconnected endografts (Fig. 5).

Stenosis

Stenosis can occur at the proximal or the distal border of the stent graft. It is usually caused by intimal hyperplasia. In our series, about 8% of cases presented with a variable degree of stenosis. The patients who had significant stenoses were successfully treated by PTA.

Type II Endoleak

Continuous flow in the aneurysm sac after open repair with a bypass graft is described in approximately 30% of the cases (13–16). In a report of 26 PAAs treated by proximal and distal ligation and bypass grafting, continuous intrasac flow was diagnosed in 38% of the cases with an increase in the aneurysm diameter in 35% of the cases (13). Persistent flow within the sac through collaterals may also occur after endovascular exclusion of the aneurysm, which is easily visualized by a duplex examination. If duplex ultrasound shows either a Type II endoleak or an enlarging aneurysm sac without an endoleak, patients should undergo either conventional angiography or CT angiography. We have seen two Type II endoleaks in our series of 66 stented aneurysms and one enlarging sac without an endoleak (17). In the two cases of Type II endoleak, successful treatment by thrombin injection was undertaken. In one case, the endoleak disappeared and the aneurysm reduced in size. In the other case, treatment by thrombin injection was technically successful, but there is no available follow-up information for this patient.

Stent Fracture

Stent grafts that are placed around the knee joint are prone to material failure. In our published series, two stent fractures were described out of the 57 treated aneurysms (11). Since then, as our series increased to 66 treated aneurysms, one more stent-graft fracture has been diagnosed. All of the stent fractures were situated at or near to the major hinge point of the PA. To avoid stent fractures it is wise to keep overlap zones away from this major hinge point. In healthy individuals the major hinge point is usually situated at the level of the medial supracondylar tubercle which corresponds to the upper border of the patella (with the leg in extension) (18). However, atherosclerosis or the presence of an aneurysm may alter the position of this major

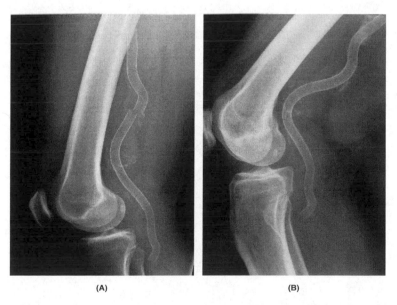

(A) (B)

FIGURE 5 (A) X-ray of the knee showing migration in the overlap zone with a disconnection and (B) after correction with a bridging stent graft.

hinge point. Therefore, a preoperative dynamic angiogram may help to assess the exact location of the popliteal hinge points. This may enable improved planning for the positioning of the overlap zones to avoid kinking and fractures.

Outcomes

Endovascular Repair

The published data on the results of endovascular repair of PAAs are limited (Table 1) (11,12,19–23). The largest prospective study was published in 2005 by our group (11). A prospective consecutive cohort of 67 aneurysms was described, of which 57 (85% inclusion rate) were treated with Gore Excluder Hemobahn or Viabahn stent grafts. Primary and secondary patency rates were 80% and 90% at one year, and 77% and 87% at two years of follow-up, respectively. Twelve stent grafts (21%) occluded after a mean follow-up of 24 months. The reintervention rate was 29% and limb survival was 100%.

Open Surgery

A review of recent surgical series is presented in Table 2 (12,13,15,24–29). The vast majority of the data are retrospective. In most series, the results of venous bypass are better than prosthetic bypass, and elective repair has improved outcomes compared with emergent procedures for acute limb ischemia. Primary patency rates from mixed populations of bypass grafts and elective/emergency procedures range from 73% to 95% at one year follow-up, and from 60% to 71% at five years. In a series of 100 elective PAA repairs, Bourriez et al. reported a one-year primary patency rate of 96% for the group with a saphenous vein graft and 83% for the group with a polytetrafluoroethylene (PTFE) bypass graft (29).

Endovascular Repair vs. Open Surgery

In the only prospective randomized trial, Antonello et al. compared venous bypass versus endografting (12). In this series 30 PAAs with a mean diameter of 3.4 cm were randomized to endovascular repair or bypass. Patients had to be suitable for either treatment, so that all patients had proximal and distal landing zones of at least 1 cm, which resulted in an inclusion rate of 73%. Open repair was performed through a medial approach and total aneurysm excision was performed in two cases (13.3%). Eleven (73%) patients were treated with a venous bypass. Four patients (27%) were treated with a PTFE bypass graft. Endovascular repair was performed with a nitinol-ePTFE stent graft (Hemobahn) in all 15 cases. The mean follow-up was 46 months for both groups. Primary patency at one and two years was 100% for open repair and 87% and 80% for endovascular repair, respectively. The authors acknowledged that the study was underpowered and that the difference in patency between open and endovascular groups had no statistical relevance. Patients in the endovascular group had a significantly lower operation time and hospital stay.

TABLE 1   Series of Endovascular Popliteal Artery Aneurysms Repair as Published from 2000

Author	Publication year	No. of aneurysms	Type of stent graft (no. per type)	No. treated emergently for acute ischemia	Follow-up period (mo; mean)	Occlusions (no. per type)
Henry (19)	2000	10	P(7); CORV(3)	—[a]	—	5 (3CORV; 2P) (50%)
Ihlberg (20)	2000	1	HB	0	5	0
Howell (21)	2002	13	WG	0	12	4
Gerasimidis (22)	2003	9	HB(6); WG(2); P(1)	0	14	4 (3HB; 1WG) (44%)
Tielliu (23)	2003	22	HB	1 (5%)	15	5 (23%)
Tielliu (11)[b]	2005	57	HB; VB[c]	5 (9%)	24	12 (21%)
Antonello (12)	2005	15	HB	0	46	1 (7%)

[a] Not stated in the article.
[b] This series is an update of the previous series by the same author.
[c] In some cases both Hemobahn and Viabahn stent grafts were used according to available diameters.
Abbreviations: CORV, Corvita; HB, Hemobahn; P, Passager; VB, Viabahn; WG, Wallgraft.

TABLE 2 Series of Open Popliteal Artery Aneurysms Repair as Published From 2000

Author	Publication year	No. of aneurysms (LSV/prosthetic graft)	No. treated emergently for acute ischemia	Follow-up period mo; mean	Primary patency (%) at				
					1 yr	2 yr	3 yr	4 yr	5 yr
Galland (24)	2002	55 (30/25)	36 (65%)	—[a]	—	—	75	—	—
Blanco (25)	2003	70 (53/17)	18 (26%)	53	89	—	—	79	71
Mahmood (26)	2003	50 (48/2)	17 (34%)	—	73	—	—	69	—
Jones (15)	2003	36 (34/2)	4 (11%)	46	—	—	—	86	—
Aulivola (27)	2004	51 (47/4)	14 (27%)	48	95	—	—	85	—
Laxdal (28)	2004	57 (51/6)	28 (49%)	42	—	—	—	—	60
Mehta (13)	2004	26 (24/2)	13 (50%)	38	—	—	81	75	—
Bourriez (29)	2005	80 (80/0)	0	—	96	94	94	—	—
		20 (0/20)	0	—	83	61	51	—	—
Antonello (12)	2005	15 (11/4)	0	46	100	—	91	—	—

[a] Not stated in the article.
Abbreviation: LSV, longer saphenous vein.

SUMMARY

Aneurysms of the lower limb are uncommon. The treatment of PA aneurysms by open repair with a bypass or an interposition graft remains the gold standard. Experience with endovascular repair is currently limited. Complications of endovascular repair include endograft occlusion, migration, stenoses, and stent fractures. These complications suggest that stent-graft design needs further study and improvement. On the basis of the limited evidence available, patency rates seem lower than for open repair.

Until there are more data from larger series supporting endovascular repair, open surgery should be considered as the main treatment option. Endovascular repair could prove a useful alternative, particularly in older and less active patients, or in cases where autologous venous material is not available.

REFERENCES

1. Dawson I, Sie R, van Baalen JM, et al. Asymptomatic popliteal aneurysm: elective operation versus conservative follow-up. Br J Surg 1994; 81:1504–7.
2. Galland RB. Popliteal aneurysms: controversies in their management. Am J Surg 2005; 190:314–8.
3. Marty B, Wicky S, Ris HB, et al. Success of thrombolysis as a predictor of outcome in acute thrombosis of popliteal aneurysms. J Vasc Surg 2002; 35:487–93.
4. Dorigo W, Pulli R, Turini F, et al. Acute leg ischaemia from thrombosed popliteal artery aneurysms: role of preoperative thrombolysis. Eur J Vasc Endovasc Surg 2002; 23:251–4.
5. Steinmetz E, Bouchot O, Faroy F, et al. Preoperative intraarterial thrombolysis before surgical revascularization for popliteal artery aneurysm with acute ischemia. Ann Vasc Surg 2000; 14:360–4.
6. Lowell RC, Gloviczki P, Hallett JW, Jr., et al. Popliteal artery aneurysms: the risk of nonoperative management. Ann Vasc Surg 1994; 8:14–23.
7. Duffy ST, Colgan MP, Sultan S, et al. Popliteal aneurysms: a 10-year experience. Eur J Vasc Endovasc Surg 1998; 16:218–22.
8. Sarcina A, Bellosta R, Luzzani L, et al. Surgical treatment of popliteal artery aneurysm: a 20 year experience. J Cardiovasc Surg 1997; 38:347–54.
9. Shortell CK, DeWeese JA, Ouriel K, et al. Popliteal artery aneurysms: a 25-year surgical experience. J Vasc Surg 1991; 14:771–9.
10. Gouny P, Bertrand P, Duedal V, et al. Limb salvage and popliteal aneurysms: advantages of preventive surgery. Eur J Vasc Endovasc Surg 2000; 19:496–500.
11. Tielliu IF, Verhoeven EL, Zeebregts CJ, et al. Endovascular treatment of popliteal artery aneurysms: results of a prospective cohort study. J Vasc Surg 2005; 41:561–7.
12. Antonello M, Frigatti P, Battocchio P, et al. Open repair versus endovascular treatment for asymptomatic popliteal artery aneurysm: results of a prospective randomized study. J Vasc surg 2005; 42:185–93.
13. Mehta M, Champagne B, Darling RC, III, et al. Outcome of popliteal artery aneurysms after exclusion and bypass: significance of residual patent branches mimicking type II endoleaks. J Vasc Surg 2004; 40:886–90.
14. Kirkpatrick UJ, McWilliams RG, Martin J, et al. Late complications after ligation and bypass for popliteal aneurysm. Br J Surg 2004; 91:174–7.
15. Jones WT, III, Hagino RT, Chiou AC, et al. Graft patency is not the only clinical predictor of success after exclusion and bypass of popliteal artery aneurysms. J Vasc Surg 2003; 37:392–8.
16. Ebaugh JL, Morasch MD, Matsumura JS, et al. Fate of excluded popliteal artery aneurysms. J Vasc Surg 2003; 37:954–9.
17. Tielliu IF, Verhoeven EL, Zeebregts CJ, et al. Experience with endovascular repair of popliteal aneurysms. In: Becquemin J-P, Alimi YS et al, eds. Controversies and Updates in Vascular Surgery. Torino: Edizioni Minerva Medica, 2006:206–11.
18. Diaz JA, Villegas M, Tamashiro G, et al. Flexions of the popliteal artery: dynamic angiography. J Invasive Cardiol 2004; 16:712–5.
19. Henry M, Amor M, Henry I, et al. Percutaneous endovascular treatment of peripheral aneurysms. J Cardiovasc Surg 2000; 41:871–83.
20. Ihlberg LH, Roth WD, Albäck NA, et al. Successful percutaneous endovascular treatment of a ruptured popliteal artery aneurysm. J Vasc Surg 2000; 31:794–7.
21. Howell M, Krajcer Z, Diethrich EB, et al. Wallgraft endoprosthesis for the percutaneous treatment of femoral and popliteal artery aneurysms. J Endovasc Ther 2002; 9:76–81.
22. Gerasimidis T, Sfyroeras G, Papazoglou K, et al. Endovascular treatment of popliteal artery aneurysms. Eur J Vasc Endovasc Surg 2003; 26:506–11.

23. Tielliu IF, Verhoeven EL, Prins TR, et al. Treatment of popliteal artery aneurysms with the Hemobahn stent-graft. J Endovasc Ther 2003; 10:111–6.
24. Galland RB, Magee TR. Management of popliteal aneurysm. Br J Surg 2002; 89:1382–5.
25. Blanco E, Serrano-Hernando FJ, Moñux G, et al. Operative repair of popliteal aneurysms: effect of factors related to the bypass procedure on outcome. Ann Vasc Surg 2004; 18:86–92.
26. Mahmood A, Salaman R, Sintler M, et al. Surgery of popliteal artery aneurysms: a 12-year experience. J Vasc Surg 2003; 37:586–93.
27. Aulivola B, Hamdan AD, Hile CN, et al. Popliteal artery aneurysms: a comparison of outcomes in elective versus emergent repair. J Vasc Surg 2004; 39:1171–7.
28. Laxdal E, Amundsen SR, Dregelid E, et al. Surgical treatment of popliteal artery aneurysms. Scand J Surg 2004; 93:57–60.
29. Bourriez A, Mellière D, Desgranges P, et al. Elective popliteal aneurysms: does venous availability has an impact on indications? J Cardiovasc Surg 2005; 46:171–5.

43 | Endovascular Treatment of Aneurysms of the Extracranial Carotid Arteries and Upper Limb Arteries

P. Bergeron, M. Boukhris, G. B. Tshiombo, M. L. Wang, Y. Y. Zhang, and J. Gay
Department of Thoracic and Cardiovascular Surgery, Hôpital Saint-Joseph, Marseille, France

EXTRACRANIAL CAROTID ARTERY ANEURYSMS

Extracranial carotid artery aneurysms (ECAAs) are rare. They may be fusiform, saccular in morphology, and either true or false. Causes of ECAAs include trauma (which may cause aneurysmal dissections), iatrogenic, atherosclerosis, vasculitis such as Takayasu's arteritis, and infection. Traumatic and iatrogenic aneurysms are the most common causes of ECAAs in the Western world. Atherosclerotic aneurysms are generally located around the carotid bifurcation, and aneurysmal dissections usually occur more distally in the internal carotid artery (ICA).

ECAAs may expand so that they compress adjacent structures in the neck or they may rupture. Typical patients are usually middle-aged or elderly and present with a pulsatile neck swelling or a sensation of a lump in the throat. Pain is a common symptom and suggests continuing expansion and some patients exhibit transient ischemic attacks or strokes secondary to distal embolization (1).

The indications for treatment of carotid artery aneurysms are lesions, which are symptomatic; aneurysms larger than 2 cm diameter; aneurysms that are increasing in size; and painful aneurysms. Small asymptomatic aneurysms can be followed by periodic duplex ultrasound.

Until recently, conventional surgery has been the only method of treatment available for ECAAs. In the last decade, reports of endovascular repair of ECAAs have appeared, although the published experience remains very limited.

Surgical excision and vein grafting is the accepted treatment method for carotid aneurysms (2,3). Although surgery for aneurysms close to the carotid bifurcation has a low morbidity, access to the distal portion of the ICA is much more challenging (4,5). Complications of distal carotid surgery are not uncommon and include transient or fixed cranial nerve palsy, and deafness (6–8).

The attractions of endovascular techniques for aneurysms in the distal ICA are obvious. Two main methods have been described, placement of an uncovered stent followed by embolization of the aneurysm with the stent in place, and exclusion of the aneurysm by stent grafts. Although endovascular techniques are particularly suited to the distal ICA, they may also be used for more proximal ICA lesions.

Uncovered Stents and Embolization

This involves placing a bare stent in the parent artery across the aneurysm. As the extracranial carotid artery is relatively superficial, self-expanding stents should be used to prevent permanent deformation of the stent, which might occur if a balloon-expandable stent is used. With the stent in place, the lumen of the aneurysm is filled with embolic material. The embolic material may be delivered through microcatheters placed in the aneurysm through the mesh of the stent or left in the aneurysm before deployment of the self-expanding stent. Most reports have used coils as the embolic material, although newer agents such as Onyx® (Micro Therapeutics, Irvine, California, U.S.A.) may also be used. With the improvement in technology, this procedure has been largely superseded by stent grafts, although there are no data comparing the two procedures.

Stent Grafts

Modern stent grafts are available in a wide range of diameters, lengths and delivery catheters, some of which can be used in the extracranial carotid artery. Stent grafts should be of the self-expanding type, e.g., Viabahn® (W.L. Gore, Flagstaff, Arizona, U.S.A.), Fluency® (Bard Angiomed, Karlsruhe, Germany), Wallgraft® (Boston Scientific Corp., Galway, Ireland). The diameter and length of the stent to be used is selected on the basis of measurements obtained from the duplex ultrasound and computed tomography (CT) or magnetic resonance (MR) angiography. The endograft is generally oversized relative to the native artery by 10% to 15% and at least 15 mm of stent graft must be placed in the normal artery either side of the aneurysm (landing zones).

The procedure is performed under local anesthesia and intravenous sedation. Similar to carotid stenting procedures for occlusive disease, it is sensible to have an anesthetist present during the procedure for patient monitoring. Facilities to perform transcranial Doppler ultrasound are also helpful.

Percutaneous femoral artery access is used and a guiding sheath is manipulated into the common carotid artery. Heparin is administered and the activated clotting time should be monitored to ensure that the patient is adequately heparinized. Angiography is performed in several projections to ascertain the best projection to visualize the aneurysm and the parent artery. A catheter and guidewire are advanced across the aneurysm into the normal artery beyond the aneurysm. Many operators use a cerebral protection device to prevent distal embolization during the procedure. The stent graft and delivery catheter are advanced to the site of the aneurysm. A roadmap is helpful to enable accurate placement of the device. After the endograft has been deployed, balloon dilatation to the normal size of the native vessel is performed. The puncture site should be closed with an arterial closure device to prevent a groin hematoma. Most operators prescribe dual antiplatelet medication in the form of clopidogrel and aspirin. Clopidogrel is commenced the same day and is continued for at least three months. Low-dose aspirin therapy is continued indefinitely. Patients are followed up by duplex ultrasound.

We have treated five patients with aneurysms of the extracranial carotid arteries [one female patient with an atheromatous aneurysm who underwent a redo intervention due to an endoleak and four patients with aneurysmal dissections (one patient had bilateral lesions); seven procedures in total] (Table 1). All of the lesions were in the distal ICAs (Figs. 1 and 2). Polytetrafluoroethylene-covered stents (Jostent®, Abbott Vascular, Santa Clara, California, U.S.A.) were used in six of seven procedures (86%), A Wallgraft was used in one patient. Distal cerebral protection was employed during four procedures (distal balloon occlusion in three cases; distal filter protection in one case).

Technical success was achieved in all five patients and there were no procedural complications. During an average follow-up period of 67 ± 31 months, there were no strokes or transient ischemic events. Duplex ultrasound examinations showed patent endografts in all patients. A Type I endoleak was observed four months after the procedure in one patient and was successfully treated by an additional endograft (Fig. 3). There was no in-stent stenosis in any patient, and all aneurysms remained thrombosed.

In summary, although there is limited evidence in terms of procedural results and durability, stent grafts should be considered as a treatment option for ECAAs, particularly aneurysms involving the distal ICA.

ANEURYSMS OF THE UPPER EXTREMITY ARTERIES

Aneurysms involving the arteries supplying the arms are unusual. Their most common sites are the brachiocephalic and subclavian arteries. Compared with the aorta, iliac and popliteal arteries, aneurysms of the upper extremities have a variety of causes in addition to atherosclerosis. The most frequent causes of these aneurysms are trauma due to penetrating

TABLE 1 Personal Series of the Endovascular Treatment of Extracranial Carotic Artery Aneurysms

Patient number	Sex	Disease	Age	Risk factors	Symptoms	Site of lesion	Cerebral protection	Length of follow-up	Aneurysm exclusion	Complications	Comments
1	F	Aneurysm	71	Coronary disease	None	Left ICA	None	7.4 yr	Yes	None	Secondary extension at 4 mo for an endoleak
2	M	Dissection	39	None	TIA	Bilateral ICA	Distal balloon	7 yr	Yes	None	1 wk delay between the 2 interventions
3	F	Dissection	54	None	TIA	Right ICA	None	6.6 yr	Yes	None	
4	M	Dissection	80	Hypertension Smoker Cardiopulmonary failure	None	Left ICA	None	3.8 yr	Yes	None	Underwent stenting of the right carotid bifurcation 2 mo earlier
5	F	Dissection	57	Hypertension Smoker Arteriopathy	Dysarthria	Right ICA	Filter	4 mo	Yes	None	

Abbreviations: ICA, internal carotid artery; TIA, transient ischemic attack.

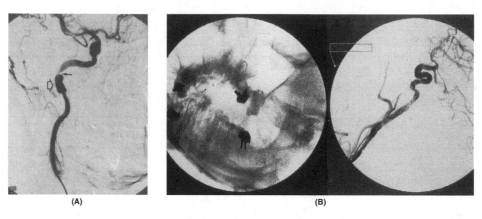

FIGURE 1 (**A**) Patient presenting an acute spontaneous dissection of the distal right internal carotid artery. (**B**) Exclusion of the aneurysm after the placement of a Wallgraft® stent (Boston Scientific Corp., Galway, Ireland).

or blunt injury, iatrogenic, vasculitis such as Takayasu's arteritis, thoracic outlet syndrome, atherosclerosis, and congenital anomalies. Pseudoaneurysms are usually caused by inadvertent catheterization of the artery during insertion of a central venous catheter or following brachial or radial angiography. Aneurysms may occur as poststenotic dilatations immediately distal to stenoses associated with thoracic outlet syndrome.

Many aneurysms involving the proximal arteries are found as incidental findings on CT or MR imaging scans. More distal aneurysms are usually palpable and may cause swelling, pain or compression of adjacent veins or nerves. Similar to the carotid arteries, the main imaging methods are duplex ultrasound for peripheral lesions and CT and MR angiography for more central lesions.

Treatment

Peripheral pseudoaneurysms can be treated by the percutaneous injection of thrombin if they have a narrow neck. The main treatment options for fusiform and saccular aneurysms are between conventional surgical bypass and exclusion of the aneurysm by endografts.

Whether aneurysms are suitable for treatment with stent grafts depends to some extent on their location. Central aneurysms close to the aortic arch are inside the thorax and are impossible to treat surgically without recourse to a thoracotomy. These aneurysms are well

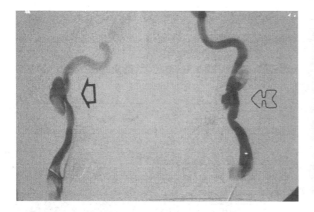
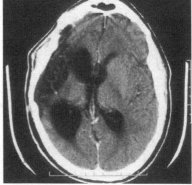

FIGURE 2 Patient with a traumatic carotid artery aneurysm.

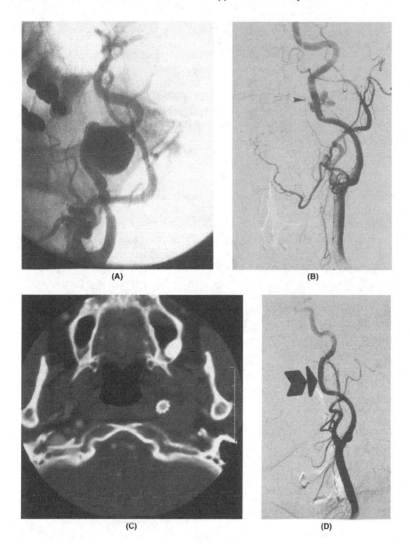

FIGURE 3 (**A**) An atheromatous carotid artery aneurysm located to the distal part of internal carotid artery. (**B**) Persisting endoleak one month after the placement of a Jomed® (Jomed International AB, Helsingborg, Sweden) stent. (**C,D**) Computer tomography scan and angiographic imaging of the complete exclusion of the aneurysm after the placement of a second Jomed stent.

suited for stent grafts, which are usually inserted into the vascular system, from femoral artery access. Either balloon-expandable or self-expanding endografts can be used because endografts are not subject to external forces in this deep-seated location.

Aneurysms at the thoracic inlet where the first rib is located close to the clavicle are less suited for endografts due to the potential for deformation and trauma to the stent by apposition of the first rib and clavicle during movement of the shoulder joint. However, removal of the first rib prior to endograft placement avoids this potential problem. In addition, stent grafts should probably not be used at joints such as the elbow joint, and possibly also the shoulder joint, although there are no data to support this statement.

If endografts are placed in the distal subclavian artery, the axillary artery or brachial artery, self-expanding rather than balloon-expandable stent grafts should be used. The vessels below the elbow joint are of narrow caliber and should be considered unsuitable for treatment by endografts.

The principles of endograft selection and deployment are similar to those for use in the carotid artery described previously. The question of which method (endografting vs. surgery) is the better treatment for upper extremities aneurysms is difficult to determine because of the limited available evidence. The results of treatment, either surgical or endovascular, are summarized below.

Results of Treatment: Endovascular vs. Surgery

A literature review revealed 33 papers from 1991 to 2005, involving a total number of 147 lesions treated in the upper limb arteries (Table 2) (9–41). Only eight studies reported more than five cases, and the largest report contained 23 patients, of which 15 patients were treated surgically.

Atheromatous Aneurysms

There were 53 aneurysms involving the subclavian arteries in 37 patients, the axillary arteries in two patients: one brachial artery and one innominate artery. The locations of 12 lesions were not specified. The aneurysms were treated by surgical resection in 77.4% of cases (41 lesions), and endovascular repair using stent grafts in 11 cases. One case report did not mention the procedure used to treat the aneurysm. Major complications after surgery were four graft occlusions and two amputations (major adverse events rate: 14.6%). No major events occurred after endovascular stent-grafting. Reported secondary complications were one local hematoma requiring surgical management, one asymptomatic strut dislocation, and one asymptomatic endograft thrombosis. The follow-up data were negligible in the majority of the papers.

TABLE 2 Published Reports of the Treatment of Upper Extremity Aneurysms

Author	Year	Number of lesions	Treatment
Assali (2)	2001	1	Stent plus coils
Bates (3)	2005	1	Stent grafts
Clark (4)	1991	10	Surgery
Cormier (5)	2001	23	8 Stent grafts, 15 surgery
Du Toit (6)	2000	8	Stent grafts
Gruss (7)	1997	18	Surgery
Jayle (8)	2002	1	Surgery
Kasirajan (9)	2003	2	Stent grafts
Komorowska-Timek (10)	2004	2	PTI
Kurimoto (11)	2003	1	Stent grafts
Levey (12)	1991	13	TCE
Maleux (13)	2000	1	TCE
Marin (14)	1995	7	Stent grafts
Marston (15)	1995	1	Stent grafts
Martinez (16)	1999	1	Stent grafts
May (17)	1993	1	Stent grafts
Michalakis (18)	2003	1	Not available
Nehler (19)	1997	12	Surgery
Oktar (20)	2002	1	Stent grafts
Patel (21)	1996	6	Stent grafts
Puech-Leao (22)	2001	1	Stent grafts
Reus (23)	2003	1	PTI
Romero Campos (24)	1991	1	Surgery
Sanada (25)	2003	1	Stent grafts
Schneider (26)	1999	1	Not available
Schoder (27)	2003	12	Stent grafts
Sitsen (28)	1999	1	Stent grafts
Siu (29)	2005	7	Surgery
Sullivan (30)	1996	3	Stent grafts
Todd (31)	1998	2	Not available
Vijayvergiya (32)	2005	1	Stent grafts
Vlychou (33)	2001	1	TCE
Waggershauser (34)	2000	4	Stent grafts

Abbreviations: PTI, percutaneous thrombin injection; TCE, transcatheter embolization.

TABLE 3 Etiologies of Iatrogenic and Post-traumatic
Arterial Lesions in the Literature

Traumatic arterial injuries	27
Post-irradiation lesions	23
Pseudoaneurysms	17
Pseudoaneurysms after drug abuse	7
Arterial injury after misplaced central venous catheter	7
Aneurysms in highlevel sportive patients	4
Emergency hemorrhages	4
Mycotic pseudoaneurysms	2
Traumatic pseudoaneurysms	2
Fistulae	1
Total	94

Traumatic Aneurysms

There were 94 posttraumatic and iatrogenic lesions (Table 3). Fifty-nine aneurysms were located in the subclavian or axillary arteries, and 13 aneurysms were distal to the axillary arteries. Twenty-two locations were not specified. The treatment method was not stated in three cases. Surgical repair was performed in 23 aneurysms (24%); 15 of these were located proximal to and 8 aneurysms were located distal to the origin of the circumflex humeral artery. At follow-up, there was only one reported case of venous bypass occlusion and no reports of recurrent symptoms. Seventy-one false aneurysms and traumatic injuries were treated by endovascular repair which consisted of stent grafts in 49 patients (69%), transcatheter embolization (TCE) in 15 patients, percutaneous thrombin injection (PTI) in 3 patients and stent deployment followed by transstent coil embolization in the remaining patients. Procedural complications in the endovascular group consisted of one stroke and one brachial artery access-related stenosis requiring an angioplasty. Late complications consisted of one in-stent restenosis at five months, which was treated by angioplasty, one compressed covered stent and one stent fracture.

The majority of the pseudoaneurysms and arterial injuries distal to the origin of the circumflex humeral artery were treated by PTI or TCE: 8 surgical repairs and 17 endovascular repairs (14 TCEs + 3 PTIs). The only complication in this group of patients was migration of a coil from an arteriovenous fistula to the pulmonary circulation, which did not require intervention, although the fistula was subsequently repaired surgically. Once again, the follow-up data are very limited.

In summary, endovascular repair of aneurysms of the upper extremity is feasible, has a high technical success rate and low complication rate. However, the limited evidence provides no useful follow-up data on the durability of stent grafts to enable a comparison to be made with the long-term outcomes of surgery. Intuitively, endografts seem less suited for aneurysms close to the first rib, the shoulder and the elbow joint; and surgery should probably remain the method of choice for aneurysms in these locations, until better quality data on durability are available.

REFERENCES

1. Goldstone J. Aneurysms of the extracranial carotid artery. In: Rutherford RB, ed. Vascular Surgery. 2nd ed. Philadelphia, PA: WB Saunders, 1984:1279.
2. Assali AR, Sdringola S, Moustapha A, et al. Endovascular repair of traumatic pseudoaneurysm by uncovered self-expandable stenting with or without transstent coiling of the aneurysm cavity. Catheter Cardiovasc Interv 2001; 53(2):253–8.
3. Bates MC, Aburahma AF, Crotty B. Successful urgent endovascular surgery for symptomatic subclavian artery aneurysmal compression of the trachea. Catheter Cardiovasc Interv 2005; 64(3):291–5.
4. Clark ET, Mass DP, Bassiouny HS, Zarins CK, Gewertz BL. True aneurysmal disease in the hand and upper extremity. Ann Vasc Surg 1991; 5(3):276–81.

5. Cormier F, Korso F, Fichelle JM, Gautier C, Cormier JM. Post-irradiation axillo-subclavian arteriopathy: surgical revascularization. J Mal Vasc 2001; 26(1):45–9.
6. du Toit DF, Strauss DC, Blaszczyk M, de Villiers R, Warren BL. Endovascular treatment of penetrating thoracic outlet arterial injuries. Eur J Vasc Endovasc Surg 2000; 19(5):489–95.
7. Gruss JD, Geissler C. Aneurysms of the subclavian artery in thoracic outlet syndrome. Zentralbl Chir 1997; 122(9):730–4.
8. Jayle C, Corbi P, Lanquetot H, Godet C, Menu P. Radial artery aneurysm: an unusual complication of radial artery catheterization. Ann Chir 2002; 127(8):631–3.
9. Kasirajan K, Matteson B, Marek JM, Langsfeld M. Covered stents for true subclavian aneurysms in patients with degenerative connective tissue disorders. J Endovasc Ther 2003; 10(3):647–52.
10. Komorowska-Timek E, Teruya TH, Abou-Zamzam AM, Jr., Papa D, Ballard JL. Treatment of radial and ulnar artery pseudoaneurysms using percutaneous thrombin injection. J Hand Surg [Am] 2004; 29(5):936–42.
11. Kurimoto Y, Tsuchida Y, Saito J, Yama N, Narimatsu E, Asai Y. Emergency endovascular stent-grafting for infected pseudoaneurysm of brachial artery. Infection 2003; 31(3):186–8.
12. Levey DS, Teitelbaum GP, Finck EJ, Pentecost MJ. Safety and efficacy of transcatheter embolization of axillary and shoulder arterial injuries. J Vasc Interv Radiol 1991; 2(1):99–104.
13. Maleux G, Stockx L, Brys P, et al. Iatrogenic pseudoaneurysm in the upper arm: treatment by transcatheter embolization. Cardiovasc Intervent Radiol 2000; 23(2):140–2.
14. Marin ML, Veith FJ, Cynamon J, et al. Initial experience with transluminally placed endovascular grafts for the treatment of complex vascular lesions. Ann Surg 1995; 222(4):449–65.
15. Marston WA, Criado E, Mauro MA, Keagy BA. Transbrachial endovascular exclusion of an axillary artery pseudoaneurysm with PTFE-covered stents. J Endovasc Surg 1995; 2(2):172–6.
16. Martinez R, Lermusiaux P, Podeur L, Bleuet F, Delerue D, Castellani L. Endovascular management of axillary artery trauma. J Cardiovasc Surg (Torino) 1999; 40(3):413–5.
17. May J, White G, Waugh R, Yu W, Harris J. Transluminal placement of a prosthetic graft-stent device for treatment of subclavian artery aneurysm. J Vasc Surg 1993; 18(6):1056–9.
18. Michalakis D, Lerais JM, Goffette P, Royer V, Brenot R, Kastler B. True isolated atherosclerotic aneurysm of the axillary artery. J Radiol 2003; 84(9):1016–9.
19. Nehler MR, Taylor LM, Jr., Moneta GL, Porter JM. Upper extremity ischemia from subclavian artery aneurysm caused by bony abnormalities of the thoracic outlet. Arch Surg 1997; 132(5):527–32.
20. Oktar GL, Balkan ME, Akpek S, Ilgit E. Endovascular stent-graft placement for the management of a traumatic axillary artery pseudoaneurysm-a case report. Vasc Endovascular Surg 2002; 36(4):323–6.
21. Patel AV, Marin ML, Veith FJ, Kerr A, Sanchez LA. Endovascular graft repair of penetrating subclavian artery injuries. J Endovasc Surg 1996; 3(4):382–8.
22. Puech-Leao P, Orra HA. Endovascular repair of an innominate artery true aneurysm. J Endovasc Ther 2001; 8(4):429–32.
23. Reus M, Vazquez V, Alonso J, Morales D, Rodriguez JM. Treatment of a radial artery pseudoaneurysm with ultrasound-guided percutaneous thrombin injection in a patient with Behcet's syndrome. J Clin Ultrasound 2003; 31(8):440–4.
24. Romero Campos R, Abellan Cubel ML, Lerma Gonce M, Camacho L. Aneurysm of the humeral artery. Angiologia 1991; 43(3):130–1.
25. Sanada J, Matsui O, Terayama N, et al. Stent-graft repair of a mycotic left subclavian artery pseudoaneurysm. J Endovasc Ther 2003; 10(1):66–70.
26. Schneider K, Kasparyan NG, Altchek DW, Fantini GA, Weiland AJ. An aneurysm involving the axillary artery and its branch vessels in a major league baseball pitcher. A case report and review of the literature. Am J Sports Med 1999; 27(3):370–5.
27. Schoder M, Cejna M, Holzenbein T, et al. Elective and emergent endovascular treatment of subclavian artery aneurysms and injuries. J Endovasc Ther 2003; 10(1):58–65.
28. Sitsen ME, Ho GH, Blankensteijn JD. Deformation of self-expanding stent-grafts complicating endovascular peripheral aneurysm repair. J Endovasc Surg 1999; 6(3):288–92.
29. Siu WT, Yau KK, Cheung HY, et al. Management of brachial artery pseudoaneurysms secondary to drug abuse. Ann Vasc Surg 2005; 19(5):657–61.
30. Sullivan TM, Bacharach JM, Perl J, Gray B. Endovascular management of unusual aneurysms of the axillary and subclavian arteries. J Endovasc Surg 1996; 3(4):389–95.
31. Todd GJ, Benvenisty AI, Hershon S, Bigliani LU. Aneurysms of the mid axillary artery in major league baseball pitchers-a report of two cases. J Vasc Surg 1998; 28(4):702–7.
32. Vijayvergiya R, Kumar RM, Ranjit A, Grover A. Endovascular management of isolated axillary artery aneurysm-a case report. Vasc Endovascular Surg 2005; 39(2):199–201.
33. Vlychou M, Spanomichos G, Chatziioannou A, Georganas M, Zavras GM. Embolisation of a traumatic aneurysm of the posterior circumflex humeral artery in a volleyball player. Br J Sports Med 2001; 35(2):136–7.
34. Waggershauser T, Herrmann K, Reiser M. Reconstructive endovascular treatment procedures in the area of the a. subclavia and its branches. Radiologe 2000; 40(9):821–5.

35. Thévenet A. Chirurgie des lésions non athéromateuses carotidiennes. In: Kieffer E, Natali J, eds. Actualités de Chirurgie Vasculaire. AERCV: Paris, 1987:219–39.
36. Moreau P, Albat B, Thevenet A. Traitement des anévrysmes de l'artère carotide interne extra-crânienne. Ann Chir Vasc 1994; 8:409–16.
37. Mercier C, Tournigand P, Piquet P, et al. Chirurgie de l'artère carotide interne juxta-crânienne. In: Kieffer E, Natali J, eds. Actualités de Chirurgie Vasculaire. Paris: AERCV, 1987:241–8.
38. Purdue GF, Pellegrini RV, Arena S. Aneurysms of the high internl carotid artery: a new approach. Surgery 1981; 89:68–270.
39. Rosset E, Albertini J-N, Magnan P-E, Ede B, Mathieu J-P, Branchereau A. In Branchereau A, Jacobs M eds. Nouveautés en Pathologie Carotidienne; Traitement chirurgical des Anévrysmes de l'Artère Carotide Interne Extra-crânienne. Armonk, NY: Futura Publishing Company, Inc., Vol. 17. 1995:177–89.
40. Ruotolo C, Kieffer E. Anévrysmes disséquants chroniques de la carotide interne: place du traitement chirurgical. In: Kieffer E, Bousser MG, eds. Actualités de Chirurgie Vasculaire. Paris: AERCV, 1988:253–8.
41. D'Anglejan Chatillon J, Ribeiro V, Mas J-L, Bousser M-G. Dissections carotidiennes extra-crâniennes spontanées chez l'adulte: 47 cas. In: Kieffer E, Bousser MG, eds. Actualités de Chirurgie Vasculaire. Paris: AERCV, 1988:245–52.

44 | Endovascular Treatment of Visceral Artery Aneurysms

Paul J. Burns and R. T. A. Chalmers
Department of Vascular Surgery, Royal Infirmary of Edinburgh, Edinburgh, U.K.

INTRODUCTION

Aneurysms involving the arteries supplying the abdominal viscera are much less common than aneurysms of the aorta and peripheral arteries. However, rupture of these aneurysms is associated with significant mortality, and therefore their management is important. Due to their relative rarity, the natural history, the indications for treatment and the optimal treatment method of visceral artery aneurysms (VAAs) are poorly defined.

The aim of this chapter is to describe the management of patients with VAAs. For the purposes of this chapter, aneurysms involving the arteries supplying the gastrointestinal tract (VAAs) and renal artery aneurysms (RAAs) are dealt with separately.

ANEURYSMS OF THE CELIAC AND MESENTERIC ARTERIES (VAAs)

Epidemiology

VAAs and pseudoaneurysms are uncommon. The splenic artery is the most commonly involved vessel followed by the hepatic artery and the superior mesenteric artery (SMA). Splenic artery aneurysms are usually secondary to pancreatitis, but are also associated with trauma, atherosclerosis and pregnancy. Hepatic artery pseudoaneurysms are usually traumatic and are secondary to blunt hepatic trauma or to invasive biliary procedures. Splenic and hepatic artery aneurysms are also associated with polyarteritis nodosa (PAN), when they may be multiple. SMA and celiac artery aneurysms are the least common splanchnic aneurysms and are usually due to atherosclerosis, trauma, or infection, although they are also found rarely in PAN (1–10).

VAAs are usually asymptomatic which causes difficulty in estimating their incidence. The incidence may be rising due to the rise in iatrogenic pseudoaneurysms caused by invasive biliary procedures and increased diagnosis of VAAs visualized as incidental findings on cross-sectional imaging studies. Postmortem studies indicate that the prevalence lies between 0.01% and 0.2% of the population (1).

Natural History

The main concern regarding VAAs is the potential for enlargement and rupture, although this is not inevitable. Follow-up of small aneurysms (<2 cm) suggests that many do not increase in size, and require no intervention (11). Aneurysms larger than 2 cm diameter tend to be treated soon after diagnosis and there are no useful data on the rupture risk of these larger aneurysms.

Clinical Features

The majority of VAAs are occult until they rupture when patients may present with severe abdominal or back pain and shock. Pain or symptoms related to a mass effect of the aneurysm are rare. Spontaneous thrombosis of VAAs occurs in some patients. If this occurs, acute thrombosis of the aneurysm and the parent vessel may give rise to end-organ ischemia. The clinical effect of acute thrombosis of the aneurysm and parent vessel depends on the site of the aneurysm. For example, occlusion of an aneurysm involving the proximal SMA could lead to ischemia of the entire small bowel, or a limited splenic infarct if the aneurysm involved a branch of the splenic artery.

Management

To Intervene or Not?

Symptomatic VAAs are considered to be at risk of imminent rupture and should be treated. However, the management of asymptomatic VAA is controversial, largely because the natural history is unknown. In a series of 25 patients, all of the VAAs that ruptured were over 2 cm, while the asymptomatic aneurysms were all between 1.5 and 3 cm (5). A conservative approach to small SMA aneurysms was advocated by Stone et al. They reported the results of conservative management of a small cohort of patients with aneurysms of the SMA, 1 to 2.4 cm in diameter. At a mean follow-up of 67 months, none of the patients had developed any complications related to their aneurysm. Furthermore, no growth of their aneurysms was detected, and no new aneurysms developed (12).

On the basis of the limited available evidence, most interventionalists treat VAA if they are 2 cm or more in diameter. Aneurysms smaller than 2 cm diameter are usually followed by imaging, usually by computed tomography.

Endovascular Techniques

Until recently, open surgery has been the treatment of choice for VAAs. In the last 10 to 15 years, endovascular techniques have substantially improved and are usually considered before open surgery in the treatment algorithm. The main endovascular methods used to treat VAAs are embolization or the insertion of stent grafts (Figs. 1–5).

Embolization

Coils are the most common embolic agent used to treat VAAs. Other alternatives are liquid embolic agents such as glue and Onyx® (Micro Therapeutics, Irvine, California, U.S.A.). Coil embolization usually involves occlusion of the vessel, which gives rise to the aneurysm. Occasionally it is possible to embolize only the aneurysm if the aneurysm is saccular with a relatively narrow neck, with preservation of the parent artery. However, such aneurysms are unusual. Moreover, the action of packing an aneurysm with multiple coils may actually cause

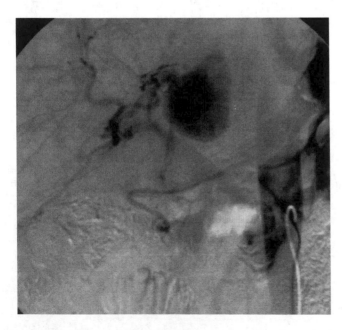

FIGURE 1   Large hepatic artery aneurysm demonstrated on angiography.

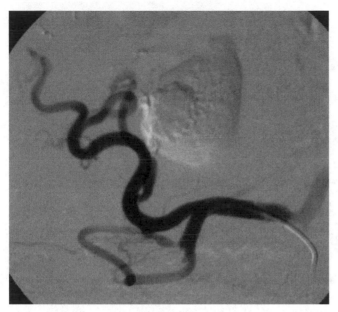

FIGURE 2 The hepatic artery aneurysm seen in Fig. 1 after coil embolization.

rupture of the aneurysm either by pressure of the coils or due to catheter and guidewire manipulations within the aneurysm sac. As a result, many interventionalists advise against packing the aneurysm itself with coils.

The aim of coil embolization is to occlude the afferent and the efferent parent artery. This involves passing a catheter through the aneurysm into the vessel beyond. This maneuver can be problematic because the catheter and guidewire tend to coil themselves within the aneurysm rather than pass beyond into the efferent vessel. However, blocking the efferent vessel ("the back door") is important, because if the efferent artery is not occluded, the aneurysm will usually continue to fill by retrograde flow from distal communications. The efferent vessel is occluded by placing multiple coils to form a nest. Once the efferent vessel is occluded, the catheter is withdrawn and the afferent vessel is blocked by multiple coils.

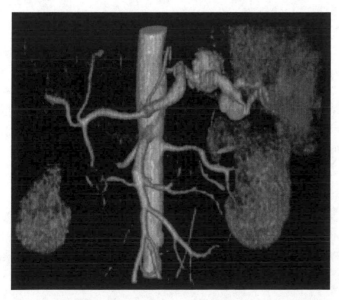

FIGURE 3 Multiple splenic artery aneurysms demonstrated on reconstructed computed tomography.

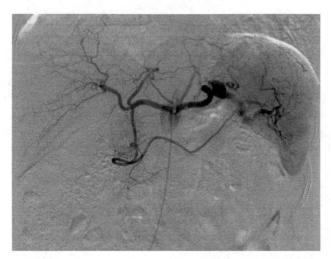

FIGURE 4   Multiple splenic artery aneurysms demonstrated on angiography.

Stent Grafts

Exclusion of the aneurysm by placement of a small stent graft across the aneurysm is the preferred endovascular method for treating VAAs because this method preserves the patency of the parent artery. The main limitations of this method are difficulties in the availability of the correct equipment for this procedure, difficulties in obtaining access to the aneurysm and the presence of important arterial branches close to the aneurysm. Few departments carry the range of guiding sheaths, guidewires, catheters and stent grafts required to treat the whole range of VAAs with stent grafts. Therefore, if this procedure is to be undertaken, it is important to plan ahead and order in the appropriate equipment. Visceral aneurysms can be difficult to access to enable placement of a stent graft. For example, while it should be feasible to place a small stent graft in the common or proper hepatic artery because of their relative proximity to the celiac artery and the straight course of these vessels, aneurysms in the distal hepatic, splenic or mesenteric circulations are much more difficult to gain access for stent-graft deployment.

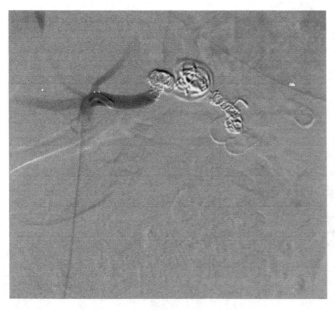

FIGURE 5   Splenic artery aneurysm after coil embolization.

Finally, if the aneurysm is very close to an important branch, endografting should generally not be undertaken because of the potential ischemic sequelae of occluding the branch vessel.

OUTCOMES

Endovascular Treatment

Whichever technique is used, endovascular treatment has a high success rate and low morbidity and mortality. Endovascular treatment of VAAs also seems to be durable with recurrence rates of 4% and 9% (4,5,7). Gabelmann et al. achieved technical success in 92% (23 of 25) of patients with VAA treated by coil embolization (5). Saltzburg et al. reported technical success in 94% of patients (15 coil embolizations, 3 stent grafts) over a 13-year period (7). The group from the Cleveland Clinic treated 48 patients with VAAs (3 celiac axis, 2 left gastric arteries, 1 SMA, 12 hepatic arteries, 20 splenic arteries, 7 gastroduodenal arteries, 1 middle colic artery, and 2 pancreaticoduodenal arteries) by embolization with technical success in 98%. The 30-day mortality was 8.3% with three of the four patients who died succumbing to causes unrelated to the procedure. At a mean follow-up of 16 months, complete exclusion of the aneurysm persisted in 97% of the patients' follow-up (13).

There is no question that endovascular treatment of VAAs is technically challenging and the impressive results of larger centers have not been replicated in smaller less experienced centers (6,14). Endovascular treatment either by means of coil embolization or by stent-grafting should only be undertaken by experienced operators who are confident in the use of fine catheter and guidewire manipulations and embolization techniques.

The mortality and morbidity rates of endovascular treatment are low. The main complication of coil embolization is thrombosis of the parent vessel, although as described above, this is often unavoidable.

Open Surgery

The options for open surgical repair include either simple ligation of the vessel supplying the aneurysm or resection of the aneurysm followed by placement of an interposition graft. One relative advantage of open repair is that it allows assessment of end-organ perfusion following simple ligation. Thus at the same operation it can be determined whether a portion of small bowel requires resection after ligation of an SMA aneurysm or splenectomy is needed after splenic artery aneurysm ligation. Although this appears attractive, in practice it seems end-organ resection is rarely required (4).

Open Surgery or Endovascular Treatment

In view of the lower complication rates of endovascular treatment together with its less invasive nature, most clinicians consider endovascular treatment to be the method of first choice. Moreover, many VAAs are very inaccessible to the surgeon, e.g., deep within the liver or spleen so that surgical treatment of these aneurysms can only be undertaken if resection of all or part of the organ is undertaken.

RENAL ARTERY ANEURYSMS

RAAs are rare, occurring in less than 1% of renal angiograms (15). Similar to other locations, they may be true or false aneurysms. RAAs may be extrarenal or intrarenal. Extrarenal aneurysms are usually caused by degeneration, trauma, fibromuscular hyperplasia, arteritis, infection or congenital abnormality. The aneurysm sac has an adverse effect on renal blood flow and many patients have associated hypertension as a result. However, hypertension is also common in conditions such as fibromuscular dysplasia, and it may be difficult to know whether the hypertension caused the aneurysm or vice versa.

The most common causes of intrarenal aneurysms are the arteritides such as PAN and illegal drug use such as cocaine or amphetamines. The aneurysms may rupture, thrombose, or may compress the collecting system leading to hydronephrosis. Clearly the most worrying complication is rupture, which is uncommon, although the potential for rupture appears to be increased by pregnancy.

RAAs may be single or multiple, unilateral or bilateral and have a propensity to occur at arterial bifurcations. The aneurysms may be saccular or fusiform and calcification in larger aneurysms is common. Similar to VAAs, published data are limited, although most aneurysms are treated if they are 2 cm or more in diameter (16).

With the improvement in endovascular techniques and equipment, most patients are considered for endovascular treatment before surgery. Similar to the treatment of VAAs, the main options are exclusion of the aneurysm with preservation of the renal arteries with small stent grafts, or embolization using coils, glue, or one of the newer embolic agents such as Onyx. Unless, the aneurysm occurs in the main renal artery with suitable landing zones between the renal artery origin and the renal artery bifurcation, stent grafts cannot be used unless physicians and patients are willing to accept sacrifice of one or more of the normal vessels.

Although technically very difficult, some patients with aneurysms at main vessel bifurcations can be treated by embolization using Onyx, with preservation of the parent arteries (17). In most centers, open surgery is associated with significant renal morbidity and should be reserved for patients who cannot be treated by endovascular methods.

SUMMARY

Aneurysms of the visceral and renal arteries are uncommon and the evidence on their incidence, the indications for treatment and the optimal treatment method is limited. With the improvement in endovascular techniques and equipment over the last decade or so, many patients can now be treated by minimally invasive therapy either with stent grafts or by embolization with increasing technical rates and durability of the results. Open surgery has higher complications than endovascular treatment and should be reserved for patients who are not suitable or who fail embolization or endografting.

REFERENCES

1. Rokke O, Sondenaa K, Amundsen S, Bjerke-Larssen T, Jensen D. The diagnosis and management of splanchnic artery aneurysms. Scand J Gastroenterol 1996; 31:737–43.
2. Carr SC, Mahvi DM, Hoch JR, Archer CW, Turnispeed WD. Visceral artery aneurysm rupture. J Vasc Surg 2001; 33:806–11.
3. Wagner WH, Allins AD, Treiman RL, et al. Ruptured visceral artery aneurysms. Ann Vasc Surg 1997; 11(4):342–7.
4. Sessa C, Tinelli G, Porcu P, Aubert A, Thony F, Magne J-L. Treatment of visceral artery aneurysms: description of a retrospective series of 42 aneurysms in 34 patients. Ann Vasc Surg 2004; 18:695–703.
5. Gabelmann A, Görich J, Merkle EM. Endovascular treatment of visceral artery aneurysms. J Endovasc Ther 2002; 9:38–47.
6. Carmeci C, McClenathan J. Visceral artery aneurysms as seen in a community hospital. Am J Surg 2002; 179:486–9.
7. Saltzberg SS, Maldonado TS, Lamparello PJ, et al. Is endovascular therapy the preferred treatment for all visceral artery aneurysms? Ann Vasc Surg 2005; 19:507–15.
8. Parfitt J, Chalmers RTA, Wolfe JHN. Visceral aneuryms in ehlers-danlos syndrome: case report and review of the literature. J Vasc Surg 2002; 31:1248–51.
9. Ko SF, Hsien MJ, Ng SH. Superior mesenteric artery aneurysm in systemic lupus erythematosus. Clin Imaging 1997; 21:13–6.
10. Hossain A, Reis ED, Dave SP, Kerstein MD, Hollier LH. Visceral artery aneurysms: experience in a tertiary-care center. Am Surg 2001; 67:432–7.
11. Mattar SG, Lumsden AB. The management of splenic artery aneurysms: experience with 23 cases. Am J Surg 1993; 169:580–4.
12. Stone WM, Abbas M, Cherry KJ, Fowl RJ, Gloviczki P. Superior mesenteric artery aneurysms: is presence an indication for intervention. J Vasc Surg 2002; 36:234–7.
13. Tulsyan N, Kashyap VS, Greenberg RK, et al. The endovascular management of visceral artery aneurysms and pseudoaneurysms. J Vasc Surg 2007; 45:276–83.
14. Chiesa R, Astore D, Guzzo G, et al. Visceral artery aneurysms. Ann Vasc Surg 2005; 19:42–8.
15. Hageman JH, Smith RF, Szilagyi E, Elliott JP. Aneurysms of the renal artery: probems of prognosis and surgical management. Surgery 1987; 84:563–72.

16. Renal arteries and veins. In: Karim V, ed. Vascular and Interventional Radiology. Saunders Elsevier, 2006:204–39.
17. Bratby MJ, Lehmann ED, Bottomlley J, et al. Endovascular embolization of visceral artery aneurysms with ethylene-vinyl alocohol (Onyx): a case series. Cardiovasc Intervent Radiol 2006; 29(6):1125–8.

Part VIII | **VASCULAR MALFORMATIONS**

45 | Vascular Malformations

Peter Rowlands
Royal Liverpool University Hospital, Liverpool, U.K.
Andrew Edward Healey
Alder Hey Children's Hospital and Royal Liverpool University Hospital, Liverpool, U.K.

INTRODUCTION

Vascular malformations are uncommon but important lesions, with a significant morbidity, wide spectrum of appearance and symptoms and occasional mortality. They occur in all parts of the body and may present at almost any age. Misdiagnosis and mismanagement of these conditions is common and few vascular centers encounter sufficient cases to allow confident treatment protocols to develop. Presentation to a particular speciality depends on the symptoms involved. Many vascular specialists, dermatologists, plastic, and orthopedic surgeons will however encounter the occasional case and it is important that appropriate initial assessment is performed. We believe that a multidisciplinary approach to patient management leads to optimal outcome.

It is most important that ill-advised treatment is not undertaken, as this is often ineffective, may significantly hamper subsequent therapeutic efforts, and has the potential to worsen symptoms.

The key to correct diagnosis is a detailed history with a clinical examination directing tailored radiological investigation. Treatment is multipronged and is tailored very specifically to the individual patient and lesion. Often conservative treatment with a watch and wait policy is the most effective. Cure is possible but symptom control is the aim of treatment and the patient may need intermittent treatment throughout their life.

Worsening of symptoms as a result of treatment is to be avoided at all costs. Rigorous use of precise nomenclature aids correct management and avoids confusion between the many clinicians involved in the patient's management.

Symptoms occur as a result of local pressure effects; pain related to thrombosis and venous stasis, adverse cosmetic appearance, spontaneous hemorrhage and occasionally high-output cardiac failure.

Vascular malformations commonly arise within the central nervous system; these are outside the scope of this discussion and will not be considered further.

CLASSIFICATION

Nomenclature of vascular malformations was previously confusing and inconsistent. Obsolete terms are still often used, both in clinical practice and in publications.

Mulliken et al. initially developed the classification currently adopted by the International Society for the Study of Vascular Malformations (1).

Lesions that Show Cell Proliferation

These lesions are true neoplasms.

Benign
Hemangiomas
Lesions are usually present at birth, grow soon after birth, enter a quiescent phase and then spontaneously regress (usually between the ages of three and eight years). Hemangiomas may leave a fibrofatty residue after regression that can be seen in adults.

Hemangioendothelioma
A variant of hemangioma associated with the Kasabach–Merritt syndrome.

Malignant

- Kaposi's sarcoma
- Angiosarcoma

Lesions Without Cell Proliferation

These are vascular malformations and are considered to represent a focal area of persistence of primitive vascular elements. The type of malformation depends on the level of abnormal communication and varies from capillary to arterial connections. The level of the communication is thought to be related to the timing of the developmental failure. They are usually evident at birth and grow with the child.

- Arterial (high flow connected to the vascular tree)
- Venous (low flow connected to the vascular tree)
- Capillary (fine network of vascular spaces)
- Lymphatic (containing tissue fluid)
    - Macrocystic (visible cystic spaces on imaging)
    - Microcystic (predominantly cystic spaces visible only on microscopy)
- Mixed (containing a mixture of two or more of the elements above)

Misnomers that Add to Confusion

- Aneurysmal bone cyst—this is an expansile venous malformation of bone.
- Vertebral hemangioma—this is a low-flow venous malformation that is nonexpansile.
- Visceral hemangioma in adults—these are low-flow venous malformations.
- Cystic hygroma—this is a macrocystic lymphatic malformation of the neck present at birth.
- Maffucci syndrome—as described below and not multiple cutaneous hemangiomas with enchondromas.

There are a number of syndromes in whom a vascular malformation forms part of the clinical features. Some of the more common examples are listed below.

Syndromes Associated with Vascular Malformations

Syndrome	Findings	Manifestations
Klippel–Trénaunay	Port wine stain Persistent embryonal leg vein Deep vein hypoplasia	Lymphoedema Hemihypertrophy
Parkes Weber	Diffuse microscopic arteriovenous fistulous malformations	Limb overgrowth
Sturge–Weber	Port wine stain Abnormal cerebral vessels	Epilepsy
Kasabach–Merritt	Hemangioendothelioma	Consumptive platelet coagulopathy
Maffucci syndrome	Multiple venous malformations and enchondromas	Deformity and disability

There is often an associated neuronal developmental abnormality, which may be seen as localized hyperhidrosis (autonomic dysfunction) or café-au-lait spots, whose origin is neuroectodermal cells (2).

Literature Review

Research is ongoing into other causative associations of vascular malformations. Eerola et al. (4) have described an association between KREV1 interaction trapped 1 protein and hyperkeratotic cutaneous capillary–venous malformation, due to a gene mutation. Boon et al. (4,5) have described a familial venous malformation associated with a mutation on the 9p chromosome.

It is likely, however, that most vascular malformations are sporadic and are part of a spectrum involving one or many cell types in a disorganized hamartomous abnormality in which the vascular component causes the predominant symptoms.

CLINICAL APPROACH

History

Venous Malformation

This usually presents with swelling and pain. The degree of swelling is often variable and is influenced by factors such as ambient temperature, dependency or elevation. The pain may be worsened by pressure from clothes or furniture. Exercise involving the affected muscle may lead to an increase in pain. Episodes of acute pain may be associated with areas of spontaneous thrombosis. Pregnancy frequently exacerbates symptoms, particularly in lower limb venous malformations. Lesions around joints particularly the knee frequently give rise to intra-articular hemorrhage. This can be very disabling with significant loss of limb function, especially in children. Limb length inequality may be seen, although less commonly than in arteriovenous malformation (AVM).

Facial venous malformations are common. Sites that are often involved include the tongue, lip, and buccal mucosa, but they may involve deeper structures such as the parotid gland and masseter muscle. They present with a cosmetic deformity: either skin discoloration (due to dilated veins, subcutaneous hemorrhage or venous hypertension) or a mass. Lesions related to the oro-pharynx may present with recurrent hemorrhage, which may be significant.

The lesion may increase in size as a result of compression of the proximal veins, dependency or by a Valsalva maneuvre. It is usual that the extent of the lesion on radiological imaging studies is much larger than the visible component.

AVM

Most lesions that are not visceral are noted at birth or in the first year. They present as a firm mass that may pulsate or have a palpable or audible bruit. There is often prominence of the supplying artery and fullness of draining veins. Distal ischemic changes, atrophy, skin ulceration and oedema may all be seen. The atrophy and ischemic change seen in the periphery are usually the result of a steal phenomenon, where the periphery is deprived of blood that is instead shunted through the AVM.

Often there is an associated growth abnormality, most usually hypertrophy of an affected limb. The hypertrophy is often apparent both in length and bulk.

AVMs may suddenly increase in size, so that previously stable and asymptomatic lesions may change and produce adverse effects on the patient's wellbeing and lifestyle. Hormonal changes of puberty and pregnancy may accelerate growth, and occasionally trauma may lead to a change in activity.

Cardiac failure is often mistakenly thought to be a frequent feature of AVM. In a series of 100 AVMs seen at New York University, only three had a significant high-output state (4–6). The two settings in which this is generally seen are in lesions of infancy and in large pelvic or abdominal lesions in adults.

Lymphatic Malformation

The distribution of lymphatic malformations is similar to that of venous malformation with craniofacial or limb involvement. The lymphatic malformations of the periphery are very similar to venous malformations. Indeed the two lesions often coexist in one limb, and are similar on imaging criteria.

Capillary Malformation

This condition may involve the head and neck and limbs also. It manifests as a flat dark patch, often termed port wine stain. The malformation is usually of cosmetic importance only, as pain or other complications are uncommon. It may be associated with venous malformation and is seen almost invariably in Klippel–Trénaunay syndrome (KTS). Facial capillary malformation is associated with epilepsy and cerebral hemorrhage secondary to dural vascular malformation in Sturge–Weber syndrome.

Patients can generally be reassured that vascular malformations are

1. not neoplastic
2. genetically isolated
3. rarely genetically transmitted
4. often stable lesions requiring no specific treatment (6)

Any lesion that does not conform to the expected clinical or radiological findings or follows an unusual course should be biopsied. Unfortunately the confusion with nomenclature endemic in radiology also affects pathology with imprecise use of terminology and vague, generic, colloquial, and outdated terminology. While evidence of any malignant features should be taken very seriously, the proffered pathological diagnosis arrived at is of less concern.

Klippel–Trénaunay Syndrome

This is mentioned as a separate condition as it is relatively common and has a typical constellation of signs and symptoms (4–7). These are:

1. Cutaneous port wine naevi. Histologically they are capillary malformations
2. Soft tissue and bony hypertrophy
3. Vascular anomalies

Previous workers had described AVM in association with the above; this is felt to be extremely rare. There is a combined lymphatic, venous, and capillary malformation. Ninety percent of KTS patients have abnormalities present at birth. Ten percent of KTS is limited to the upper limb, whilst 70% is in the lower limb only. Other congenital anomalies are present in a third of the patients.

The vascular anomalies are complex. There is frequent aplasia or hypoplasia of the deep veins of the calf and knee. Rarely the femoral or iliac vein is absent. There are often persisting embryological veins, which include the lateral vein of the thigh and the sciatic vein. These veins are often very large and produce swelling and heaviness of the limb. Severe reflux may be seen in the anomalous vein. Suprapubic veins are seen in a fifth of patients.

As well as poor function, the anomalous veins are prone to venous thrombosis. Thrombophlebitis is also common, and cellulitis is also frequently seen.

Limb hypertrophy is the least common of the three main features. It is caused by overgrowth of bone and soft tissue and may be exacerbated by venous or lymphatic dysfunction.

INVESTIGATIONS

A clinical history and examination by an experienced clinician is accurate at making a diagnosis in the majority of cases. Imaging investigations are more often used to determine the extent of a lesion rather than make a specific diagnosis as many entities have similar appearances. An assessment of high versus low flow can be made clinically, with hand-held Doppler probe or with Doppler ultrasound.

Hematological and biochemical investigations are usually normal. In rare cases there may be evidence of hemolysis or platelet destruction, and sequestration in large vascular lesions.

Plain Films

Plain films are rarely required in the assessment of vascular malformations. Bony involvement may be seen in venous and AVM. Pressure erosion may be seen and there is often periosteal new bone (that can lead to misdiagnosis and anxiety) associated with proximity to these lesions. Phleboliths are commonly seen within venous malformations. Leg length discrepancy may be associated with hemihypertrophy in AVM, and KTS.

Ultrasound

Sonography, combined with color duplex is useful in the initial assessment of vascular malformation. It is easy to differentiate high and low-flow lesions. Ultrasound also gives the best information available about the size of vascular spaces within the malformation. This allows a decision about the potential use of percutaneous sclerotherapy to be made. This is generally only successful with vascular spaces visible on ultrasound. Ultrasound is also useful in guiding the site of puncture during sclerotherapy (Fig. 1).

The major advantage of sonography is that it may be combined with the clinical examination in the outpatient department to allow informed decisions on treatment and further investigation to be made instantly.

Limitations of sonography are related to the deep extent of a lesion. It may not be possible to assess involvement of deep structures such as muscles and bones, to accurately determine the maximum extent. It would be unwise to plan major intervention without additional cross-sectional imaging. Ultrasound is very useful in follow-up, enabling a good assessment of the amount of a lesion that has been successfully occluded.

Computed Tomography

There is little role for computed tomography (CT) in the assessment of vascular malformations. Generally the ability of magnetic resonance (MR) to demonstrate vascular structures and involvement of soft tissues is much superior and is preferred. This is particularly true in the young patient where avoidance of ionizing radiation is paramount.

The higher resolution of multidetector vascular CT is promising in the assessment of the anatomy of complex AVMs. The ability to perform multiplanar reconstructions might well prove useful in the planning of complex embolization but it is unlikely that CT will replace angiography and it may lead to a further investigation with little actual gain.

Magnetic Resonance

This is the single most useful diagnostic modality in the assessment of vascular malformations. It provides, in a noninvasive fashion, exquisitely detailed information about the

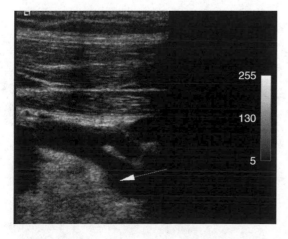

FIGURE 1 An ultrasound scan of a deep venous malformation in the thigh. Venous channels (marked) are present deep to the quadriceps muscle.

extent of lesions. It allows detailed examination of vascular supply and drainage in AVMs. The most useful sequences are T1 for detailed anatomy and fat-suppressed T2, which allows maximum contrast between malformation, which demonstrates high-intensity signal, and other tissues which are dark. MR angiography can be utilized to delineate the normal vascular anatomy.

An entire limb can be examined within a reasonable length of time; this is especially important in venous malformations where several areas in a single limb may be involved. The multiplanar nature of MR allows an anatomical demonstration of the malformation which may be easily understood by referring clinician and indeed by the patient (Fig. 2). Intravenous contrast is rarely necessary as the inherent tissue contrast of MR is sufficient to provide all necessary information.

Venography

Ascending venography is not generally helpful as vascular malformations are rarely filled by this technique. It may be useful if there is a history of venous thrombosis as it is important to avoid sclerotherapy of superficial lesions if there is occlusion of deep veins. Venography may be of value in demonstrating the abnormal venous anatomy in KTS and may be of value in demonstrating normal veins in other extensive malformations. Generally MR will provide enough information about deep venous structures.

Direct puncture phlebography is important to demonstrate the extent and connections of vascular structures within venous malformation. The direct puncture study is usually combined with the sclerotherapy treatment (Fig. 3).

Arteriography

Arteriography is rarely required to establish a diagnosis of venous malformation. Clinical assessment and noninvasive imaging do this. Angiography is required for the assessment of AVM. This may be done as part of the pre-procedure evaluation or may be the initial stage of an embolization episode. The technique used for arteriography needs to be meticulous, with high frame rates and multiple projections. Selective and superselective catheterization is necessary. It is essential that the location and supply of the nidus is clearly demonstrated, as this is critical for the successful embolization of the AVM. It is recommended that only noninvasive imaging is performed prior to referral to a specialist center as invasive imaging does not aid the diagnosis and is often repeated at the specialist center.

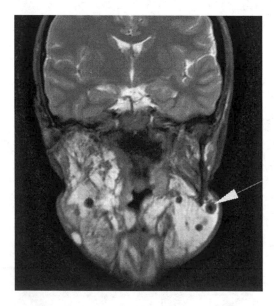

FIGURE 2 T2 weighted fat-suppressed magnetic resonance image of extensive facial venous malformation. A phlebolith is marked (*arrow*).

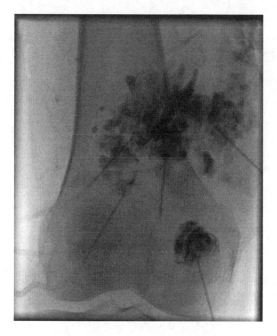

FIGURE 3 Multiple needles have been placed in a venous malformation of the knee during injection of sclerosant/contrast mixture.

TREATMENT

It is rare for a vascular malformation to present urgently. When they do it is almost always a high-flow lesion and as a result of hemorrhage or high-output cardiac failure. Both complications may be treated by endovascular embolization. Low-flow lesions that bleed can be treated by compression. Embolization is rarely required.

It is usually possible to assess and image the patients in a relaxed setting. Discussion of each case can be carried out in depth, and should lead to a rational decision about a management protocol.

It is very important to recognize that a significant proportion of patients attending such a clinic do not require any invasive treatment at all. Frequently, patients will attend a specialist center having had invasive and noninvasive imaging, and surgery or endovascular procedures, but not knowing the diagnosis nor an idea of prognosis. If the symptoms caused by the malformation are not particular severe, active intervention may not be indicated. Following an explanation of the nature and cause of the vascular malformation, and an opportunity to see the MR images, with time to ask questions, many patients are reassured and happy to live with minor or moderate symptoms.

Many of the techniques that are subsequently discussed have the potential for moderate or severe complications. It is very unsatisfactory if a patient with a benign condition with symptoms that do not interfere with day-to-day life ends up after treatment with worsening of their condition. Conversely patients with highly symptomatic lesions are prepared to accept significant risk of complications if a truly informed consent is obtained.

Conservative Management

Peripheral vascular malformations are seldom life-threatening and limb loss is rare. Often lesions grow along with the child and stabilize in early adulthood. If the lesion is not particularly symptomatic, and the patient understands cause and outlook, it might be left alone. Advice about early treatment of cellulitis in lymphatic malformations is important. If there is recurrent acute pain and tenderness in a malformation that is otherwise quiescent, areas of thrombosis are likely. An anti-platelet drug might be considered in this setting.

Surgery

Surgical treatment may be appropriate in certain situations. If a lesion is small and superficial on imaging, and can be completely resected, operative management is ideal. However the vast majority of symptomatic lesions are too large to resect and involvement of deep structures risks an outcome that is worse than if the lesion is left untreated. The recurrence rate of attempted curative surgery in venous and AVM is close to 100%. The resultant scarring is often as symptomatic as the original lesion. Better cure rates can be obtained in cervical lymphatic malformation, although the surgery is not without risk, with injury to collateral structures. Intralesional suturing, the Popescu technique (8) has some advocates in the management of venous malformation, although other authors question its effectiveness.

Ligation of supplying vessels in AVM is occasionally performed as part of a surgical approach. This is to be avoided at all costs as it may lead to difficulty in access for endovascular techniques.

Radiotherapy

This was occasionally used in the past and is referred to in a few current papers. It is of limited effectiveness and the cosmetic changes induced by radiotherapy and potential secondary malignancies are unacceptable.

Laser

Laser therapy can be very effective in reducing the intensity of color in the "port wine" stains that are frequently associated with vascular malformations (9). Pulsed light systems or flashlamp-pumped pulsed dye laser can treat these in several treatment episodes with minimal complications. Pink colored lesions respond better than purple ones. Superficial lesions tend to respond better than deeper ones, although newer systems with higher penetration show some promise. Most vascular malformations are situated in subcutaneous fat or muscle and as such are well beyond the reach of conventional lasers. Bare laser fibers have been inserted into hemangiomas; this is not likely to prove more effective than sclerotherapy (10).

Sclerotherapy and Embolization

Most lesions are not amenable to surgery or laser and will present to the interventional radiologist. The application in each lesion type is discussed below.

Venous Malformation

Sclerosant agents are effective in the management of venous malformation. They are likely to produce a significant improvement in pain, and sometimes in lesion bulk. The two most widely used agents are sodium tetradecyl sulphate (STD) and absolute alcohol. The technique used involves a preliminary direct venogram (Fig. 3). The lesion is filled with contrast and then the contrast is replaced with either neat sclerosant (STD or alcohol) or foam (STD, air, and contrast mix). If there is significant overspill into deep veins, the drainage can be occluded manually or by using a tourniquet if the lesion is within a limb. Experts differ as to the relative effectiveness of the two agents, Jackson (11) states that they are of equal effectiveness whilst Yakes (12) believes alcohol to be more effective. There is a significant difference in the ease of use. Alcohol is very painful and always requires general anesthesia, while STD can be tolerated using local anesthesia/sedation.

Risks and complications are relatively low. Deep venous thrombosis is very rare and there is a small risk of skin necrosis. Temporary neurological dysfunction has been described using alcohol.

The treatment is effective, but often several treatment episodes are required. Large series of patients having sclerotherapy have not entered the literature yet, but many operators report high rates of patient satisfaction with the technique. Pappas (13) reported significant clinical improvement in over 90% of venous malformations in the head and neck. More importantly, 95% of patients were satisfied with the outcome of treatment.

Lymphatic Malformation
Sclerotherapy using alcohol or OK432 is very effective at treatment and has become the primary treatment for the condition (8,12,14,15).

Lymphoedema treatment with external graduation compression garments may help the symptoms of limb heaviness; massage can also be effective. The use of pneumatic compression pumps has been disappointing in most cases. Debulking surgery has also met with indifferent results but can be helpful.

The patient must be aware of the signs of infection and should use antibiotics at an early stage, as the infection may be very slow to resolve.

Klippel–Trénaunay Syndrome
Much of the management of KTS patients is supportive. It is most important for the patient or carer to have a realistic understanding of the nature of the condition.

Limb swelling is usually a combination of limb overgrowth and lymphoedema. Limb length inequality up to 2 cm is usually of no significance. It is uncommon that the inequality is larger than this; referral for epiphyseal surgery is recommended above this level.

Cutaneous lesions are common in KTS and are usually capillary port wine type lesions. If they are of cosmetic concern, they often respond to laser therapy. Cellulitis is common in KTS.

Intervention in the venous system is the most difficult decision in KTS. Deep veins are usually hypoplastic and there may be varicose veins or commonly a persistent embryonic lateral vein. These veins are often very large and functionally poor. There may be marked reflux into the abnormal veins.

Management should be minimalist. A good duplex examination and MR scan will indicate the extent of the venous abnormality and localize reflux. Targeted surgery to prevent reflux may be very successful. Ligation or excision of anomalous veins may be helpful but care should be taken, as the native deep veins have limited functionality. Exclusion and sclerotherapy of anomalous veins has been reported but is to be performed with great care (16).

Arteriovenous Malformations
The management of AVM is the biggest challenge in this group of conditions. Potential for significant complications is highest and the outcome for ill-advised or poorly planned intervention is also very high. In many cases, if symptoms are minor or absent, an explanation of the condition to the patient and occasional review is the best management. Intervention may be considered if there is significant pain or cutaneous involvement, or if there is peripheral ischemia due to shunting.

The key to the successful management of these lesions is a clear understanding of the nature of the anatomy that is present and of the location of the nidus, or arteriovenous connection(s). The work of Houdart allows (17) the anatomy to be divided into three types. The first type is *arteriovenous*, in which no more than three arteries shunt to the initial venous component. The second is *arteriolovenous*, in which there are multiple arteries shunting to a single vein. The third is *arteriolovenulous*, in which multiple arterioles shunt to multiple draining venules.

Permanent embolic agents that can be used include coils, cyanoacrylate, and alcohol copolymer/tantalum (Onyx, EV3, Irvine, California). Absolute alcohol can also be used. Particle agents include polyvinyl alcohol.

Arteriovenous lesions can be treated either via an arterial or venous route or by direct puncture. The former is convenient, as arterial access is required to image the AVM. Embolic agent is introduced at the level of the shunt to close the arteriovenous connections. It is very important that the embolization is limited to the smallest possible area to avoid collateral damage.

Arteriolovenous lesions have a single venous component and it is convenient to treat them via a venous approach, or by direct puncture if not feasible. Embolic agents can be introduced at the level of the fistulae. It is frequently necessary to mechanically occlude the

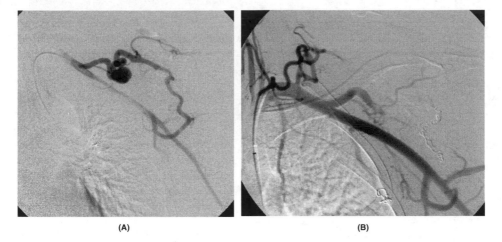

(A)   (B)

FIGURE 4 (**A**) Arteriovenous malformation arising from proximal subclavian artery with a further feeding vessel arising from the distal subclavian artery. (**B**) The distal feeding vessel was embolized using coils to avoid distal flow of embolic material. The nidus was catheterized and filled with alcohol copolymer (Onyx, EV3, Irvine, California) with ablation of flow.

venous outflow to reduce flow and allow the embolic agent prolonged contact with the nidus. An alternative approach is to pack the venous outflow with coils, to occlude the flow through the lesion.

Arteriolovenulous lesions are very resistant to treatment due to the multiplicity of supplying and draining vessels. The results of embolization are poor and palliation is often all that can be achieved. Particle embolization may be effective at reducing flow and bulk of these lesions. Particle embolization may also be used in devascularization prior to surgical debulking or resection. Figure 4 demonstrates endovascular treatment of a high-flow vascular malformation.

Complications of Embolization
The number of potential complications of embolization in AVM is much higher than venous or lymphatic malformation. Agents and devices such as coils and balloons can pass through the fistulae if incorrectly sized. This should be rare. With liquid agents there is a risk of overspill into other vessels that are not part of the AVM. This is a particular fear with alcohol as cases of tissue necrosis and nerve damage have been reported (12). The advances in imaging and the development of superior catheter technologies should allow accurate deployment of embolic materials.

SUMMARY

Although they are uncommon, clinicians should be familiar with the wide spectrum of disease and symptoms, the morbidity, and the optimal management of vascular malformations. Achieving a correct diagnosis is essential to provide the correct management of these lesions. Management is multidisciplinary and should occur in centers of expertise, with wide experience in the treatment of vascular malformations. The goal of treatment is control of symptoms and cure is rarely possible. If there is any doubt about the possibility of malignancy, lesions should be biopsied, although the results of biopsy rarely lead to a definitive diagnosis if the lesion is a malformation.

For the majority of patients, conservative management is often optimal.

If lesions require intervention, the results of treatment are as variable as the lesions involved. Perseverance with an unsuccessful technique time after time is of no benefit. Most patients require episodic treatment over their entire life as symptoms wax and wane and their lifestyle and expectations alter. The majority of patients derive most benefit from with a combination approach of laser, sclerotherapy, and conservative measures. More complex tailored techniques beyond the scope of this text can be applied to individual lesions that are refractory to the techniques described above.

REFERENCES

1. Mulliken JB, Glowacki J. Classification of pediatric vascular lesions. Plast Reconstr Surg 1982; 70(1):120–1.
2. Rosen R, Riles T. Arteriovenous malformations. In: Strandness E, Van Breda A, eds. Vascular Diseases: Surgical and Interventional Therapy. New York: Churchill Livingstone, 1993.
3. North PE, Waner M, Mizeracki A, et al. A unique microvascular phenotype shared by juvenile hemangiomas and human placenta. Arch Dermatol 2001; 137(5):559.
4. Eerola I, Plate KH, Spiegel R, Boon LM, Mulliken JB, Vikkula M. KRIT1 is mutated in hyperkeratotic cutaneous capillary-venous malformation associated with cerebral capillary malformation. Hum Mol Genet 2000; 9(9):1351–5.
5. Boon L, Mulliken JB, Vikkula M. Assignment of a locus for dominantly inherited venous malformations to chromosome 9p. Hum Mol Genet 1994; 3:1583–7.
6. Rosen R, Riles T. Arteriovenous malformations. In: Strandness E, Van Breda A, eds. Vascular Diseases: Surgical and Interventional Therapy. New York: Churchill Livingstone, 2004.
7. Jacob A, Driscoll DJ, Shaughnessy WJ, Stanson AW, Clay RP, Gloviczki P. Klippel–Trenaunay syndrome: spectrum and management. Mayo Clin Proc 1998; 73:28–36.
8. Popescu V. Intratumoral ligation in the management of orofacial cavernous haemangioomas. J Maxillofac Surg 1985; 13:99–107.
9. Raulin C, Schroeter CA, Weiss RA, Keiner M, Werner S. Treatment of port-wine stains with a noncoherent pulsed light source: a retrospective study. Arch Dermatol 1999; 135(6):679.
10. Glaessl A, Schreyer AG, Wimmershoff MB, Landthaler M, Feuerbach S, Hohenleutner U. Laser surgical planning with magnetic resonance imaging-based 3-dimensional reconstructions for intralesional Nd:YAG laser therapy of a venous malformation of the neck. Arch Dermatol 2001; 137(10):1331.
11. Jackson J. Vascular malformations. In: Beard J, ed. Vascular and Endovascular Surgery. 2nd ed. Saunders, 2001:515–28.
12. Yakes WF, Haas DK, Parker S. Symptomatic vascular malformations: ethanol embolotherapy. Radiology 1989; 170:1059–66.
13. Pappas DC, Jr., Persky MS, Berenstein A. Evaluation and treatment of head and neck venous vascular malformations. Ear Nose Throat J 1998; 77(11):914.
14. Burrows P. Personal Communication, 2003.
15. Jackson J. Vascular malformations. In: Gaines PA, Beard J, eds. Vascular and Endovascular Surgery. 2nd ed. Elsevier, 2000:515–28.
16. Burrows P. Effectiveness of sclerotherapy in multilocular lymphatic malformation. Personal Communication, 2003.
17. Houdart E, Gobin YP, Casasco A, Aymard A, Herbreteau D, Merland JJ. A proposed classification of intracranial arteriovenous fistulae and malformations. Interv Neuroradiol 1993; 35:381–5.

46 | Role of Endovascular Procedures in Management of Extremity and Cervical Vascular Trauma

Alan B. Lumsden
Methodist DeBakey Heart Center, Houston, Texas, U.S.A.
Carlos F. Bechara
Baylor College of Medicine, Houston, Texas, U.S.A.
Eric K. Peden and Michael J. Reardon
Methodist DeBakey Heart Center, Houston, Texas, U.S.A.

INTRODUCTION

The use of endovascular surgery in the trauma patient is becoming more popular and superior to conventional surgery in certain situations. Like open surgery, endovascular surgery can be both diagnostic and therapeutic. This chapter focuses on the role of endovascular therapy in the management of vascular injuries to the neck and extremities. Peripheral injuries account for 80% of all cases of vascular trauma.

The decision to pursue an endovascular strategy or the conventional open approach is dependent on the expertise of the trauma surgeon, availability of imaging and the condition of the patient. Many centers now have access to hybrid operating suites which offer excellent imaging facilities within a traditional surgical environment.

With the evolution of portable, high-quality imaging, the opportunity exists to perform point of service angiography, to initiate vascular control, or even provide definitive endoluminal management. This has numerous potential advantages: shortening of time from admission to definitive open or endoluminal therapy, and avoidance of complex transportation issues in injured patients. Clearly this must be accomplished without compromising the quality of patient care.

Arterial injuries can present in a variety of ways: ischemia, bleeding (external when associated with significant soft tissue damage, or internal associated with signs of hypovolemic shock) or as a pulsatile mass. The injuries can result from either penetrating or blunt trauma, causing frank disruption of the vessel, dissection, pseudoaneurysm, occlusion or arteriovenous fistula. Most patients who are unstable at the time of presentation or have non-controllable external or internal bleeding should undergo an urgent conventional open operative repair. There are however, selective situations where even hemodynamically unstable patients are best stabilized using endovascular techniques. Pelvis fractures with bleeding from torn hypogastric branches are such an example. But as a general rule, open exploration, in these patients, has the benefit of exploring other injuries, mainly associated venous injury.

Hard clinical signs of vascular injury include ischemia, absent distal pulses, active external hemorrhage, pulsatile or expanding hematoma, paresthesia, paralysis, poikilothermia, bruit or a thrill. Soft signs include diminished distal pulses, proximity of vessels to injury, significant bleeding at the scene and peripheral neurologic deficit.

GENERAL TECHNICAL CONSIDERATIONS

The advantage of angiography is it can evaluate different vascular beds in the same setting. Furthermore, it permits imaging of the arterial intima and allows the evaluation of an injury without exploration through an existing hematoma. However, many of these benefits can also be provided by computed tomographic (CT) angiography. The key benefit of diagnostic angiography is the possibility to immediately progress to either endoluminal vascular control or definitive endoluminal repair. Key findings during angiography are intraluminal filling defects, contrast extravasation, dilation of arterial contrast, arteriovenous fistula, narrowing of vessels and occlusion of the vessel. The type of vascular lesion determines the type of intervention required.

BASIC ENDOVASCULAR TECHNIQUES FOR VASCULAR TRAUMA

Embolization Techniques

Active bleeding in a non-critical vessel is usually managed with vessel sacrifice using catheter delivery of embolic agents. Generally a catheter should be placed as close to the target vessel as possible. Ideally, occlusion both proximal and distal to the bleeding site should be performed. Gelfoam embolization is useful in treating small bleeding vessels. The gelfoam is manually rolled into a bullet shaped pellet, which can be injected through a catheter delivered to the bleeding vessel. Polyvinyl alcohol particles of appropriate diameter are selected to occlude small parenchymal vessels. Larger bleeding vessels should be embolized using coils. There are a variety of such coils, which essentially consist of a metal core with Dacron fibers attached, to induce vessel thrombosis.

Embolization of pelvic and parenchymal (spleen, kidney and liver) injuries after blunt and penetrating trauma is increasingly being utilized as first-line therapy.

Bare Stents and Stent-Grafts

Bare stents have a limited role in trauma which may be limited to repairing an intimal dissection. There are an increasing number of covered stents, which have the ability to completely seal a vessel. Covered stents are mainly used to treat arterial injuries in the trauma patient. There are only sporadic case reports of their use in the venous system.

Endoluminal Vascular Control

In a patient with active bleeding in a vessel, which cannot be sacrificed, positioning and inflation of a compliant occlusion balloon can provide immediate control to permit patient resuscitation to proceed. Similarly, such a technique can also be used to minimize the magnitude of an open operation by providing proximal control in an area where open surgical control may be challenging.

VASCULAR INJURIES IN THE NECK

Trauma to the cervical vasculature usually results in significant morbidity and mortality since the brain is less tolerant of ischemia compared to other end organs. The expeditious diagnosis and management of these injuries is crucial but sometimes difficult in the comatose patient. Vascular injuries of the neck make up 5% of all civilian vascular injuries. These vascular injuries can occur with both penetrating and blunt trauma. Penetrating trauma causes almost 95% of all neck vascular injuries. Classically, traumatic injuries to the neck are classified according to three anatomic zones (1):

- Zone 1: The anatomic area between the sternal notch and the cricoid cartilage.
- Zone 2: The anatomic area between the cricoid cartilage and the angle of the mandible.
- Zone 3: The anatomic area between the angle of the mandible and the base of the skull.

This classification helps guide the diagnostic workup of these injuries as well as the operative approach.

Carotid Artery Injuries

Carotid artery injuries constitute 6% of all penetrating neck injuries and 22% of all cervical vascular injuries (2). The common carotid artery is the most injured vessel followed by the internal carotid artery (ICA) then by the external carotid artery. Mortality rates of 5% to 20% have been reported (3,4) along with a stroke rate of 28%. The presence of a neurologic deficit on presentation, along with the severity and duration of shock was reported to be the main determinants of worse outcome and survival (4).

The recognition of blunt carotid artery injury is increasing due to more vigilant screening of the trauma patient. Half of these patients present with no overt signs of cervical trauma or neurologic deficit. Blunt carotid artery injury accounts for 3% to 5% of all carotid injuries (3,5). The distal ICA accounts for more than 90% of blunt injuries. This injury carries a mortality rate of 5% to 43% and a poor neurologic outcome in more than half of these patients (5). Penetrating and blunt injury to the carotid artery can result in thrombosis, pseudoaneurysm formation, intimal flap formation, dissection, arteriovenous fistula, or complete disruption (3).

Patients who present with hard signs of vascular injury in the neck should be immediately explored in the operating room. Most, if not all, data on the role of endovascular surgery in carotid artery injury in the literature describe its use in treating aneurysms, dissections and fistulas. Endovascular techniques have been used more frequently in treating injuries to zones 1 and 3; surgically inaccessible lesions; lesions that require extensive surgical dissection; or when excessive bleeding is anticipated due to venous hypertension, as in fistula formation.

Penetrating Injuries

Covered and bare stents have been used to treat carotid artery pseudoaneurysms or arteriovenous injuries (6–14). Bare stents have been used successfully to treat carotid aneurysms (9–12) in association with embolization coils, which are placed through the interstices of the stent into the aneurysm sac (Fig. 1A,B). Only aneurysms with a relatively narrow neck can be treated using this technique and it has been suggested that this technique should be reserved for high cervical carotid pseudoaneurysms, not amenable to surgical exposure (12).

Covered stents can be used to completely exclude carotid aneurysms (Fig. 2A,B). However, these stents require a much larger delivery system and a catheter length of 120 cm

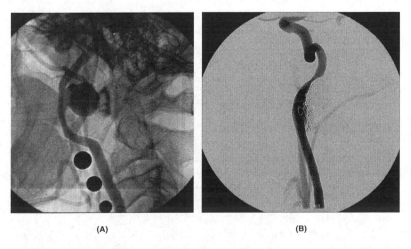

(A)   (B)

FIGURE 1 (**A**) Traumatic pseudoaneurysm of high internal carotid artery, with narrow-based communication. This was a result of a blunt trauma to the neck. (**B**) The entrance to the pseudoaneurysm has been covered with a stent and detachable micro-coils placed via a microcatheter into the pseudoaneurysm.

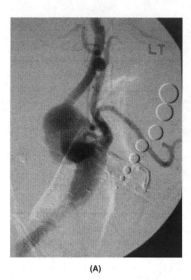
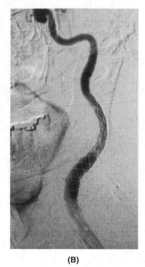

(A)   (B)

FIGURE 2 (A,B) Broad-based traumatic pseudoaneurysm close to origin of internal carotid artery, treated with placement of a covered stent (Wallgraft, Boston Scientific, Natick, Massachusettes U.S.A.). This also resulted in exclusion of the external carotid artery.

may be needed to reach the distal ICA. Some groups have successfully used Wallgrafts to repair Zone 3 ICA injuries (6,7,13). The "homemade" Palmaz balloon-expandable stent covered with polytetrafluoroethylene (PTFE) graft has been used in the treatment of an ICA pseudoaneurysm located at the skull base (8) and for an arteriovenous fistula with a pseudoaneurysm at the skull base (6). Parodi (14) used vein-covered stents in two patients with penetrating trauma. One patient presented with an HIV-associated pseudoaneurysm and another patient had an infected false aneurysm. Vein was utilized as it might be more resistant to infection than prosthetic material.

Blunt Injuries

Blunt carotid dissections and thrombosis have been traditionally managed by anticoagulation (15,16). However, this strategy is not without complications and some polytrauma patients have contraindications for anticoagulation. Covered stents have been used successfully to treat carotid artery dissection or pseudoaneurysm formation following blunt trauma (17–20). In one report (17), all patients were successfully treated with no sequelae and without the use of anticoagulation. However, in another report (20), three patients suffered complications due to stent deployment, two suffered acute stent thrombosis and one had transient ischemic attacks.

In another study (21) 10 patients with ICA dissection and contraindication for anticoagulation underwent stent placement. At 7 to 28 month follow-up, all stents were patent, all patients were neurologically intact and the mean dissection stenosis was reduced from 69% to 8%. All patients were treated with antiplatelet therapy only.

There are no current studies evaluating the role and long-term outcome of endovascular surgery in treating cervical vascular injuries. Zhou et al. showed that endovascular surgery is being increasingly used in treating carotid artery aneurysms. This study also demonstrated that patients treated with stents had shorter convalescence and less procedure related complications compared to conventional open repair (22).

Vertebral Artery Injuries

Vertebral artery (VA) injuries are rare and can be caused by penetrating or blunt trauma. The incidence is less than 5% of all cervical vascular injuries, and most are due to penetrating injuries. The recognition of these injuries is also increasing due to improved diagnostic imaging. These patients usually present with no neurologic deficit or evidence of arterial trauma. Posterior cerebral circulation ischemia rarely occurs if the contralateral VA is patent. However, VA injury should be suspected in patients with cervical spine injuries and/or cervical vertebral injuries. Arteriovenous fistulas seem to occur more frequently in this location due to the rich venous plexus. Mortality related to VA injury alone is approximately 5% but, in practice, is usually higher because of the association with other cervical injuries.

Because of the difficult anatomic location of the VA, catheter-based interventions are becoming more popular. VA trauma can be treated endovascularly with either embolization or stent placement. Coil embolization of the distal and proximal VA has been successful in treating arteriovenous fistulas and pseudoaneurysms (23,24). With more expertise, stents and small stent-grafts have been used with success (23,24). In cases of complete disruption of the VA, there is always a risk of rebleeding, and close follow up is recommended. A concomitant retrograde and antegrade approach can be used to embolize the injured VA (25,26).

Technical Considerations

The mid to distal extracranial VA is extremely tortuous, making endovascular placement of a covered stent difficult. Most commercially available stent-grafts are too large. The GraftMaster (Jostent®, Jomed M.V., Germany) for use in the coronary arteries is an expanded PTFE covered stent which provides an appropriate size match. The dorsal cervical musculature is supplied by branches off the VA. Care must be taken not to perforate these branches during catheter manipulation. Arterial access via radial or brachial artery rather than common femoral artery is sometimes preferable because of the angulation of the VA origin of the subclavian artery.

Venous Injuries in the Neck

Most cervical venous injuries are managed in the setting of arteriovenous fistulae. Traditionally, most cervical venous injuries can be ligated with limited morbidity. In general, when there is bilateral venous injury, then attempted repair is advised to avoid the superior vena cava syndrome. A case report of successful endovascular management of right internal jugular vein injury has been reported in the literature (27). This was a zone 3 injury treated by acrylate cylinder embolization using a retrograde approach.

VASCULAR INJURIES IN THE EXTREMITY

Peripheral arterial injuries account for 90% of all vascular injuries, most of them occurring in the upper extremities. Most of these injuries are due to penetrating trauma. Patients with hard sings of extremity arterial injury should be explored immediately. Blunt injuries are usually associated with other extremity injuries, e.g., dislocations and fractures.

Subclavian and Axillary Artery Injuries

Most of these injuries are related to penetrating trauma (Fig. 3A–C). Blunt injuries occur with abrupt deceleration and should be suspected in first rib and clavicle fractures. Unfortunately,

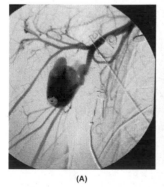 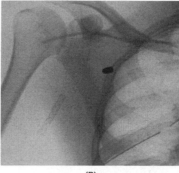 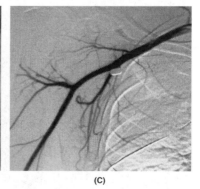

| (A) | (B) | (C) |

FIGURE 3 (**A**) Complex pseudoaneurysm of proximal axillary artery as a result of a gun shot wound. In view of the massive axillary hematoma, it was opted to treat this with a covered stent. (**B**) Stent graft has been successfully placed into the artery via a transfemoral approach. (**C**) Follow-up angiography demonstrates a normal luminal contour.

most of these patients do not survive transfer to the hospital due to severe uncontrolled hemorrhage (28). Open surgical approaches to these injuries may result in significant bleeding and morbidity even in hemodynamically stable patients (29). The difficulty of open surgical control has made the endovascular approach an attractive option. Endovascular surgery has been used with success to treat hemodynamically stable patients with pseudoaneurysms, arteriovenous fistula and thrombosis of the subclavian–axillary arterial system (14,30–35). In one report, a combined endovascular and open repair was used to treat an embolizing traumatic subclavian artery aneurysm. The aneurysm was covered with nitinol stent and a vein bypass of the occluded brachial artery was performed (36). Short-term results are promising, but long-term data are needed to compare endovascular surgery with conventional open techniques. In one report where nine subclavian artery injuries were treated with stent-grafts, follow up at 29 months demonstrated one stenosis and one thrombosis (37). The technical success for placing a subclavian or axillary stent for trauma, was 94%, with 85% primary patency rate at a mean follow-up of 18 months (38).

Technical Considerations

Stent grafting the subclavian artery near the vertebral orifice, which is the first branch of the subclavian, could result in vertebrobasilar embolization or even direct occlusion. The presence of a contralateral patent VA should be determined prior to sacrifice of the ipsilateral artery. There remain significant concerns about placing stent-grafts through the thoracic outlet. Balloon expandable devices should not be placed in this location since they will be compressed by the pinchcock effect of the clavicle and fist rib. Concerns exist also for self-expanding stent-grafts in this location since stent fracture may also occur because of repetitive compression and motion. The ideal location for use of a stent-graft in subclavian injury is a left subclavian proximal injury, not involving the aorta.

Subclavian and Axillary Vein Injuries

These injuries carry a high mortality rate, even higher than arterial injuries, possibly because the vein does not contract as well as the artery and there is the additional risk of an air embolus. Penetrating injuries cause 65% of subclavian vein injuries, which also have an arterial component in 20% (28). There are no data available discussing the role of endovascular surgery in this type of injury. There is a single case report of a successful placement of a covered stent to occlude a proximal left subclavian vein pseudoaneurysm after a blunt trauma (39). The stent was patent one year later.

Brachial, Radial, and Ulnar Vascular Injuries

These injuries rarely manifest with signs of ischemia due to the rich collateral supply in the upper limb. Brachial artery injuries could be the result of penetrating, blunt or even iatrogenic injury. Arteriovenous fistula is detected by the presence of a bruit and palpable thrill (Fig. 4).

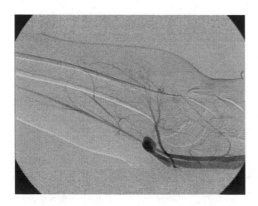

FIGURE 4 Arteriovenous fistula between the axillary artery and vein.

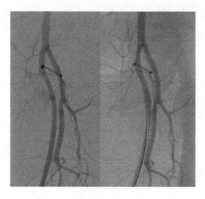

FIGURE 5 Pseudoaneurysm of proximal superficial femoral artery pre- and post-exclusion with covered stent.

Fistulae are best treated by open surgery, but covered stents can be used to exclude the entrance point from the artery (Fig. 4), if there is a contraindication to open repair.

There are two case reports where brachial artery transections after blunt trauma were repaired successfully with a covered stent (40). In one case, a retrograde and an antegrade approach was used to cross the transected lesion. This clearly shows that more technically challenging injuries can be repaired by endovascular means with increased expertise.

Stent placement to treat radial or ulnar injuries is not feasible due to the smaller vessel caliber. However, embolization of bleeding arterial or venous branches could be achieved if clinically warranted.

Femoral, Popliteal, and Tibial Vascular Injuries

Femoral artery injuries are most commonly seen with penetrating injuries (Fig. 5). Due to the expansion in endovascular procedures and cardiac catheterization, an increasing number of iatrogenic femoral artery injuries are seen. These usually manifest as either pseudoaneurysms or arteriovenous fistulae.

Most of the data on endovascular treatment of femoral artery injuries are related to catheterization resulting in pseudoaneurysms or fistulae. These lesions could be treated endovascularly with stents or coil embolization, but complications appear to be common (41). Stent thrombosis is a potential problem and was reported in 17% of patients in one series (41). This option might be feasible for the high-risk patients, but young trauma patients would be

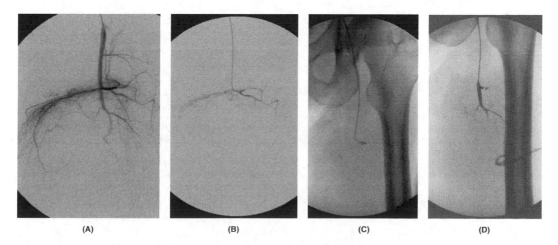

(A) (B) (C) (D)

FIGURE 6 (A) Extravasation from a branch of the profunda femoris artery following a stab wound. (B) Selective catheterization of the branch prior to coil embolization. (C) Coils being placed into the bleeding artery. (D) A post-embolization angiogram showing the stump of the vessel which has been successfully occluded.

better served with an open repair. The role of catheter-based treatment in lower limb trauma has a role in embolizing branches that are difficult to access surgically. A good example would be branches of the profunda femoris artery (Fig. 6).

Popliteal artery blunt injuries should be suspected with knee dislocations. Popliteal artery injuries can also be repaired by endovascular means (42). A case of popliteal arteriovenous fistula from gunshot wound with tibial osteomyelitis was successful treated with a covered stent (43). Ligation or embolization of a single injured tibial artery is usually well tolerated, and so stent placement has no place in treating injured tibial arteries.

Venous injuries of the lower extremity are not uncommon but no data are available using endovascular treatment except in the setting of arteriovenous fistula.

CONCLUSION

The traditional and recommended treatment of the injured vessel in the trauma patient is still open surgical repair. The most widely used endovascular utility remains selective diagnostic angiography. However, since CT angiography is very accurate for vascular diagnosis, we increasingly believe that use of angiography should be closely tied to the potential of therapeutic intervention. These techniques can be adjunctive or definitive. Adjunctive techniques such as endoluminal vascular control should augment and facilitate open repair. Definitive catheter-based techniques have found a role in treating high-risk patients, challenging anatomically located lesions and certain injuries in hemodynamically stable patients. Long-term data are not yet available to evaluate stent-grafts used in the trauma patients.

REFERENCES

1. Monson DO, Saletta JD, Freeark RJ. Carotid and vertebral artery trauma. J Trauma 1969; 9(12):987–99.
2. Demetriades D, Asensio JA, Velmahos G, et al. Complex problems in penetrating neck trauma. Surg Clin North Am 1996; 76(4):661–83.
3. Byrne MP, Welling RE. Penetrating and blunt extracranial carotid artery injuries. In: Ernst CB, Stanely JC, eds. Current Therapy in Vascular Surgery. St. Louis: Mosby-Year Book, 1995:598–603.
4. Ramadan F, Rutledge R, Oller D, et al. Carotid artery trauma: a review of contemporary trauma center experiences. J Vas Surg 1995; 21(1):46–55.
5. Biffl WL, Moore EE, Ryu RK, et al. The unrecognized epidemic of blunt carotid arterial injuries: early diagnosis improves neurologic outcome. Ann Surg 1998; 228(4):462–70.
6. Duane TM, Parker F, Stokes GK, et al. Endovascular carotid stenting after trauma. J Trauma 2002; 52(1):149–53.
7. McNeil JD, Chiou AC, Gunlock MG, et al. Successful endovascular therapy of a penetrating zone III internal carotid injury. J Vasc Surg 2002; 36(1):187–90.
8. Reiter BP, Marin ML, Teodorescu VJ, et al. Endoluminal repair of an internal carotid artery pseudoaneurysm. J Vasc Interv Radiol 1998; 9(2):245–8.
9. Hurst RW, Haskal ZJ, Zager E, et al. Endovascular stent treatment of cervical internal carotid artery aneurysms with parent vessel preservation. Surg Neurol 1998; 50(4):313–7.
10. Ditmars ML, Klein SR, Bongard FS. Diagnosis and management of zone III carotid injuries. Injury 1997; 28(8):515–20.
11. Horowitz MB, Miller G, Meyer Y, et al. Use of intravascular stents in the treatment of internal carotid and extracranial vertebral artery pseudoaneurysms. Am J Neuroradiol 1996; 17(4):693–6.
12. Marks MP, Dake MD, Steinberg GK, et al. Stent placement for arterial and venous cerebrovascular disease: preliminary experience. Radiology 1994; 191(2):441–6.
13. Ellis PK, Kennedy PT, Barros D'Sa AA. Successful exclusion of a high internal carotid pseudoaneurysm using the wallgraft endoprosthesis. Cardiovasc Intervent Radiol 2002; 25(1):68–9.
14. Parodi JC, Schonholz C, Ferreira LM, et al. Endovascular stent-graft treatment of tramatic arterial lesions. Ann Vasc Surg 1999; 13(2):121–9.
15. Fabian TC, Patton JH, Croce MA, et al. Blunt carotid injury. Importance of early diagnosis and anticoagulant therapy. Ann Surg 1996; 223(5):513–22.
16. Miller PR, Fabian TC, Bee TK, et al. Blunt cerebrovascular injuries: diagnosis and treatment. J Trauma 2001; 51(2):279–85.
17. Duke BJ, Ryu RK, Coldwell DM, et al. Treatment of blunt injury to the carotid artery by using endovascular stents: an early experience. J Neurosurg 1997; 87(6):825–9.
18. Coldwell DM, Novak Z, Ryu RK, et al. Treatment of posttraumatic internal carotid artery pseudoaneurysms with endovascular stents. J Trauma 2000; 48(3):470–2.

19. Kerby JD, May AK, Gomez CR, et al. Treatment of bilateral blunt carotid injury using percutaneous angioplasty and stenting: case report and review of the literature. J Trauma 2000; 49(4):784–7.
20. Biffl WL, Moore EE, Offner PJ, et al. Blunt carotid and vertebral arterial injuries. World J Surg 2001; 25(8):1036–43.
21. Cohen JE, Ben-Hur T, Rajz G, et al. Endovascular stent-assisted angioplasty in the management of traumatic internal carotid artery dissections. Stroke 2005; 36(4):45–7.
22. Zhou W, Lin PH, Bush RL, et al. Carotid artery aneurysm: evolution of management over two decades. J Vasc Surg 2006; 43(3):493–6.
23. Beaujeux RL, Reizine DC, Casasco A, et al. Endovascular treatment of vertebral arteriovenous fistula. Radiology 1992; 183(2):361–7.
24. Halbach VV, Higashida RT, Dowd CF, et al. Endovascular treatment of vertebral artery dissections and pseudoaneurysms. J Neurosurg 1993; 79(2):183–91.
25. Miller RE, Hieshima GB, Giannotta SL, et al. Acute traumatic vertebral arteriovenous fistula: balloon occlusion with the use of a contralateral approach. Neurosurgery 1984; 14(2):225–9.
26. Cohen JE, Rajz G, Itshayek E, et al. Endovacular management of exsanguinating vertebral artery transection. Surg Neurol 2005; 64(4):331–4.
27. Sanabria A, Jimenez CM. Endovascular management of an exsanguinating wound of the right internal jugular vein in zone III of the neck: case report. J Trauma 2003; 55(1):158–61.
28. Demetriades D, Asensio JA. Subclavian and axillary vascular injuries. Surg Clin North Am 2001; 81(6):1357–73.
29. Degiannis E, Velmahos G, Krawczykowski D, et al. Penetrating injuries of the subclavian vessels. Br J Surg 1994; 81(4):524–6.
30. Marin ML, Veith FJ, Panetta TF, et al. Transluminally placed endovascular stented graft repair for arterial trauma. J Vasc Surg 1994; 20(3):466–72.
31. Patel AV, Marin ML, Veith FJ, et al. Endovascular graft repair of penetrating subclavian artery injuries. J Endovasc Surg 1996; 3(4):382–8.
32. Gomez-Jorge JT, Guerra JJ, Scagnelli T, et al. Endovascular management of a traumatic subclavian arteriovenous fistula. J Vasc Interv Radiol 1996; 7(4):599–602.
33. May J, White G, Waugh R, et al. Transluminal placement of a prosthetic graft-stent device for treatment of subclavian artery aneurysm. J Vasc Surg 1993; 18(6):1056–9.
34. Strauss DC, Du Toit DF, Warren BL. Endovascular repair of occluded subclavian arteries following penetrating trauma. J Endovasc Ther 2001; 8(5):529–33.
35. Xenos ES, Freeman M, Stevens S, et al. Covered stents for injuries of subclavian and axillary arteries. J Vasc Surg 2003; 38(3):451–4.
36. Meyer T, Merkel S, Lang W. Combined operative and endovascular treatment of a post-traumatic embolizing aneurysm of the subclavian artery. J Endovasc Surg 1998; 5(1):52–5.
37. Hilfiker PR, Razavi MK, Kee ST, et al. Stent-graft therapy for subclavian artery aneurysms and fistulas: single center mid term results. J Vasc Interv Radiol 2000; 11(5):578–84.
38. Ohki TO, Veith FJ, Marin ML, et al. Endovascular approaches for traumatic arterial lesions. Semin Vasc Surg 1997; 10(4):272–85.
39. Jeroukhimov I, Altshuler A, Peer A, et al. Endovascular stent-graft is a good alternative to traditional management of subclavian vein injury. J Trauma 2004; 57(6):1329–30.
40. Maynar M, Baro M, Qian Z, et al. Endovascular repair of brachial artery transection associated with trauma. J Trauma 2004; 56(6):1336–41.
41. Thalhammer C, Kirchherr AS, Uhlich F, et al. Postcatheterization pseudoaneurysms and arteriovenous fistulas: repair with percutaneous implantation of endovascular covered stents. Radiology 2000; 214(1):127–31.
42. Burger T, Meyer F, Tautenhahn J, et al. Initial experiences with percutaneous endovascular repair of popliteal artery lesions using a new PTFE stent-graft. J Endovasc Surg 1998; 5(4):365–72.
43. Criado E, Marston WA, Ligush J, et al. Endovascular repair of peripheral aneurysms, pseuodoaneurysms and arteriovenous fistulas. Ann Vasc Surg 1997; 11(3):256–63.

47 | The Role of Endovascular Therapy in Injuries to the Thorax, Abdomen, and Pelvis

Brian G. Peterson
Division of Vascular Surgery, Saint Louis University School of Medicine, St. Louis, Missouri, U.S.A.
Jon S. Matsumura
Division of Vascular Surgery, Department of Surgery, Northwestern University Feinberg School of Medicine, Chicago, Illinois, U.S.A.
Albert A. Nemcek
Section of Interventional Radiology, Northwestern University Feinberg School of Medicine, Chicago, Illinois, U.S.A.

THE ROLE OF ENDOVASCULAR THERAPY IN INJURIES TO THE THORAX

Historical Perspective and Evolution of Treatment

As Parmley first reported in 1958, 85% of thoracic aortic injuries in the setting of blunt trauma result in death at the scene of the accident. For the remaining 15% of patients arriving to a medical facility, subsequent mortality rates are 1% per hour for the first 48 hours in patients not undergoing surgical intervention with most of the deaths occurring within the first week (1). In a more recent review, aortic injury accounted for the second most common cause of death in the setting of blunt trauma, second only to head injury (2). The worldwide magnitude of this problem is evident when one considers that in North America alone, approximately 7500 to 8000 cases of blunt aortic injury occur each year (3,4). Efficient patient transport, early diagnosis, and appropriate intervention are paramount.

In 1959, Passaro described the first successful primary repair of a traumatic aortic transection by Klassen the year before (5), and since that time open surgical repair has been the mainstay of treatment. However, despite improvements in anesthesia, surgical technique, and postoperative critical care, contemporary studies have reported mortality rates from 5% to 28% and paraplegia rates secondary to spinal cord ischemia from 2% to 18% following open repair of blunt aortic injuries (6–11). In an effort to avoid the complications of early surgical repair some investigators began to advocate delayed surgical repair. Despite close surveillance and strict blood pressure control, 2% to 5% of their patients developed secondary rupture, usually within a week of the initial injury, thus mitigating the advantages of delayed repair (11–13) (see chap. 29 for more detail regarding the rationale and results with delayed surgical repair).

An alternative to open surgical repair of blunt aortic injury came about during the endovascular era of aortic aneurysm repair. Shortly after Dake and colleagues described the use of endoluminally placed stent grafts for the treatment of thoracic aortic aneurysms (14), this same group reported the use of endovascular techniques for the treatment of thoracic aortic transection (15). Since that time, there have been several small reports demonstrating the technical feasibility of endovascular repair of traumatic aortic transections (16–22). Early reports utilizing off-label, custom-made devices and abdominal aortic extension cuffs (Fig. 1) for the treatment of traumatic aortic transections have more recently been replaced by reports utilizing the now commercially available thoracic endoprostheses (see chap. 29).

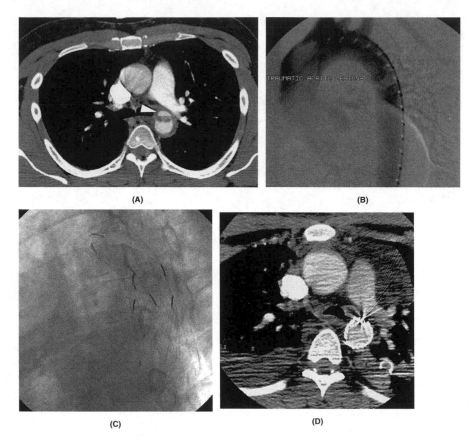

(A)   (B)

(C)   (D)

FIGURE 1   34-year-old male unrestrained driver in a motor vehicle accident. (**A**) Initial contrast enhanced computed tomography (CT) scan demonstrating a traumatic transection of the descending thoracic aorta. Contrast (*arrowhead*) is seen in the mediastinum external to the disrupted aortic wall. (**B**) Digital subtraction aortogram demonstrating an extraluminal contrast collection indicating traumatic transection of the thoracic aorta. (**C**) Radiograph after thoracic endovascular aortic repair (TEVAR) for traumatic transection of the thoracic aorta using abdominal aortic extension cuffs. (**D**) Follow-up CT scan demonstrating coverage of a traumatic thoracic aortic transection after TEVAR. Also shown is a left-sided chest tube needed to evacuate a large hemothorax.

Advantages of Endovascular Repair over Standard Open Repair

Thoracic endovascular aortic repair (TEVAR) of thoracic aortic injuries possesses clear advantages over open surgery. Thoracic aortic injuries in the setting of blunt trauma are rarely isolated. These injuries are commonly associated with injuries to other organ systems making care for this patient population particularly complex. In Fabian's prospective study of patients with blunt aortic injury, 62% had additional chest injury, half suffered brain injury, 34% had pelvic or long-bone fractures, and 22% had intraabdominal injury accounting for a mean injury severity score of 42 (11). Clearly with this high incidence of concomitant intracranial and intraabdominal injury, standard open repair with the use of systemic heparinization is not ideal. TEVAR can be performed quickly with minimal to no anticoagulation allowing associated injuries to be dealt with expediently.

The avoidance of thoracotomy and single-lung ventilation is of particular importance when considering that most of these patients have significant pulmonary contusion and fractures of the thoracic cage. TEVAR is tolerated well, and patient convalescence is largely determined by associated injuries rather than the aortic injury. Additionally, aortic cross-clamping can be avoided with endovascular repair. Prolonged aortic cross clamp times in the setting of open repair of thoracic aortic transections have been associated with an increased incidence of paraplegia (7,23–26). The lack of aortic cross-clamping not only preserves flow to the spinal cord, but also to the viscera and kidneys decreasing fluid shifts, coagulopathy, and risk of renal insufficiency.

When femoral access is adequate for the introduction of sheaths necessary to deliver the endoprostheses into the thoracic aorta, TEVAR can be performed using local anesthetic. This avoids the hypotension seen during induction of general anesthesia. Additionally, the potential for shorter operative times and blood loss as compared to conventional, open surgical repair makes TEVAR quite appealing. The importance of these advantages in multiply injured patients, particularly when they are hemodynamically unstable, cannot be overstated.

Endovascular Techniques and Troubleshooting

Injuries to the thoracic aorta in the setting of blunt trauma typically occur in the proximal descending aorta, just distal to the left subclavian artery necessitating the use of relatively long delivery systems for TEVAR. Prior to the commercial availability of devices specifically designed for treatment of thoracic aortic lesions, the off-label use of aortic extension cuffs designed for the treatment of infrarenal aortic aneurysms was an option. However, abdominal aortic extension cuff delivery catheter length was an issue when trying to reach the area of injury, in many cases necessitating iliac artery access via a retroperitoneal approach, or even direct aortic puncture via laparotomy. Depending on the aortic extender manufacturer, delivery system shaft length varies from 55 to 63 cm in length, making access to the injury from the standard femoral artery approach particularly difficult in taller patients. Estimations of the device delivery system length needed to treat lesions in the proximal thoracic aorta can be obtained from preoperative CT scans or more rudimentarily by measuring the distance from the sternal notch to the inguinal skin crease (21). Using the latter measurement, one group reported 100% accuracy in determining whether iliac access as opposed to femoral access was required (16). Additionally, the short stent-graft length (range 3.3–7.5 cm) may require placement of several components to treat the aortic lesion.

To combat the problem of inadequate delivery system shaft length, device accessibility, device length, and device diameter limitations, custom-made devices fabricated from woven polyester grafts and larger diameter stents have been used to treat thoracic aortic disruptions (27). The devices are assembled and back-loaded into large diameter sheaths used to deliver them into the proximal descending aorta. Some of the problems encountered with these devices included large, stiff delivery systems and difficulty de airing the devices prior to deployment, that may increase the risk for stroke from air embolization. Additionally, the relative slow deployment of these devices requires pharmacologic bradycardia, fibrillation, or even cardiac arrest for accurate deployment. The extra time necessary to assemble these devices makes their use in the setting of an acute thoracic aortic injury cumbersome. These issues, as well as the stiff device construct have relegated these custom-made devices as "last resort" options. In the years before commercially available devices, the site of aortic rupture posed some challenges for delivery sheath length and device size (16,21).

In the present climate of commercially available devices, cost may appear to prohibit keeping a large stock of variously sized device diameters and lengths. However, this is often less expensive than preparing for a ruptured aneurysm considering the fact that traumatic aortic injuries are typically focal, and extensive coverage of the aorta is unnecessary making 10-cm device lengths adequate. A smaller variety of different device diameters are required when considering treatment for thoracic aortic injury as the pathology involves otherwise normal aortas. In fact, device diameter can be an issue for a different reason. The smallest commercially available thoracic device is 28-mm in diameter. According to the instructions for use, this device is only to be used in patients with at least a 23-mm aorta. Many of the patients with traumatic aortic injuries have aortic diameters smaller than this cutoff, and when large diameter devices are placed within this otherwise normal aorta, significant oversizing can result. This oversizing prevents device expansion, leads to graft infolding, and can lead to device collapse (28). Device collapse may be a clinical catastrophe and significant oversizing should be avoided when possible.

Paraplegia is one of the most devastating complications following thoracic aortic surgery, and an incidence as high as 18% has been reported following open repair of blunt thoracic aortic injuries (11). Paraplegia remains a risk in the setting of TEVAR, especially when considering that the intercostal vessels cannot be reimplanted. Because aortic lesions following blunt trauma are usually focal, obviating the need for extensive coverage of the aorta, the risk of paraplegia is theoretically lower than endoluminal treatment for aneurysms of the thoracic aorta. Various maneuvers can be implemented in an effort to reduce the risk of paraplegia following TEVAR including lumbar drainage catheters, maintaining mean arterial blood pressures above 90 mmHg, and preserving collateral spinal cord arterial supply by transposing the left subclavian artery to the common carotid artery when coverage of the left subclavian orifice is needed to ensure an adequate proximal seal zone (29). A low threshold for lumbar drainage catheters and chemically induced hypertension is indicated in patients undergoing endovascular treatment of thoracic aortic transection who have had prior infrarenal aortic surgery, or absent hypogastric artery flow. Spinal cord perfusion is optimized by using these techniques, but like open repair, the paraplegia risk cannot be completely eliminated with TEVAR.

Because the use of endografts in the setting of blunt aortic injuries is in its infancy, the long-term outcome and durability of these thoracic endovascular devices has yet to be proven. Follow-up with regular physical examinations, radiographs, and surveillance computed tomography scans is warranted. While there have been few reports of endoleak, stent migration, stent fracture, or late pseudoaneurysm formation, close monitoring is required until long-term data are available. If device related problems do occur in follow-up, TEVAR for traumatic thoracic aortic transections may evolve into "bridging therapy" in the acute setting with more definitive open surgical repair being performed under elective circumstances, in healthier, more stable patients.

Current Literature and Comparison Studies

Since the first report of endovascular treatment of blunt thoracic aortic injuries appeared in 1997 (15), several case reports have reported similar success using endoluminal techniques (18,21,22,30–39). Table 1 summarizes the current literature by providing technical success rates, device-related mortality rates, and paraplegia rates by groups reporting at least ten cases of TEVAR for thoracic aortic injuries since 2002. While definitive conclusions cannot be made without randomized, controlled clinical trials and long-term follow-up, early results are promising. Most groups report technical success rates near 100% with no incidence of paraplegia. Mortality in these reports is rarely directly related to the aortic injury, but is more commonly due to concomitant injuries in these multiply injured patients. The experience published from Northwestern consists of 11 patients with a mean follow-up of 21 months using TEVAR for traumatic aortic injuries and similarly demonstrates 100% technical success and no device-related mortality or paraplegia in multiply injured patients.

TABLE 1 Published Reports Containing at Least 10 Cases of Thoracic Endovascular Aortic Repair for Traumatic Thoracic Aortic Transection Since 2002

Investigator	Year	Cases	Technical success (%)	Stent-related mortality	Paraplegia
Bortone (30)	2002	10	100	0	0
Fattori (31)	2002	11	100	0	0
Lachat (32)	2002	12	100	1	0
Orend (33)	2002	11	92	1	0
Karmy-Jones (34)	2003	11	100	3	0
Dunham (18)	2004	16	100	1	0
Melnitchouk (35)	2004	15	100	1	0
Neuhauser (36)	2004	10	92	0	0
Scheinert (37)	2004	10	100	0	0
Peterson (21)	2005	11	100	0	0
Rousseau (22)	2005	29	100	0	0
Hoornweg (38)	2006	28	100	0	0
Tehrani (39)	2006	30	100	0	0
Total		204	99	7	0

There have been a few reports that have compared endovascular repair to standard open repair of thoracic aortic injuries. In 2003, Kasirajan et al. (40) compared open controls with five patients undergoing TEVAR and reported significantly lower mean procedural times, hospital length of stay, and mortality rates in the endovascular group. Later Ott et al. (41) demonstrated similar encouraging results as to the benefits of endovascular repair, reporting their findings of a 17% mortality rate and 16% paraplegia rate following open repair, with no deaths or paraplegia in the endovascular group. More recently, Rousseau et al. (22) reported their experience of 70 patients with traumatic aortic injury treated over a 12-year period. Patients were divided into three groups: a surgical group in which patients received immediate treatment or delayed intervention, an endovascular group, and a group treated medically when injuries were deemed to be stable. Patients treated with immediate surgical intervention had mortality and paraplegia rates of 21% and 7%, respectively, while there were no deaths or paraplegia in the TEVAR arm.

While long term results are lacking, the short term success of TEVAR with markedly reduced mortality and paraplegia strongly suggests it will be a preferred initial treatment for patients with acute thoracic aortic trauma.

THE ROLE OF ENDOVASCULAR THERAPY IN INJURIES TO THE ABDOMEN AND PELVIS

Epidemiology

Abdominal Trauma

In an analysis of 2471 cases of arterial injuries suffered during World War II, DeBakey et al. reported an incidence of abdominal arterial trauma of only 2% (42). Similarly, Rich et al. describing 1000 arterial injuries inflicted during the Vietnam conflict, demonstrated an incidence of abdominal arterial injuries of only 2.9% (43). These numbers are in stark contrast to contemporary studies of civilian trauma in which Demetriades et al. report a 14.3% incidence of abdominal arterial trauma in the setting of abdominal penetrating injuries (44).

Most patients suffering penetrating abdominal trauma with concomitant major abdominal vascular injury suffer lethal injuries. However, those patients who survive the initial insult have been found to have various types of abdominal arterial injuries which may be amenable to repair. These lesions include false aneurysm formation, arteriovenous fistulae, lacerations, and arterial dissections. These types of lesions may be treated with a variety of endovascular strategies. Likewise, catheter-based interventions may be used to treat abdominal arterial injuries in the setting of blunt trauma (Fig. 2). Those lesions most amenable to endoluminal techniques in the setting of blunt trauma include arterial dissections, pseudoaneurysm formation, and arteriovenous fistulae.

Pelvic Trauma

Despite the mechanism of injury, mortality rates following pelvic fracture range from 10% to 50% and are largely determined by the severity of concomitant injuries and pelvic bleeding (45–48). In 1973, Huittinen et al. (49) performed postmortem angiography and hypogastric artery dissections on patients succumbing to traumatic injuries. All of these patients suffered pelvic fractures. This report demonstrated that the most frequent site of hemorrhage following pelvic fracture was bone edge bleeding and injury to venous structures of the pelvis. Unlike their arterial counterparts, bone edge bleeding and venous bleeding tend to stop secondary to tamponade provided by the limited retroperitoneal space. When death occurred in the setting of pelvic fracture, they found the most common etiology to be arterial bleeding from the internal iliac artery. Specifically, lacerations in the superior gluteal and pudendal arteries were the source of this lethal hemorrhage (Fig. 3). If patients remain hemodynamically unstable following pelvic fixation or transcatheter therapy to address arterial bleeding, major pelvic venous injury must be considered. In this setting, venography has been shown to be useful in diagnosing iliac vein injuries and catheter-based techniques have been used to treat these lesions as well (50).

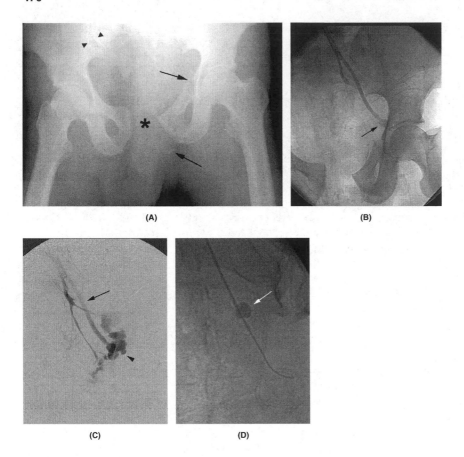

FIGURE 2   39-year-old male who presented with crush injury after large scaffolding fell on him. The patient was hypotensive on arrival and underwent pelvic angiography. (**A**) Plain radiograph of the pelvis shows significant bony injury including diastasis of the pubic symphysis (*asterisk*), widening of the right sacroiliac joint (*arrowheads*) and fractures of the left pubis (*arrows*). (**B**) Selective left iliac digital arteriogram shows abrupt truncation of the left external iliac artery with extravasation of contrast (*arrow*). (**C**) Selective left digital subtraction arteriogram; further extravasation (*arrowhead*) is noted arising from the external iliac artery (*arrow*). The distal external iliac artery is not visualized. (**D**) A balloon occlusion catheter (*arrow*), contrast filled inflated balloon was placed in the distal external iliac artery to tamponade the extravasation, allowing the patient to be transferred to the operating room for surgical reconstruction of the left external iliac artery.

Other Injuries

Aside from the utility of endovascular techniques in the setting of both blunt and penetrating abdominopelvic trauma, endovascular surgery also has a role in treating complications of complex orthopedic surgery, or other types of iatrogenic injuries following complex procedures (Fig. 4). While the incidence of arterial injury in the setting of orthopedic surgery is quite low and ranges from 0.005% to 0.5% (51,52), serious vascular injuries may occur during complex procedures leading to lesions amenable to endoluminal intervention. In the early 1980s, Miller et al. reported on the use of arteriographic embolization to treat excessive bleeding during revision of total hip arthroplasty (53). Since that time, numerous papers have described the use of endoluminal technology to treat various arterial complications following orthopedic surgery ranging from arterial laceration to postoperative pseudoaneurysm formation (54–57).

At times, patients with abdominopelvic trauma and associated bleeding are particularly difficult to stabilize, and while open exploration and packing in a damage control fashion remain an option in unstable patients, a diagnostic angiogram with the potential for therapeutic intervention offers several advantages over an attempt at open surgical control of ongoing hemorrhage.

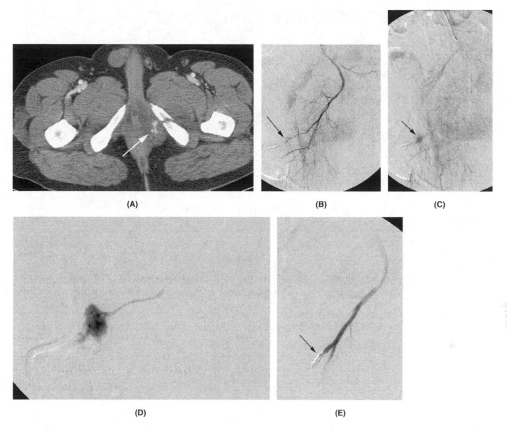

FIGURE 3 35-year-old male unrestrained passenger in a motor vehicle accident. (**A**) Contrast-enhanced computed tomography shows focal extravasation of contrast in the left ischiorectal fossa (*arrow*) adjacent to a pubic fracture. (**B**) Superselective left internal pudendal digital subtraction arteriogram, mid-arterial phase shows irregularity of a small internal pudendal branch (*arrow*). (**C**) Late-arterial phase, a focus of contrast extravasation is identified (*arrow*). (**D**) Utilizing a coaxial microcatheter, the bleeding branch was catheterized. Contrast injection confirms the site of bleeding. (**E**) Arteriogram obtained after embolization of the bleeding artery with gelfoam and fibered microcoils (*arrow*), deployed through the microcatheter, resulting in successful hemostasis.

Advantages of Endovascular Therapy

Whether isolated abdominopelvic vascular injury or vascular injury in the setting of concomitant solid organ or hollow viscus injury is encountered, several advantages exist for treating these injuries using endovascular techniques as opposed to open surgical control and repair. With retroperitoneal or pelvic bleeding leading to large hematomas, open exposure to obtain proximal and distal arterial control can be quite burdensome. Landmarks are distorted, soft tissues are blood-stained, and dissection planes may be difficult to recognize. Similarly, large pseudoaneurysms can distort the anatomy making exposure quite difficult. When traumatic arteriovenous fistulae are present as a result of traumatic injury, venous hypertension can make dissection troublesome and cause added blood loss. In these settings, remote arterial access and vessel control using catheter-based interventions provides a significant advantage over open exposure.

When arterial injuries are associated with concomitant bowel injury and potential contamination, specific arterial injuries may be better addressed using endoluminal intervention rather than open repair. Specifically, when stents are used to treat intraluminal defects caused by trauma, repair is achieved expediently without exposure to the contamination. Another inherent advantage of endovascular repair over open repair in the setting of

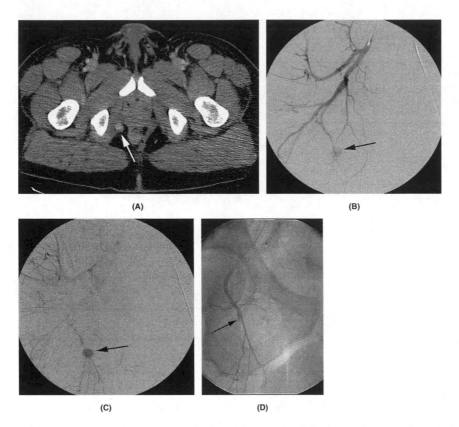

FIGURE 4 40-year-old woman who developed hypotension following total proctocolectomy for rectal cancer. (**A**) Contrast-enhanced computed tomography shows focal pooling of contrast in the right ischiorectal fossa. (**B,C**) Selective right internal iliac digital subtraction arteriogram in the mid- and late-arterial phase show a pseudoaneurysm arising from an anterior division arterial branch (*arrows*). (**D**) Unsubtracted digital arteriogram following super-selective catheterization and Gelfoam embolization of the branch giving rise to the pseudoaneurysm. The branch is truncated (*arrow*) and the pseudoaneurysm no longer fills.

abdominal and pelvic trauma lies in the fact that angiography serves as both a diagnostic and therapeutic modality. The precise location of the arterial injury can be determined angiographically and most times can be accessed with a combination of catheters and wires without much difficulty, regardless of where the lesion is located. Some areas, such as the distal branches of the internal iliac artery, are difficult to expose surgically because of their anatomic location deep within the pelvis. These lesions can be reached relatively easily using catheter based interventions.

There are few limitations to endovascular therapy in the setting of abdominal and pelvic arterial injuries. Besides the standard risks of vessel access and the use of potentially nephrotoxic contrast, the angiography suite may not be an ideal location to resuscitate and warm a severely hemodynamically unstable patient. Angiography suites based in the operating room with fixed fluoroscopy units could enable teams to work in concert to address these multiply injured patients.

Endovascular Techniques

As improvements are made in imaging equipment and new techniques and devices are developed, the variety of traumatic lesions being treated by catheter-based interventions continues to expand. The following is a brief description of the most commonly employed endovascular techniques used in the trauma setting and a synopsis of the specific types of lesion each technique is best suited to treat.

Balloon Occlusion

Since the original description of using balloons to control hemorrhage in the 1970s (58), the technique of temporary balloon occlusion has been applied to various settings. Remote arterial access away from the site of injury provides quick vascular control without decompressing hematomas and restarting massive bleeding. Additionally, balloon occlusion is ideal when vessel control is needed emergently in areas of difficult access, and vessel reconstruction is necessary to avoid tissue ischemia. In this manner, balloon occlusion serves as a "bridge" to definitive therapy, allowing for immediate control of hemorrhage, followed by resuscitation and controlled vascular reconstruction of essential vessels.

Stenting

Endovascular stenting has played an important role in treating arterial injuries following trauma. Lesions most suitable for stenting have included intimal flaps and dissections. Several groups have reported technical success in treating dissections of the aorta (59), renal arteries (60,61), and iliac arteries (62) with stents following abdominal trauma. Following stent placement, anti-platelet regimens are usually implemented when bleeding risk from concomitant traumatic injuries allows. Complications following stent placement in the setting of trauma are no different than when they are used to treat atherosclerotic lesions or nontraumatic dissections. These complications include stent fracture and thrombosis. In general, endoluminal treatment of traumatic dissections with stents is technically feasible and should be used when dissections are hemodynamically significant or when patients are not able to tolerate anticoagulation given their associated injuries.

Covered Stents

With the introduction of covered stents, traumatic lesions previously addressed by open surgical repair can now be addressed endoluminally. Specifically, traumatic abdominopelvic pseudoaneurysms and arteriovenous fistulae can be treated with stent grafts, as can arterial lacerations if the lesion is able to be crossed by a wire (63). The use of covered stents has even been technically successful in the treatment of a renal arteriovenous fistula (64). One of the drawbacks associated with stent-graft use includes the fact that slightly larger sheaths are currently needed for delivery in comparison to their bare metal counterparts. Additionally, because graft material is used, covered stents are theoretically at greater risk of becoming infected than are bare metal stents. This may become significant when associated traumatic injuries lead to fecal contamination. Finally, the concern for long-term patency is present when stent-grafts are used, and standard anticoagulation protocols should be employed when bleeding risk from associated injuries is negligible.

Embolization

The most commonly used catheter-based therapeutic intervention in the setting of abdominal or pelvic trauma is embolization. Embolization can be used to treat vessel lacerations, solid organ injury, pseudoaneurysms, and arteriovenous fistulae. One of the most important points to remember before embolizing a bleeding vessel, fistula, or pseudoaneurysm is to make sure that the artery being embolized is a nonessential vessel. Along similar lines, the anatomy must clearly be defined angiographically at the time of embolization because collateral vessels may supply the source of bleeding leading to ongoing hemorrhage despite embolization. Superselective catheterization is often necessary to pinpoint the source of bleeding and deliver the embolic material—whether it is gelatin foam, polyvinyl alcohol, any variety of coils, or various combinations of these materials. Complications seen with embolization include migration or nontarget embolization and tissue ischemia leading to pain or infection. Overall, embolization is extremely effective at treating a variety of traumatic injuries and complication can be reduced with clear delineation of the anatomy and superselective catheterization techniques.

SUMMARY/CONCLUSION

A variety of endovascular techniques have been applied to treat various vascular lesions seen in the setting of thoracic, abdominal and pelvic trauma. With continuous improvements in endovascular technology and creative applications of this technology, an increasing number of traumatic arterial and venous lesions are amenable to catheter-based interventions. These minimally invasive techniques will certainly benefit this often difficult to manage patient population.

REFERENCES

1. Parmley LF, Mattingly TW, Manion WC, et al. Nonpenetrating traumatic injury of the aorta. Circulation 1958; 17:1086.
2. Smith RS, Chang FC. Traumatic rupture of the aorta: still a lethal injury. Am J Surg 1986; 152:660.
3. Jackson DH. Of TRAs and ROCs. Chest 1984; 85:585.
4. Mattox KL. Fact and fiction about management of aortic transection. Ann Thorac Surg 1989; 48:1.
5. Passaro E, Pace WG. Traumatic rupture of the aorta. Surgery 1959; 41:787.
6. Lobato AC, Quick RC, Phillips B, et al. Immediate endovascular repair for descending thoracic aortic transection secondary to blunt trauma. J Endovasc Ther 2000; 7:16–20.
7. Cowley RA, Turney SZ, Hankins JR, et al. Rupture of thoracic aorta caused by blunt trauma: a fifteen-year experience. J Thorac Cardiovasc Surg 1990; 100:652–60.
8. Gott VL. Heparinized shunts for thoracic vascular operations. Ann Thorac Surg 1972; 14:219–20.
9. Verdant A. Traumatic rupture of the thoracic aorta. Ann Thorac Surg 1990; 49:686–7.
10. von Oppell UO, Dunne TT, De Groot MK, Zilla P. Traumatic aortic rupture: twenty-year meta-analysis of mortality and risk for paraplegia. Ann Thorac Surg 1994; 58:585–93.
11. Fabian TC, Richardson JD, Croce MA, et al. Prospective study of blunt aortic injury: multicenter trial of the American Association for the Surgery of Trauma. J Trauma 1997; 42:374–80.
12. Pierangeli A, Turinetto B, Galli R, et al. Delayed treatment of isthmic aortic rupture. Cardiovasc Surg 2000; 8:280–3.
13. Holmes JH, Bloch RD, Hall RA, et al. Natural history of traumatic rupture of the thoracic aorta managed non operatively: a longitudinal analysis. Ann Thorac Surg 2002; 73:1149–54.
14. Dake MD, Miller DC, Semba CP, et al. Transluminal placement of endovascular stent-grafts for the treatment of descending thoracic aortic aneurysms. N Engl J Med 1994; 331:1729–34.
15. Kato N, Dake MD, Miller DC, et al. Traumatic thoracic aortic aneurysm: treatment with endovascular stent-grafts. Radiology 1997; 205:657–62.
16. Sam A, II, Kibbe M, Matsumura J, et al. Blunt traumatic aortic transection: endoluminal repair with commercially available aortic cuffs. J Vasc Surg 2003; 38:1132–5.
17. Wellons ED, Milner R, Solis M, et al. Stent-graft repair of traumatic thoracic aortic disruptions. J Vasc Surg 2004; 40:1095–100.
18. Dunham MB, Zygun D, Petrasek P, et al. Endovascular stent grafts for acute blunt aortic injury. J Trauma 2004; 56:1173–8.
19. Semba CP, Kato N, Kee ST, et al. Acute rupture of the descending thoracic aorta: repair with use of endovascular stent-grafts. J Vasc Interv Radiol 1997; 8:337–42.
20. Ahn SH, Cutry A, Murphy TP, Slaiby JM. Traumatic thoracic aortic rupture: treatment with endovascular graft in the acute setting. J Trauma 2001; 50:949–51.
21. Peterson BG, Matsumura JS, Morasch MD, et al. Percutaneous endovascular repair of blunt thoracic aortic transection. J Trauma 2005; 59(5):1062–5.
22. Rousseau H, Dambrin C, Marcheix B, et al. Acute traumatic aortic rupture: a comparison of surgical and stent-graft repair. J Thorac Cardiovasc Surg 2005; 129:1050–5.
23. Hunt JP, Baker CC, Lentz CW, et al. Thoracic aorta injuries: management and outcome of 144 patients. J Trauma 1996; 40:547.
24. Higgins RSD, Sanchez JA, DeGuidis L, et al. Mechanical circulatory support decreases neurologic complications in the treatment of traumatic injuries of the thoracic aorta. Arch Surg 1992; 127:516.
25. Katz M, Blackstone E, Kirklin J, et al. Incremental risk factors for spinal cord injury following operation for acute traumatic aortic transection. J Thorac Cardiovasc Surg 1981; 81:669.
26. Zeiger A, Clark DE, Morton JR. Appraisal of surgical treatment of traumatic transection of the thoracic aorta. J Cardiovasc Surg 1990; 31:607.
27. Peterson BG, Longo GM, Matsumura JS, et al. Endovascular repair of thoracic aortic pathology with custom-made devices. Surgery 2005; 138(4):598–605.
28. Idu MM, Reekers JA, Balm R, Ponsen KJ, de Mol BA, Legemate DA. Collapse of a stent-graft following treatment of a traumatic thoracic aortic rupture. J Endovasc Ther 2005; 12(4):503–7.
29. Peterson BG, Eskandari MK, Gleason TG, Morasch MD. Utility of left subclavian artery revascularization in association with endoluminal repair of acute and chronic thoracic aortic pathology. J Vasc Surg 2006; 43:433–9.
30. Bortone AS, DeCillis E, D'Agostino D, et al. Stent graft treatment of thoracic aortic diseases. Surg Technol Int 2004; 2:189–93.

31. Fattori R, Napoli G, Lovato L, et al. Indications for, timing of, and results of catheter-based treatment of traumatic injury to the aorta. Am J Roentgenol 2002; 179:603–9.
32. Lachat M, Pfammatter T, Witzke H, et al. Acute traumatic aortic rupture: early stent-graft repair. Eur J Cardiothorac Surg 2002; 21:959–63.
33. Orend KH, Pamler R, Kapfer X, et al. Endovascular repair of traumatic descending aortic transection. J Endovasc Ther 2002; 9:573–8.
34. Karmy-Jones R, Hoffer E, Meissner MH, et al. Endovascular stent grafts and aortic rupture: a case series. J Trauma 2003; 55:805–10.
35. Melnitchouk S, Pfammatter T, Kadner A, et al. Emergency stent-graft placement for hemorrhage control in thoracic aortic rupture. Eur J Cardiothorac Surg 2004; 25:1032–8.
36. Neuhauser B, Czermak B, Jaschke W, et al. Stent-graft repair for acute traumatic thoracic aortic rupture. Am Surg 2004; 70:1039–44.
37. Scheinert D, Krankenberg H, Schmidt A, et al. Endoluminal stent-graft placement for acute rupture of the descending thoracic aorta. Eur Heart J 2004; 25:694–700.
38. Hoornweg LL, Dinkelman MK, Goslings C, et al. Endovascular management of traumatic ruptures of the thoracic aorta: a retrospective multicenter analysis of 28 cases in The Netherlands. J Vasc Surg 2006; 43:1096–102.
39. Tehrani HY, Peterson BG, Katariya K, et al. Endovascular repair of thoracic aortic tears. Ann Thorac Surg 2006; 82:873–8.
40. Kasirajan K, Heffernan D, Langsfeld M. Acute thoracic aortic trauma: a comparison of endoluminal stent-grafts with open repair and nonoperative management. Ann Vasc Surg 2003; 17:589–95.
41. Ott MC, Stewart TC, Lawlor DK, et al. Management of blunt thoracic aortic injuries: endovascular stents versus open repair. J Trauma 2004; 56:565–70.
42. DeBakey ME, Simeone FA. Battle injuries of the arteries in World War II: an analysis of 2,471 cases. Ann Surg 2000; 123:534–79.
43. Rich NM, Baugh JH, Hughes CW. Acute arterial injuries in Vietnam: one thousand cases. J Trauma 1970; 10:359–69.
44. Demetriades D, Velmahos G, Cornwell EE, et al. Selective non-operative management of gunshot wounds of the anterior abdomen. Arch Surg 1997; 132:178–83.
45. Baylis TB, Norris BL. Pelvic fractures and the general surgeon. Curr Surg 2004; 61:30–5.
46. Cydulka RK, Parreira JG, Coimbra R, et al. The role of associated injuries on outcome of blunt trauma patients sustaining pelvic fractures. Injury 2000; 31:677–82.
47. Demetriades D, Karaiskakis M, Toutouzas K, et al. Pelvic fractures: epidemiology and predictors of associated abdominal injuries and outcomes. J Am Coll Surg 2002; 195:1–10.
48. Poole GV, Ward EF. Causes of mortality in patients with pelvic fractures. Orthopedics 1994; 17:691–969.
49. Huittinen VM, Slatis P. Postmortem angiography and dissection of the hypogastric artery in pelvic fractures. Surgery 1973; 73:454–62.
50. Kataoka Y, Maekawa K, Nishimaki H, et al. Iliac vein injuries in hemodynamically unstable patients with pelvic fracture caused by blunt trauma. J Trauma 2005; 58:704–10.
51. Wilson JS, Miranda A, Johnson BL, et al. Vascular injuries associated with elective orthopaedic procedures. Ann Vasc Surg 2003; 17:641–4.
52. Nachbur B, Meyer RP, Verkkala K, et al. The mechanisms of severe arterial injury in surgery of the hip joint. Clin Orthop 1979; 141:122–33.
53. Miller ME, Niemann KMW, Meyer RD, et al. Arteriographic embolization for control of excessive blood loss complicating revision of total hip arthroplasty. J Bone Joint Surg Am 1983; 65:848–50.
54. Carlin RE, Papenhausen M, Farber MA, et al. Sural artery pseudoaneurysm after knee arthroplasty: treatment with transcatheter embolization. J Vasc Surg 2001; 33:170–3.
55. Plagnol P, Diard N, Bruneteau P, et al. Pseudoaneurysm of popliteal artery complicating a total knee replacement: a successful percutaneous endovascular treatment. Eur J Vasc Endovasc Surg 2001; 21:81–3.
56. Noorpuri BSW, Maxwell-Armstrong CA, Lamerton AJ. Pseudo-aneurysm of the geniculate collateral artery complicating total knee replacement. Eur J Vasc Endovasc Surg 1999; 18:534–5.
57. Kickuth R, Anderson S, Kocovic L, et al. Endovascular treatment of arterial injury as an uncommon complication after orthopedic surgery. J Vasc Interv Radiol 2006; 17:791–9.
58. Sheldon GF, Winestock DP. Hemorrhage from open pelvic fracture controlled intraoperatively with balloon catheter. J Trauma 1978; 18:68–70.
59. Marty-Ane CH, Alric P, Prudhomme M, et al. Intravascular stenting of traumatic abdominal aortic dissection. J Vasc Surg 1996; 23:156–61.
60. Lee JT, White RA. Endovascular management of blunt traumatic renal artery dissection. J Endovasc Ther 2002; 9:354–8.
61. Villas PA, Cohen G, Putnam SG. Wallstent placement in a renal artery after blunt abdominal trauma. J Trauma 1999; 46:1137–9.

62. Lyden SP, Srivastava SD, Waldman DL, et al. Common iliac artery dissection after blunt trauma: case report of endovascular repair and literature review. J Trauma 2001; 50:339–42.
63. Balogh Z, Voros E, Suveges G, et al. Stent-graft treatment of an external iliac artery injury associated with pelvic fractures: a case report. J Bone Joint Surg Am 2003; 85:919–22.
64. Sprouse LR, II, Hamilton IN, Jr. The endovascular treatment of a renal arteriovenous fistula: placement of a covered stent. J Vasc Surg 2002; 36:1066–8.

48 | Arterial Pseudoaneurysm (Indications, Technical Aspects, Troubleshooting, and Current Results)

Elias N. Brountzos
Second Department of Radiology, National and Kapodistrian University of Athens, Medical School, Attikon University Hospital, Haidari, Athens, Greece

INTRODUCTION

Pseudoaneurysms are caused by arterial wall defects, allowing extravasation of blood into the surrounding tissues at arterial pressure. Presenting as a pulsating, encapsulated hematoma in direct communication with the lumen of a "feeding" artery, synonyms include "false aneurysm" and "pulsatile or communicating hematoma." Histologically, early in development the surrounding capsule is composed of outer arterial layers and perivascular tissues; but over time a layer of reactive fibrosis develops (1–11). According to etiology, pseudoaneurysms are classified as traumatic, anastomotic, dissecting, or infective (1,3).

This chapter will discuss the management of pseudoaneurysms occurring as a complication of vascular reconstruction and percutaneous arterial access (4).

Anastomotic Pseudoaneurysms

Anastomotic pseudoaneurysms (APAs) have traditionally been attributed to faulty surgical technique, fatigue of suture material, graft degeneration, or progressive disease of the host vessel. Disruption of the suture line leads to pseudoaneurysm formation, with blood flowing outside of the native vessel or graft wall (4–7). Developments in the manufacture of suture and graft materials have led to decreased incidence of APAs (6), though it has been suggested that this represents a delay in formation rather than a true reduction in incidence (8). Recently, chronic obstructive pulmonary disease, current smoking, and postoperative wound infection have been identified as independent predictors of femoral APA development after aortobifemoral reconstruction (7). Graft infection is also recognized as an important causative factor. In one study, positive cultures were obtained from explanted graft material in 60% of 45 femoral APAs with no overt signs of infection (5).

Femoral Anastomotic Pseudoaneurysms

The most common site for APAs is the femoral artery, with an incidence of between 14% and 44%, though the majority of these are of no clinical significance. Presentation ranges from 2 months to 19 years after bypass surgery, with a mean graft age of 6.2 years (4,7–10). Complications include nerve and venous compression, skin necrosis, thrombosis, distal embolization, and rupture (4–11). The most useful diagnostic tool is Color-Doppler ultrasonography with a sensitivity and specificity of 94% and 97% respectively. This characteristically shows a swirling motion of blood entering and exiting the sac (1,4,11). Computerized tomography angiography (CTA) may also be useful in providing detailed anatomical information of the aneurysm and surrounding vasculature (11–13). CTA is non-operator dependent and has a sensitivity and specificity of 95.1% and 98.7% (13). Gadolinium-enhanced three-dimensional magnetic

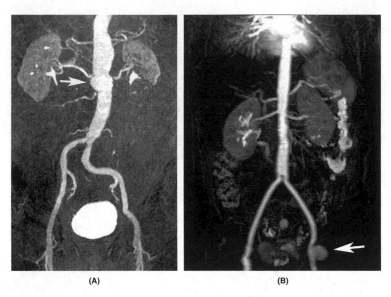

(A)   (B)

FIGURE 1 **(A)** Maximum intensity projection of a gadolinium-enhanced 3-D magnetic resonance angiogram in a patient treated with a tube graft for abdominal aortic aneurysm. This depicts a juxta-renal anastomotic pseudoaneurysm (*arrow*). **(B)** Maximum intensity projection of a gadolinium-enhanced 3-D magnetic resonance angiogram in a patient treated with bifurcated aortobifemoral graft. This depicts a femoral anastomotic pseudoaneurysm (*arrow*).

resonance angiography has similar advantages to CTA, with the additional benefit of avoiding exposure to radiation and nephrotoxic contrast media (11,14) (Fig. 1). Some still consider transcatheter angiography to be the gold standard despite these recent developments in imaging (1,11,12). However, the procedure is invasive, requires exposure to radiation and contrast, and provides no information regarding aneurysm size (1,11,12).

Indications for Treatment
Treatment of femoral APAs is primarily surgical. Elective surgery has a mortality rate of less than 4%, though emergency procedures are associated with a much higher risk (4,10,15). In the presence of infection, the mainstay of treatment is resection of the infected material and extra-anatomic bypass. Occasionally adequate collaterals enable vessel ligation in isolation, without threat to limb viability (4,11,16).

Endovascular treatment is not usually considered an alternative to surgery for femoral APAs (5,17). Involvement close to the femoral bifurcation precludes aneurysm exclusion because of the threat to branch vessels and risk of stent-graft failure inherent upon deploying across the inguinal ligament. Stent-graft treatment of femoral APAs, though reported, should therefore only be considered in selected non-surgical candidates (18).

Aortic and Iliac Anastomotic Pseudoaneurysms
APAs may also occur at aortoiliac anastomoses. These may pose diagnostic difficulties in differentiating between pseudoaneurysms and true degenerative disease (19–26). The reported incidence is probably an under-estimate since many are asymptomatic, and no routine postoperative imaging is performed for aortoiliac reconstructive surgery (20). Life-table analysis suggests an incidence as high as 22.8% at 15 years (19,22). Potential complications include thrombosis or distal embolization leading to acute limb ischemia, or rupture into the peritoneal cavity or adjacent structures (21–23).

Detailed imaging is essential in the management of patients with aortoiliac APAs (20–26). Ultrasonography has a more limited role especially in obese patients. CTA and magnetic resonance angiography have a key role in evaluating the complex anatomy, especially with the use of image post-processing (1,11,20). Angiography or intravascular ultrasonography may be used, especially when endovascular techniques are employed (21–27). Magnetic resonance imaging and labeled white blood cell scans can be helpful for excluding infection (28).

Indications for Treatment

Treatment is indicated for aortoiliac APAs regardless of size. Though mortality rates for elective surgical repair approach 17%, mortality and morbidity rates for emergency operations have been reported at 24% to −70%, and 70% to 83% respectively (21–27). Patients are often elderly with complex co-morbidity, presenting on average 109 months after aortic surgery (24). Conventional surgical repair is challenging, particularly dissection and cross clamping through dense scar tissue. Recently, endovascular treatment of aortoiliac APAs has been described and is an attractive option (21–29). The risk associated with endovascular treatment appears lower than that of open repair (21–29). However the global experience is small, with a few case reports and small series (3 to 33 patients) reported (21–27). Coil embolization of aortic APA is only anecdotally reported (30).

Technical Aspects

For device delivery, the common femoral artery, external iliac artery or limb of the bifurcated graft should be exposed under general or loco-regional anesthesia. For aortic APAs, or true anastomotic aneurysms, bifurcated, tubular, or aortouniiliac prostheses may be used (Fig. 2A,B) (Table 1). In the case of proximal APA, at least 10 mm infrarenal aortic neck is mandatory for stent graft fixation. If distal, the graft represents an ideal proximal attachment site (24). Tubular endoprostheses can be deployed in an overlapping fashion to exclude the APA (26). However, there is less columnar stability associated with tube endografts, and late rupture has occurred in two patients treated with this configuration (22). Bifurcated endografts provide better stability and sealing, but the deployment of the iliac limbs may be problematic within a narrow prosthetic graft. Aortouniiliac grafts may be a good compromise for the management of distal aortic APAs. In addition, aortouniiliac grafts are indicated for iliac APAs. In this case embolization of the contralateral iliac limb with a vascular plug, or ligation of the graft limb or native artery is also performed (Fig. 2C). In the later case, embolization of one internal iliac artery may be necessary if the APA involves the iliac bifurcation (23). In more simple cases, a tubular stent graft may be satisfactory (Figs. 2D and 3). Care should be taken to preserve one internal iliac artery if possible. Endovascular treatment of APAs after surgical reconstruction of the thoracic aorta is technically feasible with the use of thoracic aortic endografts (31–33).

Troubleshooting

The presence of a suitable proximal and distal attachment site is fundamental for successful endovascular treatment. Cross sectional imaging, with detailed measurements of the diameters of the aorta, graft and native iliac arteries is essential. A 25% over sizing of device diameter is recommended to achieve a seal (21–29).

Aortouniiliac and bifurcated endografts have better columnar strength than tubular grafts, and maybe better suited for aortic APAs (22). If bifurcated endografts are chosen, the surgical graft must be of adequate diameter to allow contralateral limb deployment and to prevent limb trapping.

All efforts should be taken to rule out the presence of infection. Surgical repair is usually advocated when there is evidence of infection (4,29), though endovascular treatment is reported in emergent cases as a bridge to open surgery (29).

Results

Considering the limited global experience, the results of endovascular treatment are encouraging, with technical success approaching 100%. In the small published series, procedural mortality is zero, with morbidity rates similar to elective aortic endovascular aneurysm repair (EVAR). Similarly, short-term durability of the method is identical to that of EVAR (Table 1) (21–29).

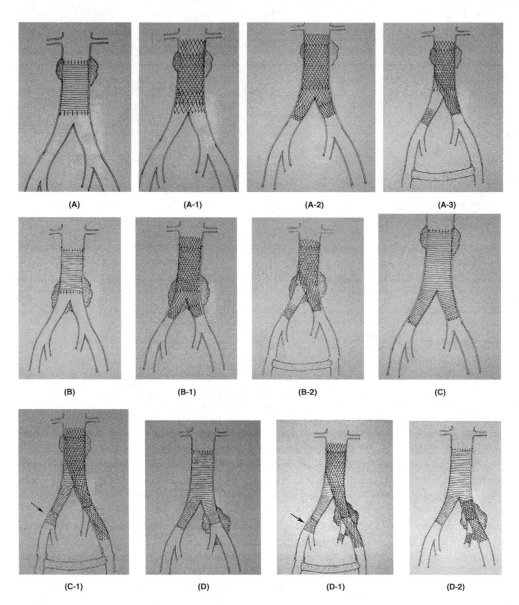

FIGURE 2 Endovascular treatment of anastomotic pseudoaneurysms (APAs): (**A**) Proximal aortic APA following surgically placed tube graft. (**A-1**) A tube endograft is deployed at an infrarenal position to exclude the APA; (**A-2**) An infrarenal bifurcated endograft is deployed if adequate space exists within the surgical graft to expand the two limbs; (**A-3**) An aortouniiliac graft is deployed, the contralateral iliac artery is occluded using an iliac occluder, while arterial flow to both legs is maintained using a femorofemoral bypass. (**B**) Distal aortic APA following surgically placed tube graft. (**B-1**) An infrarenal bifurcated endograft is deployed if adequate space exists within the surgical graft to expand the two limbs; (**B-2**) An aortouniiliac graft is deployed, the contralateral iliac artery is occluded using an iliac occluder, while arterial flow to both legs is maintained using a femorofemoral bypass. (**C**) Proximal aortic APA following surgery with a bifurcated graft. (**C-1**) Endovascular treatment with aortouniiliac graft, iliac graft limb occlusion with occluder (*arrow*), and femoro-femoral bypass. In such a case bifurcated endografts may be impossible to deploy because of space limitations. (**D**) Distal aortoiliac APA following surgery with a bifurcated graft. (**D-1**) Endovascular treatment with aortouniiliac graft, iliac graft limb occlusion, and femorofemoral bypass. Embolization of one internal iliac artery may be necessary if the iliac APA involves the iliac artery bifurcation; (**D-2**) If there is adequate proximal attachment zone a tube stent graft, such as an iliac limb from a bifurcated endograft, may effectively exclude the APA.

TABLE 1   Endovascular Treatment of Aortoiliac Anastomotic Pseudoaneurysms, and True Anastomotic Aneurysms After Aortic Reconstruction Surgery

Author/yr (Refs.)	No aortic APAs	No true aortic AAs	No iliac APAs	No true iliac AAs	Graft configuration	Mortality	Follow-up (mo)	Outcome
Tiesenhausen, 2001 (21)	3				1 tube, 1 bifurcated, 1 uniiliac	0	16	1 endoleak I (tube graft)
Curti, 2001 (23)			11	2	Tube	0	28	Success
Faries, 2003 (24)	12[a]		21[a]		Tube, uniiliac, bifurcated	0	10.6	1 endoleak II, 2 late occlusions
Van Herwaarden, 2004 (22)	6		2	6	3 tube, 11 bifurcated	0	12	2 tube grafts failed
Magnan, 2003 (25)	10				8 uniiliac, 2 tube	0	17.7	1 uniiliac graft occlusion
Zhou, 2006 (26)	5				Tube grafts overlapping	0	10	Success

[a] No distinction between AAs and APAs was made.
Abbreviations: AAs, anastomotic true aneurysms; APAs, anastomotic pseudoaneurysms.

Summary

APAs after aortoiliac reconstruction are common with serious potential complications, so elective treatment is advocated regardless of size. Open surgical resection with or without vascular reconstruction is the treatment of choice for femoral APAs. Imaging surveillance is recommended after aortic surgery to detect aortic and iliac APAs. Because of the inherent

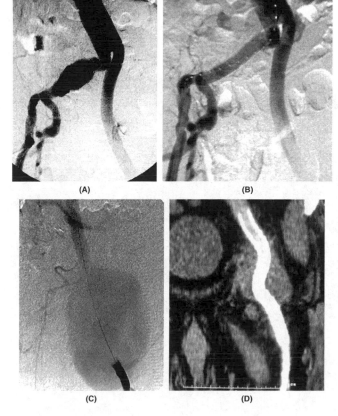

(A)   (B)

(C)   (D)

FIGURE 3   Bilateral anastomotic pseudoaneurysms in a patient treated with a bifurcated graft for aortic occlusive disease. (**A**) Digital subtraction angiogram depicts a pseudoaneurysm at the right iliac anastomosis. (**B**) Digital subtraction angiography after endovascular treatment with placement of a tubular stent graft depicts complete exclusion of the pseudoaneurysm. (**C**) Digital subtraction angiography depicts a large pseudoaneurysm at the left femoral anastomosis. (**D**) Curved multiple projection reconstruction of a computer tomographic angiography at the left groin after endovascular treatment with stent grafts depicts exclusion of the pseudoaneurysm. *Source*: From Ref. 18.

difficulties with operative treatment of aortoiliac APAs, endovascular treatment offers an encouraging alternative.

Post-Catheterization Pseudoaneurysms

Post-catheterization pseudoaneurysms (PCPAs) occur after arterial cannulation for diagnostic or therapeutic procedures, related to failure to achieve hemostasis at the puncture site (4,11,34). The most common site is the femoral artery; occurring less frequently in the brachial, axillary, and subclavian arteries (4,34). The incidence of PCPAs varies in the reported literature from 0.05% to 7.7% (2,4,34) with an apparent rise over time probably related to the increased use and sensitivity of ultrasound (US) in diagnosis (2,34,35).

Endovascular procedures are more frequently associated with the development of PCPAs than diagnostic catheterization. Risk factors include anticoagulation, use of large bore catheters, arterial hypertension, obesity, and calcified arteries (2,4,34–37). Operator-dependent factors include insufficient manual compression after the procedure. Puncture of the superficial femoral or profunda femoris artery, instead of the common femoral artery, has been associated with more frequent PCPA formation, because of the lack of posterior bony elements to support manual compression (34,37).

In summary, the incidence of PCPAs is high and is anticipated to rise with the increase in endovascular techniques, the use of large (>10 F) delivery devices, and perioperative use of anticoagulation.

Clinically, PCPAs present with pain, swelling, bruising, and a pulsatile mass at the arterial puncture site. The most feared complication is rupture, which is size related. Others complications include distal embolization, compression of adjacent veins and nerves, skin necrosis, and infection, though this is unusual (2,4,34).

US is the mainstay of diagnosis, with 94% sensitivity and 97% specificity (1,11,34). Gray-scale scans depict a hypoechoic structure adjacent to the artery which may be uni- or multi-lobular (simple or complex), and can determine the length and width of the neck. Duplex and Color Doppler ultrasonography can help establish the diagnosis by identifying the typical swirling motion within the sac (the "yin-yang" sign), the neck and the communication of the sac with the parent artery producing a "to and fro" waveform (Fig. 4) (11).

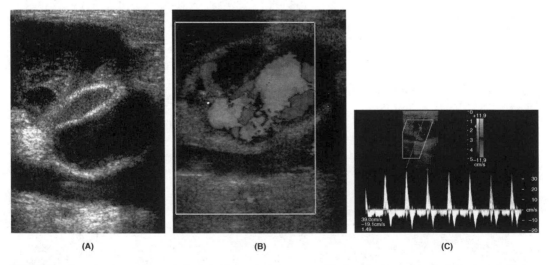

(A)   (B)   (C)

FIGURE 4 Complex femoral post catheterization pseudoneurysm. (**A**) Gray-scale ultrasonographic image depicts a complex structure; the anechoic area represents the patent lobe, while the hyperechoic area is the thrombosed lobe. (**B**) Color Doppler ultrasonography depicts the typical swirling motion in the patent lobe. (**C**) Typical waveform at the pseudoaneurysm neck with "to and fro" flow pattern.

Indications for Treatment

There is no universal consensus as to the size at which PCPAs should be treated. Most PCPAs of less than 2 cm diameter will spontaneously thrombose and some recommend a conservative approach with US surveillance (34). Others have suggested that smaller diameter aneurysms should be treated (38).

Treatment options include surgery, US-guided compression, and US-guided thrombin injection. Compression was first described in 1991 (39). Surgery is complicated by problematic wounds and permanent femoral neuralgias in between 19% to 32% of cases, and with lymphatic leaks in 40% (40) but is indicated in the presence of infection; rapid enlargement; skin necrosis; limb ischemia or neuropathy; and when less invasive measures have failed (4,11,34).

US-Guided Compression

Technical Aspects

Prior to compression, an US examination is performed to evaluate the size and geometry of the lesion, and to demonstrate the pseudoaneurysm neck. Pressure is applied over the neck with the US probe until flow in the PCPA is eliminated. Alternatively pressure may be applied over the sac itself. The pressure is maintained for 10 minutes, and released to evaluate thrombosis. If there is still flow a new pressure cycle starts for 10 more minutes. If the PCPA fails to thrombose after three or four cycles, most operators discontinue the procedure. After successful thrombosis, overnight bed rest is recommended. A follow-up US examination is useful in revealing early recurrences, though others limit these to patients with recurrent symptoms.

Troubleshooting

Compression can be a lengthy and painful procedure. Mean time to achieve thrombosis ranges from 37 to 75 minutes (Table 2). Pain, obesity, or the presence of a large hematoma may interfere with the efficiency of the pressure applied on the neck, predisposing to failure. PCPAs extending above the inguinal ligament cannot be adequately compressed. Complications, though uncommon (2.4–4.3%), may be significant, including rupture, distal embolization, and femoral vein thrombosis (34–37,39,41,43–46,50).

Results

The procedure is technically successful in 63% to 88% of cases (34–37,39,41). Anticoagulation is the main factor affecting successful thrombosis and should be reversed prior to compression whenever possible (34,41,44,46,50). Pseudoaneurysm size is also inversely related to successful compression: Coley reported a 100% success for PCPA diameter of 2 cm or smaller, but only 67% for diameter of 4 to 6 cm (41). Dean and coworkers published a 78% success for PCPA

TABLE 2 Ultrasound-Guided Compression for Post-Catheterization Pseudoaneurysms

Author/yr (Ref.)	N	Initial success (%)	Final success (%)	Compression time	Complications (%)
Coley, 1995 (41)	126		86		0
Hajarizadeh, 1995 (50)	57	83	95 anticoagulation only risk factor		0
Dean, 1996 (43)	77	<4 cm: 78 >4 cm: 42	73		
Chatterjee, 1996 (44)	41	Anticoagulation 70 Without 97			
Ugurluoglu, 1997 (45)	134		Symptomatic 78 Asymptomatic 100		
Hertz, 1997 (42)	41		88		
Eisenberg, 1999 (46)	281	72.1	74	44 min	2.1
Taylor, 1999 (47)	40		63	37 min	0
Paulson, 2000 (48)	281		74	41.5 min	0
Weimann, 2002 (49)	30		87	75 min	0

diameter less than 4 cm, and 42% for PCPA diameter greater than 4 cm, in anticoagulated patients (43). Other factors that may affect outcome include neck length and width, the size of the arterial sheath, the chronicity of the PCPA, and whether simple or complex (34,39,41, 43–46,50).

US-Guided Thrombin Injection

Percutaneous thrombin injection was first described in 1998 (34,38,40,47–49,51–61). Thrombin is derived from prothrombin, a circulating zymogen precursor, and its role is fundamental in thrombosis through conversion of fibrinogen to fibrin, and activation of prothrombin by positive feedback and through several other coagulation factors (61).

Technical Aspects

Bovine thrombin is frequently used because it is widely available and relatively inexpensive. It is provided as a powder and reconstituted with normal saline solution containing 1000 or 500 U/mL (34,38,40,47–49,51–61). Human thrombin is preferred by some, with the advantage of a lower risk of anaphylactic reactions. Commercially available preparations include Beriplast® P (Aventis, Behring, Marburg, Germany), and Tisseel® (Baxter, Glendale, California). Both consist of a fibrinogen component and a thrombin component in separate vials. The thrombin component is reconstituted with calcium chloride. The fibrinogen component contains human fibrinogen, human factor XIII, and bovine aprotinin. Although simultaneous infusion of both components results is fast thrombosis, most operators use the thrombin component in isolation (34,62).

Thrombin is directly injected into the PCPA lobe through a fine needle (21–23-G) using US guidance (38,40,47–49,51–62). Some recommend the use of balloon occlusion of the neck from a contralateral groin puncture (53), though this is deemed unnecessary by many and has not gained widespread acceptance (38,40,47–49,51–62). An alternative technique involves transar-terial injection of thrombin after selective catheterization of the pseudoaneurysm through the aneurysm neck (63,64).

Prior to thrombin injection, a detailed US assessment is essential, as for manual compression. Sterile conditions should be used and local anesthesia is advocated by some authors (40), though intravenous analgesia and sedation are rarely required. A 21 to 23 guage spinal needle, preloaded with thrombin (500–1000 U/mL),is connected to a 1 mL syringe of reconstituted thrombin.

The US probe (5.0–7.5-MHz linear array, or curved linear array) is covered with a sterile drape, and the needle is directed into the PCPA using free-hand technique, or with the aid of a biopsy-guide. In the case of complex PCPAs the more proximal to the neck is preferentially punctured if possible (38,48). The color mode is turned off during insertion, to facilitate needle visualization, and turned on during thrombin injection. Thrombin is injected at aliquots of 0.1 to 0.3 mL, and may be seen as "jets" on color doppler exiting the needle tip (Fig. 5). If thrombosis is incomplete, a second injection is performed. Residual flow in the neck is often observed but does not warrant additional injection as most stop spontaneously (40,61). Peripheral pulses and ankle-brachial index are evaluated. Bed rest for six hours is recommended. Follow-up US at 24 hours and one week is advised to check for reperfusion, which may require further treatment (34,38,40,48,61).

Troubleshooting

Thrombin injection is simple, though experience with US-guided techniques is required. Thrombin should not be injected before secure needle position is achieved within the PCPA lobe, to avoid thromboembolic complications, which occur in up to 2% of cases (34,38, 40,47–49,51–62). Although most resolve spontaneously, operators should be prepared to perform angiography, suction thrombectomy, intraarterial thrombolyzis, or surgical throm-bectomy. There is indirect evidence that thrombin does enter the circulation, though in small volumes that do not cause downstream thrombosis (34,40,61). However, thrombin binds to antithrombin III, and these complexes have antithrombin action that may cause severe coagulopathy.

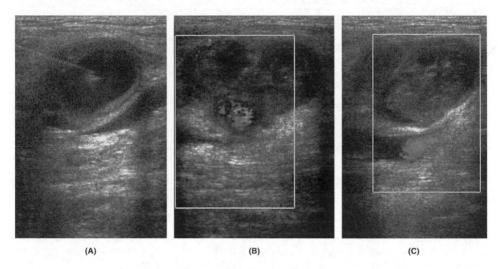

(A)   (B)   (C)

FIGURE 5 Ultrasound-guided thrombin injection treatment of a complex femoral post-catheterization pseudo-aneurysm. (**A**) Under gray-scale ultrasonographic guidance a 21-G needle is introduced into the patent distal lobe of the pseudoaneurysm. (**B**) Partial thrombosis of the pseudoaneurysm after percutaneous injection of 350 units of thrombin. (**C**) Complete thrombosis of the pseudoaneurysm after 600 units of thrombin.

Failure of thrombosis, or reperfusion of a successfully thrombosed aneurysm may occur. In a recent review, Krueger reported a 2.1% reperfusion rate. Repeat thrombin injection is recommended, though failure may be due to large arterial defects not amenable to this mode of treatment and surgery may be required (65). Other complications include pain, sometimes for up to three weeks, infection and rupture (40).

Results
Thrombin injection has a high success rate (Table 3). In Krueger's series of 240 patients, the primary and secondary success rates were 93.8% and 99.6%, respectively, and these have been replicated in other reports (34,38,40,47–49,51–62). Success rates are lower for complex PCPAs,

TABLE 3 Ultrasound-Guided Thrombin Injection for Post Catheterization Pseudoaneurysms

Author/yr (Ref.)	N	Primary success (%)	Final success (%)	Complication (%)
Paulson, 2001 (38)	114		96	4
Khoury, 2002 (59)	131		96	3
Kang, 1998 (51)	21		95	0
Kang, 2000 (52)	83		98	1.2
Owen, 2000 (53)	25		100 (with balloon protection)	0
Pezzullo, 2000 (54)	23		96	0
Sackett, 2000 (55)	30		90	3
Friedman, 2002 (57)	40		98	2.5
Elford, 2002 (58)	14 (human thrombin)		100	0
Etemad-Rezai, 2003 (60)	61	90	100	1.6
Krueger, 2003 (61)	50	Simple 97, complex 61	100	0
Sheinman, 2003 (65)	54		91	
La Perna, 2000 (56)	70	37 required 2nd injection	94	
Krueger, 2005 (40)	240 (44.6% anti-coagulation)	93.8 (simple 95.8, complex 89)	99.6 (simple 100, complex 99)	1.25

which require more injections (1.17 vs. 1.04), and greater thrombin dose (520.33 vs. 382.12 U) than simple PCPAs. The outcome is not adversely affected by anticoagulation (34,38,40,47–49, 51–62). Comparing thrombin injection with compression, though with non-randomized historic controls (47–49), the latter takes longer and has a lower success rate.

Other Methods for PCPA Treatment

Stainless steel coils have been used successfully to occlude 17 PCPAs after failed compression. The coils were introduced via direct puncture (66). Some have raised concerns about the risk of rupture, and the presence of coils which may prevent aneurysm shrinkage.

Gehling described a method of saline injection beneath the communication tract to achieve rapid thrombosis in six patients, avoiding the risk of thromboembolic and allergic complications (67). Further experience is required to validate this treatment modality.

Stent grafts have been used in one series of 16 patients with PCPAs and 10 with arteriovenous fistulas. The procedure was successful in all patients but 17% were occluded at one year, probably related to flexion at the hip kinking the devices (68).

In summary, thrombin injection is relatively easy, with high success and low complication rates and is the first-line treatment for PCPAs.

REFERENCES

1. Sueyoshi E, Sakamoto I, Nakashima K, et al. Visceral and peripheral arterial pseudoaneurysms. Pictorial essay. Am J Roentgenol 2005; 185:741–9.
2. Katzenschlager R, Ugurluoglu A, Ahmadi A, et al. Incidence of pseudoaneurysms after diagnostic and therapeutic angiography. Radiology 1995; 195:463–6.
3. Glikman BS, Rehm JP, Baxter BT. Arterial aneurysms: etiologic considerations. In: Rutherford RB, ed. Vascular Surgery, Vol. 1. Philadelphia, PA: W.B. Saunders Company, 2000:373–86.
4. Schwartz LB, Clark ET, Gewertz BL. Anastomotic and other pseudoaneurysms. In: Rutherford RB, ed. Vascular Surgery. 5th ed., Vol. 1. Philadelphia, PA: W.B. Saunders Company, 2000:752–63.
5. Seabrook GR, Schmitt DD, Bandyk DF, et al. Anastomotic femoral pseudoaneurysm: an investigation of occult infection as an etiologic factor. J Vasc Surg 1990; 11:629–34.
6. Biancari F, Ylonen K, Anttila V, et al. Durability of open repair of infrarenal abdominal aortic aneurysm: a 15-year follow-up study. J Vasc Surg 2002; 35:87–93.
7. Ylonen K, Biancari F, Leo E, et al. Predictors of development of anastomotic femoral pseudoaneurysms after aortobifemoral reconstruction for abdominal aortic aneurysm. Am J Surg 2004; 187:83–7.
8. Levi N, Schroeder TV. Anastomotic femoral aneurysms: increase in the interval between primary operation and aneurysm formation. Eur J Vasc Endovasc Surg 1996; 11:207–9.
9. Sieswerda C, Skotnicki SH, Barentz JO, et al. Anastomotic aneurysms-an underdiagnosed complication after aorto-iliac reconstructions. Eur J Vasc Surg 1989; 3:233–9.
10. Ernst CB, Elliott JP, Jr., Ryan CJ, et al. Recurrent femoral anastomotic aneurysms: a 30-year experience. Ann Surg 1988; 208(4):401–9.
11. Saad NEA, Saad WEA, Davies MG, et al. Pseudoaneurysms and the role of minimally invasive techniques in their management. Radiographics 2005; 25:S173–89.
12. Munera F, Soto JA, Palacio D, Velez SM, Medina E. Diagnosis of arterial injuries caused by penetrating trauma to the neck: comparison of helical CT angiography and conventional angiography. Radiology 2000; 216:356–62.
13. Soto JA, Munera F, Morales C, et al. Focal arterial injuries of the proximal extremities: helical CT arteriography as the initial method of diagnosis. Radiology 2001; 218:188–94.
14. Glockner JF. Three-dimensional gadolinium-enhanced MR angiography: applications for abdominal imaging. Radiographics 2001; 21:357–70.
15. Dennis JW, Littooy FN, Griesler HP, et al. Anastomotic pseudoaneurysms: a continuing late complication of vascular reconstructive procedures. Arch Surg 1986; 121:314–7.
16. Reddy DJ, Smith RF, Elliott JP, Jr., et al. Infected femoral artery false aneurysms in drug addicts: evolution of selective vascular reconstruction. J Vasc Surg 1986; 3:718–24.
17. Criado E, Marston WA, Ligush J, et al. Endovascular repair of peripheral aneurysms, pseudoaneurysms, and arteriovenous fistulas. Ann Vasc Surg 1997; 11:256–63.
18. Brountzos EN, Malagari K, Gougoulakis A, et al. Common femoral artery anastomotic pseudoaneurysm: endovascular treatment with Hemobahn stent-grafts. J Vasc Interv Radiol 2000; 11:1179–83.
19. Edwards JM, Teefey SA, Zierler RE, et al. Intraabdominal paraanastomotic aneurysms after aortic bypass grafting. J Vasc Surg 1992; 15:344–53.

20. Bastounis E, Georgopoulos S, Maltezos C, et al. The validity of current vascular imaging methods in the evaluation of aortic anastomotic aneurysms developing after abdominal aortic aneurysm repair. Ann Vasc Surg 1996; 10:537–45.

21. Tiesenhausen K, Hausegger KA, Tauss J, et al. Endovascular treatment of proximal anastomotic aneurysms after aortic prosthetic reconstruction. Cardiovasc Intervent Radiol 2001; 24:49–52.

22. van Herwaarden JA, Waasdorp EJ, Bendermacher BLW, et al. Endovascular repair of paraanastomotic aneurysms after previous open aortic prosthetic reconstruction. Ann Vasc Surg 2004; 18:280–6.

23. Curti T, Stella A, Rossi C, et al. Endovascular treatment as first-choice treatment for anastomotic and true iliac aneurysms. J Endovasc Ther 2001; 8:139–43.

24. Faries PL, Won J, Morrissey NJ, et al. Endovascular treatment of failed prior abdominal aortic aneurysm repair. Ann Vasc Surg 2003; 17:43–8.

25. Magnan PE, Albertini JN, Bartoli JM, et al. Endovascular treatment of anastomotic false aneurysms of the abdominal aorta. Ann Vasc Surg 2003; 17:365–74.

26. Zhou W, Bush RL, Bhama JK, et al. Repair of anastomotic abdominal aortic pseudoaneurysm utilizing sequential AneuRx aortic cuffs in an overlapping configuration. Ann Vasc Surg 2006; 20(1):17–22 (Epub ahead of print).

27. White RA, Donayre CE, Walot I, et al. Endoluminal graft exclusion of a proximal para-anastomotic pseudoaneurysm following aortobifemoral bypass. J Endovasc Surg 1997; 4:88–94.

28. Abou-Zamzam AM, Jr., Ballard JL. Management of sterile para-anastomotic aneurysms of the aorta. Semin Vasc Surg 2001; 14:282–91.

29. Curti T, Freyrie A, Mirelli M, et al. Endovascular treatment of an ilioenteric fistula: a bridge to aortic homograft. Eur J Vasc Endovasc Surg 2000; 20:204–6.

30. Fann JI, Samuels S, Slonim S, et al. Treatment of abdominal aortic anastomotic pseudoaneurysm with percutaneous coil embolization. J Vasc Surg 2002; 35:811–4.

31. Smayra T, Otal P, Soula P, et al. Pseudoaneurysm and aortobronchial fistula after surgical bypass for aortic coartation: management with endovascular stent-graft. J Endovasc Ther 2001; 8:42–428.

32. Munneke G, Loosemore T, Smith J, et al. Pseudoaneurysm after aortic coarctation repair presenting with an aortobronchial fistula successfully treated with an aortic stent graft. Clin Radiol 2006; 61:104–8.

33. Eskandari MK, Resnick SA. Salvage of endoluminal exclusion of an anastomotic arch aneurysm with a "kissing" carotid stent. J Vasc Interv Radiol 2004; 15:1317–21.

34. Morgan R, Belli A-M. Current treatment methods for postcatheterization pseudoaneurysms. J Vasc Interv Radiol 2003; 14:697–710.

35. Eichlisberger R, Frauchiger B, Schmitt II, et al. Pseudoaneurysm after femoral artery catheterization: diagnosis and follow-up using duplex ultrasound. Ultrashall Med 1992; 13:54–8.

36. Wyman RM, Safian RD, Portway V, et al. Current complications of diagnostic and therapeutic cardiac catheterization. Am Coll Cardiol 1988; 12:1400–6.

37. Rapoport S, Sniderman KW, Morse SS, et al. Pseudoaneurysm: a complication of faulty technique in femoral artery puncture. Radiology 1985; 154:529–30.

38. Paulson EK, Nelson RC, Mayes CE, et al. Sonographically guided thrombin injection of iatrogenic femoral pseudoaneurysms: further experience of a single institution. Am J Roentgenol 2001; 177:309–16.

39. Fellmeth BD, Roberts AC, Bookstein JJ, et al. Postangiographic femoral artery injuries: nonsurgical repair with US-guided compression. Radiology 1991; 178:671–5.

40. Krueger K, Zaehringer M, Strohe D, et al. Postcatheterization pseudoaneurysm: results of US-guided percutaneous thrombin injection in 240 patients. Radiology 2005; 236:1104–10.

41. Coley BD, Roberts AC, Fellmeth BD, et al. Postangiographic femoral artery pseudoaneurysms: further experience with US-guided compression repair. Radiology 1995; 194:307–11.

42. Hertz SM, Brener BJ. Ultrasound-guided pseudoaneurysm compression: efficacy after coronary stenting and angioplasty. J Vasc Surg 1997; 26:913–6.

43. Dean SM, Olin JW, Piedmonte M, et al. Ultrasound-guided compression closure of postcatherization pseudoaneurysms during concurrent anticoagulation: a review of seventy-seven patients. J Vasc Surg 1996; 23:28–34.

44. Chatterjee T, Do DD, Kaufman U, et al. Ultrasound-guided compression repair for treatment of femoral artery pseudoaneurym: acute and follow-up results. Cathet Cardiovasc Diagn 1996; 38:335–40.

45. Ugurluoglu A, Katzenschlager R, Ahmadi R, et al. Ultrasound guided compression therapy in 134 patients with iatrogenic pseudo-aneurysms: advantage of routine duplex ultrasound control of the puncture site following transfemoral catheterization. Vasa 1997; 26:110–6.

46. Eisenberg L, Paulson EK, Kliewer MA, et al. Sonographically guided compression repair of pseudoaneurysms: further experience from a single institution. Am J Roentgenol 1999; 173:1567–73.

47. Taylor BS, Rhee RY, Muluk S, et al. Thrombin injection versus compression of femoral artery pseudoaneurysms. J Vasc Surg 1999; 30:1052–9.

48. Paulson EK, Sheafor DH, Kliewer MA, et al. Treatment of iatrogenic femoral arterial pseudoaneurysms: comparison of US-guided thrombin injection with compression repair. Radiology 2000; 215:403–8.

49. Weinmann EE, Chayen D, Kobzantzev ZV, et al. Treatment of postcatheterization false aneurysms: ultrasound-guided compression vs. ultrasound-guided thrombin injection. Eur J Vasc Endovasc Surg 2002; 23:68–72.

50. Hajarizadeh H, LaRosa CR, Cardullo P, et al. Ultrasound-guided compression of iatrogenic femoral pseudoaneurysm failure, recurrence, and long-term results. J Vasc Surg 1995; 22:425–30.

51. Kang SS, Labropoulos N, Mansour MA, et al. Percutaneous ultrasound guided thrombin injection: a new method for treating postcatheterization femoral pseudoaneurysms. J Vasc Surg 1998; 28:1120–1.

52. Kang SS, Labropoulos N, Mansour MA, et al. Expanded indications for ultrasound-guided thrombin injection of pseudoaneurysms. J Vasc Surg 2000; 31:289–98.

53. Owen RJ, Haslam PJ, Elliott ST, et al. Percutaneous ablation of peripheral pseudoaneurysms using thrombin: a simple and effective solution. Cardiovasc Intervent Radiol 2000; 23:441–6.

54. Pezzullo JA, Dupuy DE, Cronan JJ. Percutaneous injection of thrombin for the treatment of pseudoaneurysms after catheterization: an alternative to sonographically guided compression. Am J Roentgenol 2000; 175:1035–40.

55. Sackett WR, Taylor SM, Coffey CB, et al. Ultrasound-guided thrombin injection of iatrogenic femoral pseudoaneurysms: a prospective analysis. Am Surg 2000; 66:937–40.

56. La Perna L, Olin JW, Goines D. Ultrasound-guided thrombin injection for the treatment of postcatheterization pseudoaneurysms. Circulation 2000; 102:2391–5.

57. Friedman SG, Pellerito JS, Scher L, et al. Ultrasound-guided thrombin injection is the treatment of choice for femoral pseudoaneurysms. Arch Surg 2002; 137:462–4.

58. Elford J, Burrell C, Freeman S, et al. Human thrombin injection for the percutaneous treatment of iatrogenic pseudoaneurysms. Cardiovasc Intervent Radiol 2002; 25:115–8.

59. Khoury M, Rebecca A, Greene K, et al. Duplex scanning-guided thrombin injection for the treatment of iatrogenic pseudoaneurysms. J Vasc Surg 2002; 35:517–21.

60. Etemad-Rezai R, Peck DJ. Ultrasound-guided thrombin injection of femoral artery pseudoaneurysms. Can Assoc Radiol J 2003; 54:118–20.

61. Krueger K, Zaehringer M, Soehngen F-D, et al. Femoral pseudoaneurysms: management with percutaneous thrombin injections-success rates and effects on systemic coagulation. Radiology 2003; 226:452–8.

62. Vazquez V, Reus M, Pinero A, et al. Human thrombin for treatment of pseudoaneurysms: comparison of bovine and human thrombin sonogram-guided injection. Am J Roentgenol 2005; 184:1665–71.

63. Walker TG, Geller SC, Brewster SC. Transcatheter occlusion of a profunda femoral artery pseudoaneurysm using thrombin. Am J Roentgenol 1987; 149:185–6.

64. Brountzos EN, Malagari K, Papathanasiou MA, et al. Internal iliac artery aneurysm embolization with fibrin sealant: a simple and effective solution. Cardiovasc Intervent Radiol 2003; 26:76–80.

65. Sheiman RG, Mastromatteo M. Iatrogenic femoral pseudoaneurysms that are unresponsive to percutaneous thrombin injection: potential causes. AJR Am J Roentgenol 2003; 181:1301–4.

66. Kobeiter H, Lapeyre M, Becquemin JP, et al. Percutaneous coil embolization of postcatheterization arterial femoral pseudoaneurysms. J Vasc Surg 2002; 36:127–31.

67. Gehling G, Ludwig J, Schmidt A, et al. Percutaneous occlusion of femoral artery pseudoaneurysm by para-aneurysmal saline injection. Catheter Cardiovasc Interv 2003; 58:500–4.

68. Thalhammer C, Kirchherr AS, Uhlich F, et al. Postcatheterization pseudoaneurysms and arteriovenous fistulas: repair with percutaneous implantation of endovascular covered stents. Radiology 2000; 214:127–31.

49 | Percutaneous Closure of Large Vessels

Lakshmi A. Ratnam and Graham J. Munneke
Department of Radiology, St. George's Hospital, London, U.K.

INTRODUCTION

Previously, manual compression was the only method of achieving hemostasis following percutaneous vascular intervention (1,2). But more recently mechanical compression and arterial closure devices have become available. The aim of this chapter is to provide an overview of closure devices available including indications, contraindications, and evidence for efficacy and safety of the different products.

Manual compression requires 10 to 15 minutes of groin compression, and entails patient discomfort and 4 to 8 hours bed rest. This often necessitates an overnight hospital stay. Complications include hemorrhage, infection, thrombosis, pseudoaneurysm formation, arteriovenous fistula, arterial dissection and distal embolization (3–5). With advances in the fields of interventional radiology, vascular surgery and cardiology, the complexity of cases treated percutaneously have increased. Bigger sheath sizes, prolonged sheath indwelling times and the use of anticoagulation and antiplatelet therapy during procedures have all added to the risks involved and resulting access site complications (6). Large scale trials using manual compression have found that the incidence of major vascular complications following cardiac catheterizations range between 0.3% and 1.0% (7,8). More recent studies have reported a higher rate of complications for complex interventional procedures (9,10).

A variety of mechanical compression devices have been introduced. Though reducing the need for manual compression, these devices do not necessarily provide improved patient safety. In the 1990s, closure devices were introduced with the aim of reducing time to hemostasis, time to ambulation, patient discomfort and complication rates (11–13). Although recommendations vary from device to device, in general, mobilization after two hours is possible. The ability to reduce time to ambulation and therefore time to discharge also allows for more procedures to be performed on a day case basis with significant cost implications (14). Studies of the initial designs demonstrated improved time to hemostasis and ambulation, though complication rates were comparable to manual compression, and in some cases higher (5,10,15).

A large variety of closure devices are now available. Hemostasis is achieved primarily via four mechanisms as shown in Table 1.

COLLAGEN PLUG DEVICES

Following arterial puncture, the contact of blood with the exposed arterial wall smooth muscle cells and collagen initiates platelet aggregation. Bovine collagen plugs augment this process by providing greater surface area for the adherence and activation of platelets. The resulting mass of hemostatic plug provides a mechanical seal of the vessel and tissue tract. Bovine collagen is degraded by granulocytes and macrophages and reabsorbed within four weeks in an animal model (16).

Angio-Seal®

The Angio-Seal® is one of the more widely used devices, and consists of four components: an insertion sheath, an arteriotomy locator, a 70-cm J-tipped guidewire and the closure device

TABLE 1 Closure Devices

Collagen plug devices
1. Angio-Seal™ (St. Jude Medical, St. Paul, Minnesota, U.S.A.)
2. Vasoseal Extravascular Security (ES) (Datascope Corporation, Montvale, New Jersey, U.S.A.)
3. Duett (Vascular Solutions, Minneapolis, Minnesota, U.S.A.)

Suture-mediated devices
1. Closer S (Abbott Vascular, Abbott Park, Illinois, U.S.A.)
2. Perclose (Abbott Vascular, Abbott Park, Illinois, U.S.A.)
3. Sutura superstitch (Sutura, Fountain Valley, California, U.S.A.)
4. X-Press™ (X-Site Medical, Blue Bell, Pennsylvania, U.S.A.)
5. Surestitch (Sutura, Fountain Valley, California, U.S.A.)
6. Prostar-techstar (Abbott Vascular, Abbott Park, Illinois, U.S.A.)

Staple/clip device
1. Starclose (Abbott Vascular, Abbott Park, Illinois, U.S.A.)
2. Expanding Vascular Stapling (EVS™) Vascular Closure System (Angiolink, Danvers, Massachusetts)

Patch technology
1. Syvek® Patch (Marine Polymer Technologies, Danvers, Massachusetts)
2. Clo-Sur™ Pad (Scion Cardio-Vascular, Miami, Florida, U.S.A.)
3. Chito-Seal® Pad (Abbott Vascular, Abbott Park, Illinois, U.S.A.)
4. D-Stat® (Vascular Solutions, Minneapolis, Minnesota, U.S.A.)

itself (Fig. 1). The device consists of an anchor composed of a polylactide and polyglycolide polymer, a collagen plug and a suture, contained within a special carrier system. When inserted, it achieves hemostasis by compressing the arterial puncture site between the anchor and the collagen plug (17). Use of the device has a short learning curve, it can consistently be deployed within one minute and the components are thought to be completely bioabsorbable. The manufacturer recommends no repuncture at the site of Angioseal closure within 90 days, though several studies have shown that repuncture slightly above or below the initial puncture can be performed safely within one to seven days (14,18).

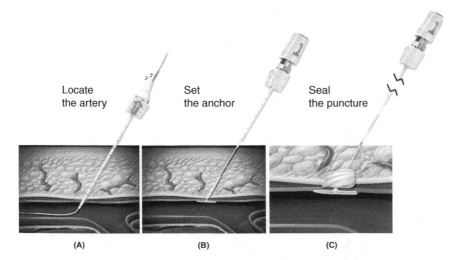

FIGURE 1 The Angio-Seal device. (**A**) The sheath with the vessel locator is inserted through the arteriotomy. The vessel locator enables correct positioning of the sheath just distal to the arteriotomy. (**B**) The footplate is advanced through the sheath. Upward traction on the sheath locates the anchor against the arteriotomy and unsheaths the collagen plug within the tract. (**C**) While maintaining traction on the suture, the tamper tube is used to sandwich the arteriotomy between the collagen sponge and the anchor.

Complications such as infection, hemorrhage, and vessel occlusion are uncommon, ranging from 0.5% to 1.9% of cases (19,20). The device, in common with most other closure devices, should not be used in the superficial femoral or profunda femoris artery, or above the inguinal ligament. A specific disadvantage of Angio-Seal is the presence of a large intravascular suture anchor, which can act as a nidus for platelet aggregation. Also, the collagen plug induces a significant subcutaneous inflammatory reaction. Angio-Seal should not be used in patients who may require imminent surgical exposure of the femoral artery for bypass or stent-graft placement, because the retention suture may be cut leading to embolization of the intravascular anchor (17).

Vasoseal®

The Vasoseal® device places one or more collagen plugs in the puncture tract external to the artery. It employs an 8-F tubular delivery sheath but does not increase the size of the arterial puncture. The number of collagen plugs positioned depends on the depth of the artery from the skin surface. After positioning the plugs, only slight pressure should be applied at the puncture site, allowing blood and collagen to interact and form an occlusive thrombus. According to the manufacturer there is no contraindication to the use of this device in patients with peripheral vascular disease (21). The Vasoseal is simple and effective to use with a reported high technical success rate and a low major complication rate of 0.6% (22,23).

Duett®

The Duett® device delivers a mixture of bovine collagen and thrombin using a balloon positioning catheter. The mixture is delivered through a 3-F catheter system with a distal occlusion balloon, positioned inside the artery through the sheath. The balloon is inflated within the artery, retracted initially against the sheath and subsequently the whole system against the vessel wall. An attempt at aspiration through the sheath is made when the balloon reaches the arterial puncture site. As the sheath lies outside the artery, blood should not be aspirated. At this point, injection of the procoagulant mixture takes place. If blood is aspirated through the sheath, the balloon is deflated, the system repositioned deeper, and the steps repeated. The mixture is injected while removing the sheath to cover the external surface of the artery and seal the tract. At the end of injection, the balloon is deflated and removed through the sealed tract. The device can be used with 5- to 9-F sheath sizes. The Duett is contraindicated in peripheral vascular disease due to intraluminal balloon inflation and is indicated for femoral arteriotomy closure only (21,24).

Studies evaluating the use of Duett have shown reduced time to hemostasis and ambulation, and a comparable complication rate to manual compression. Complications include device failure, inadvertent injection of procoagulant into the arterial system, pseudoaneurysm formation, and allergy to bovine-derived procoagulant components (25,26).

SUTURE MEDIATED, CLIP, AND STAPLE DEVICES

The use of suture-mediated, clip and staple devices result in complete apposition of the tissue, allowing closure independent of clot formation, and reducing time to hemostasis. They have a particular role in patients on antiplatelet and anticoagulant therapy, and those in whom larger vascular sheaths are used (27).

Closer S® and Perclose®

The Perclose® is designed to perform a percutaneous surgical closure of an arterial puncture using braided polyester sutures (Fig. 2). Its primary sealing is not dependent on clot formation and can be used on patients who are anticoagulated or have undergone thrombolysis. The original devices were Techstar 6-F, and Prostar 8-F and 10-F. The Closer S®, a 6-F device, has replaced the Techstar 6-F device and can be used to close punctures sites up to 8-F. Larger sheath sizes can be accommodated if the device is deployed prior to arteriotomy dilatation. A further modification is the Perclose A-T (auto-tie) in which the slipknot is created within the device, allowing quicker, easier and single-handed operation (28).

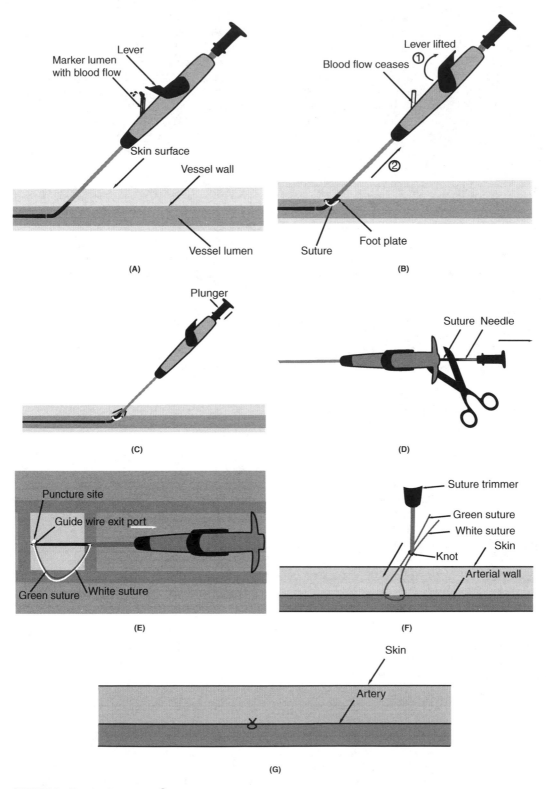

FIGURE 2 The Perclose device®. (Caption on facing page)

While applying pressure, the device shaft is rotated through the subcutaneous tissue and positioned in the artery. Once arterial placement is confirmed by pulsatile blood flow from a marker lumen, the needles of the device are deployed which capture the sutures. The device is removed, the suture externalized and the knot advanced onto the artery (29).

The Closer S has a relatively complicated deployment mechanism, resulting in a longer learning curve. The major complication rate in one study showed Angio-Seal to be 0.3% and Closer S to be 0.6%. The nonabsorbable suture material used in the Closer S system remains within the arterial lumen and may induce foreign body reactions, vascular inflammation and necrosis (29).

Although the newer Perclose A-T with its pretied knot is easier to use, the Perclose still remains more difficult to deploy compared to some of the other devices available. One distinct advantage of the Perclose is that it can be used to close large arteriotomies including after percutaneous placement of a stentgraft. One device is deployed for sheath sizes of up to 12-F and two devices are used for sheath sizes greater than 12-F (30).

Starclose

The Starclose system features a star-shaped 4-mm diameter Nitinol clip which is positioned against the outside arterial wall at the puncture site, then released (Fig. 3). The device has small pins which engage the arterial tissue from the outside, and fold inwards, causing it to pucker and seal the puncture, providing extravascular closure. The clip applier is attached to the introducer sheath which is left in place after the primary procedure and the clip is deployed at the arteriotomy site through a peel-away sheath.

Starclose has shown reduced time to hemostasis and time to ambulation with a minor complication rate comparable to manual compression. No major vascular complications have been reported in the two published studies to date. Technical success is high. Follow-up ultrasound after two weeks in one study showed no compromise of the vessel lumen (31,32).

The device is easy to use, but there is a small incidence of the delivery system failing to disconnect from the patient after deployment. The situation can usually be resolved by traction on the device while applying pressure to the arteriotomy site with the other hand after ensuring the safety release button is down.

EVS Vascular Closure System

The EVS Vascular Closure System comprises an introducer assembly, biocompatible titanium staple and a trigger activated staple deployment device. Following removal of the arterial introducing sheath, the EVS dilator and introducer are advanced as a unit over a guidewire, through overlying tissues, until brisk blood response from the dilator arterial marking lumen is achieved. The guidewire is removed. The stabilization feet are then deployed intraluminally and retracted until there is tactile feedback against the anterior wall of the artery. The dilator is then removed and the staple device advanced through the introducer until resistance against the anterior wall of the artery is encountered. The staple is then trigger-activated. There are no relative or absolute contraindications to the device and the major complication rate reported is less than that of manual compression. The use of staples and clips for varied surgical procedures over the years have demonstrated minimal biological

---

FIGURE 2 (*Facing page*) (**A**) The Perclose device is inserted over the guidewire into the arterial lumen. Satisfactory position is confirmed by blood flow through the marker lumen. (**B**) The lever is lifted to deploy the footplate (*1*) the device is then withdrawn until the footplate is apposed to the arterial wall (*2*) and blood flow through the marker lumen should cease. (**C**) The plunger is depressed, deploying the needles which capture the suture. (**D**) The plunger is removed, revealing the green suture which is then cut. The lever is pushed down to park the footplate. (**E**) The device is withdrawn until the guidewire exit port is visible. The two suture ends (green and white) are removed from the device. (**F**) While maintaining constant tension on the green suture, the device is removed. The suture trimmer is loaded on the green suture and the knot advanced to the arteriotomy. Traction on the white suture locks the knot. (**G**) The suture trimmer is advanced over both sutures which are then cut just above the arteriotomy.

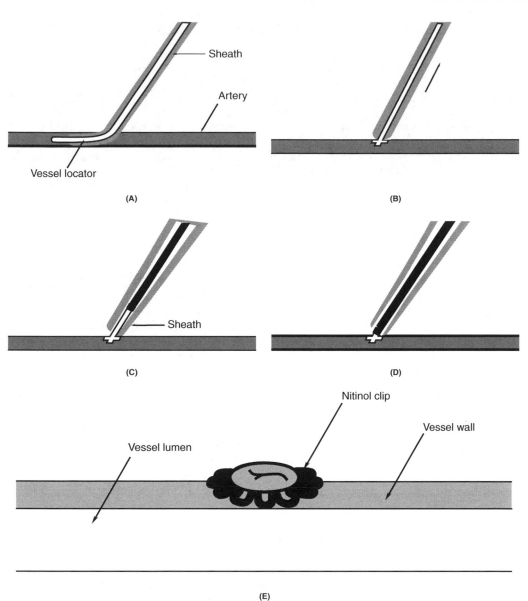

FIGURE 3 The Starclose device. (**A**) The vessel locator is inserted through its sheath. (**B**) The vessel locator is deployed and withdrawn until it is apposed to the arteriotomy. (**C**) The clip is advanced to the arteriotomy. This process results in splitting of the sheath. (**D**) When the clip reaches the arteriotomy, it is deployed and the vessel locator simultaneously retracts. (**E**) The clip apposes the edges of the arteriotomy providing rapid hemostasis.

response. The mechanism of the staple activation is simple allowing for reduced operator error (33).

PATCHES AND PADS

Noninvasive hemostatic patches and pads were developed to assist closure at percutaneous puncture sites by accelerating the hemostatic process. They have several advantages, including use over a broad range of puncture sites and sizes, no foreign material is left, they allow immediate reaccess to the puncture site and are easy to use (34).

Syvek® Patch

Introduced in 1999, the Syvek® Patch employs a high molecular weight polysaccharide, poly-*N*-acetyl glucosamine, formulated into a solid matrix material making up the patch. It is applied topically to the puncture site after catheter removal. Once in contact with blood, the patch acts as a catalytic surface, enhancing the rate of local hemostasis via the acceleration of normal clotting mechanisms. No foreign material is left behind at the puncture site or in the tissue tract, reducing the potential for infection and localized inflammatory response. The protocol recommends 10 minutes of manual compression for diagnostic cases and 20 minutes for interventional cases. The rate of bleeding and pseudoaneurysm complications have been reported to be less than manual compression alone and much less than invasive mechanical devices (34,35).

Clo-Sur™ Pad

The Clo-Sur™ pad is applied topically to accelerate puncture site hemostasis. The pad contains chitosan, a composite marine products polymer that is cationically charged. When placed over the puncture site, it works as a cell-binding agent of positively charged chitosan molecules that attract negatively charged red blood cells and platelets. Initial reports indicate that this product requires a 10 to 15 minutes hold time, with a 3.7% complication rate for diagnostic patients and a 5% complication rate for interventional patients (34).

Chito-Seal® Pad

Also based on chitosan, the Chito-Seal® pad is backed with a cellulose coating. The puncture site is covered with the moistened pad and pressure applied for two to three minutes or until hemostasis is achieved. The pad is left in place and covered with a dressing. Within 24 hours, the pad is soaked with water and removed. There are no current reports on its effectiveness.

D-Stat® Dry/D-Stat® Radial

This hemostatic pad uses thrombin to accelerate coagulation. As with other pads it works in combination with manual compression. The pad is left in situ for two hours then removed. A version designed specifically for radial artery punctures is also available. This was designed to eliminate occlusive compression of the radial artery and to prevent compression of the ulnar artery.

It should be noted that the patches do not allow quicker ambulation and require comparable length of compression to manual compression alone.

SUMMARY

There are a variety of commercially available arterial closure devices, designed to reduce time to hemostasis and ambulation, free operator time and improve patient comfort. Unfortunately, they are not without complications. The FDA Center for the Devices of Radiological Health has proposed several recommendations to help avoid complications with the use of vascular hemostatic devices (17)

- Should not be used in cases of suspected double wall arterial puncture.
- Should be used with caution in patients with bleeding disorders or patients taking glycoprotein IIb/IIIa receptor inhibitors.
- Puncture site should be carefully monitored as a standard practice after manual compression.
- Postprocedure management and ambulation guidelines should be strictly adhered to based on the specific device used.

Most existing data are based on comparing the safety and efficacy of individual devices with manual compression. A study with 705 subjects compared the safety and efficacy of the three main collagen based devices (Angio-Seal, Vasoseal and Duett). In the diagnostic group, the device deployment rates and ambulation times were similar, though Angioseal was significantly slower to achieve hemostasis. In angioplasty patients, deployment rates and ambulation times were similar and, again, time to hemostasis was longer for Angioseal. Ambulation times were longer than for diagnostic patients. The three devices had similar major complication rates. The concurrent use of abciximab, which inhibits platelet aggregation, led to an increase in severe complications (36).

In a further study comparing Angio-Seal, Perclose and manual compression, times to hemostasis and ambulation were shorter for the Angio-Seal group compared to those treated with Perclose and manual compression. The complication rates were significantly less with Angio-Seal compared to Perclose, and patients treated with Angio-Seal reported greater overall satisfaction, better wound healing and less discomfort (37).

Despite individual trials suggesting comparability or equivalence to manual compression in terms of safety and efficacy, a meta-analysis suggests that many trials are undersized and that adverse trends may approach significance (38). This emphasizes the importance of careful patient selection for closure devices and adherence to manufacturer guidelines. It should also be noted that most of the published literature is with reference to first generation devices and may not be representative of current versions (39).

Although many of the devices have similar indications and contraindications, choice of device should be tailored to individual cases. For example, the Perclose device can be used for larger arteriotomies, and hemostatic patches may have a role in radial and brachial artery punctures. Closure devices may be particularly helpful in cases of patients at high risk for vascular access site complications, in particular hypertensive, anticoagulated patients and those in whom prolonged bed rest is not feasible, such as the confused or restless patient, and those with cardiorespiratory distress (40). In day-case patients, early ambulation can improve patient satisfaction and have cost implications. Overall, arterial closure devices have a safety profile comparable to that of manual compression and are a useful adjunct in the field of percutaneous vascular intervention.

REFERENCES

1. Semler HJ. Transfemoral catheterization: mechanical versus manual control of bleeding. Radiology 1985; 154:235.
2. Prayck JB, Wall TC, Longabaugh P, et al. A randomized trial of vascular haemostasis techniques to reduce femoral vascular complications after coronary intervention. Am J Cardiol 1998; 81:970–6.
3. Gardiner GA, Meyerovitz MF, Stokes KR, et al. Complications of transluminal angioplasty. Radiology 1986; 159:201–8.
4. Ricci MA, Trevisani GT, Pilcher DB. Vascular complications of cardiac catheterization. Am J Surg 1994; 167:375–8.
5. Waksman R, King SB, Douglas JS, et al. Predictors of groin complications after balloon and new-device coronary intervention. Am J Cardiol 1995; 75:886–9.
6. EPILOG Investigators. Platelet glycoprotein IIb/IIIa receptor blockade and low-dose heparin during percutaneous coronary revascularization. N Engl J Med 1997; 336:1689–96.
7. Babu SC, Piccorelli GO, Shah PM. Incidence and results of arterial complications among 16,350 patients undergoing cardiac catheterization. J Vasc Surg 1989; 10:113–6.
8. Johnson LW, Lozner EC, Johnson S. Coronary arteriography 1984–1987: a report of the Registry of the Society for Cardiac Angiography and Interventions: results and complications. Catheter Cardiovasc Diag 1989; 17:5–10.
9. Khoury M, Bantra S, Berg R, et al. Influence of arterial sites and interventional procedures on vascular complications after cardiac catheterization. Am J Surg 1992; 164:205–10.
10. Muller DW, Shamir KJ, Ellis SG, et al. Peripheral vascular complications after conventional and complex percutaneous coronary interventional procedures. Am J Cardiol 1992; 69:63–8.
11. Sanborn TA, Gibbs HH, Brinker JA, et al. A multicenter randomized trial comparing a percutaneous collagen hemostasis device with conventional manual compression after diagnostic angiography and angioplasty. J Am Col Cardiol 1993; 22:1273–9.
12. Kussmaul WG, Buchbinder M, Whitlow PL, et al. Rapid arterial hemostasis and decreased access site complications after cardiac catheterization and angioplasty: results of a randomized trial of a novel hemostatic device. J Am Coll Cardiol 1995; 25:1685–92.

13. Gerckens U, Cattelaens N, Lampe EG, et al. Management of arterial puncture site after catheterization procedures: evaluating a suture-mediated closure device. Am J Cardiol 1999; 83:1658–63.
14. Abando A, Hood D, Weaver F, et al. The use of the Angioseal device for femoral artery closure. J Vasc Surg 2004; 40:287–90.
15. Wagner SC, Gonsalves CF, Eschelman DJ, et al. Complications of a percutaneous suture-mediated closure device versus manual compression for arteriotomy closure: a case-controlled study. J Vasc Interv Radiol 2003; 14:735–41.
16. Hoffer EK, Bloch RD. Percutaneous arterial closure devices. J Vasc Interv Radiol 2003; 14:865–86.
17. Rilling WS, Dicker M. Arterial puncture using a collagen plug, I. (Angio-Seal). Tech Vasc Interv Radiol 2003; 6(2):76–81.
18. Applegate RJ, Rankin KM, Little WC, et al. Restick following initial Angioseal use. Catheter Cardiovasc Interv 2003; 58:181–4.
19. Shammas NW, Rajendran VR, Alldredge SG, et al. Randomised comparison of Vasoseal and Angioseal closure devices in patients undergoing coronary angiography and angioplasty. Catheter Cardiovasc Interv 2002; 55:421–5.
20. Cremonesi A, Castriota F, Tarantino F, et al. Femoral arterial haemostasis using the Angio-Seal system after coronary and vascular percutaneous angioplasty and stenting. J Invasive Cardiol 1998; 10:464–9.
21. Silber S. Rapid haemostasis of arterial puncture sites with collagen after diagnostic and interventional cardiac catheterization. Clin Cardiol 1997; 20:981–92.
22. Cleveland G, Hill S, Williams S. Arterial puncture closure using a collagen plug II (VasoSeal). Tech Vasc Interv Radiol 2003; 6(2):82–4.
23. Shrake K. Comparison of major complication rates associated with four methods of arterial closure. Am J Cardiol 2000; 85:1024–5.
24. Dickey K. Arterial hemostasis using the Duett sealing device. Tech Vasc Interv Radiol 2003; 6(2):85–91.
25. The SEAL Trial Study Team. Assessment of the safety and efficacy of the DUETT vascular hemostasis device: final results of the Safe and Effective Vascular Hemostasis (SEAL) trial. Am Heart J 2002; 143:612–9.
26. Silber S, Tofte AJ, Kjellevand TO, et al. Final report of the European multi-center registry using the DUETT vascular sealing device. Herz 1999; 24:620–3.
27. Facchini FR. Percutaneous arterial access: redefining the possibilities using suture-mediated closure (Perclose). Tech Vasc Interv Radiol 2003; 6(2):72–5.
28. D'Souza S. Closure devices: indications and results. In: Wyatt MG, Watkinson AF, eds. Endovascular Intervention-Current Controversies. Shrewsbury, U.K.: TFM publishing, 2004:205–16.
29. Park Y, Roh HG, Choo SW, et al. Prospective comparison of collagen plug (Angio-Seal) and suture-mediated (the Closer S) closure devices at femoral access sites. Korean J Radiol 2005; 6:248–55.
30. Quinn SF, Kim J. Percutaneous femoral closure following stent-graft placement: use of the Perclose device. Cardiovasc Interv Radiol 2004; 27:231–6.
31. Hermiller J, Simonton C, Hinohara T, et al. Clinical experience with a circumferential clip-based vascular closure device in diagnostic catheterization. J Invasive Cardiol 2005; 17(10):504–51.
32. Ruygrok PN, Ormiston JA, Steward JT, et al. Initial experience with a new femoral artery closure device following percutaneous coronary intervention with glycoprotein IIb/IIIa inhibition. Catheter Cardiovasc Interv 2005; 66:185–91.
33. Caputo RP, Ebner A, Grant W, et al. Percutaneous femoral arteriotomy repair- initial experience with a novel staple closure device. J Invasive Cardiol 2002; 14:652–6.
34. Hirsch JA, Reddy SA, Capasso WE, et al. Non-invasive hemostatic closure devices: "Patches and Pads." Tech Vasc Interv Radiol 2003; 6(2):92–5.
35. Carey D, Martin JR, Moore CA, et al. Complications of femoral artery closure devices. Catheter Cardiovasc 2001; 52:3–7.
36. Michalis LK, Rees MR, Patsouras D. A prospective randomized trial comparing the safety and efficacy of three commercially available closure devices (Angioseal, Vasoseal and Duett). Cardiovasc Interv Radiol 2002; 25:423–9.
37. Duffin DC, Muhlestein JB, Allisson SB, et al. Femoral arterial puncture management after percutaneous coronary procedures: a comparison of clinical outcomes and patient satisfaction between manual compression and two different vascular closure devices. J Invasive Cardiol 2001; 13:354–62.
38. Vaitkus PT. A meta-analysis of percutaneous vascular closure devices after diagnostic catheterization and percutaneous coronary intervention. J Invasive Cadiol 2004; 16:243–6.
39. Aggarwal K, Murtaza M. Commentary: vascular closure device complications: the case is not closed yet. J Invasive Cardiol 2004; 16:251.
40. O'Sullivan GJ, Buckenham TM, Belli AM. The use of the Angio-Seal haemostatic puncture closure device in high risk patients. Clinical Radiology 1999; 54:51–5.

50 | Percutaneous Intervention for Acute Deep Venous Thrombosis of the Lower Extremities

Eric M. Walser and Andrew H. Stockland
Department of Radiology, Mayo Clinic, Jacksonville, Florida, U.S.A.

HISTORY AND BACKGROUND

Deep venous thrombosis (DVT) of the lower extremities and its most feared complication, pulmonary embolus (PE), are conditions that have affected mankind for centuries and are collectively known as venous thromboembolic disease (VTE) (1). After the pioneering study of Barritt and Jordan in 1960 (2), anticoagulation became the mainstay of treatment for VTE.

CLINICAL SIGNIFICANCE AND PREVALENCE

Factors predisposing to DVT are well known and include acquired factors (smoking, immobility, extended air travel, obesity), medications (oral contraceptives, hormone replacements), post-surgical conditions and congenital hypercoagulable states. Patients with DVT usually present with acute swelling, warmth and dull pain in the lower extremity occasionally with palpable tenderness over the course of deep veins in the thigh or behind the knee. Sometimes, there is increased resistance and pain on dorsiflexion of the foot (Homans' sign). This straightforward clinical picture can be muddied in debilitated patients with partially occlusive thrombosis or minimal clot burden and only mild lower extremity edema (Fig. 1). On the other extreme end of clinical presentation is phlegmasia cerulea dolens (PCD), which consists of severe swelling, decreased strength and violaceous discoloration of the affected leg due to near complete deep venous obstruction. This condition is an emergency and may lead to phlegmasia alba dolens, where there is loss of arterial pulses to the affected extremity and limb-threatening ischemia (3,4).

CURRENT TREATMENT FOR DVT

DVT is an extremely common medical condition occurring in one out of every thousand Americans annually (5), with a lifetime risk of 2.2% to 5% (6). From the patient's perspective, acute DVT is most significant for the swelling and pain that it provokes. To the physician, the risk of PE is the most troubling prospect, estimated to occur in 50% of patients with untreated proximal DVT (7,8). Fortunately, the time-tested application of anticoagulation, including intravenous heparin and oral warfarin has drastically improved the outcome of patients with acute DVT. The risk of PE drops to 2% with anticoagulation treatment (9–11). The pain and swelling is not affected by anticoagulation, but rather by the patient's natural fibrinolytic activity and venous collateral formation, which eventually diminishes these symptoms. Occluded veins are gradually recannalized with the duration and amount of clot resolution depending on patients' genetic fibrinolytic mechanisms, the presence of risk factors, and ongoing anticoagulation. One study showed that almost all occluded veins recannalize by three years, although 50% of patients have residual chronic thrombus (12). Standard therapy for DVT today is use of compression stockings with intravenous heparin therapy or subcutaneous low-molecular weight heparin therapy for a short period with conversion to oral warfarin therapy for

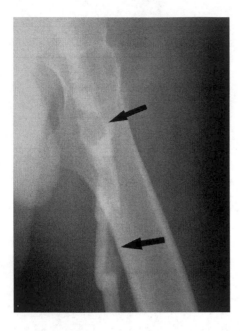

FIGURE 1   Early deep venous thrombosis (DVT) is non-occlusive and originates in the valve cusp regions (*arrows*). Pulmonary embolus occurred in this patient who had no symptoms of DVT.

three months or longer if significant risk factors remain. The addition of compression stockings to the treatment for DVT further decreases venous stasis and subcutaneous edema formation and studies show a 50% reduction in post-thrombotic syndrome (PTS) with their use (13).

However, in the long term a large proportion of patients develop chronic venous disease in the lower extremities, known as PTS. This disorder is caused by faulty venous valve function and residual venous obstruction despite anticoagulation therapy. Such patients develop varicosities, chronic leg swelling, pain, skin hyperpigmentation and fibrosis and they may eventually develop venous ulceration which is resistant to conventional therapy (Fig. 2).

Since a huge volume of patients treated for DVT with conventional therapy are released into the community with variable and inconsistent follow-up, it is probably an underestimate

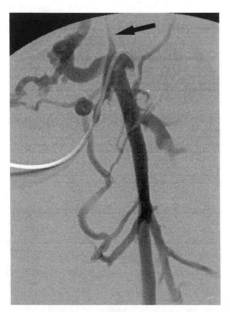

FIGURE 2   Venogram through a catheter placed into the saphenous vein shows findings of post-thrombotic syndrome with reflux of contrast past incompetent venous valves into the superficial femoral vein, large venous collateral formation, and scarred, atrophic external iliac vein from old deep venous thrombosis (*arrow*).

that 10% of patients with acute DVT treated conventionally develop PTS and 6% of patients with DVT may go on to develop venous ulceration (14,15). One study suggested that 50% of people may have symptoms of PTS two years after treatment for acute DVT (13). A recent report suggested that PTS leads to chronic disability in 4% of patients (16). Additionally, the quality of life, scored by questionnaires, is significantly lower in patients with PTS (17,18).

Early Days: Systemic Thrombolytic Therapy for DVT

With the appearance of streptokinase in the 1970s, systemic thrombolytic therapy was proposed as treatment for DVT. Early attempts to treat DVT involved systemic administration of streptokinase and, later, urokinase. Although cost and bleeding complications were significant, systemic therapy produced interesting preliminary data as to the effectiveness of clot dissolution versus anticoagulation alone. The partial to complete clot resolution rates were near 50% for patients receiving systemic lytic therapy compared to only 4% for anticoagulated patients (19). PTS symptoms were also less in the lytic group at 5% compared to 21% of the anticoagulated groups, although these data derive from a small study of 78 patients (20,21). A meta-analysis involving larger patient cohorts, however, derived a PTS rate of 65% in anticoagulated patients versus 48% for those treated with systemic thrombolysis (22). Additionally, some groups reported more disappointing results from systemic lytic therapy with one study showing only a 29% rate of significant clot reduction using systemic tissue plasminogen activator (tPA) with one patient suffering an intracranial hemorrhage (ICH) (23). Despite very careful patient selection, the major hemorrhage rate was 13.2% in the lytic group compared to only 3.5% in the anticoagulation group (24). Patients were excluded frequently in these early studies of systemic lytic therapy, with one study rejecting 93% of eligible candidates (25), primarily due to recent surgery. Due to early formation of pelvic venous collaterals, iliac vein thrombosis responded poorly to systemic lytic administration as the drug simply did not perfuse the thrombosed segment (26).

Catheter-Directed Thrombolytic Therapy

With the successes of catheter-directed arterial thrombolysis, it proved relatively easy to apply these techniques to the venous circulation. The rationale was straightforward—infuse thrombolytics directly within the thrombus to increase the volume of clot exposed to lytic action and reduce systemic levels of lytic drugs. Early efforts were confined to patients with limb-threatening venous thrombosis (PCD), but indications begin to relax when it became apparent that CDT opened the thrombosed segments better than conventional therapy, and that there was an earlier decrease in leg edema and pain (14,27,28).

Basic research in vein thrombosis revealed several critical factors for lytic therapy. Firstly, valvular incompetence is the earliest sign of impending PTS (29) and total thrombosis predisposes to valvular dysfunction (30–33). Secondly, earlier lysis leads to preserved valvular function and fewer symptoms (34). Lastly, plasminogen-bound fibrin diminishes within the thrombus of DVT and the success rate of lytic therapy drops considerably after about one week (14). The above factors strongly suggested that CDT, by quickly restoring flow and reducing clot burden, should reduce the incidence of PTS over conventional therapy. Moreover, in the correct patient and circumstances, CDT is necessary within a week of the acute thrombotic event or venous thrombolysis is unlikely to provide significant impact on the acute course of DVT or the more chronic complications. Unfortunately, these theoretical advantages of CDT in preventing PTS remain unproven due to the lack of firm evidence from properly randomized and controlled clinical studies.

A recent study from 2004 showed that 44% of CDT patients preserve valve function compared to only 13% of those receiving systemic lytics although the clinical outcome was the same at three years (35). There was also suggestive evidence from a recent series of 45 patients with ileofemoral DVT who had tPA CDT. Only 2 of 41 patients developed venous reflux with an average two-year follow-up (36). Another recent retrospective study involved a venous registry composed of 287 patients who received CDT for acute lower extremity DVT and were followed for one year. Greater than 50% lysis was achieved in 83% of patients and venous reflux developed in 58% overall but only in 28% of those patients who had complete lysis of their thrombosis (37,38). Since only 31% of patients in this study experienced complete lysis, it may prove that CDT reduces PTS only in this subset of patients with complete response to lytic therapy. To address this deficiency of good clinical data, a multidisciplinary panel of venous experts convened in 2004 and determined that a prospective randomized trial of CDT versus anticoagulation be undertaken with the specific intent to determine the relative incidence of PTS (39). This trial (acute venous thrombosis: thrombus removal with adjunctive catheter–directed thrombolysis) should begin recruiting patients in 2007.

Surgical Thrombectomy for DVT

Surgical techniques for acute DVT are limited currently and are generally confined to patients with iliofemoral DVT and phlegmasia. Due to the low flow rates in the venous system, surgical thrombectomy is generally coupled with an arteriovenous fistula to increase flow across the operated segment. A surgical series with both 5- and 10-year follow-up showed that patients with iliofemoral DVT had a patent iliac vein in 83% of cases compared to only 41% of patients who received anticoagulation therapy only. Venous function and PTS symptoms were worse in the conventionally treated group (40,41).

CDT TECHNIQUE

The current preferred method to treat symptomatic proximal DVT is CDT, which rapidly replaced systemic lytic administration due to improved recannalization rates and increased efficacy in iliac venous thrombosis. Patient selection is crucial since current data are scant for the long-term clinical benefits of lysis over anticoagulation and the increased cost and bleeding complications inherent in lytic therapy warrant a conservative approach. Elderly patients or those with poor life expectancy are poor candidates for CDT (Fig. 3). Young patients with symptomatic proximal DVT or any patient with PCD should be considered for CDT. In fact, since younger patients (less than 40 years) with DVT are more likely to develop PTS later, this

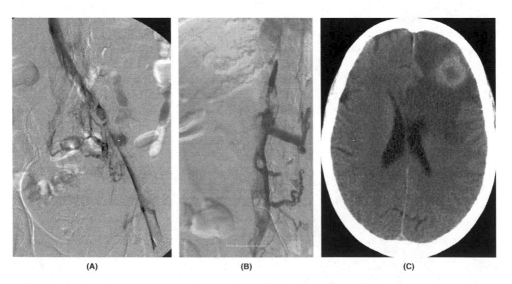

(A)   (B)   (C)

FIGURE 3   (**A,B**) Elderly patient with extensive ileocaval deep venous thrombosis and lung cancer. She did not have phlegmasia cerulea dolens clinically, but had severe edema in the lower extremity. Catheters were inserted into the acute thrombus via a popliteal approach. Due to her cancer history, a non-enhanced head computed tomography (CT) was done prior to lytic administration. (**C**) The CT revealed a left frontal metastatic lesion and no catheter-directed thrombolytic therapy (CDT) was performed. Patients with cancer, advanced age or chronic conditions should be very carefully selected for CDT due to their increased risk of complications and lack of firm data about the long-term benefits of CDT.

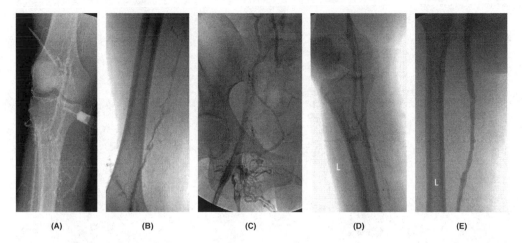

(A) (B) (C) (D) (E)

FIGURE 4 **(A–C)** Extensive ileofemoral and tibiopopliteal deep venous thrombosis approached via popliteal vein access. **(D)** "Criss-crossed" popliteal catheters advanced inferiorly into the popliteal and tibial veins and **(E)** superiorly into the ileofemoral segments allowed infusion of tPA into long segments of acute thrombus. Notice the good response to lytic therapy on the 48 hours follow-up venography.

group is a perfect target for CDT (42). This topic continues to be controversial and The American College of Chest Physicians is one of several groups that recommend CDT be confined to patients with PCD and an ischemic, threatened extremity (43,44).

Percutaneous approaches for DVT include the contralateral femoral vein, ipsilateral popliteal vein, or internal jugular vein. A popliteal vein approach is preferred by our group as it provides the most direct access to clot while the other routes involve the use of long catheters with an increased risk of dislodgement or buckling. Regional lytic administration is delivered directly into the thrombus and can be supplemented with infusion via a foot vein (flow-directed thrombolytic administration), particularly if significant tibial thrombosis is present. Lytic agents can be infused into the infrapopliteal veins via a foot vein with one or two tourniquets applied at the ankle and knee to "drive" the drug infusion into the deep venous circulation. Alternatively, two catheters entering the popliteal vein in a "criss-cross" fashion can allow infusion above and below the knee (Fig. 4). While the ideal situation is to clear all thrombus from the deep venous system and provide straight line flow from the foot to the inferior vena cava (IVC), infrapopliteal venous lysis is sometimes difficult and there is some debate as to its importance.

CDT should be planned keeping in mind the superficial and deep venous network of the lower extremity and their communications. Opening the femoral vein and leaving occluded infrapopliteal veins may be ineffective if there is extensive and preferential venous drainage via the superficial venous system since deep venous inflow is not provided to the reopened segment, and it remains at risk for re-thrombosis. Furthermore, thrombolytic therapy in the venous system frequently suffers from stagnant flow so that a typical concentration of tPA (0.01 mg/mL or 10 mg tPA in 1 L normal saline) can be delivered at 0.5 to 1.0 mg and augmented with a piggybacked normal saline infusion of 20 to 100 cc/hr to flush the lytic through thrombosed areas with slow flow. Infusion volumes can be reduced as venous patency is restored. If tourniquets are used to divert superficial venous flow of lytic into the deep system, they should be loosened for 10 to 15 minutes every hour. Due to the long segments of clot formation in DVT, coaxial lytic administration through multiside-hole catheters and infusible guidewires enables 20 to 60 cm of clot "coverage" by lytic drugs (Fig. 5). For tPA, 0.5 to 1.0 mg tPA/hr is the suggested dose that can be split between coaxial infusions and flow-directed therapy via a foot vein. Dosing and piggybacked saline infusion rates can be customized so that higher concentrations and flow are delivered to areas of stasis and high clot burden. While full systemic anticoagulation with heparin was the norm during the administration of urokinase, the use of recombinant tPA is now more common and systemic

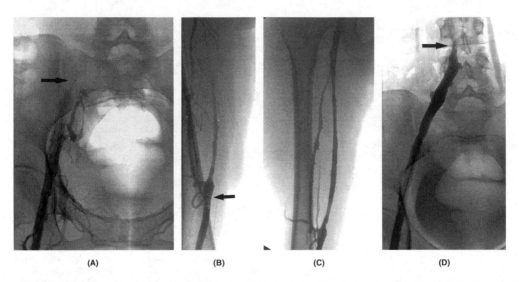

FIGURE 5   Ileofemoral deep venous thrombosis (DVT) treated with catheter-directed thrombolytic therapy (CDT). (**A**) An infusible guidewire (Prostream®, Microtherapeutics, Inc., Irvine, California, U.S.A.) with 12 cm sidehole coverage was positioned in the iliac clot (*arrow*) in distal sidehole. (**B**) A 5 Fr catheter with 20 cm of sideholes (Cragg-McNamara®, Microtherapeutics, Inc., Irvine, California, U.S.A.) was positioned in the femoral segment in a proximal sidehole (*arrow*) enabling over 30 cm of clot infusion capacity. (**C,D**) After 48 hours tissue plasminogen activator (tPA) CDT, there was complete clot lysis and visualization of the left common iliac venous stenosis associated with May–Thurner syndrome (*arrow*).

heparinization tends to be less aggressive. Our group tends to infuse heparin at a low rate of 300 units/hr. Recent studies suggest an increased risk of ICH with the use of tPA and one study showed that ICH was tPA dose-independent (45,46). Therefore, minimal anticoagulation in the setting of tPA use for venous lysis is warranted. Some suggested algorithms for CDT are outlined in Figure 6. As long as venous lysis is progressing without patient complications or severe drop in fibrinogen levels, the lytic drug can be continued. However, most interventionalists are hesitant to continue venous lysis beyond three days.

As venous lysis tends to progress slower than arterial cases, daily follow-up angiography is not crucial and we will often wait 48 hours before checking a venogram if we are treating extensive DVT and no complications arise. The follow-up venogram will show where remaining thrombus is clustered and degree of flow restoration, which serves as a guide to catheter repositioning and lytic dose distribution. The degree of lysis will depend on the age and extent of the thrombus. When there is no further progression of clot dissolution and venous flow has been restored, attention is directed to balloon dilation or stenting of persistent venous stenoses to complete the course of CDT (Fig. 7).

OUTCOME AND COMPLICATIONS OF CDT

Multiple small series evaluating the use of CDT and comparison with conventional anti-coagulation therapy are promising. However, these are all retrospective studies. A single randomized control trial was performed showing partial to complete resolution of clot in groups receiving CDT with streptokinase, versus none of the anticoagulated patients (47). This study was hampered by inclusion of a small number (34) of patients due to stringent exclusion criteria. Several subsequent larger studies seem to validate the claim of improved clot clearance with CDT claiming partial to complete thrombus dissolution in 92% to 97% of cases (27,48)—results much better than with anticoagulation or even systemic lytic therapy. The Achilles heel of CDT remains the increased bleeding complications due to lytic administration with major bleeding complications estimated at 11% in the venous registry report (37) versus only 2% for conventional anticoagulation. Additionally, many patients with DVT have comorbidities such as metastatic carcinoma or chronic debilitation (Fig. 3). The expected decrease in bleeding

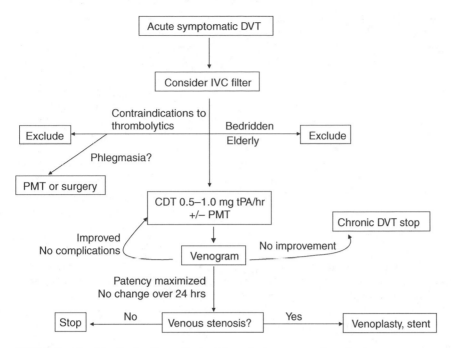

FIGURE 6   Algorithm for treating patients with acute deep venous thrombosis.

complications from local, rather than systemic, delivery of lytic drugs has not been realized and this may be partially due to less strict exclusion criteria in many CDT studies. The 5% major bleed occurrence in Grunwald's 2004 CDT study suggests that the goal of reducing hemorrhage with CDT is achievable (48).

Other disadvantages of CDT include the necessity for intensive care unit (ICU) monitoring during lytic administration, prolonged hospitalization compared to conventional therapy, and cost. The expense of a five-day course of intravenous heparin is about $47 and about $500 for five days of low-molecular weight heparin compared to the cost of a typical 72 hours CDT case using 1 mg/hr tPA of $2000. Follow-up venography, ICU expenses, laboratory and procedural costs add a more substantial investment of about $60,000 (49). In comparison, the cost of graded compression stockings is insignificant and is proven to

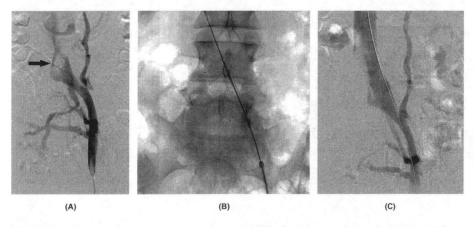

FIGURE 7   **(A,B)** Left iliac venogram in prone patient after ileofemoral catheter-directed thrombolytic therapy shows typical left common iliac vein stenosis due to compression from the right common iliac artery (*arrow*). **(C)** Metal stent placement restored venous flow and abolished the venous gradient.

reduce the incidence of PTS by 50% when added to anticoagulation therapy for DVT (13). Clearly, CDT should not be universally applied to patients with acute DVT. In fact, one study looking at 209 patients with acute DVT judged that only 7% were appropriate candidates (25). These issues again point to the need for controlled studies evaluating CDT and its application to the wide variety of patients presenting with acute DVT.

As time goes on, it is apparent that patients with DVT traditionally treated with conservative therapy have a fairly high incidence of iliac lesions. Most studies with CDT have found the need to perform iliac venoplasty or stent placement in 33% to 60% of cases (36,37,50,51). Therefore, the incidence of significant iliofemoral venous stenoses is probably higher than was once imagined when the cause of DVT was not specifically investigated. May–Thurner's syndrome is increasingly recognized and treated with the advent of CDT (Fig. 7) (52,53). Post-stent iliac venous patency is acceptable with series reporting 54% to 80% primary patency over one year with better patency rates in those patients who had complete lysis initially (37,54,55).

PHARMACOMECHANICAL THROMBOLYTIC THERAPY

In an effort to reduce the ICU time, lytic dose, and bleeding complications, newer devices were developed to clear clot mechanically, without the use of thrombolytics. In practice, these devices are used in conjunction with lytic therapy, and this technique is known as pharmacomechanical thrombolysis (PMT). One type of mechanical clot removal device is a rheolytic catheter which utilize the suction effect of high speed retrograde saline jets within a lumen. These devices include the Angiojet® (Possis Medical, Inc., Minneapolis, Minnesota, U.S.A.), the Oasis® (Boston Scientific, Natick, Massachusetts, U.S.A.), and the Hydrolyzer® thrombectomy catheter (Cordis, J&J Medical Systems, Florida, U.S.A.) (Fig. 8). Non-rheolytic fragmentation devices use rotating baskets or propellers to mechanically break up thrombus and include the Amplatz® thrombectomy device (Microvena, White Bear Lake, Minnesota, U.S.A.) and the Arrow-Trerotola® Over-the-Wire Percutaneous Thrombolytic device (Arrow International, Reading, Pennsylvania, U.S.A.) (Fig. 9). Low-technology and low-cost thromboaspiration through catheters or sheaths have also been used as an adjunct with lytic administration (56). All of these devices perform the function of rapid restoration of a lumen through an occluded venous segment, increasing the surface area of the clot available for lytic therapy, and reducing the time and lytic dose needed to clear DVT.

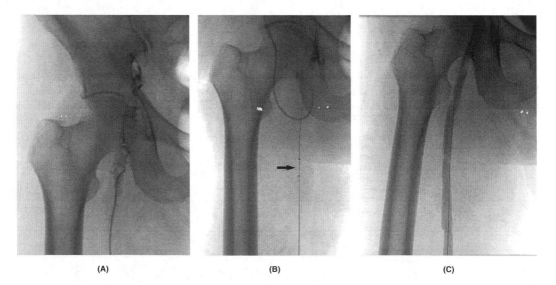

(A) (B) (C)

FIGURE 8 (A) Acute ileofemoral deep venous thrombosis, (B) initially treated via a popliteal venous approach using an Angiojet® catheter (*arrow*). (C) This procedure was followed by catheter-directed thrombolytic therapy with eventual near-complete clot clearance.

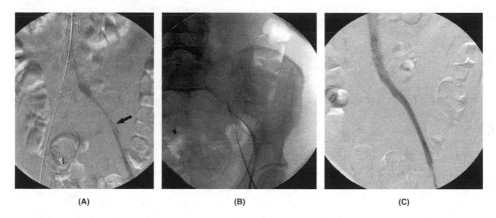

(A)   (B)   (C)

FIGURE 9 (**A**) Residual thrombus (*arrow*) in the right common iliac vein (patient prone) post-iliac stent placement bilaterally for venous stenoses extending into the inferior vena cava. (**B**) An Arrow-Trerotola® device was used to remove this thrombus (**C**) with restoration of venous flow afterwards.

Recent investigations into the combined use of PMT and CDT show a significant reduction in lytic dose (from 6 million to about 2.7 million of urokinase) and decreased duration of infusion from about 40 to 20 hours (57,58). Procedural success (restoration of patency with less than 30% residual venous stenosis) was obtained in 82% of patients in one retrospective series of PMT using a variety of lytic drugs and mechanical devices. In this study, mechanical thrombectomy alone provided only 26% thrombus removal compared to 62% when it was used after a course of CDT (58). Thrombolysis and mechanical clot removal can also be performed concurrently with thrombolytic drug infused forcefully and directly into thrombus using the Angiojet device ("power pulse-spray technique").

One could also argue for mechanical clot therapy first to establish a flow channel, with the thought being that thrombolytic drugs work better flowing through partial, rather than sitting in complete occlusions. Thus, currently, mechanical devices are more used as an adjunctive technique with lytic therapy rather than stand-alone devices. This situation may change as devices improve. Despite these obvious advantages, major hemorrhage occurred in 14% in Vedantham's study (58), although no major hemorrhage was reported in another series of 20 patients treated with Angiojet/tPA PMT. This study also reported an impressive 90% partial to complete clot clearance rate and immediate (<24 hours) clinical improvement in 74% of patients (50). As this technique matures, the acute and long-term patency rates will likely approach that of CDT. If hemorrhage rates and lytic dose and duration diminish as expected, the risk/benefit ratio and cost of PMT should propel this technique ahead of CDT.

Concerns over mechanical devices focus on possible endothelial vein damage and iatrogenic pulmonary embolism. No significant venous valve injury was discovered with the use of the ATD in a canine model if the vein lumen was greater than 6 mm in diameter (59). Similarly, the Arrow-Trerotola device did not damage veins or induce valvular incompetence in veins over 7 mm in diameter (60). Initial studies of CDT were suggestive of an increased risk of PE (one study suggested 4.5% incidence versus 2% of patients receiving standard anticoagulation therapy) (26). However, the venous registry in 1999 noted an incidence of PE during CDT of only 1% which is similar to that of routine anticoagulation (37).

Initially, some operators placed IVC filters prior to CDT. However, trapped thrombus was seen rarely, and many centers discontinued routine filter placement during CDT (51). However, when mechanical thrombectomy devices became available, the situation changed slightly and the risk of PE became more concerning (Fig. 10). Trerotola noted pulmonary emboli and increases in pulmonary artery pressures in all 14 dogs subjected to mechanical thrombectomy of IVC thrombosis with the Arrow-Trerotola device (61). Early human use of the ATD for caval thrombosis resulted in a large PE in one case report (62) and another series using mechanical thrombectomy noted episodes of oxygen desaturation and embolic material trapped in temporary IVC filters (63).

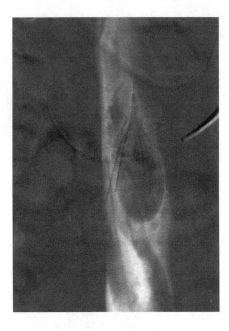

FIGURE 10   Trapped thrombus in a retrievable inferior vena cava filter after pharmacomechanical thrombolytic therapy for iliac deep venous thrombosis.

A comparison of available mechanical thrombectomy devices showed similar abilities to fragment thrombus, although the ATD showed the highest peripheral embolization of particles over 1 mm (64) The rheolytic devices, which are more adept at clot removal, are probably less prone to significant embolization. In fact, a series from 2002 had 14 patients treated with an Angiojet device with good lysis in over half the patients and no clinical pulmonary emboli (65). Given the availability of retrievable IVC filters, a reasonable approach would be to use them in PMT cases, especially when using the ATD or any mechanical device in the absence of thrombolytic administration. Additionally, some investigators recommend, when using mechanical thrombectomy devices, removing the more distal clot first and then clearing the proximal segment in the IVC last, so that optimum clot maceration can be performed before flow is restored into the right atrium (63).

FUTURE DIRECTIONS

New mechanical devices are continually tested for use in arterial or venous occlusions. One innovative type of mechanical device for DVT is ultrasound-accelerated CDT, in which an ultrasound catheter (EKOS Lysus® Peripheral System, EKOS Corporation, Bothell, Washington) transmits sound waves into thrombus creating cavitation and increasing the surface area available for the action of lytic drugs (66). Data from a recent 13-center, open enrollment registry over a nine-month period indicated approximately 70% complete clot dissolution in an average treatment time of 23.3 hours and a major bleeding rate of 5.5%. A possible advantage of this technique lies in the ability of ultrasonic catheters to insonate clot located behind venous valves—an area where PMT and CDT are less effective due to poor flow and the relative inaccessibility of clot hidden behind valve cusps (Fig. 11) (67). Advances in thrombolytic agents may also improve success and diminish bleeding risks associated with CDT or PMT. In particular, some newer agents, such as alfimeprase, may allow true local clot dissolution without significant systemic lytic effects (68).

CONCLUSIONS

Current status of CDT and PMT for DVT is that it is an acceptable method to treat patients with either limb-threatening venous occlusions (phlegmasia), and probably as an effective frontline therapy for younger patients with symptomatic DVT with the goal of preventing or at least

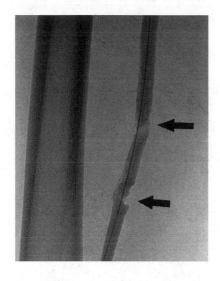

FIGURE 11 After pharmacomechanical thrombolytic therapy, some residual thrombus remains around venous valve cusps (*arrows*). Ultrasonic thrombolysis may improve clot removal from these difficult areas.

reducing the incidence of PTS in these patients with relatively long life expectancies. This is an extremely important, yet unproven, outcome in such patients since the available treatments for PTS are rather limited. The combination of chronic venous occlusion and venous valve disease is difficult to treat surgically or percutaneously due to the diffuse nature of the venous abnormality. Surgical placement of transposed arm veins and placement of artificial or porcine venous valves remains unproven and restricted to specialized centers. As such, preventing the chronic debilitating course of PTS in a younger patient is important.

REFERENCES

1. Mannucci PM. Venous thrombosis: the history of knowledge. Pathophysiol Haemost Thromb 2002; 32(5–6):209–12.
2. Barritt DW, Jordan SC. Anticoagulant drugs in the treatment of pulmonary embolism: a controlled trial. Lancet 1960; 1·1309–12.
3. Rakel RE, Bope ET. Conn's Current Therapy. 55th ed. Philadelphia, PA: WB Saunders, 2003.
4. Marx J, Hockerberger R, Walls R. Rosen's Emergency Medicine: Concepts and Clinical Practice. 5th ed. St. Louis, MO: Mosby, 2002.
5. Heit JA, Silverstein MD, Mohr DN, et al. The epidemiology of venous thromboembolism in the community. Thromb Haemost 2001;86–452-63.
6. Browse NL, Burnand KG, Lea TM. Diseases of the Veins. 2nd ed. London: Edward Arnold, 1999.
7. Buller HR, Agnelli G, Hull RD, et al. Approach to the diagnosis and therapy of suspected deep vein thrombosis. Chest 2004; 126(Suppl. 3):401S–28.
8. Hirsh J, Lee AY. How we diagnose and treat deep vein thrombosis. Blood 2002; 99(9):3102–10.
9. Hyers TM, Agnelli G, Hull RD, et al. Antithrombotic therapy for venous thromboembolic disease. Chest 2001; 119:S176–93.
10. Green D, Hirsh J, Heit J, et al. Low molecular weight heparin: a critical analysis of clinical trials. Pharmacol Rev 1994; 46:89–109.
11. Krishnan JA, Segal JB, Streiff MB, et al. Treatment of venous thromboembolism with low-molecular weight heparin: a synthesis of the evidence published in systematic literature reviews. Respir Med 2004; 98:376–86.
12. Markel A, Meissner M, Manzo RA, et al. Deep venous thrombosis: rate of spontaneous lysis and thrombus extension. Int Angiol 2003; 22:376–82.
13. Brandjes DP, Buller HR, Heijboer H, et al. Randomised trial of effect of compression stockings in patients with symptomatic proximal-vein thrombosis. Lancet 1997; 349(9054):759–62.
14. Janssen MCH, Wollersheim H, Schultze-Kool LJ, et al. Local and systemic thrombolytic therapy for acute deep venous thrombosis. J Med 2005; 63(3):81–90 (Van Zuiden Communications)..
15. Johnson BF, Manzo RA, Bergelin RO, et al. Relationship between changes in the deep venous system and the development of the postthrombotic syndrome after an acute episode of lower limb deep vein thrombosis: a one-to-six year follow- up. J Vasc Surg 1995; 21(2):307–13.
16. Eichlisberger R, Widmer MT, Frauchiger B, et al. The incidence of post-thrombotic syndrome. Wien Med Wochenschr 1994; 144(10-11):192–5.

17. Beyth RJ, Cohen AM, Landefeld CS. Long-term outcomes of deep-vein thrombosis. Arch Intern Med 1995; 155:1031–7.
18. Launois R, Reboul-Marty J, Henry B. Construction and validation of a quality of life questionnaire in chronic lower limb venous insufficiency (CIVIQ). Qual Life Res 1996; 5:539–54.
19. Comerota AJ, Aldridge SC. Thrombolytic therapy for deep venous thrombosis: a clinical review. Can J Surg 1993; 36:359–64.
20. Elliot MS, Immelman EJ, Jeffery P. A comparative randomized trial of heparin versus streptokinase in the treatment of acute proximal venous thrombosis: an interim report of a prospective trial. Br J Surg 1979; 66:838–43.
21. Arnesen H, Hoiseth A, Ly B. Streptokinase of heparin in the treatment of deep vein thrombosis. Follow-up results of a prospective study. Acta Med Scand 1982; 211:65–8.
22. Watson LI, Armon MP. Thrombolysis for acute deep vein thrombosis. Ovid/Watson/The Cochrane Library, Vol. 4, 2005.
23. Goldhaber SZ, Meyerovitz MF, Green D, et al. Randomized controlled trial of tissue plasminogen activator in proximal deep venous thrombosis. Am J Med 1990; 88:235–40.
24. Hirsh J, Lensing AW. Thrombolytic therapy for deep vein thrombosis. Int Angiol 1996; 5:S22–5.
25. Markel A, Manzo RA, Strandness DE, Jr. The potential role of thrombolytic therapy in venous thrombosis. Arch Intern Med 1992; (152):1265–7.
26. Schweizer J, Kirch W, Koch R, et al. Short- and long-term results after thrombolytic treatment of deep venous thrombosis. J Am Coll Cardiol 2000; 36:1336–43.
27. Semba CP, Dake MD. Iliofemoral deep venous thrombosis: aggressive therapy with catheter-directed thrombolysis. Radiology 1994; 191:487–94.
28. Verhaeghe R, Stockx L, Lacroix H, et al. Catheter-directed lysis of iliofemoral vein thrombosis with use of rt-PA. Eur Radiol 1997; 7:996–1001.
29. Haenen JH, Jannsen MC, Wollersheim H, et al. The development of postthrombotic syndrome in relationship to development of postthrombotic syndrome in relationship to venous reflux and calf muscle pump dysfunction at 2 years after the onset of deep venous thrombosis. J Vasc Surg 2002; 35:1184–9.
30. Haenen JH, Janssen MC, van Langen H, et al. Duplex ultrasound in the hemodynamic evaluation of the late sequelae of deep venous thrombosis. J Vas Surg 1998; 27:472–8.
31. Markel A, Manzo RA, Bergelin RO, et al. Incidence and time occurrence of valvular incompetence following deep vein thrombosis. Wien Med Wochenschr 1994; 144:216–20.
32. Van Haarst EP, Liasis N, van Ramshorst B, et al. The development of valvular incompetence after deep vein thrombosis: a 7 year follow-up study with duplex scanning. Eur J Vasc Endovasc Surg 1996; 12:295–9.
33. Van Ramshorst B, van Bemmelen PS, Hoeneveld H, et al. The development of valvular incompetence after deep vein thrombosis: a follow-up study with duplex scanning. J Vasc Surg 1994; 19:1059–66.
34. O'Shaughnessy AM, Fitzgerald DE. Natural history of proximal deep vein thrombosis assessed by duplex ultrasound. Int Angiol 1997; 16:45–9.
35. Laiho MK, Oinonen A, Sugano N, et al. Preservation of venous valve function after catheter-directed and systemic thrombolysis for deep venous trombosis. Eur J Vasc Endovasc Surg 2004; 28:391–6.
36. Sillesen H, Just S, Jorgensen M, et al. Catheter directed thrombolysis for treatment of ilio-femoral deep venous thrombosis is durable, preserves venous valve function and may prevent chronic venous insufficiency. Eur J Vasc Endovasc Surg 2005; 30(5):556–62.
37. Mewissen MW, Seabrook GR, Meissner MH, et al. Catheter-directed thrombolysis for lower extremity deep venous thrombosis: report of a national multicenter registry. Radiology 1999; 211:39–49.
38. Meissner MH. Thrombolytic therapy for acute deep vein thrombosis and the venous registry. Rev Cardiovasc Med 2002; 3(Suppl. 2):S53–60.
39. Vedantham S, Rundback JH, Comerota AJ, et al. Development of a research agenda for endovascular treatment of venous thromboembolism: proceedings from a multidisciplinary consensus panel. J Vasc Interv Radiol 2005; 16:1567–73.
40. Plate G, Akesson H, Einarsson E, et al. Long-term results of venous thrombectomy combined with a temporary arterio-venous fistula. Eur J Vasc Surg 1990; 4:483–9.
41. Plate G, Eklof B, Norgren L, et al. Venous thrombectomy for iliofemoral vein thrombosis—10 year results of prospective randomized study. Eur J Vasc Endovasc Surg 1997; 14:367–74.
42. Mohr DN, Silverstein MD, Heit JA, et al. The venous stasis syndrome after deep venous thrombosis or pulmonary embolism: a population-based study. Mayo Clin Proc 2000; 75:1249–56.
43. Buller HR, Hull RD, Hyers TM, et al. Antithrombotic therapy for venous thromboembolic disease. The seventh ACCP conference on antithrombotic and thrombolytic therapy. Chest 2004; 126(Suppl.):S401–28.
44. Bates SM, Ginsberg JS. Treatment of deep-vein thrombosis. N Engl J Med 2004; 351:268–77.
45. Ouriel K, Gray B, Clair DG, et al. Complications associated with the use of urokinase and recombinant tissue plasminogen activator for catheter-directed peripheral arterial and venous thrombolysis. J Vasc Interv Radiol 2000; 11:295–8.

46. Thomas SM, Gaines P. Vascular surgery society of Great Britain and Ireland: avoiding the complications of thrombolysis. Br J Surg 1999; 86:710.
47. Elsharawy M, Elzayat E. Early results of thrombolysis vs anticoagulation in iliofemoral venous thrombosis. A randomized clinical trial. Eur J Vasc Endovasc Surg 2002; 24(3):209–14.
48. Grunwald MR, Hofmann LV. Comparison of urokinase, alteplase, and reteplase for catheter-directed thrombolysis of deep venous thrombosis. J Vasc Interv Radiol 2004; 15:347–52.
49. Navarro F, Dean S. Young patients with iliofemoral deep venous thrombosis should receive thrombolytic therapy. Med Clin N Am 2003; 87:1165–77.
50. Bush RL, Lin PH, Bates JT, et al. Pharmacomechanica thrombectomy for treatment of symptomatic lower extremity deep venous thrombosis: safety and feasibility study. J Vasc Surg 2004; 40(5):965–70.
51. Dake MD, Semba CP. Thrombolytic therapy in venous occlusive disease. J Vasc Interv Radiol 1995; 6:S73–7.
52. Rilinger N, Gorich J, Mickley V, et al. Endovascular stenting in patients with iliac compression syndrome. Experience in three cases. Invest Radiol 1996; 31(11):729–33.
53. Kwak HS, Han YM, Lee YS, et al. Stents in common iliac vein obstruction with acute ipsilateral deep venous thrombosis: early and late results. J Vasc Interv Radiol 2005; 16(8):1120.
54. Jackson LS, Wang XJ, Dudrick SJ, et al. Catheter-directed thrombolysis and/or thrombectomy with selective endovascular stenting as alternatives to systemic anticoagulation for treatment of acute deep vein thrombosis. Am J Surg 2005; 190(6):864–8.
55. Bjarnason H, Kruse JR, Asinger DA, et al. Iliofemoral deep venous thrombosis: safety and efficacy outcome during 5 years of catheter–directed thrombolytic therapy. J Vasc Interv Radiol 1997; 8:405–18.
56. Roy S, Laerum F. Transcatheter aspiration: the key to successful percutaneous treatment of deep venous thrombosis? Acad Radiol 1999; 6(12):730–5.
57. Johnson SP, Cutts S, Durham JD, et al. Initial experience with percutaneous mechanical thrombectomy using the Amplatz thrombectomy device for the treatment of deep venous thrombosis. J Vasc Interv Radiol 2000; 11:196–7.
58. Vedantham S, Vesely TM, Parti N, et al. Lower extremity venous thrombolysis with adjunctive mechanical thrombectomy. J Vasc Interv Radiol 2002; 13:1001–8.
59. Sharafuddin MJ, Gu X, Han YM, et al. Injury potential to venous valves from the Amplatz thrombectomy device. J Vasc Interv Radiol 1999; 10(1):64–9.
60. McLennan G, Trerotola SO, Davidson D, et al. The effects of a mechanical thrombolytic device on normal canine vein valves. J Vasc Interv Radiol 2001; 12:89–94.
61. Trerotola SO, McLennan G, Davidson D, et al. Preclinical in vivo testing of the arrow Trerotola percutaneous thrombolytic device for venous trombosis. J Vasc Interv Radiol 2001; 12(1):95–103.
62. Uflacker R. Mechanical thrombectomy in acute and subacute thrombosis with use of the Amplatz device: arterial and venous applications. J Vasc Interv Radiol 1997; 8:923–32.
63. Delomez M, Beregi J, Willotezux S, et al. Mechanical thrombectomy in patients with deep venous thrombosis. Cardiovasc Intervent Radiol 2001; 24:42–8.
64. Muller Hulsbeck S, Grimm J, Leidt J, et al. Comparison of in vitro effectiveness of mechanical thrombectomy devices. J Vasc Interv Radiol 2001; 12:1185–91.
65. Kasirajan K, Gray B, Ouriel K. Percutaneous Angiojet thrombectomy in the management of extensive deep venous thrombosis. J Vasc Interv Radiol 2001; 12:179–85.
66. Blinc A, Francis CW, Trudnowski JL, et al. Characterization of ultrasound-potentiated fibrinolysis in vitro. Blood J 1993; 81(10):2636–43.
67. Accessed March 1, 2006 at http://www.ekoscorp.com/pdEK_prod.html.
68. Ouriel K, Cynamon J, Weaver FA, et al. A phase I trial of alfimeprase for peripheral arterial thrombolysis. J Vasc Interv Radiol 2005; 16:1075–83.

51 | Chronic Benign Lower Limb Venous Insufficiency and Occlusion (Indications, Technical Aspects, Troubleshooting, and Current Results)

Matthew Matson
Department of Radiology, Royal London Hospital, Barts and the London NHS Trust, Whitechapel, London, U.K.

INTRODUCTION

Chronic venous disease of the lower limbs is defined as an abnormally functioning venous system, which may be congenital or acquired, for example after previous deep venous thrombosis (DVT). It is a common condition, with an estimated prevalence in the general population of 10% to 15% (1). The hallmark is venous hypertension and the mainstay of therapy is aimed at relieving this. Traditionally, the pathophysiology was thought to be mainly related to superficial and deep reflux secondary to incompetent venous valves.

More recently, venous outflow obstruction has also been shown to be a significant contributory factor in lower limb chronic venous disease (2,3). It is the predominant factor in up to one-third of post-thrombotic limbs and may coexist with venous reflux in over a half of symptomatic limbs. Indeed the combination of outflow obstruction and reflux has been shown to produce worse symptoms and higher ambulatory venous pressures than either patho-physiological mechanism alone. For this reason, there has been interest in treating the obstructive component in symptomatic patients. While open surgical bypass may yield reasonable results in carefully selected patients (4), it has not been uniformly successful, and highly specialized techniques such as venous valve reconstruction and venous bypass techniques have tended to be limited to a few specialized centers. An endovascular approach offers an attractive alternative treatment strategy.

CLINICAL PRESENTATION OF LOWER LIMB CHRONIC VENOUS DISEASE

Patients typically present with symptoms of pain, swelling or skin changes in the lower limb. Venous claudication may mimic arterial intermittent claudication, though it typically takes longer to subside after stopping exercise, can be bursting in nature and may be associated with limb swelling on exercise. Clinical examination may reveal telangiectases, venous flares or evidence of varicose veins; limb edema indicates more severe disease. Skin changes include discoloration, venous eczema, lipodermatosclerosis or, in advanced cases, venous ulceration.

Chronic venous disease of the lower limb may be classified using the Clinical–Etiology–Anatomic–Pathophysiologic system (Table 1) (5). Clinical signs (C), are graded on a scale from zero, with no visible sign of disease, to six, reflecting active skin ulceration. Etiology (E) may be congenital; primary, not congenital but due to an unknown cause; or secondary, due to previous venous thrombosis or trauma for example. Anatomic sites (A) are deep, superficial or perforating veins, although a combination of affected sites may be present. Underlying pathophysiology (P) may be reflux, venous outflow obstruction or both, as described above.

TABLE 1   Classification of Chronic Lower Extremity Venous Disease

C	Clinical signs supplemented by (a) for asymptomatic and (s) for symptomatic presentation
E	Etiologic classification (congenital, primary or secondary)
A	Anatomical distribution (superficial, deep or perforator, alone or in combination)
P	Pathophysiological dysfunction (reflux or obstruction, alone or in combination)

INVESTIGATION OF LOWER LIMB CHRONIC VENOUS DISEASE

Historically, a number of investigations have been introduced to investigate lower limb venous function, including plethysmography, infra-red photography, thermography, foot volumetry and nuclear medicine techniques such as isotope plethysmography, fibrinogen uptake test and radioactive plasmid uptake test.

Venography, or phlebography, has remained the gold standard for demonstration of deep venous anatomy since its first description by Dos Santos in 1938 (6). The standard technique involves injection of contrast into a pedal vein while the patient is semierect on a tilting table, with a tourniquet at the ankle to encourage preferential filling of the deep venous system and another at the lower thigh to delay emptying of the calf veins. For more detailed views of the iliac veins, direct femoral vein puncture can be used for venogaphy. Demonstration of collateral vessels adds weight to the functional significance of any stenoses seen. However, it is recognized that short, web-like stenoses and *en face* lesions may be missed on venography.

Ascending venography also allows the opportunity for measuring femoral venous pressures. In a normal individual, vigorous calf exercise with repeated plantar flexion will produce a symmetrical rise of 2 to 4 mmHg in the femoral veins. A pressure rise of more than 10 mmHg indicates significant outflow obstruction (7).

Descending phlebography is a variation of the technique to demonstrate venous reflux. Contrast is injected into the femoral vein while the patient performs a Valsalve manoeuvre. Reflux is demonstrated by flow of contrast towards the periphery and can be numerically graded for severity. In practice, it has been generally superseded by duplex ultrasound.

In recent years duplex ultrasonography has emerged as the primary investigation of chronic venous disease. Duplex can reliably detect deep venous reflux in the femoral and popliteal veins, as evidenced by reversal of flow in the vein on vasalva manoeuvre or release of manual compression. The sapheno-femoral and sapheno-popliteal junctions may be evaluated for incompetence and other significant sites of perforation and reflux identified. Duplex is less sensitive in reliably detecting post phlebitic change and will also easily miss iliac vein and inferior vena cava (IVC) stenoses and occlusions. Ascending venography is more sensitive than duplex in the evaluation of iliac segment stenoses. Intravascular ultrasound (IVUS) has been found to be useful by some authors during endovascular stenting of veins in identifying stenoses not appreciable on venography (8). It can be used intraprocedurally to detect stenoses that otherwise may not be appreciable on other imaging modalities and may also be used to evaluate the efficacy of stenting. The routine use of IVUS may be limited by cost considerations.

Magnetic resonance imaging is also gaining acceptance as technique for investigation of iliac venous disease (9). Three-dimensional contrast-enhanced gradient echo sequences such as venous enhanced peak arterial (VESPA) sequences can be used to evaluate both the arterial and venous vessels by obtaining a number of acquisitions and use of post-processing subtraction techniques (10). Magnetic resonance direct thrombus imaging can be used to detect or exclude the presence of clot in the veins.

The CT appearance of acute and chronic venous thrombosis in the iliofemoral veins was reported as far back as the late 1980s (11,12). Direct computed tomography (CT) venography was subsequently described and shown to have a sensitivity and specificity comparable to ascending venography (13), but still required cannulation of a pedal vein. With faster scanners came the development of indirect CT venography, performed as an adjunctive examination to CT pulmonary angiography using delayed scans following a single injection, as first described by Loud in 1988 (14). As well as being able to demonstrate thrombus or occlusion of the iliofemoral veins, CT venography can demonstrate any compression of pelvic veins from, for example, a pelvic mass. It is also able to detect iliocaval compression syndrome of venous compression from the adjacent iliac artery (*vide infra*) (15).

ENDOVASCULAR TREATMENT OF CHRONIC OCCLUSIVE LOWER LIMB OCCLUSIVE DISEASE

Inferior Vena Caval Disease

Although occlusion of the IVC may be asymptomatic, a number of patients will suffer back pain and signs of venous disease in the lower limbs, including lower limb pain and weakness, edema and ulceration, sometimes known as the IVC syndrome.

While thrombolysis has been used in the acute setting (see chap. 50), the treatment options for chronic disease are limited. Anticoagulation is generally not effective for symptom relief. Surgery includes femorocaval, iliocaval and cavoatrial bypass grafts, with published results of secondary patency around 50% at two years in selected patients (4).

Reports of successful balloon angioplasty of IVC occlusive disease are mostly concerned with treatment of membranous obstruction of the hepatic vena cava, in which it is a successful enduring treatment, although repeated dilatations may be required (16). However, membranous obstruction of the IVC is a rare cause of occlusive IVC disease in the West and the good results of primary angioplasty without stent use in this specific condition cannot be generally inferred.

Chronic IVC occlusion is most commonly due to previous venous thrombosis. This may be related to caval compression due to abdominal lymphadenopathy, retroperitoneal fibrosis, abdominal tumors or aortic aneurysms (17). IVC thrombosis may also be precipitated by trauma, the presence of an IVC filter or hypercoagulable states such as factor V Leiden or unusual conditions like Behçet's Syndrome.

If the occlusion can be crossed, endovascular stents may be used to maintain patency. Successful recanalization of long chronic occlusions may be difficult. A combined superior and inferior approach from femoral and jugular access with snaring of the wire can be useful and sharp recanalization may be necessary. Reestablishing patency of a chronically occluded IVC can result in dramatic immediate relief of symptoms (18). In the largest published series to date of endovascular stenting for chronic IVC occlusion, Razavi and colleagues treated 17 patients, of whom 13 were treated for benign disease (19). They were able to achieve technical success in 15 out of 17 patients (88%), who were treated with Wallstents (Boston Scientific) and Palmaz stents (Fig. 1). In those 15 patients, there was a primary patency rate of 80% (12/15) and a primary assisted patency rate of 87% (13/15) after a mean period of 19 months. Regrettably the authors do not give the clinical outcomes of the patients treated.

Iliac Vein Disease

Like IVC occlusion, iliac vein occlusion is most commonly related to previous iliac vein thrombosis, and IVC and iliac vein occlusion may coexist. Whereas iliac vein stenoses are relatively straightforward to treat with stents, long occlusions may be technically much more challenging. A combination of curved catheters and hydrophilic wires is generally used to enter the obstructed segment, following which it is usually easier to progress along a plane within the obstruction. It is crucial to ensure that the free end of the wire is intraluminal before ballooning or stenting, by passing a catheter over the wire and demonstrating free aspiration of blood and injection of contrast into the lumen.

Chronic iliac vein occlusion as a result of previous DVT will not uncommonly involve the common femoral venous segment. Percutaneous access for treating these lesions is usually through the thigh into the superficial femoral vein or the popliteal vein under ultrasound guidance. The popliteal vein is more superficial for access but requires that the patient is placed prone. Accessory access from the internal jugular vein can also be useful and, in cases where the superficial femoral vein is occluded, ultrasound guided puncture of the deep femoral vein has been used (20).

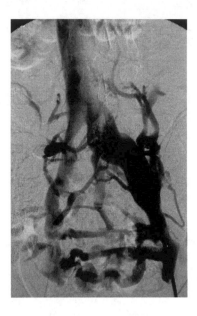

FIGURE 1 Injection into the left common femoral vein demonstrates an impression at the origin of the left common iliac vein and numerous collateral veins.

Involvement of the common femoral vein may also necessitate extending stents down below the inguinal ligament. This raises hypothetical concerns of compression of the stent by the inguinal ligament and stent fatigue from placement across a joint. In fact, the point of maximum flexion of the hip joint is several centimeters below the inguinal ligament and animal studies have shown Wallstents® (Boston Scientific, Natick, Massachusetts, U.S.A.) placed across the hip joint to be resistant to fractures, although susceptible to more neointimal hyperplasia (21). The group from Jackson, Mississippi have reported using Wallstents in this manner without significant complication. It may be that some of the newer flexible nitinol stents may be even better suited for implantation at this site, as they may be more resistant to fractures, which, at least in the femoral arterial segments, are known to predispose to restenosis and thrombosis (22). Extension down into the superficial femoral vein is not generally necessary so long as a good profunda vein provides inflow to the stent. Even if the extent of the diseased iliac segment does not extend into the IVC, some authors advocate extending stents into the IVC, having found a high rate of restenosis at the iliocaval junction in patients treated with stents confined to the iliac veins. The theoretical concern is interruption of flow on the contralateral side. One solution might be to place "kissing stents" at the iliac vein confluence, but one group has reported no problems with placing a stent across the contralateral iliac vein in over 500 cases (23).

Iliac venous dilatation can be painful, which has prompted some authors to recommend that it is always undertaken under general anesthesia, while other groups have found local anesthesia with sedation acceptable.

One problem of stenting of venous stenoses is the development of in-stent restenosis. This appears to occur to some degree in most stents; in one study 80% of stents developed some degree of in-stent restenosis at three and a half years, although less than 20% of treated veins had greater than 50% stenosis. Thrombotic disease, a thrombophilic diathesis and the presence of long stents crossing the inguinal ligament appeared to be risk factors for restenosis. Restenosis appears to be related to neointimal hyperplasia and may not be progressive. It is, however, difficult to treat, being generally resistant to balloon angioplasty, while further stenting may stimulate further the reactive process.

Clinical Results of Iliac Venous Stenting

Regrettably, much of the literature on iliac venous stenting for chronic venous insufficiency relies on vessel patency as the primary endpoint. The group from Jackson has reported on the clinical results of stenting of 304 iliac veins in 292 patients. The majority of lesions were stenoses; the authors included 17 successfully stented occlusions but excluded technical failures for stenting. Pain was measured on a visual analog scale from 0 to 10 and decreased from a median level of four preprocedurally to zero postprocedurally, with the percentage of patients reporting no pain increasing from 17% before stenting to 71% after. Similarly, the degree of limb swelling decreased in the population treated, with the proportion of limbs with no swelling increasing from 12% to 47% after treatment.

Iliocaval Compression Syndrome (May–Thurner Syndrome/Cockett Syndrome)

Classic iliocaval compression syndrome arises as a result of compression of the left common iliac vein by the overlying right common iliac artery. Virchow noted the increased incidence of DVT on the left side compared to the right in 1851. May and Thurner described spurs within the left iliac vein in 1957 and postulated that these were caused by compression of the vein between the right common iliac artery and the fifth lumbar vertebra and the repeated pulsation (Fig. 2). These webs are thought to pre-dispose to left-sided iliofemoral deep vein thrombosis, classically in young or middle-aged women after a period of immobilization or pregnancy, and the syndrome should therefore be actively looked for as a cause of DVT in patients presenting in this way. Endovascular treatment of the acute condition with thrombolytics and stents has been described with good results (24).

The syndrome may also present as a chronic condition. Cockett, a British vascular surgeon, and Thomas, a radiologist, from St. Thomas' Hospital, London, described the clinical syndrome of pain, swelling and venous stasis in the left lower limb. The left iliac vein may be occluded due to previous DVT, or stenosed but patent as a result of the compression and venous webs.

As well as the classical form of iliocaval compression syndrome, the St. Thomas' group also described compression of the right iliac vein by the right iliac artery. More distal compression of the left iliac vein by the left internal iliac artery has also been described.

Not all workers however have accepted iliocaval compression syndrome as a true pathological entity, but have suggested that it is essentially a normal variant. One study of CT examinations from patients with no symptoms of lower limb thrombosis or swelling found a 24% incidence of 50% or greater compression of the left iliac vein and a 66% incidence of 25% or more compression (25). These results are in concordance with post mortem studies showing a 22% to 32% incidence of obstructing lesions. Given the incidence of DVT is only 0.1% per annum, clearly other factors are at work. Nevertheless, the finding of iliocaval compression not only in patients presenting with acute thrombosis but also in those with chronic venous disease

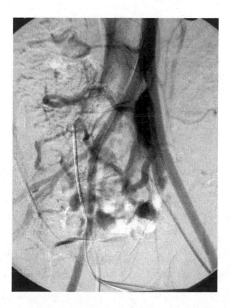

FIGURE 2 Arteriography performed simultaneously confirms the right common iliac artery is the cause of the left common iliac vein compression.

has led some workers to employ a tactic of aggressive iliac vein stenting in both patients with an obstructive pattern and those with predominantly reflux (26).

O'Sullivan et al. described the treatment of 39 patients with iliocaval compression syndrome at Stanford, of whom 20 presented with chronic symptoms (median duration 270 days) (27). Patients were treated using local anesthetic with an ultrasound-directed popliteal vein puncture using a micropuncture technique with subsequent dilatation to five French.

The first 12 patients in the chronic group of patients were treated in the same way as patients in the acute group with initial thrombolysis before attempting to cross the lesion with a wire and place a stent. However, they achieved technical success in only eight patients (67%) and abandoned thrombolysis in the subsequent eight patients who were treated with primary stenting with a 100% technical success rate. In those patients who received a stent, the patency rate at one year was 94%. In the group treated with primary stenting without thrombolysis, there was clinical improvement in all eight patients, with six reporting complete relief of symptoms.

Hurst et al. reported on the treatment of 18 patients with iliocaval compression syndrome (28). Six were found to have acute thrombus and seven had chronic thrombus. Seventeen patients were treated with iliac vein stenting and one with angioplasty alone. Six patients received thrombolysis. Similar to O'Sullivan's study, patients were generally treated with Wallstents or Palmaz stents (Fig. 3), though in this series the left common femoral vein was the primary access site. In contrast to the group from Jackson, the authors report that they are careful in positioning stents within the left common iliac vein such that the proximal end of the stent does not overlap into the IVC. Using these methods, the authors achieved a primary patency rate of 79% at one year.

Femoral Veins

Experience of stents placed within the infrainguinal veins is limited compared to the iliofemoral segments. Results from a multicenter national registry of patients who had venous stents placed following transcatheter thrombolysis for DVT demonstrated that, while stents placed in the iliac veins had acceptable patency rates, 80% of the five stents placed in the infrainguinal veins were occluded by day 42 (29). The authors recommend against placing infrainguinal venous stents. However, the number of patients treated, even in this national registry, is very small. Further developments in stent technology may alter the feasibility of infrainguinal venous placement, but this will be best evaluated by controlled trials.

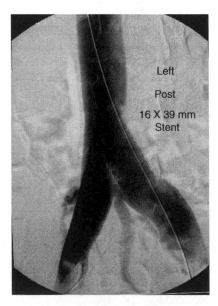

FIGURE 3   Appearance after treatment with a Palmaz® stent (Cordis, Johnson & Johnson, Miami Lakes, Florida, U.S.A.).

PERCUTANEOUS PROSTHETIC VENOUS VALVES AS ENDOVASCULAR TREATMENT OF CHRONIC LOWER LIMB VENOUS REFLUX

The possibility of treating venous reflux with percutaneously delivered transcatheter prosthetic valves was first postulated by Charles Dotter in 1981. Subsequently, there have been many attempts to develop prosthetic or bioprosthetic venous valves for percutaneous transcatheter deployment. The devices have generally consisted of an artificial or bioprosthetic membrane supported on a metallic stent with a variable number of cusps, designed to allow unidirectional flow through them.

Animal experiments in the 1990s gave encouraging results for patency and competency in the short term. However, the first feasibility study in humans of implantation of prosthetic valves implanted into femoral veins for reflux resulted in an unacceptably high rate of early occlusion, with four out of five valves occluded at follow up. A more recent pilot study saw bioprosthetic venous valves implanted into three patients with lower limb venous reflux and followed up to one year, at which time two patients had improvement in clinical symptoms (30). From these initial studies it is apparent that accurate sizing of the valves to the recipient vein is important, which may be achieved with careful ultrasound. Tilting of the valve may also decrease valve function and a second generation valve with less tendency to tilt has been trialed in the short term on an animal model (31).

Stents have been designed for esophageal cancer involving the cardia that combine radial strength for dilation with an anti-reflux mechanism (32). It can be hoped that manufactured reliable implantable valves will be available for larger scale clinical trials in the near future.

CONCLUSION

Chronic venous disease is a common condition, affecting 10% to 15% of the general population. The hallmark of therapy for deep venous insufficiency has been compression stockings; specialized techniques such as valve reconstruction or venous bypass have only been undertaken by specialist centers and the results have not been universally encouraging. Venous outflow obstruction is being increasingly recognized as a major factor in chronic venous insufficiency in addition to venous reflux, and the two pathophysiological mechanisms are synergistic. Iliofemoral venous stenting has an excellent technical success rate in venous stenosis. Occlusions are technically more challenging, but the majority can be successfully treated. Technically successful results of stenting have been shown to exhibit good midterm patency rates and encouraging clinical results, with improvement in the major symptoms experienced such as pain and swelling. Technical failures and restenoses can be treated with traditional surgical bypass techniques.

Implantable transcatheter percutaneous prosthetic or bioprosthatic valves are currently experimental therapy but may develop into a valuable tool for the treatment of chronic deep venous insufficiency.

REFERENCES

1. Da SA, Navarro MF, Batalheiro J. The importance of chronic venous insufficiency. Various preliminary data on its medico-social consequences. Phlebologie 1992; 45(4):439–43.
2. Neglen P, Thrasher TL, Raju S. Venous outflow obstruction: an underestimated contributor to chronic venous disease. J Vasc Surg 2003; 38(5):879–85.
3. Neglen P, Raju S. Proximal lower extremity chronic venous outflow obstruction: recognition and treatment. Semin Vasc Surg 2002; 15(1):57–64.
4. Jost CJ, Gloviczki P, Cherry KJ, Jr., et al. Surgical reconstruction of iliofemoral veins and the inferior vena cava for nonmalignant occlusive disease. J Vasc Surg 2001; 33(2):320–7.
5. Porter JM, Moneta GL. Reporting standards in venous disease: an update. International Consensus Committee on Chronic Venous Disease. J Vasc Surg 1995; 21(4):635–45.
6. Dos Santos J. La phlebographie directe. Conception, technique, premier resultats. J Int Chir 1938; 107:582.
7. Negus D, Cockett FB. Femoral vein pressures in post-phlebitic iliac vein obstruction. Br J Surg 1967; 54(6):522–5.

8. Neglen P, Raju S. Intravascular ultrasound scan evaluation of the obstructed vein. J Vasc Surg 2002; 35(4):694–700.
9. Wolpert LM, Rahmani O, Stein B, Gallagher JJ, Drezner AD. Magnetic resonance venography in the diagnosis and management of May–Thurner syndrome. Vasc Endovascular Surg 2002; 36(1):51–7.
10. Fraser DG, Moody AR, Martel A, Morgan PS. Re-evaluation of iliac compression syndrome using magnetic resonance imaging in patients with acute deep venous thromboses. J Vasc Surg 2004; 40(4):604–11.
11. Bauer AR, Jr., Flynn RR. Computed tomography diagnosis of venous thrombosis of the lower extremities and pelvis with contrast material. Surg Gynecol Obstet 1988; 167(1):12–5.
12. Lomas DJ, Britton PD. CT demonstration of acute and chronic iliofemoral thrombosis. J Comput Assist Tomogr 1991; 15(5):861–2.
13. Baldt MM, Zontsich T, Stumpflen A, et al. Deep venous thrombosis of the lower extremity: efficacy of spiral CT venography compared with conventional venography in diagnosis. Radiology 1996; 200(2):423–8.
14. Loud PA, Grossman ZD, Klippenstein DL, Ray CE. Combined CT venography and pulmonary angiography: a new diagnostic technique for suspected thromboembolic disease. AJR Am J Roentgenol 1998; 170(4):951–4.
15. Oguzkurt L, Tercan F, Pourbagher MA, Kizilkilic O, Turkoz R, Boyvat F. Computed tomography findings in 10 cases of iliac vein compression (May–Thurner) syndrome. Eur J Radiol 2005; 55(3):421–5.
16. Sato M, Yamada R, Tsuji K, et al. Percutaneous transluminal angioplasty in segmental obstruction of the hepatic inferior vena cava: long-term results. Cardiovasc Intervent Radiol 1990; 13(3):189–92.
17. Sonin AH, Mazer MJ, Powers TA. Obstruction of the inferior vena cava: a multiple-modality demonstration of causes, manifestations, and collateral pathways. Radiographics 1992; 12(2):309–22.
18. Robbins MR, Assi Z, Comerota AJ. Endovascular stenting to treat chronic long-segment inferior vena cava occlusion. J Vasc Surg 2005; 41(1):136–40.
19. Razavi MK, Hansch EC, Kee ST, Sze DY, Semba CP, Dake MD. Chronically occluded inferior venae cavae: endovascular treatment. Radiology 2000; 214(1):133–8.
20. Akesson H, Lindh M, Ivancev K, Risberg B. Venous stents in chronic iliac vein occlusions. Eur J Vasc Endovasc Surg 1997; 13(3):334–6.
21. Andrews RT, Venbrux AC, Magee CA, Bova DA. Placement of a flexible endovascular stent across the femoral joint: an in vivo study in the swine model. J Vasc Interv Radiol 1999; 10(9):1219–28.
22. Scheinert D, Scheinert S, Sax J, et al. Prevalence and clinical impact of stent fractures after femoropopliteal stenting. J Am Coll Cardiol 2005; 45(2):312–5.
23. Raju S, McAllister S, Neglen P. Recanalization of totally occluded iliac and adjacent venous segments. J Vasc Surg 2002; 36(5):903–11.
24. Kwak HS, Han YM, Lee YS, Jin GY, Chung GH. Stents in common iliac vein obstruction with acute ipsilateral deep venous thrombosis: early and late results. J Vasc Interv Radiol 2005; 16(6):815–22.
25. Kibbe MR, Ujiki M, Goodwin AL, Eskandari M, Yao J, Matsumura J. Iliac vein compression in an asymptomatic patient population. J Vasc Surg 2004; 39(5):937–43.
26. Raju S, Neglen P. High prevalence of nonthrombotic iliac vein lesions in chronic venous disease: a permissive role in pathogenicity. J Vasc Surg 2006; 44(1):136–44.
27. O'Sullivan GJ, Semba CP, Bittner CA, et al. Endovascular management of iliac vein compression (May–Thurner) syndrome. J Vasc Interv Radiol 2000; 11(7):823–36.
28. Hurst DR, Forauer AR, Bloom JR, Greenfield LJ, Wakefield TW, Williams DM. Diagnosis and endovascular treatment of iliocaval compression syndrome. J Vasc Surg 2001; 34(1):106–13.
29. Seabrook GR, Mewissen MW, Schmitt DD, et al. Percutaneous intraarterial thrombolysis in the treatment of thrombosis of lower extremity arterial reconstructions. J Vasc Surg 1991; 13(5):646–51.
30. Pavcnik D, Machan L, Uchida B, Kaufman J, Keller FS, Rosch J. Percutaneous prosthetic venous valves: current state and possible applications. Tech Vasc Interv Radiol 2003; 6(3):137–42.
31. Pavcnik D, Kaufman J, Uchida B, et al. Second-generation percutaneous bioprosthetic valve: a short-term study in sheep. J Vasc Surg 2004; 40(6):1223–7.
32. Dua KS. Antireflux stents in tumors of the cardia. Am J Med 2001; 111(Suppl. 8A):190S–6.

52 | Endovenous Techniques for the Treatment of Varicose Veins

Ian M. Loftus, Peter Holt, and Matt M. Thompson
St. George's Vascular Institute, St. George's Hospital, London, U.K.

BACKGROUND

Varicose veins are extremely common, though only a minority seek treatment, either for cosmetic reasons or related symptoms. Despite this varicose veins represent a significant financial burden on health services and the largest single cause of medicolegal claims against surgeons (1,2). Patient satisfaction, with both symptom relief and cosmetic result, is essential.

The primary problem in lower extremity venous insufficiency is non-functional valvular disease with associated vein wall abnormalities. The cornerstone in treatment of venous problems is to eliminate the source of the venous hypertension, often the long saphenous vein. Traditional surgery for venous hypertension involving the long saphenous vein entails ligation of the saphenofemoral junction including the tributaries, stripping of the vein and multiple phlebectomies. Despite being a relatively minor procedure, varicose vein surgery is one of the commonest reasons for litigation. Approximately 5% of cases experience a cutaneous nerve injury and up to 10% develop wound infections and/or hematomas (3). Rarer, but potentially tragic complications include pulmonary embolus, and ligation of the femoral artery or vein.

Various minimally invasive techniques have been introduced for the treatment of varicose veins in recent years to achieve the primary aim of preventing reflux in the long or short saphenous vein (4). The most widely accepted of these novel techniques are endovenous laser ablation and radiofrequency ablation. The methods and evidence base for these endovenous treatment modalities will be discussed.

ENDOVENOUS LASER ABLATION

Introduction

Endovenous laser techniques employ an 810 nm-diode laser to heat the long or short saphenous vein (or major tributaries), inducing a combination of endothelial damage, focal coagulative necrosis, shrinkage of the vein and thrombotic occlusion.

Endovenous laser ablation (EVLA) is a relatively simple and quick technique which can be performed under a local anesthetic. Many proponents of the technique now perform this as an outpatient ambulatory service, without the use of theatre space or equipment. This has potentially significant cost implications, and the technique itself has many potential advantages over conventional surgery. No groin incision is required, and the trauma associated with stripping of the long saphenous vein is avoided. These advantages should reduce the risk of nerve damage, groin infection, bleeding and bruising complications. Potential disadvantages include initial failure rates, concerns regarding long-term recanalization and recurrent veins from the groin tributaries which are traditionally ligated during conventional surgery, risks of burns and deep vein thrombosis. The initial costs of the equipment and recurrent disposable costs also need to be considered.

The Technique of EVLA

Initial assessment must be performed with a duplex ultrasound scan to elicit the site and magnitude of venous reflux and the diameter of the affected vein. Most technicians experienced in laser therapy would consider truncal varicosities ranging from 4 to 1.4 mm in size as suitable for treatment.

The patient should be placed initially in the reverse Trendelenburg position to distend the vein. The vein may be marked on the skin as a guide for treatment. Under ultrasound control the vein is punctured with a 19-gauge percutaneous entry needle, through which a 0.035-in. guidewire is manipulated. If performed under a local anesthetic, a small amount should be infiltrated at the planned site of puncture. The guidewire should pass without resistance up through the saphenofemoral junction, and should be followed with ultrasound to ensure that it does not pass through a perforator into the deep veins. Once positioned through the junction, a small incision is made in the skin at the entry point to allow for the passage of a 5 F introducer sheath using the Seldinger technique. Having removed the dilator and guidewire, the laser fiber is introduced and positioned 2 cm proximal to the saphenofemoral junction. This can be clearly visualized on ultrasound (Figs. 1 and 2). The fiber is then connected to the laser console. Tumescent local anesthetic (usually 0.1% lignocaine with adrenaline) should then be delivered to the perivenous area, again using ultrasound to guide the needle. This manoeuvre compresses the vein wall to ensure apposition to the fiber, acts as a heat sink to prevent thermal damage to surrounding tissues and provides analgesia. The patient is then placed in the Trendelenburg position, safety glasses donned and the laser activated while withdrawing the fiber in the sheath at a steady and constant pace (Fig. 3). Compression hosiery or bandaging should be applied at the end of the procedure.

The power of the laser should be set at between 10 and 14 W. The author's preference is to treat both long and short saphenous veins at 10 W, withdrawing the laser at 80 J/cm for the long saphenous, and 40 J/cm for the short saphenous. Compression hosiery is prescribed for two weeks following the ablative procedure.

The Results of EVLA

The most extensive results of EVLA have been published by Min and co-workers in New York (5). Their early results were published in 2001, a series of 84 patients in which 90 long saphenous veins were treated using laser therapy followed by clinical and ultrasound evaluation at one, three, six and nine months. It should be noted that this was a nonrandomized study in which patients were offered a choice of surgery, sclerotherapy, radiofrequency ablation or laser therapy. In the group treated with laser, injection sclerotherapy was offered for residual veins at 6 to 12 weeks following initial treatment.

In this early study, successful placement and laser application were achieved in all patients, and all were well tolerated under local anesthetic. Only three patients showed flow in the long saphenous vein after one week and all underwent successful repeat laser treatment.

Sapheno-femoral junction

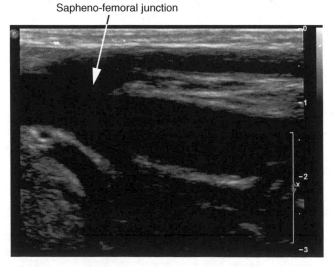

FIGURE 1 The sapheno-femoral junction should be clearly visualized prior to both laser and radiofrequency treatment.

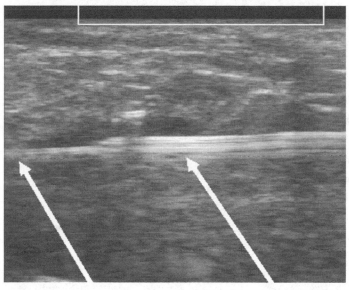

Tip of laser fibre   Outer sheath

FIGURE 2 The tip of the laser fiber is clearly visible on ultrasound and should be positioned 2 cm back from the sapheno-femoral junction.

The authors stated that most patients experienced mild bruising and discomfort along the long saphenous vein for one to two weeks, but only five patients required analgesia for up to two weeks. A single patient reported localized paraesthesia which resolved by six weeks.

The same group published longer-term results in 2003 (6). Over a three-year period, 499 long saphenous veins were treated in 423 subjects. Successful occlusion was demonstrated in all but nine patients at one week, and 113 of 121 limbs followed up to three years had remained closed. Interestingly, most of the recurrences occurred very early after the initial treatment. Bruising was noted in 24% and tightness in 90%. There were no cases of skin burns, deep vein thrombosis or long-term paraesthesia.

These results are in line with reports from other single centers' experience. In the authors' own early series of 174 limbs in 135 patients, technical failure occurred in two cases with no early recanalization, no major complications, temporary paraesthesia in 2% and pain for more than one week requiring analgesia in 3%.

In a review of the first 1000 cases submitted to an Italian Endovenous Laser Working Group, initial occlusion rates of 99%, and 36 month occlusion rates of 97% were demonstrated (7). Again, there were no reports of major complications, including burns or deep vein thrombosis. This registry also demonstrated reduced postoperative pain, shorter duration off work and faster resolution to normal activities, than conventional surgery.

On a more cautionary note, in a series of 145 veins in 136 patients from Belfast, primary failure was somewhat higher at 14.5%, largely due to problems with cannulation and passage of the guidewire (8). This group also documented one episode of saphenous nerve injury and a single skin burn. Despite this, patient satisfaction with the technique was high.

Comparative Data

There are no controlled studies to compare the effectiveness of endovenous laser treatment with conventional surgery, leading to calls for a randomized trial (9). The published results of laser treatment are from single center series and the Italian Registry. It does appear, even from this low-level evidence, that EVLA offers significant advantages over conventional surgery in terms of cosmesis, postoperative pain, early return to normal activities and complications. The feared incidences of skin burns and deep vein thromboses have not materialized in the published

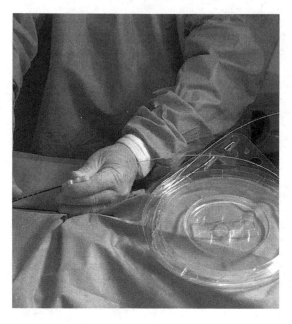

FIGURE 3 Having performed tumescent local anesthesia around the vein, the sheath and laser fiber are locked together and withdrawn at a constant rate from the vein while delivering energy to the vein. Treatment should cease 5 cm or more proximal to the puncture site.

series. Longer-term fears of recanalization and recurrence associated with tributaries also seem, at present, unfounded, though further studies are required.

RADIOFREQUENCY ABLATION

Introduction

The technique of radiofrequency ablation is very similar to that described above for laser therapy. It can be performed under local or general anesthesia and consideration in choosing the type of anesthesia must take into account the length of the procedure, which is significantly longer than laser ablation.

The Technique of Radiofrequency Ablation

Elimination of reflux is achieved with the use of radiofrequency heating rather than laser. The VNUS vein treatment system using the Closure® catheter (VNUS Medical Technologies, Sunnyvale, California, U.S.A.) is the most widely used system, employing electrodes which monitor the electrical and thermal effects of the catheter. The manufacturers recommend treatment of non-tortuous veins of less than 12 mm in diameter. The technique is often performed under a general anesthetic, though it can be performed under a local anesthetic.

   The long saphenous vein is cannulated at the level of the knee with a 5- or 8-F gauge catheter. This is advanced to the saphenofemoral junction. The device produces heat from bipolar sheathed electrodes to provide precise vein wall destruction with minimal thrombus formation. The generator connects directly to the intraluminal catheter within the saphenous vein. Tumescent anesthesia is performed as described above, and duplex guidance used throughout to ensure position and successful vein obliteration as the catheter is slowly withdrawn.

The Results of Radiofrequency Ablation

In the first large series to be reported, early long saphenous closure was documented in 93% of 141 veins, with a two-year closure rate of over 90%. This compares well with historical data regarding recurrence following conventional surgery (10,11).

Sybrandy and Wittens followed up subjects for one year after treatment of 26 limbs and revealed that, while 31% of junctions demonstrated reflux, the vein remained closed in 88%. Recanalization of the main trunk occurred in one patient (12). Even higher rates of junction reflux have been demonstrated in larger studies, but rarely associated with truncal reflux. Pichot published a series of 63 limbs followed up for a median of 25 months and demonstrated reflux at the junction in 82% but in the trunk in only 8% (13). No groin revascularization was demonstrated. Merchant et al. demonstrated a rather higher recanalization rate of 11.3% (14). Some have advocated vein ablation with concomitant high saphenous ligation, though there is no evidence to support this in routine practise (15).

In the Closure registry, three patients demonstrated deep vein thrombosis (0.57% of a total 522 patients) (16). Pulmonary embolism occurred in one patient. The risk of saphenous nerve injury appears high however, demonstrated in 12.5% at one week, 2.75% at 12 months and 3.6% at 24 months.

Comparative Data

There have been two randomized controlled trials comparing radiofrequency ablation with conventional surgery. In the Endovenous Radiofrequency Obliteration (Closure) versus Ligation and Vein Stripping study, 81 patients were randomized, and 81% closure rates were demonstrated in the VNUS group (17). The duration of the procedure was shorter in the ablation group, as was the recovery period. There was a lower (though non-significant) complication rate in the ablation group though paraesthesia was more common (16% vs. 6% in the surgical group). While supporting a potential role in the management of varicose veins, this trial has been criticized for differences in anesthesia, adjunctive procedures and for being under powered.

In a second, even smaller, trial Rautio randomized 28 patients to radiofrequency ablation or surgery, all with concurrent phlebectomies and all under general anesthesia (18). Successful occlusion was demonstrated in all patients. There were no differences in quality of life or symptom score, though a lower pain score was demonstrated in the ablation group. In the VNUS group, there were three burns, and three episodes of thrombophlebitis. There were similar rates of paraesthesia. The value of this study is severely limited by its size.

SUMMARY

Conventional surgery for varicose veins does relieve symptoms and has a role on the prevention of chronic venous ulceration. Minor complications are common. Novel minimally invasive "endovenous" techniques have emerged over the last five years, the most promising of which are radiofrequency ablation and EVLA.

Outcome data on these techniques is less extensive than for conventional surgery, and is limited to small randomized trials, single-center series and registries. Despite this, both techniques now have many proponents, and the National Institute for Clinical Excellence has approved their use in the U.K. in standard clinical practice (19).

In the absence of randomized trials, it is difficult to directly compare the techniques, though they seem comparable in terms of long saphenous occlusion. Both, particularly laser ablation, have relatively low complication rates. The issue regarding the fate of tributaries remains unanswered, though many proponents of a minimally invasive approach would suggest that, should tributaries form recurrences in the future, these could be treated with ultrasound guided foam sclerotherapy (see chap. 53).

REFERENCES

1. Evans CJ, Fowkes FG, Ruckley CV, Lee AJ. Prevalence of varicose veins and chronic venous insufficiency in men and women in the general population: Edinburgh Vein Study. J Epidemiol Community Health 1999; 53:149–53.
2. Campbell WB, France F, Goodwin HM. Research and Audit Committee of the Vascular Surgical Society of Great Britain and Ireland. Medico-legal claims in vascular surgery. Ann R Coll Surg Engl 2002; 84:181–4.

3. Rudstrom H, Bjorck M, Bergqvist D. Iatrogenic vascular injuries in varicose vein surgery: a systematic review. World J Surg 2007; 31(1):228–33.

4. Beale RJ, Gough MJ. Treatment options for primary varicose veins—a review. Eur J Vasc Endovasc Surg 2005; 30:83–95.

5. Min RJ, Zimmet SE, Isaacs MN, Forrestal MD. Endovenous laser treatment of the incompetent greater saphenous vein. J Vasc Interv Radiol 2001; 12:1167–71.

6. Min RJ, Khilnani N, Zimmet SE. Endovenous laser treatment of saphenous vein reflux: long term results. J Vasc Interv Radiol 2003; 14:991–6.

7. Agus GB, Mancini S, Magi G, Italian Endovenous Laser Working Group. The first 1000 cases of Italian Endovenous-laser Working Group. Rationale and long term outcomes of the 1999–2003 period. Int Angiol 2006; 25:209–15.

8. Sharif MA, Soong CV, Lau LL, Corvan R, Lee B, Hannon RJ. Endovenous laser treatment for long saphenous vein incompetence. Br J Surg 2006; 93:831–5.

9. Mundy L, Merlin TL, Fitridge RA, Hiller JE. Systematic review of endovenous laser treatment for varicose veins. Br J Surg 2005; 92:1189–94.

10. Manfrini S, Gasbarro V, Danielsson G, et al. Endovenous management of saphenous vein reflux. J Vasc Surg 2000; 32:330–43.

11. Kabnick LS, Merchant RF. Twelve and twenty-four month follow up after endovenous obliteration of saphenous vein reflux: a report from the multicentre registry. J Phlebol 2001; 1:17–24.

12. Sybrandy JEM, Wittens CHA. Initial experiences in endovenous treatment of saphenous vein reflux. J Vasc Surg 2002; 36:1207–12.

13. Pichot O, Creton D, Merchant RF, Schuller-Petroviae S, Chandler JG. Duplex ultrasound findings two years after greater saphenous vein radiofrequency endovenous obliteration. J Vasc Surg 2004; 39:189–95.

14. Merchant RF, DePalma RG, Kabnick LS. Endovenous obliteration of saphenous reflux: a multicentre study. J Vasc Surg 2002; 35:1190–6.

15. Hach-Wunderle V, Hach W. Invasive therapeutic options in truncal varicosity of the great saphenous vein. Vasa 2006; 35:157–66.

16. Nicolini P, Closure Group. Treatment of primary varicose veins by endovenous obliteration with the VNUS closure system: results of a prospective multicentre study. Eur J Vasc Endovasc Surg 2005; 29:433–9.

17. Lurie F, Creton D, Eklof B, et al. Prospective randomised study of endovenous radiofrequency obliteration (closure) versus ligation and vein stripping (EVOLVeS): two year follow up. Eur J Vasc Endovasc Surg 2005; 29:67–73.

18. Rautio T, Perala J, Ohtonen P, et al. Endovenous obliteraion versus conventional stripping operation in the treatment of primary varicose veins: a randomised controlled trial with comparison of costs. J Vasc Surg 2002; 35:958–65.

19. National Institute for Clinical Excellence. Interventional procedure overview of endovenous laser treatment of varicose veins. London: NICE, 2003; (http://www.nice.org.uk/pdf/ip/209overview.pdf).

53 | Ultrasound-Guided Foam Sclerotherapy for Chronic Venous Disease

Philip Coleridge Smith
UCL Medical School, Thames Valley Nuffield Hospital, London, U.K.

INTRODUCTION

Although surgical treatment is widely used for varicose veins, recent publications show that recurrence may be expected in 25% to 50% of patients at five years (1–4). Patients require on average two weeks away from work following treatment to allow postoperative bruising and discomfort to subside. Surgery leaves scars and may result in damage to adjacent structures including nerves, lymphatics, major arteries and veins (5). Deep vein thrombosis (DVT) and pulmonary embolism may also follow surgical treatment for varicose veins (6,7). A desire to reduce such complications has led to the development of alternative treatments which include radiofrequency obliteration (RF obliteration) (8), endovenous laser treatment (EVLT) (9) and ultrasound-guided foam sclerotherapy (UGFS).

ULTRASOUND-GUIDED SCLEROTHERAPY

Sclerotherapy has been used to treat varicose veins for 150 years. A detailed review of the history of this subject has been published recently (10). In the 1980s ultrasound was introduced for the diagnosis of venous disease of the lower limb. In France, where enthusiasm for the use of sclerotherapy was well established, Schadeck and Vin improved the efficacy of their treatment by using ultrasound imaging to guide injections into incompetent saphenous trunks (11,12). This method of treatment was found to achieve obliteration of the saphenous trunks in a substantial proportion of patients resulting in long-term relief from varices. As with conventional sclerotherapy, the problem of recanalization of veins was encountered in up to one-quarter of patients at one year (13).

Foam Sclerotherapy

In 1944 Orbach described the "air-block" technique. A small volume of air is included in the syringe with the sclerosant. The air is injected ahead of the sclerosant in order to prevent blood diluting the sclerosant and reducing its efficacy. In 1950 Orbach published a further paper that described the use of a foam created by vigorously shaking a syringe containing air and sclerosant to produce a froth (14).

The next significant advance came in 1993 when Cabrera suggested that foam could be created using carbon dioxide mixed with a polidocanol (POL), a detergent sclerosant (15). Cabrera published a further article in 1997 describing his experience in 261 limbs with great saphenous varices and eight patients with vascular malformations (16). He had used sclerotherapy with foam, guiding his injections by ultrasound imaging. Some of the varicose veins reached 20 mm in diameter. He considered that foam greatly extended the range of vein sizes which could be managed by sclerotherapy. He felt that the increased efficacy of foam was attributable to it displacing blood from the treated vein and increasing the contact time between the sclerosant and the vein. He used a "microfoam," that is a foam made of very small bubbles which was created by the use of a small rapidly rotating brush. This distinguished his foam from the "froth" made by Orbach.

Preparation of Sclerosant Foam

A series of authors have described methods of preparing "home-made" foam which may be used for ultrasound-guided sclerotherapy. Monfreux described a method necessitating a glass syringe which produced small quantities of POL foam which he used in a series of patients with truncal varicose veins (17). Sadoun described a method of preparing foam using a plastic syringe avoiding the need for reusable glass syringes (18). Subsequently Tessari has described a method of preparing foam using two disposable syringes and a three-way tap (19). This method can be used to produce large quantities of foam suitable for treating saphenous trunks and large varices. Frullini has added his own method of producing foam to this increasing list (20) based on that of Flückinger (21).

The most widely used method is that of Tessari which is readily achieved using materials available in most clinics (Fig. 1A,B). Two syringes are connected using a three-way tap. These can be either 2 or 5 mL syringes or a combination. A mixture of sclerosant and air is drawn into one syringe at a ratio of 1 part of sclerosant to 3 or 4 parts of air. The sclerosant can be sodium tetradecyl sulphate (STS) 1% to 3% (Fibrovein, STD Pharmaceuticals, Hereford, U.K.) or POL 0.5% to 3% (Sclerovein, Resinag AG, Zurich, CH). Low concentrations of POL (0.5%) make better foam when mixed 1:1 with air. The mixture is oscillated vigorously between the two syringes about 10 or 20 times. The tap can be turned slightly to reduce the aperture and increase the smoothness of the foam. The foam produced in this way is stable for about two minutes so it should be injected immediately it has been created.

Applications of Foam Sclerotherapy

Orbach suggested that sclerosant foam could be injected instead of liquid sclerosant in the management of varicose veins (14). The advantage of using foam is that more varices appear to be treated per injection and lower volumes of sclerosant are required. Since veins injected with foam have blood displaced from them and develop spasm it is usually obvious which veins have been treated without the need for ultrasound imaging.

In 1999 Henriet reported his results in 10,000 patients with reticular varices and telangiectases of the lower limb treated between the years 1995 and 1998 (22). He found that the outcome of foam treatment in small varices was excellent and that reduced volumes and concentrations of sclerosant could be employed compared to liquid sclerosants. Benigni reported the findings of a pilot study comparing liquid and foam sclerosants. He measured the outcome using a visual analogue scale to describe the improvement in appearance. He found that foam resulted in a 20% improved appearance as compared to liquid sclerosant (23).

Treatment of Saphenous Trunks

Cabrera described the use of foam sclerotherapy to treat saphenous trunks as an alternative to surgical stripping of the veins. This requires ultrasound-guided injection since the saphenous trunks cannot be readily treated safely and effectively without imaging control (Figs. 2 and 3). Cabrera described cannulation of the affected saphenous trunk followed by injection of foam

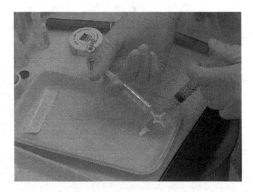

FIGURE 1 Tessari's method of creating sclerosant foam. A mixture of sclerosant (3% Fibrovein) and air is oscillated between two syringes connected by a three-way tap.

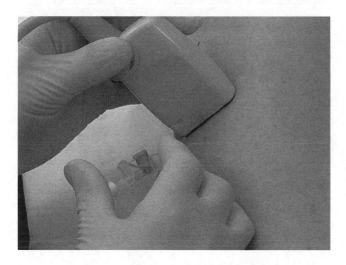

FIGURE 2 Ultrasound-guided cannulation of the small saphenous vein (SSV) during ultrasound-guided foam sclerotherapy of varices arising from the SSV. The patient is lying in the left lateral position.

until the vein has been completely filled along with its tributaries. Any unfilled tributaries were managed by injection using a Butterfly needle (Figs. 4 and 5). In France it is standard practice to inject the saphenous trunk using a needle and syringe. The complete length of the incompetent vein and tributaries are managed by several injections carried out over a number of sessions. Direct needle injection has the advantage of simplicity but in some anatomic regions, such as the popliteal fossa, a number of large arteries may lie adjacent to the small saphenous vein (SSV). Inadvertent intra-arterial injection causes disastrous results with extensive skin loss (24).

A wide range of maximum suggested volumes have been reported. Cabrera injected up to 100 mL of his foam whereas other authors have averaged 1 to 2 mL in a single session. A recent consensus document suggested that 6 to 8 mL of foam per session is the maximum appropriate amount (25).

It is conventional to apply compression following foam sclerotherapy, although scientific evidence to support this is not available, and the duration for which it should be applied has never been established. Some authors use stockings alone (15,26) and others use bandages (27). As with earlier practices in sclerotherapy, immediate ambulation and return to work are encouraged. There is little need for time away from work.

Any vein suitable for injection may be treated by foam sclerotherapy. In contrast to techniques requiring the passage of a catheter, such as RF closure or EVLT, UGFS can be used to

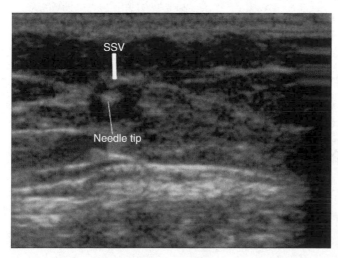

SSV

Needle tip

FIGURE 3 Transverse ultrasound image of the small saphenous vein with the bright echo of the needle tip in the lumen.

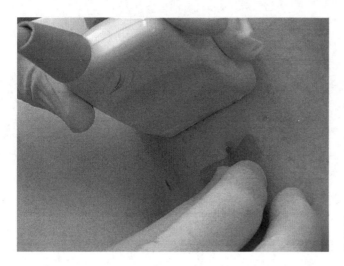

FIGURE 4 The distal small saphenous vein is canulated using a 25-gauge butterfly needle.

manage primary and recurrent varices arising in saphenous tributaries or trunks. The treatment is limited only by the skill of the sclerotherapist to inject the vein.

Outcomes

Cabrera has published a clinical series of 500 lower limbs treated by foam sclerotherapy. He reported that after three or more years 81% of treated great saphenous trunks remained occluded and 97% of superficial varices had disappeared. This required one session of sclerotherapy in 86% of patients, two in 11% and three sessions in 3% of patients. No DVT or pulmonary embolism was encountered in this series. A small number of other clinical series have been published, including those of Frullini and Cavezzi who reported a series of 453 patients (28) and Barrett who reported a series of 100 limbs (29). Cavezzi has subsequently published a detailed analysis of the efficacy of foam sclerotherapy in 194 patients, reporting a good outcome in 93% of patients (26). In fact, this technique has become widely used in southern Europe, Australia, New Zealand, South America and the U.S.A. (25). However, few surgeons in the U.K. use this method perhaps because of limited evidence of efficacy. One series has been recently reported from the U.K involving 60 patients comparing surgical treatment with foam sclerotherapy combined with saphenofemoral ligation (30).

A multicenter European randomized controlled trial has been conducted and the results presented at a scientific meeting (31). This open label trial included two separate studies:

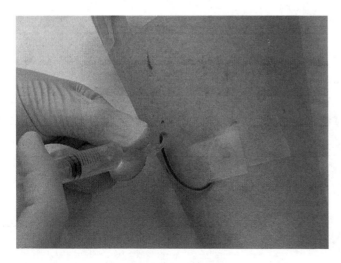

FIGURE 5 Correct function of the needle is confirmed by aspiration of blood and injection of saline.

a surgical part undertaken by surgeons who randomized patients to saphenous stripping or UGFS. Sclerotherapists randomized patients to ultrasound-guided sclerotherapy conducted using either foam or liquid sclerosant. In all, 654 patients were treated during this study. Up to four sessions of UGFS were allowed over a three-month period to obliterate the saphenous trunks. After 12 months the surgeons had eliminated truncal saphenous reflux in 130 of 176 patients (74%) by UGFS and in 84/94 (88%) by surgery. In comparison, sclerotherapists had eliminated reflux in 239 of 254 patients (91%) by UGFS and 104/125 (83%) by liquid sclerotherapy. Posttreatment pain was assessed by a visual analog scale which showed that surgery was much more painful than UGFS during the first week. Normal activities were resumed after a median of 13 days in the surgery group and two days in the UGFS group. DVT was observed in 10 patients treated by UGFS and one patient treated by liquid sclerotherapy.

Darke has recently reported the outcome of his clinical series of 192 patients managed by foam sclerotherapy for incompetence of saphenous trunks (32). A regime of up to three treatments per limb was devised which achieved occlusion of 91% of saphenous trunks at six weeks follow-up. He reported that all 23 small saphenous trunks were occluded by this regime.

My own experience of the use of UGFS is based on an analysis of all patients treated for varicose veins during the period January 2002 to August 2005 (33). A total of 808 patients (666 women, 142 men) were managed by UGFS for truncal saphenous incompetence. In all 1411 limbs were affected by varices [Clinical Etiological Anatomical Pathological Classification (CEAP) C1 $n=212$, 15%; CEAP C2 $n=1154$, 82%]. Great saphenous vein (GSV) reflux alone was present in 766 limbs (69%), SSV reflux alone in 223 limbs (20%) and combined GSV and SSV reflux in 120 (11%). A surprisingly high proportion of patients had undergone previous surgery for varicose veins in the vessel being treated ($n=267$, 30% of GSVs and $n=60$, 17% of SSVs). The median diameter of the GSVs treated was 5 mm (interquartile range, IQR 4–6 mm) and for the SSVs 5 mm (IQR 4–6 mm).

Thrombophlebitis occurred in a small number of patients (5%) and was managed by analgesia, compression and aspiration of thrombus. Calf vein thrombosis was confined to isolated gastrocnemius veins or to part of the posterior tibial vein (10 cases). All resolved with compression by stocking or bandage and exercise without use of anticoagulants. Three patients suffered partial common femoral vein thrombosis. No major systemic complication such as anaphylaxis, stroke or transient ischemic attack occurred in this series. A number of patients (14.2% of all patients treated) reported visual disturbance following treatment.

In all 457 limbs have been reviewed at six months or more following treatment, average 11 months, range 6 to 46 months. Duplex examination of the GSVs showed occlusion was obtained in 322 of 364 (88%). In the SSVs occlusion was present in 118 of 143 (83%).

The only residual adverse events still present at six months or more of follow-up were skin pigmentation and palpable lumps. Skin pigmentation was seen in 115 of 457 limbs and palpable lumps were present in 21 limbs. The skin pigmentation was almost always of a minor extent and continued to fade with the passage of time.

In the management of severe venous disease Bergan et al. have reported that UGFS was effective at healing all 27 venous ulcers treated by this method compared to only 10 of 22 ulcers managed by compression and wound dressing (34). Kakkos et al. have reported that UGFS was effective at managing 38 patients presenting with recurrent varices following previous surgery (35). All varices and residual or recurrent trunks were managed by a total of 73 injection sessions.

Safety of Foam Sclerotherapy

A large numbers of patients are treated by foam sclerotherapy throughout the world on a daily basis and the extent of recorded complications is very low. Guex et al. have reported the complication rate following 12,173 sclerotherapy sessions (36). Only 49 (0.4%) adverse events were encountered of which the most common were visual disturbances (20 cases) of which 19 involved the use of foam sclerosants. All resolved without complication within an hour. One femoral vein thrombosis was observed in this series. This treatment carries a low risk of serious adverse reactions.

Local complications include extravasation of sclerosant foam associated with skin necrosis. This is more commonly seen with STS than with POL foam which is much less likely to cause problems if it leaks from a vein during treatment. Thrombophlebitis occurs reasonably frequently following sclerotherapy but is readily managed by aspiration of thrombus. Frullini reported two cases of skin necrosis and seven of thrombophlebitis in a series of 196 patients treated by foam sclerotherapy.

DVT may occur following surgery or sclerotherapy for varicose veins. Gastrocnemius veins in the calf are at risk of exposure to sclerosant foam injected into superficial varices. Frullini also reported one case of gastrocnemius thrombosis and a further case of popliteal vein thrombosis in his series of 196 patients.

Systemic complications which have been described following both liquid and foam sclerotherapy include visual disturbance and chest symptoms, including coughing. These occur in about 1% to 2% of patients. Visual disturbance often occurs in patients with a previous history of migraine associated with a visual aura. There is some evidence that visual disturbances may be attributable to the passage of bubbles via a patent foramen ovale (PFO, which is in any case present in 20% of people). There is a rapidly expanding literature on the association of PFO and migraine in the general population (37). However, the fact that visual disturbance and other neurologic symptoms are well known following injection of liquid sclerosants suggest that this may be a simplistic explanation. A case of "stroke" following foam sclerotherapy has been reported (38). Right-sided weakness occurred following a session of foam sclerotherapy. However, there was no identifiable lesion on magnetic resonance imaging and the patient made a complete recovery. The patient was found to have a large PFO.

Severe allergic reactions to sclerosants are rare but not unknown. Anyone performing sclerotherapy of any type should be suitably equipped to deal with such an event.

CONCLUSIONS

Foam sclerotherapy offers an alternative to surgical intervention for patients with varicose veins. It can be conducted on an outpatient basis and is far less complex than EVLT or RF ablation of saphenous veins. It can also be used in primary or recurrent truncal incompetence as well as in tributaries and small varices. The recurrence rate following this treatment has yet to be established in comparison to surgery. Ultrasound imaging studies suggest that 85% to 90% of veins treated in this way remain occluded after three years although little detailed information has so far been published. This is comparable to EVLT and RF ablation and similar to rates of neovascularization reported following surgery. This technique promises to be a useful addition to the methods currently employed for managing superficial venous incompetence.

REFERENCES

1. van Rij AM, Jiang P, Solomon C, Christie RA, Hill GB. Recurrence after varicose vein surgery: a prospective long-term clinical study with duplex ultrasound scanning and air plethysmography. J Vasc Surg 2003; 38:935–43.
2. Winterborn RJ, Foy C, Earnshaw JJ. Causes of varicose vein recurrence: late results of a randomized controlled trial of stripping the long saphenous vein. J Vasc Surg 2004; 40:634–9.
3. Fischer R, Linde N, Duff C, Jeanneret C, Chandler JG, Seeber P. Late recurrent saphenofemoral junction reflux after ligation and stripping of the greater saphenous vein. J Vasc Surg 2001; 34:236–40.
4. Perrin MR, Guex JJ, Ruckley CV, et al. Recurrent varices after surgery (REVAS), a consensus document. REVAS group. Cardiovasc Surg 2000; 8:233–45.
5. Campbell WB, France F, Goodwin HM. Research and Audit Committee of the Vascular Surgical Society of Great Britain and Ireland. Medicolegal claims in vascular surgery. Ann R Coll Surg Engl 2002; 84:181–4.
6. van Rij AM, Chai J, Hill GB, Christie RA. Incidence of deep vein thrombosis after varicose vein surgery. Br J Surg 2004; 91:1582–5.
7. Srilekha A, Karunanithy N, Corbett CRR. Informed consent: what do we tell paitents aobu the risk of fatal pulmonary embolism after varicose vein surgery? Phlebology 2005; 20:175–6.

8. Merchant RF, Pichot O, Closure Study Group. Long-term outcomes of endovenous radiofrequency obliteration of saphenous reflux as a treatment for superficial venous insufficiency. J Vasc Surg 2005; 42:502–9.
9. Mundy L, Merlin TL, Fitridge RA, Hiller JE. Systematic review of endovenous laser treatment for varicose veins. Br J Surg 2005; 92:1189–94.
10. Wollmann JC. The history of sclerosing foams. Dermatol Surg 2004; 30:694–703.
11. Schadeck M, Allaert F. Echotomographie de la sclérose. Phlébologie 1991; 44:111–30.
12. Vin F. Echo-sclérothérapie de la veine saphène externe. Phlébologie 1991; 44:79–84.
13. Kanter A, Thibault P. Dermatol Saphenofemoral incompetence treated by ultrasound-guided sclerotherapy. Surg 1996; 22:648–52.
14. Orbach EJ. The thrombogenic activity of foam of a synthetic anionic detergent (sodium tetradecyl sulfate NNR). Angiology 1950; 1:237–43.
15. Cabrera Garrido JR, Cabrera Garcia Olmedo JR, Garcia Olmedo Dominguez MA. Nuevo metodo de esclerosis en las varices tronculares. Pathologica Vasculares 1993; 1:55–72.
16. Cabrera Garrido JR, Cabrera Garcia-Olmedo JR, Garcia-Olmedo Dominguez MA. Elargissement des limites de la schlérothérapie: noveaux produits sclérosants. Phlébologie 1997; 50:181–8.
17. Monfreux A. Traitement sclérosant des troncs saphènies et leurs collatérales de gros calibre par le méthode mus. Phlébologie 1997; 50:351–3.
18. Sadoun S, Benigni JP. Télangiectasies et varices réticulaires traitement par la mousse d'aetoxisclérol à 0.25% présentation d'une étude pilote. Phlébologie 1999; 52:283–90.
19. Tessari L. Nouvelle technique d'obtention de la scléro-mousse. Phlébologie 2000; 53:129.
20. Frullini A. New technique in producing sclerosing foam in a disposable syringe. Dermatol Surg 2000; 26:705–6.
21. Flückinger P. Nicht-operative retrograde Varizenverödung mit Varsylschaum. Schweizer Med Wochenschrift 1956; 86:1368–70.
22. Henriet JP. Expérience durant trois années de la mousse de polidocanol dans le traitement des varices réticulaires et des varicosités. Phlébologie 1999; 52:277–82.
23. Benigni JP, Sadoun S, Thirion V, Sica M, Demagny A, Chahim M. Télangiectasies et varices réticulaires traitement par la mousse d'aetoxisclérol à 0.25% présentation d'une étude pilote. Phlébologie 1999; 52:283–90.
24. Biegeleisen K, Neilsen RD, O'Shaughnessy A. Inadvertent intra-arterial injection complicating ordinary and ultrasound-guided sclerotherapy. J Dermatol Surg Oncol 1993; 19:953–8.
25. Breu FX, Guggenbichler S. European consensus meeting on foam sclerotherapy, April, 4–6, 2003, Tegernsee, Germany. Dermatol Surg 2004; 30:709–17.
26. Cavezzi A, Frullini A, Ricci S, Tessari L. Treatment of varicose veins by foam sclerotherapy: two clinical series. Phlebology 2002; 17:13–8.
27. Yamaki T, Nozaki M, Iwasaka S. Comparative study of duplex-guided foam sclerotherapy and duplex-guided liquid sclerotherapy for the treatment of superficial venous insufficiency. Dermatol Surg 2004; 30:718–22.
28. Frullini A, Cavezzi A. Sclerosing foam in the treatment of varicose veins and telangiectases: history and analysis of safety and complications. Dermatol Surg 2002; 28:11–5.
29. Barrett JM, Allen B, Ockelford A, Goldman MP. Microfoam ultrasound-guided sclerotherapy of varicose veins in 100 legs. Dermatol Surg 2004; 30:6–12.
30. Bountouroglou DG, Azzam M, Kakkos SK, Pathmarajah M, Young P, Geroulakos G. Ultrasound-guided foam sclerotherapy combined with sapheno-femoral ligation compared to surgical treatment of varicose veins: early results of a randomised controlled trial. Eur J Vasc Endovasc Surg 2006; 31:93–100.
31. Wright D, Gobin JP, Bradbury AW, et al. Varisolve® polidocanol microfoam compared with surgery or sclerotherapy in the management of varicose veins in the presence of trunk vein incompetence: European randomized controlled trial. Phlebology 2006; 21:180–90.
32. Darke SG, Baker SJ. Ultrasound-guided foam sclerotherapy for the treatment of varicose veins. Br J Surg 2006; 93:969–74.
33. Coleridge Smith P. Chronic venous disease treated by ultrasound guided foam sclerotherapy. Eur J Vasc Endovasc Surg 2006; 32:577–83.
34. Bergan J, Pascarella L, Mekenas L. Venous disorders: treatment with sclerosant foam. J Cardiovasc Surg (Torino) 2006; 47:9–18.
35. Kakkos SK, Bountouroglou DG, Azzam M, Kalodiki E, Daskalopoulos M, Geroulakos G. Effectiveness and safety of ultrasound-guided foam sclerotherapy for recurrent varicose veins: immediate results. J Endovasc Ther 2006; 13:357–64.
36. Guex JJ, Allaert FA, Gillet JL, Chleir F. Immediate and midterm complications of sclerotherapy: report of a prospective multicenter registry of 12,173 sclerotherapy sessions. Dermatol Surg 2005; 31:123–8.
37. Holmes DR, Jr. Strokes and holes and headaches: are they a package deal? Lancet 2004; 364:1840–2.
38. Forlee MV, Grouden M, Moore DJ, Shanik G. Stroke after varicose vein foam injection sclerotherapy. J Vasc Surg 2006; 43:162–4.

54 | Inferior Vena Cava Filters

Graham Plant
Department of Interventional Radiology, North Hampshire Hospital, Basingstoke, Hampshire, U.K.

ROLE OF INFERIOR VENA CAVAL (IVC) FILTERS

Natural History of Venous Thromboembolism

The sole aim of inferior vena caval (IVC) filters is to prevent pulmonary emboli (PE) reaching the heart and lungs from the drainage area of the IVC, which includes the deep veins of the legs, the deep veins of the pelvis, the ovarian and renal veins. The aim of use is to diminish the mortality and morbidity of pulmonary embolism.

Historically PE have been associated with a significant mortality. In the prospective investigation of pulmonary embolism diagnosis study trial, 8.3% of patients who had been diagnosed with PE and treated appropriately had recurrent emboli. Half of these occurred within one week and a third of these patients died of their PE (1).

The natural history of venous thromboembolism reveals that 90% of PE are not fatal. If untreated, however, patients with significant PE are at higher risk of death and one-fourth will die within two weeks. In a group of patients classified as having severe PE one-fourth will recur and with milder PE, 10% recurred within three months (2).

These figures are confirmed by Yonezawa who showed that 30% of patients with recurrent PE would die without therapy though this was decreased to 8% if the patients were anticoagulated and to less to 1% if a filter was inserted (3).

The guidelines issued by the Cardiovascular and Interventional Radiological Society of Europe (CIRSE) and the Society of Interventional Radiology (SIR) indicate that between 400,000 and 630,000 cases of nonfatal PE occur each year in Europe and America, causing between 50,000 and 200,000 deaths (4,5).

History and Therapy for Pulmonary Embolus

In order to diminish the epidemic of deaths due to PE, IVC ligation was first performed in 1893, anticoagulation was introduced in 1960 and the first IVC filter, the Mobin-Udin filter, was devised in 1967. The early filters were inserted surgically with percutaneous devices becoming available in 1975 (6,7).

The natural history of venous thromboembolism has been most extensively studied in the postoperative period. It is believed that thrombosis starts in the valve cusps in the calf, often intraoperatively and in the immediate postoperative period. Of these calf deep vein thromboses (DVTs), approximately half resolve within 72 hours but one in six will reach the proximal vessels and approximately half of these will become clinical DVTs (8,9).

Ninety percent of symptomatic DVT are proximal and 90% of these will start in the calf. Without anticoagulation, between 25% and 33% of symptomatic calf DVT will extend proximally. If untreated a patient with proximal DVT has a 50% chance of having a symptomatic pulmonary embolus within four months. The current evidence base favors subcutaneous low molecular weight heparin and three to six months of oral anticoagulation for the treatment of isolated DVT.

There are some risks to stopping anticoagulation after this period. If the patient has a continuing risk factor there is a 10% chance of recurrent DVT at the cessation of anticoagulation. If the risk factor for which the patient was anticoagulated was temporary, this figure drops to 3%. The patients with idiopathic thrombosis are at greater a risk than those with cancer, who, in turn, are at greater risk than those with temporary risk factors (4,10). If patients with deep vein thrombosis are treated conventionally with warfarin they have a 4% risk of recurrence on treatment during the first three months (this risk is increased three fold if the patient has cancer).

There are of course risks and costs to anticoagulation treatment, Warfarin is associated with a risk of a major bleed of 4.4% to 8.2% and will cause death at a rate of nine deaths per 100 patient years. Heparin is associated with a rate of major bleeds of 3 to 5.3 per 1000 patient days (11).

Indications for IVC Filters

The guidelines issued in a joint document by CIRSE and SIR (4,12) suggest that absolute indications for filters include patients with pulmonary embolism or thrombus in the IVC, iliac or femoral regions who also have:

- Contra indications to anticoagulation
- A complication of anticoagulation
- Failure of anticoagulation

Additional relative indications in selected patients include:

- Massive PE with a residual risk
- Free floating IVC or iliofemoral clot
- Severe cardiovascular disease and deep vein thrombosis
- Poor compliance with drug therapy
- Severe trauma
- High-risk patients including prophylactic insertion for protection prior to surgery

Large volumes of clot in the IVC and proximal iliac veins are regarded in some centers, including ours, as an indication for IVC filters. The term free floating clot has been coined to indicate clot that is only secured distally, and therefore has a higher rate of embolization. This author has always found differentiating adherent from free floating clot to be difficult or risky.

There have only been limited studies in these patients; however, Radomsky (13) showed that in a small series of patients with clot in the cava, of whom two thirds were defined as free floating, one-half presented with a pulmonary embolism (as opposed to 15% of patients with fixed thrombus). In patients with IVC thrombus who were treated with heparin, 27% of patients with free floating clot had a subsequent PE as opposed to 17% of patients with a fixed clot.

Pacuret (14) reported a group of 95 patients with DVT who had clot in the IVC. Sixty percent had free-floating clot, 25% had occlusive thrombus in the cava. The patients were treated with heparin or low molecular weight heparin and warfarin. Two thirds of the patients had presented with a pulmonary embolism, but the recurrent pulmonary embolism rate on anticoagulation was 3% (in patients with occlusive clot pulmonary embolism occurred in half and the recurrent pulmonary embolism rate was 3.7%).

The CIRSE/SIR guidelines for suprarenal placement suggest that filters should be inserted suprarenally in cases with:

- clot in the renal vein
- high IVC clot
- in patients who are pregnant (or with child bearing potential)
- if there is gonadal vein clot
- in the case of relevant anatomical variants (see below)

Technical Aspects of IVC Filters

IVC filters can be inserted from a variety of sites. The author's personal preference is to use the right common femoral vein unless there is evidence of clot between the right femoral vein and the cava. Insertion from the left common femoral is equally straightforward. If filter retrieval is being carried out this will almost always be via the neck, which may lead one to trying to avoid a jugular route in the first instance.

In our institution, the practice is to puncture the common femoral vein with a 6-F sidewinder catheter that has its primary curve reformed in the right atrium before being withdrawn into the cava. The catheter is withdrawn to engage and enter the right and left renal veins and their position is marked with a metallic clip on the patient's drape. The position of the iliac bifurcation is also identified by drawing the sidewinder down onto the bifurcation and this too is marked with a metallic clip.

Anatomical variants (see below) are rarely an issue; however, it may be worth withdrawing the catheter down the lateral aspects of the IVC to see if it will engage any large veins (which may be aberrant renal veins or may represent large paralumbar veins). These are not a problem but may require consideration when deciding where to place the filter.

The upper end of the delivery catheter is placed in the upper common iliac vein or low IVC, and a cavagram obtained. This allows sizing and also an additional check as to any defects in the contrast column created by inflow from large veins. The IVC filter, mounted on its delivery system, is inserted into the sheath, taking standard precautions to avoid air embolization. The filter is positioned in an appropriate place within the cava, and then deployed according to protocol. Different devices have differing amounts of control over this process, but in the majority of cases the filter will release from the delivery device, spring open and attach itself to the caval walls without angulation or migration (Fig. 1).

Under direct visualization the delivery system is withdrawn, ensuring that there is no snagging of the filter on the delivery device. A further cavagram is performed to confirm the position of the filter within the cava and its relationship to the walls. It is our practice to arrange an abdominal film the following day, both to act as a standardized baseline for follow-up and for also to see if there is any migration.

The choice of position of the filter has been source of some discussion. It is our practice to try and deploy the filter infrarenally with its tip level with the renal veins. One should try and avoid the fixation points of the device overlapping or entering the renal veins or other large veins entering the cava as this can cause the filter to tip.

The length of cava between the junction of the common iliacs and the insertion of the renal vein is usually long enough for all current devices. If, however, an anatomical variant

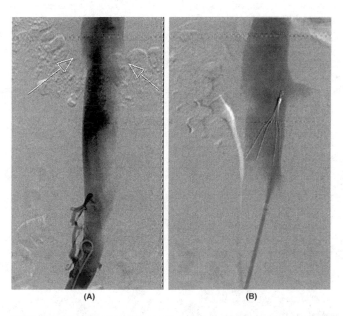

(A)   (B)

FIGURE 1 Insertion of a filter in the infrarenal inferior vena caval (IVC). (**A**) This cavogram shows a patent IVC and filling defects at the level of the renal veins (*arrows*), which signifies inflowing blood not opacified by contrast. The filter should be placed below this level. (**B**) The filter has been successfully deployed below the renal veins.

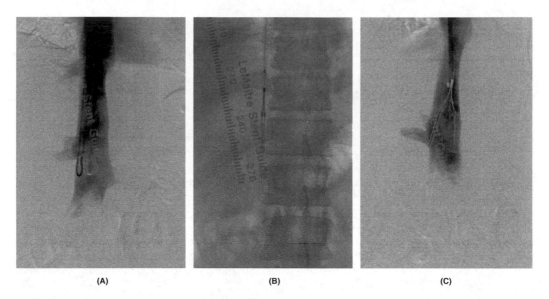

(A)   (B)   (C)

FIGURE 2   Placement of a filter above the renal veins. This patient had thrombus in the infrarenal inferior vena caval (IVC) up to the level of the renal veins. The upper veins on the right of the IVC are the hepatic veins and the vein to the right of the catheter tip is the vein draining the caudate lobe. (**A**) Cavogram prior to filter insertion. A small filling defect is visible inferiorly, which is consistent with thrombus. (**B**) A filter is advanced within its delivery sheath to the IVC above the thrombus and the renal veins. (**C**) A cavogram after insertion of the filter, which was deployed above the renal veins at the level of the caudate lobe vein.

makes the infrarenal vena cava too short, or if there is thrombus in the infrarenal IVC, then placement in the suprarenal vena cava segment is safe (Fig. 2). There is no evidence of significant risk associated with suprarenal caval placement although practical considerations, including consideration of where the cava may be surgically compressed during an operation, should be taken into account. In pregnant women, who will usually have a retrievable filter inserted, suprarenal placement is preferred (4,15,16).

Most of the deployment devices for jugular insertion have the same or increased security associated with the release of the filter via this route. Because the suprarenal IVC opens directly into the right atrium one is particularly careful about the positioning and with those devices that have the ability to release the filter legs without releasing the filter completely it may be appropriate to check the placement before the final filter release.

Deployment Problems

Deployment problems are rare but can usually be recognized and resolved during the procedure. They include the filter not releasing completely from the delivery device or becoming entangled with part of the delivery device. This can usually be resolved by judicious manipulation.

Some patients experience pain when the filter is released. This appears to occur in about 10% of patients and may be associated with either increased sensitivity of the caval wall or possibly a degree of phlebitis. This is very rarely a problem and if there are no other causes it usually disappears within 24 hours with conventional oral analgesics.

Anatomical Difficulties

Anomalies to consider include left sided duplication of the cava; these usually rejoin the main channel via the left renal vein although other configurations are possible. In these cases, consideration should be given to placing a filter in the suprarenal cava or alternatively two filters can be deployed one in each infrarenal cava.

Variants of insertion of renal veins can produce difficulties in assessing the position at which the filter should be deployed. As long as the anchoring device is not negated by tipping or angulation related to deployment across the vein entrance it is rarely a problem. The filter can usually be placed above a low insertion of a renal vein or possibly in the space between the main renal vein and a low inserting vein.

Paralumbar veins can pose difficulties, particularly in patients who have a degree of occlusion of the cava. In this instance paralumbar collateral veins tend to open and guidewires and catheters being passed up the iliacs may engage or pass into these. On occasions the cephalad tip of a filter will angle into the mouth of one of the tributaries of the cava which may be the cause of pain or cause difficulties in retrieval in the case of optional or temporary filters.

Angulation of IVC Filters

With some of the earlier devices, particularly the original Greenfield filter, angulation beyond 15° resulted in widening of the effective inter-strut distance and therefore diminution of clot trapping ability. Most modern filters are designed so that this does not happen and angulation, per se, is very rarely of clinical significance. It may cause problems in terms of retrieval of filters if the tip of the filter lies against the wall (Fig. 3). This can result in the tip becoming endothelialized and therefore, difficult to pick up, rendering retrieval problematical.

Caval Size

The majority of cava, particularly the infrarenal portion, have a maximum diameter of less than 2.8 cm. In less than 1% of cases the cava may be larger than this in which case consideration should be given to placing a specific device (the birds nest filter is available for large cavas up to a diameter of 35 mm). Most other filters have a maximum size of between 28 and 30 mm. In cases where filtration is necessary but these larger devices are not available or appropriate it may be possible to deploy two conventional filters, one in each common iliac. It should be noted that the suprarenal cava is usually 10% to 15% larger than the infrarenal portion.

Choice of IVC Filter

There are multiple devices on the market. These can be most usefully divided into those that are designed for permanent use and those that are retrievable. In the latter group, the term optional

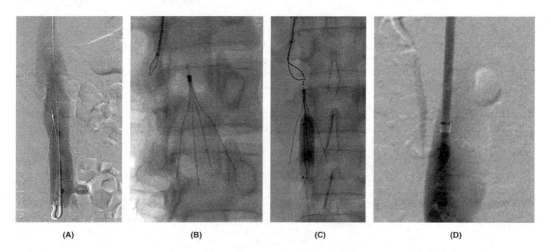

(A)   (B)   (C)   (D)

FIGURE 3 Retrieval of a filter. (**A**) Prior to retrieval of a filter, a cavogram should be performed to ensure that the filter is clear of thrombus. (**B**) A snare is advanced from a jugular vein access with the aim of catching the small hook on the top of this Gunther Tulip filter. However, the filter is tilted a little which is causing difficulty in snaring the filter. (**C**) A balloon has been passed from a femoral vein access into the filter straightening it, which enables the operator to snare the filer. (**D**) The snared filter has been pulled into the sheath and removed.

filter has been coined to indicate a filter that can be left in permanently but which can be retrieved safely at a variable time after insertion.

These optional filters have come to the market more recently than some of the permanent filters and may have additional advantages such as magnetic resonance imaging compatibility. In contrast to these newer devices, some of the longer established filters have the advantage of longer follow-up (17–20).

An ideal filter will be easy to insert, have a good safety profile with no or minimal complications, be stable in a large cava, be safe for long-term use, but be retrievable, show no evidence of migration, perforation nor IVC occlusion (except on the occasion when a large clot is caught and held by the filter in the IVC) (21–29).

Adjunctive Medication

The need for adjunctive medication, particularly anticoagulation, reflects the need of the primary disease. The presence of the filter itself is not an indication for anticoagulation. In the majority of cases in whom contra indications do not exist, we would prefer the patient to be anticoagulated for at least 12 weeks, which is usually subsumed within the proposed length of time of the treatment of the primary condition.

One very important point is that patients who have been on long-term anticoagulation and have a filter inserted, perhaps for prophylaxis prior to major surgery should be reestablished on their anticoagulation as soon as possible after surgery, probably within a few days. If this does not occur they are at significant risk of developing further deep vein thrombosis that may embolize and may lead to caval occlusion by clot, propagation of clot through the filter and pulmonary embolism.

Clinical Efficacy

The longest follow-up in the world is that reported by Greenfield and Proctor on the Greenfield filters (30–43). In our institution, we have followed up every filter inserted, with over 95% of patients followed until death or to the current day, with regular clinical assessments, abdominal x-rays and Doppler ultrasound examinations. This now extends to 20 years.

The recurrent pulmonary embolism rate in our institution is 2.5% including 2% fatal PE. Five percent suffered IVC occlusion, all of which have been asymptomatic. The cumulative DVT rate is 10.4%, i.e., 10.4% of patients in our long-term follow-up series have had a DVT since the insertion of their filter.

These figures are similar to those that have been reported in other long term series. Greenfield reported a pulmonary embolism rate of 1.5% and occlusion of 2.3% (32), Athanassoulis (44) in a 26 year single center series reported a recurrent pulmonary embolism rate of 5.6% and 2.7% occlusion and Nicholson reported a recurrent pulmonary embolism rate of 1.3% and an occlusion of 4.7% in a five year series following up Birds Nest filters (45).

An alternative view has been championed by Decousus (46,47), who suggested that although PE are decreased in the short term, there is an excess of deep vein thrombosis caused by the presence of filters.

COMPLICATIONS OF IVC FILTERS

The CIRSE/SIR filter guidelines suggest the following ranges of complications and a proposed guideline as to the maximum complication rate that should be anticipated (Table 1) (4,48).

TABLE 1   CIRSE/SIR Filter Guidelines

Complication	Incidence (%)	Guidelines (%)
Death	0.12	<1
Recurrent pulmonary embolism	0.5–6	5
IVC occlusion	2–30	10
Filter embolization	2–5	2
Access vein thrombosis	6	1

Of these complications migration or embolization are the biggest fears, with retrieval from the heart and pulmonary circulation often causing death or requiring surgery. Other rarer complications include bleeding due to perforation (49,50).

TEMPORARY FILTRATION

The position of temporary filtration has become clearer in recent years. The term temporary filter was originally used to denote a filter that it was only possible to use temporarily, often being attached permanently to an indwelling catheter. More recently the term optional filters has been used for filters that can be used for temporary filtration but are deployed in the same way as permanent filters and which can be left in place permanently if the patient's condition dictates. These optional or retrievable filters are now becoming the norm as manufacturers produce variations of these devices.

The retrieval window is important and the manufacturers are actively pursuing new designs that decrease endothelialization of the filter, without increasing risks of migration or perforation. In addition there have been attempts to elongate the retrieval window by moving the filter prior to extraction (51).

The use of the original temporary filters, permanently attached to indwelling catheters should be discouraged as they are associated with a high incidence of complications, particularly thrombosis and infection. The use of these devices is now uncommon and the optional or retrievable permanent filter is now usually used instead (52).

The place of temporary filtration includes use in patients with a short, defined period of risk especially in the case of younger patients and patients with benign disease. A defined period of risk may be centerd around an operation or during pregnancy.

The major problem with removal comes with difficulties in trying to engage or snare the upper part of the filter, which if tilted may have become endotheliolized to the caval wall. Once it has been snared it is often possible to slide a sheath down the outside with a view to disengaging the legs. This is easier with some designs than others and if significant endothelialization has occurred then a variety of manoeuvres and considerable time may be required in order to disengage the device from the caval wall (53).

CONCLUSION

Extensive clinical experience indicates that patients who have a filter inserted have a very low probability of suffering a pulmonary embolus. Filters are devices with an undoubted benefit in appropriate patients. They are associated with a small incidence of complications, although some of these are life threatening. Used appropriately these devices improve patient survival and quality of life.

REFERENCES

1. Worsley GF, Alavi A. Comprehensive analysis of the results of the PIOPED Study. Prospective Investigation of Pulmonary Embolism Diagnosis Study. J Nucl Med 1995; 36(12):2380–7.
2. Kearon C. Long-term management of patients after venous thromboembolism. Circulation 2004; 110:I-10—18.
3. Yonezawa K, Yokoo N, Yamaguchi T. Effectiveness of an inferior vena caval filter as a preventive measure against pulmonary thromboembolism after abdominal surgery. Surg Today 1999; 29:821–4.
4. Kaufman JA, Kinney TB, Streiff MB, et al. Guidelines for the use of retrievable and convertible vena cava filters: report from the Society of Interventional Radiology multidisciplinary consensus conference. J Vasc Interv Radiol 2006; 17(3):449–59.
5. Kinney TB. Update on inferior vena cava filters. J Vasc Interv Radiol 2003; 14:425–40.
6. Dodson MG, Mobin-Uddin K, O'Leary JA. Intracaval umbrella-filter for prevention of recurrent pulmonary embolism. South Med J 1971; 64(8):1017–8.
7. Crane C. The Mobin-Uddin inferior vena caval filter. Arch Surg 1971; 103(6):661.
8. Stein PD, Henry JW, Relyea B. Untreated patients with pulmonary embolism. Outcome, clinical, and laboratory assessment. Chest 1995; 107(4):931–5 (see comment).
9. Henry JW, Relyea B, Stein PD. Continuing risk of thromboemboli among patients with normal pulmonary angiograms. Chest 1995; 107(5):1375–8.

10. Dalen JE, Alpert JS. Natural history of pulmonary embolism. Prog Cardiovasc Dis 1975; 17(4):259–70.
11. Levine MN, Raskob G, Beyth RJ, et al. Hemorrhagic complications of anticoagulant treatment: The Seventh ACCP Conference on Antithrombotic and Thrombolytic Therapy. Chest 2004; 126:287S–310.
12. Siskin G, Kwan B. Inferior vena cava filters. (Accessed November 2006 at http://www.emedicine.com/Radio/topic762.htm)
13. Radomski JS, Jarrell BE, Carabasi RA, et al. Risk of pulmonary embolus with inferior vena cava thrombosis. Am Surg 1987; 53(2):97–101.
14. Pacouret G, Alison D, Pottier JM, et al. Free-floating thrombus and embolic risk in patients with angiographically confirmed proximal deep vein thrombosis: preliminary results from a long-term follow-up. Arch Intern Med 1997; 157:305–8.
15. De Swiet M. Review article: management of pulmonary embolus in pregnancy. Eur Heart J 1999; 20:1378–85.
16. Ganguli S, Tham JC, Komlos F, et al. Fracture and migration of a suprarenal inferior vena cava filter in a pregnant patient. J Vasc Interv Radiol 2006; 17(10): 1707–11.
17. Ponchon M, Goffette P, Hainaut P. Temporary vena caval filtration. Preliminary clinical experience with removable vena caval filters. Acta Clinica Belgica 1999; 54(4):223–8.
18. Zwaan M, Lorch H, Kulke C, et al. Clinical experience with temporary vena caval filters. J Vasc Interv Radiol 1998; 9(4):594–601.
19. Neuerburg JM, Gunther RW, Vorwerk D, et al. Results of a multicenter study of the retrievable Tulip vena cava filter: early clinical experience. Cardiovasc Intervent Radiol 1997; 20(1):10–6.
20. Millward SF, Oliva VL, Bell SD, et al. Günther Tulip retrievable vena cava filter: results from the registry of the Canadian Interventional Radiology Association. J Vasc Interv Radiol 2001; 12:1053–8.
21. Grande WJ, Trerotola SO, Reilly PM, et al. Experience with the recovery filter as a retrievable inferior vena cava filter. J Vasc Interv Radiol 2005; 16(9):1189–93.
22. Rousseau H, Perreault P, Otal P, et al. The 6-F nitinol TrapEase inferior vena cava filter: results of a prospective multicenter trial. J Vasc Interv Radiol 2001; 12:299–304.
23. Reekers JA, Hoogeveen YL, Wijnands M, et al. Evaluation of the retrievability of the OptEase IVC filter in an animal model. J Vasc Interv Radiol 2004; 15:261–7.
24. de Gregorio MA, Gamboa P, Gimeno MJ, et al. The Gunther Tulip retrievable filter: prolonged temporary filtration by repositioning within the inferior vena cava. J Vasc Interv Radiol 2003; 14:1259–65.
25. Bruckheimer E, Judelman AG, Bruckheimer SD, et al. In vitro evaluation of a retrievable low-profile nitinol vena cava filter. J Vasc Interv Radiol 2003; 14:469–74.
26. Oliva VL, Szatmari F, Giroux M-F, et al. The Jonas study: evaluation of the retrievability of the Cordis OptEase inferior vena cava filter. J Vasc Interv Radiol 2005; 16:1439–45.
27. Roehm JO, Jr., Gianturco C, Barth MH, et al. Percutaneous transcatheter filter for the inferior vena cava. A new device for treatment of patients with pulmonary embolism. Radiology 1984; 150(1):255–7.
28. Roehm JO, Jr. The bird's nest filter: a new percutaneous transcatheter inferior vena cava filter. J Vasc Surg 1984; 1(3):498–501.
29. Roehm JO, Jr., Johnsrude IS, Barth MH, et al. The bird's nest inferior vena cava filter: progress report. Radiology 1988; 168(3):745–9.
30. Greenfield LJ, Michna BA. Twelve-year clinical experience with the Greenfield vena caval filter. Surgery 1988; 104(4):706–12.
31. Greenfield LJ, Cho KJ, Proctor M, et al. Results of a multicenter study of the modified hook-titanium Greenfield filter. J Vasc Surg 1991; 14(3):253–7.
32. Greenfield LJ, Proctor MC. Recurrent thromboembolism in patients with vena cava filters. J Vasc Surg 2001; 33(3):510–4.
33. Greenfield LJ, Proctor MC, Saluja A. Clinical results of Greenfield filter use in patients with cancer. Cardiovasc Surg 1997; 5(2):145–9.
34. Greenfield LJ, Proctor MC, Michaels AJ, et al. Prophylactic vena caval filters in trauma: the rest of the story. J Vasc Surg 2000; 32(3):490–5 (Discussion 496–7).
35. Greenfield LJ, Proctor MC. Suprarenal filter placement. J Vasc Surg 1998; 28(3):432–8 (Discussion 438).
36. Greenfield LJ, Cho KJ, Proctor MC, et al. Late results of suprarenal Greenfield vena cava filter placement. Arch Surg 1992; 127(8):969–73.
37. Greenfield LJ, McCurdy JR, Brown PP, et al. A new intracaval filter permitting continued flow and resolution of emboli. Surgery 1973; 73(4):599–606.
38. Greenfield LJ, Zocco J, Wilk J, et al. Clinical experience with the Kim-Ray Greenfield vena caval filter. Ann Surg 1977; 185(6):692–8.
39. Greenfield LJ, Proctor MC. Twenty-year clinical experience with the Greenfield filter. Cardiovasc Surg 1995; 3(2):199–205.
40. Greenfield LJ, Proctor MC, Cho KJ, et al. Extended evaluation of the titanium Greenfield vena caval filter. J Vasc Surg 1994; 20(3):458–64 (Discussion 464–5).

41. Greenfield LJ, Savin MA. Comparison of titanium and stainless steel, Greenfield vena caval filters. Surgery 1989; 106(5):820–8.
42. Greenfield LJ, Proctor MC. Experimental embolic capture by asymmetric Greenfield filters. J Vasc Surg 1992; 16(3):436–43 (Discussion 443–4).
43. Greenfield LJ, Proctor MC, Cho KJ, et al. Limb asymmetry in titanium Greenfield filters: clinically significant? J Vasc Surg 1997; 26(5):770–5.
44. Athanasoulis CA, Kaufman JA, Halpern EF, et al. Inferior vena caval filters: review of a 26-year single-center clinical experience. Radiology 2000; 216(1):54–66.
45. Nicholson AA, Ettles DF, Paddon AJ, et al. Long-term follow-up of the Bird's Nest IVC Filter. Clin Radiol 1999; 54(11):759–64.
46. Decousus H, Leizorovicz A, Parent F, et al. A clinical trial of vena caval filters in the prevention of pulmonary embolism in patients with proximal deep-vein thrombosis. Prevention du Risque d'Embolie Pulmonaire par Interruption Cave Study Group. N Engl J Med 1998; 338(7):409–15.
47. The PREPIC Study Group. Eight-year follow-up of patients with permanent vena cava filters in the prevention of pulmonary embolism: the PREPIC (Prevention du Risque d'Embolie Pulmonaire par Interruption Cave). Circulation 2005; 112(3):416–22.
48. Ray CE, Kaufman JA. Complications of inferior vena cava filters. Abdom Imaging 1996; 21:368–74.
49. Mansour JC, Lee FT, Jr., Chen H, et al. Chronic abdominal pain and upper gastrointestinal bleeding due to duodenal perforation caused by migrated inferior vena cava filter: a case report. Vasc Endovasc Surg 2004; 38(4):381–4.
50. The MAUDE database. (Accessed November 2006 at http://www.accessdata.fda.gov/scripts/cdrh/cfdocs/cfMAUDE/search.cfm)
51. Binkert CA, Sasadeusz K, Stavropoulos SW. Retrievability of the recovery vena cava filter after dwell times longer than 180 days. J Vasc Interv Radiol 2006; 17(2):299–302.
52. Scholz KH, Just M, Buchwald AB, et al. Experiences with temporary vena cava filters in 114 at-risk patients with thrombosis or thromboembolism. Dtsch Med Wochenschr 1999; 124(11):307–13.
53. Stavropoulos SW, Solomon JA, Trerotola SO. Wall-embedded recovery inferior vena cava filters: imaging features and technique for removal. J Vasc Interv Radiol 2006; 17(2):379–82.

55 | Percutaneous Interventions for Pulmonary Embolism

Renan Uflacker
Department of Radiology, Division of Vascular and Interventional Radiology,
Medical University of South Carolina, Charleston, South Carolina, U.S.A.

Venous thromboembolism includes deep venous thrombosis and pulmonary embolism (PE). PE is the third most common cardiovascular disease and a leading cause of death (1,2). The natural history of PE is not well known and most episodes go undetected, despite recent technological advancements (3). The true incidence is unknown, though PE is a significant cause of morbidity and mortality in hospitalized patients (3–5).

The immediate mortality rate related to PE is less than 8% when the condition is recognized and treated promptly. Of the 70% of undiagnosed patients, the mortality rate approaches 30% (1,3,6). If appropriate therapy is introduced, mortality may decrease but the overall mortality has not significantly changed over 30 years. Massive PE causes a rapid increase in pulmonary arterial pressure resulting from restriction of blood flow. Respiratory changes include bronchoconstriction, increased dead space, and decreased pulmonary surfactant (7). If there is underlying cardiopulmonary disease, these risks are higher, requiring more aggressive treatment than anticoagulation (8).

Pulmonary arteriography remains the gold standard in diagnosing PE, but several other imaging modalities and blood tests have been used (3). No single noninvasive test is both sensitive and specific and choice of test should consider the probability of PE and patient characteristics (9). The most promising new technology is fast multislice spiral computed tomography angiogram (10), though imaging quality is limited by patients' inability to hold their breath (11). Cardiac troponin T monitoring identifies a high-risk group of normotensive patients with acute severe PE (12).

Traditional therapeutic options are anticoagulation, systemic thrombolysis, and surgical thrombectomy in more severe cases. Recently, several minimally invasive procedures have been introduced, including catheter-directed thrombolysis, percutaneous embolectomy, embolus fragmentation techniques, pulmonary artery stent placement or a combination of such techniques (2,13–16). Successful management of acute massive PE requires prompt risk stratification and decisive, early intervention (Table 1). At least one of the described criteria must be present to justify more aggressive treatment (14,16), in particular involvement of 50% or more of the pulmonary circulation.

TABLE 1 Risk Stratification and Indications for Aggressive Intervention to Treat Massive Pulmonary Embolism

Arterial hypotension (<90 mmHg systolic or drop of >40 mmHg)
Cardiogenic shock with peripheral hypoperfusion and hypoxia
Circulatory collapse with need for cardiopulmonary resuscitation
Echocardiographic findings indicating right ventricular afterload stress and/or pulmonary hypertension
Diagnosis of precapillary pulmonary hypertension (mean PAP >20 mmHg in presence of normal PAP occlusion pressures)
Widened arterial-alveolar O_2 gradient, >50 mmHg
Clinically severe pulmonary embolism with a contraindication to anticoagulation or thrombolytic therapy

At least one of the above criteria must be present (2,12).
Abbreviation: PAP, pulmonary artery pressure.

Assessment of pulmonary involvement and response has been performed in various ways, including Miller's "index of severity" of pulmonary artery obstruction (Fig. 1) (17). In cases of massive PE, the use of percutaneous embolectomy, catheter-directed thrombolysis and fragmentation techniques is very attractive, owing to their capacity to rapidly reestablish pulmonary blood flow, especially if systemic thrombolysis fails.

ANTICOAGULATION

Initial intravenous (IV) administration of heparin is the therapy of choice for all forms of PE.

There is consensus regarding the goals of anticoagulation therapy in pulmonary thromboembolism:

1. Immediate inhibition of the growth of the thromboembolus
2. Promotion of thromboembolic resolution
3. Prevention of recurrence

Heparin achieves the first goal, encouraging the second by allowing fibrinolytic dissolution to be achieved unopposed by thrombus growth, and it assists in preventing recurrence (18). Heparin therapy is directed at the source of embolism rather than treatment of the embolus. If the patient survives the initial episode with no treatment, there is an 18% to 30% chance of recurrent lethal PE (1,2,19). Anticoagulation may assist in reducing PE recurrence by reducing propagation of the venous thrombus in the lower extremities (1,19,20). Propagation of thrombus in the pulmonary artery may be also reduced.

The most common complication associated with heparin anticoagulation is bleeding (1.6–14%) (21). Recent evidence suggests this reduced with the use of low-molecular weight heparin (22–29).

There is evidence that severe heparin-induced thrombocytopenia (HIT) (platelet count <100,000/microliters) occurs in 1% to 10% of patients (30,31). Argatroban is currently approved in the U.S., as an injectable heparin substitute for the prophylaxis or treatment of patients with HIT (32,33).

Full anticoagulation with heparin should be maintained for 7 to 10 days. Oral anticoagulation should be started three to four days before heparin is discontinued. Oral anticoagulation with warfarin is typically used for three to six months, targeting an International Normalized Ratio range of 2.0 to 3.0.

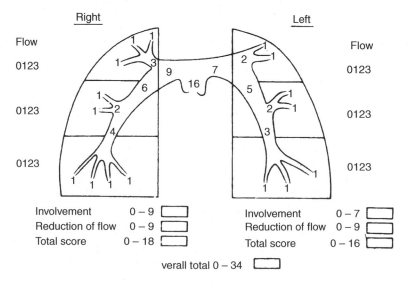

FIGURE 1 The lung arterial segments, used to grade severity of embolism on angiography before and after thrombolytic therapy or mechanical thrombectomy. Occlusion of segments and reduction of flow were scored separately. *Source*: From Ref. 17.

SYSTEMIC THROMBOLYSIS

Because anticoagulation alone does not treat the PE, there have been several trials of IV thrombolysis (34,35), demonstrating a more rapid clot lysis, reduction in pulmonary hypertension and improvement in lung perfusion scans compared with heparin alone (Fig. 2). Sometimes there is clinical improvement without significant improvement in pulmonary artery perfusion (Fig. 3). The place of thrombolytic therapy in the management of PE still remains to be defined. More recent, nonrandomized studies showed improvement of one-year survival (20) and pulmonary hemodynamics (36) after thrombolysis. A large multicenter registry of major but hemodynamically stable PE, compared thrombolysis [using recombinant tissue plasminogen activator (rt-PA), SK and UK] with heparin and demonstrated a lower mortality (4.7% vs. 11.1%), reduced PE recurrence (7.7% vs. 18.7%, $p=0.016$) but a higher incidence of major bleeding complications (21.9% vs. 7.8%) (15,37–39).

Proposed thrombolytic regimes for PE are as follows (40):

1. *Streptokinase.* 250,000 IU as a loading dose over 30 minutes followed by 100,000 IU/hr (25).
2. *Urokinase.* 2000 IU/lb loading dose over 10 minutes, followed by 2000 IU/lb/hr for 12 to 24 hours (25).
3. *rt-PA.* 100 mg, continuous peripheral IV infusion over 2 hours or 50 mg/2 hr plus an additional 40 mg/4 hr if necessary (40) or 100 mg IV over 7 hours (41).
4. *Heparin.* 5000 IU bolus followed by 1000 IU/hr (in association with the above regimens), or weight-based heparin dosing nomogram, heparin at 100 IU/kg/hr (42).

CATHETER-DIRECTED THROMBOLYSIS

Catheter-directed thrombolytic therapy with intrapulmonary artery infusion is an alternative technique advocated by many (43–45), aiming to accelerate clot lysis and pulmonary reperfusion. This requires catheterization, via femoral access, into the pulmonary artery clot, with bolus injection of thrombolytic agent followed by continuous infusion for 12 to 24 hours in association with systemic heparinization (Fig. 4). Verstraete et al. in 1988 (41) demonstrated no significant difference between peripheral IV and intrapulmonary treatment of acute massive PE with rt-PA (100 mg over a seven hours period) in a multicenter, comparative study. A prolonged infusion of rt-PA over seven hours was shown to be superior to a single infusion of 50 mg over a two-hour period. In the Verstraete study, the catheter was positioned in the main pulmonary artery, rather than close to or within the clot, as is standard today.

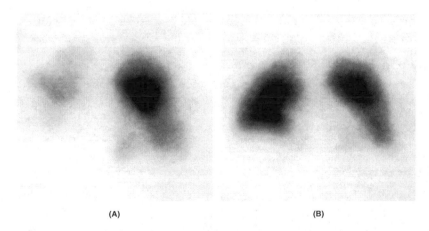

(A)   (B)

FIGURE 2   Female patient with massive pelvic vein thrombosis and pulmonary embolism. (**A**) Pulmonary perfusion scan showed occlusion of the right pulmonary artery and significant reduction of left lower lobe perfusion. Bilateral femoral vein infusion of urokinase at 100,000 IU/hr for 12 hours cleared the pelvic veins (not shown). (**B**) Follow-up lung perfusion scan showed remarkable improvement 24 hours after the infusion started.

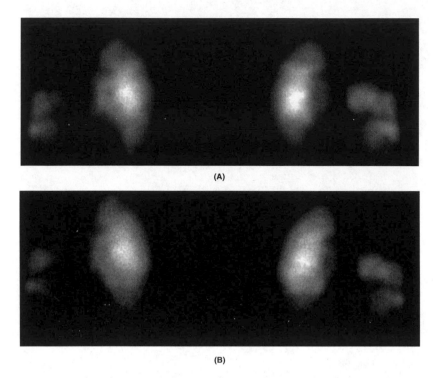

(A)

(B)

FIGURE 3   Pre- and post-thrombolytic therapy lung scan showing minimal response to peripheral thrombolysis and anticoagulation in a patient with massive pulmonary embolism. (**A**) Pretreatment perfusion lung scan (anterior and posterior views) showed massive perfusion defects in the right lung and segmental perfusion defects in the left lung. (**B**) Posttreatment lung scan (48 hours) showed mild improvement in the perfusion of the right lower lobe and left upper lobe (anterior and posterior views). Clinical improvement was observed, despite negligible perfusion improvement.

Fragmentation of a large occlusive thrombus will increase pulmonary perfusion and increase the drug/clot contact surface, accelerating the lytic process (46).

Proposed catheter-directed intrapulmonary thrombolytic regimens for PE are as follows (41,43–47):

1. *Urokinase.* Infusion of 250,000 IU/hr mixed with 2000 IU of heparin over 2 hours, followed by an infusion of 100,000 IU/hr of urokinase for 12 to 24 hours.
2. *rt-PA.* Bolus of 10 mg followed by 20 mg/hr over 2 hours (total of 50 mg), or 100 mg over 7 hours. Or a bolus of 20 mg, followed by mechanical fragmentation and 80 mg over a period of 2 hours (total of 100 mg) (13).
3. *Heparin.* Infusion of 1000 IU/hr, keeping the partial thromboplastin time at 1.5 to 2.5 times the upper normal limits (in association with the above regimens).

Fibrinogen levels should be monitored at four- to six-hour intervals, and if the level falls by 30% to 40% the infusion should be stopped or reduced. Combining thrombolysis with other techniques, such as mechanical thrombus fragmentation with pulse spray, angioplasty balloon catheter or other devices, may increase speed of lysis. Increased clot surface area contributes to improved thrombolysis in such cases (Fig. 5). Clot fragmentation causes peripheral dispersion of smaller fragments to peripheral branches, reducing pulmonary arterial pressure and increasing pulmonary flow. Though it is reasonable to assume that early reperfusion may improve long-term results, larger randomized studies will be necessary to prove this hypothesis. In a recent report using rt-PA, rapid clot lysis was obtained in 94% of patients, with pronounced lysis in 66% (47).

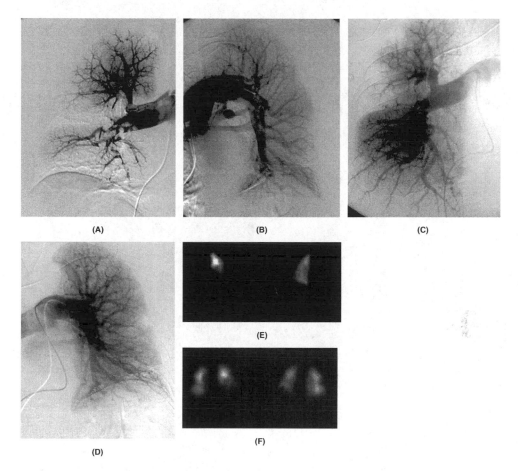

FIGURE 4 Patient with massive pulmonary embolism (PE) presented with syncope. (**A**) Massive PE of the right pulmonary artery with a large thrombus occluding most of the artery, sparing just a portion of the right upper lobe. (**B**) Left pulmonary angiogram showed large filling defect in the main left pulmonary artery. Catheter-directed thrombolytic therapy was performed. The catheter was wedged into the main thrombus in the right pulmonary artery and urokinase was started at 100,000 IU/hr for 36 hours, with alternating catheterization of the left pulmonary artery for 12 hours. (**C,D**) Posttreatment pulmonary angiography showed significant improvement in circulation to both lungs. The patient experienced dramatic recovery of the symptoms and reduction of pulmonary artery pressures. (**E,F**) Pre- and posttreatment lung perfusion scans showed marked improvement of right lung perfusion. Note some improvement on the left lower lobe.

SURGICAL EMBOLECTOMY AND THROMBOENDARTERECTOMY

Massive PE can lead to circulatory shock and irreversible damage. If thrombolysis and anticoagulation fail, until recently, surgical thrombectomy through a sternotomy and pulmonary arteriotomy was the only option (Fig. 6). This is now rarely considered because the results have not been encouraging, though recent significant improvement in mortality has been achieved (48–50).

A relatively small, carefully selected subset of patients with pulmonary hypertension and right heart failure secondary to chronic thromboembolic disease may also benefit from pulmonary thromboendarterectomy (48).

PERCUTANEOUS EMBOLECTOMY, CATHETER FRAGMENTATION, AND THROMBECTOMY

Frequently the comorbid conditions that deem patients unsuitable for thrombolysis also deem them inappropriate for open surgery (51), and less invasive options are now available, using

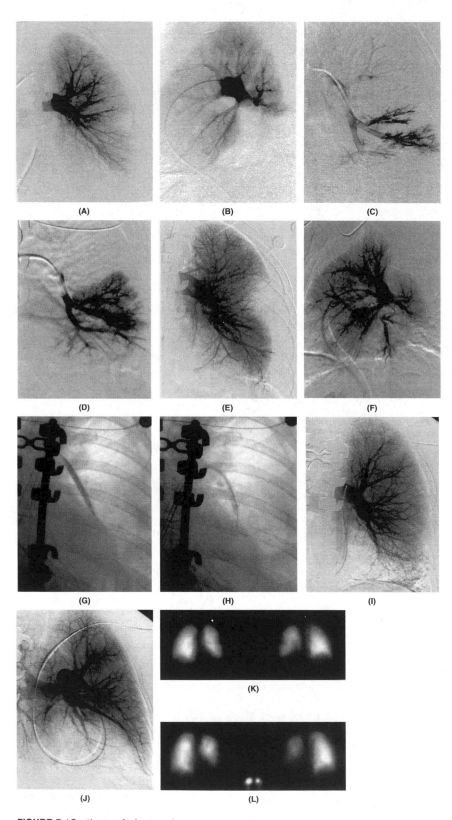

FIGURE 5 (*Caption on facing page*)

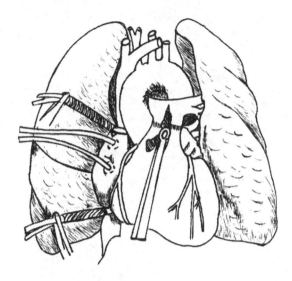

FIGURE 6 Schematic drawing of a surgical embolectomy from the main pulmonary artery with a surgical forceps. Note the circulatory bypass with catheters placed in the inferior and superior vena cava tightened up by vascular loops.

devices to remove, fragment, maceration or aspirate clot (52,53). Some of the techniques do not eliminate thrombus, but rather break it into smaller fragments that migrate peripherally, opening the main pulmonary artery and improving perfusion (54). The rationale for using these devices in the pulmonary circulation is based on the rapid relief of central obstruction. The cross-sectional area and volume of the peripheral pulmonary circulatory bed are four and two times those of the central circulation, respectively, suggesting that redistribution of larger central clots into the peripheral vasculature may acutely improve cardiopulmonary hemodynamics (Fig. 7) (46,55). Although, this rationale is disputed by some (56), there is evidence of a reduction in pulmonary pressure and improved perfusion on follow-up catheterization and pulmonary perfusion studies (46,55,57). Softening of the clot with thrombolytics facilitates the treatment (46–46). Fragmentation should be used as an adjunct to thrombolytic therapy (Fig. 5), exposing fresh surfaces for thrombolytic agents to work (Table 2) (58).

THROMBECTOMY AND EMBOLECTOMY DEVICES

Greenfield Embolectomy Device

The Greenfield embolectomy device (Boston Scientific, Natick, Massachusetts, U.S.A.) is a 10-French braided steerable catheter with a 5- or 7-mm plastic cup at the tip, and was designed to be inserted through femoral or jugular venotomy. By manual suction with a large syringe, the device pulls out non-organized clots through the venotomy, or a large valveless vascular sheath (Fig. 8). Multiple passes may be required. In experienced hands, it has been successful in extracting pulmonary thrombus in 76% of cases, with significant reduction of pulmonary artery

---

FIGURE 5 (*facing page*)   A 45-year-old female patient with lymphoma presented with chest pain and dyspnea. (**A**) Left pulmonary artery angiography showed occlusion of the posterior basal segment of the left lower lobe (LLL). (**B**) Lateral view of the arteriogram showed occlusion of the posterior basal segment. Note patency of the superior, anteromedial and lateral basal segments with a wedge of the posterior basal segment missing. (**C**) A straight catheter was advanced into the posterior basal segment artery and contrast medium injection showed extensive thrombosis. The catheter was wedged and urokinase infusion was started. (**D**) Follow-up angiography, 12 hours into the treatment, showed restored patency of the peripheral branches of the posterior basal segment with persistent proximal occlusion of the posterior basal segment artery. (**E,F**). Anterior and lateral view of the 24 hours follow-up angiogram showing persistent proximal occlusion and increased volume of pleural effusion, with further collapse of the superior segment and left upper lobe. (**G,H**) Balloon angioplasty and occlusion balloon thrombectomy was performed in the persistently occluded segment of the posterior basal segment, produced recanalization. (**I,J**). follow-up left pulmonary angiogram one month after treatment showed patent posterior basal segment. (**K**) Pretreatment perfusion showed reduced perfusion of the LLL. (**L**) Posttreatment lung perfusion scan showed persistent reduced perfusion of the left lung base, due to significant increase in pleural effusion.

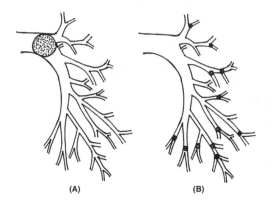

(A)   (B)

FIGURE 7 Schematic drawing demonstrating the effect of mechanical fragmentation of a total occlusive central thrombus in the pulmonary artery (**A**) before and (**B**) after mechanical fragmentation and dispersion of the smaller clots into the peripheral branches of the pulmonary artery. Fragmentation and distal dispersion is likely to reduce pulmonary artery pressure and increase total pulmonary perfusion. Note that a number of peripheral branches of the pulmonary artery are open following fragmentation of the thrombus.

pressure and increase in cardiac output (59). The same device has been less successful in the hands of other investigators (60).

Balloon Angioplasty for Clot Fragmentation

Balloon angioplasty for fragmentation of PE produce rapid restoration of pulmonary blood flow and promotes improvement of cardiac output and reduction of pulmonary pressure (46,55). Manipulation with other more conventional, pigtail catheters and latex occlusion balloons is also useful when the clots are fresh (61,62).

   Mechanical fragmentation using 6 to 16 mm angioplasty balloon catheter associated with thrombolysis (urokinase, 80,000–100,000 IU/hr for 8–24 hours) was recently shown to be very successful, with a 87.5% recovery rate for massive PE, as measured by pulmonary artery pressures, and clinical outcomes (Fig. 9) (13,46).

Kensey Dynamic Device (Trac-Wright Device)

The Kensey device (Dow Corning, Miami, Florida, U.S.A.) was made of flexible polyurethane catheter, in 5- and 8-French sizes. At the distal tip there was a high-speed rotating cam, driven at speeds of 5000 to 100,000 rpm by a direct current motor. A vortex was created at the catheter tip promoting fragmentation of thrombus (Fig. 10). A number of complications, mainly related to the unprotected rotational tip, were observed, including vessel perforation, intimal dissection, and extravasation of contrast material (63).

Hydrodynamic Thrombectomy Catheter (Hydrolyser) and Oasis Catheter

The Hydrolyser catheter system (Cordis, Warren, New Jersey, U.S.A.) is a 7-French, over-the-wire straight but flexible catheter, with a large side hole near the distal tip. The system has a double-lumen shaft, the larger one dedicated to aspiration of fragmented clots. The smaller lumen is an injection channel with a metallic tubing looped at 180° in opposite direction to the tip of the catheter (Fig. 11). High-velocity injection through the small lumen creates lower pressure dynamics in the larger lumen, and a vortex that causes fragmentation of the clots and aspiration due to the pressure gradient (64). The rigidity of the catheter causes some difficulty in advancing through the right heart to the pulmonary artery. The application of the Hydrolyser in the pulmonary circulation seems to be limited to fresh clots and more peripheral branches. However, a recently published case report described a successful thrombectomy of major branches of the pulmonary artery (65). The Oasis catheter (formerly known as the Shredding Embolectomy Thrombectomy catheter; Boston Scientific, Natick, Massachusetts, U.S.A.) also works with a Venturi-based system, creating a vortex that causes clot fragmentation and aspiration (Fig. 12) (52). Due to the design, limited power and size, it has a limited application in larger vessels.

TABLE 2 Technique and Device Listing with Current Information for the Treatment of Pulmonary Embolism

Device/technique	Advantages	Disadvantages	Size (French)	Efficacy	FDA approval/ modality	Current U.S. trial	Availability in U.S.
Anticoagulation	Reduces mortality and recurrence of PE	Does not treat existing thrombus	N/A	Effective			
Heparin	Large experience	Bleeding complications	N/A	Effective	Yes	N/A	Yes
Low-molecular weight heparin	Reduced bleeding complications	Small experience	N/A	Presumed effective	No	Unknown	Yes
Argatroban	Alternative to heparin in HIT	Small experience	N/A	Presumed effective	No	No	Yes
Systemic thrombolysis	Accelerate clot lysis, pulmonary reperfusion, improve pulmonary capillary blood volume	Bleeding complications, presumed less effective than local	N/A	Effective	Yes	N/A	Yes
Streptokinase	Effective	Small experience, allergic reactions		Effective	Yes	N/A	Yes
Urokinase	Effective large experience	Currently not available			Yes	N/A	No
Recombinant tissue plasminogen activator	Effective	Small experience			Yes	N/A	Yes
Catheter-directed thrombolysis	Accelerate clot lysis, and reperfusion	Bleeding complications	Small	Effective	No	No	Yes
Surgical embolectomy	Acute reperfusion of pulmonary circulation	High morbidity and mortality	N/A	Effective	N/A	N/A	Yes
Percutaneous embolectomy/ thrombectomy							
Greenfield	Rapid reperfusion	Difficult manipulation arrhythmias	Large	Effective	Yes	No	Yes
Balloon angioplasty and fragmentation	Rapid reperfusion	Moderate morbidity	Small	Effective	No	No	Yes
Kensey	Potential reperfusion	High mortdity	Small	Moderate	No	No	No
Hydrolyser	Potential reperfusion	High morbidity	Small	Low	No	No	Yes
Oasis	Potential reperfusion	Low power	Small	Low	No	No	Yes
Angiojet	Potential reperfusion	Effective in peripheral branches, and some central in some cases	Small	Moderate	No	No	Yes

(Continued)

TABLE 2 Technique and Device Listing with Current Information for the Treatment of Pulmonary Embolism (*Continued*)

Device/technique	Advantages	Disadvantages	Size (French)	Efficacy	FDA approval/modality	Current U.S. trial	Availability in U.S.
Impeller basket	Rapid reperfusion	Limited steerability and experience	Small	Effective	No	No	No
Thrombolizer	Rapid reperfusion	Trauma to the vessel, limited experience	Small	Moderate	No	No	
Modified impeller catheter	Rapid reperfusion	Trauma to the vessel, limited experience	Small	Moderate	No	No	
Rotatable pigtail	Rapid reperfusion	Potential trauma	Small	Effective	No	No	No
Arrow-Trerotola	Rapid reperfusion	Potential trauma, not steerable	Small	Effective	No	No	Yes[a]
Amplatz thrombectomy device	Rapid reperfusion	Potential trauma, not over the wire	Small	Effective	No	No	Yes
Lang device	Rapid reperfusion homemade	Potential trauma, limited experience	Large	Effective	No	No	Yes
Amplatz maceration aspiration thrombectomy catheter	Rapid reperfusion	Potential trauma	Small	Effective	No	No	
Rotarex	Unknown	Potential trauma for small vessels	Small	Promising	No	No	
Pulmonary artery stent Wallstent/Z-stent	Rapid reperfusion	Potential trauma, and migration	Small	Effective	No	No	Yes

[a] Available in a different configuration.

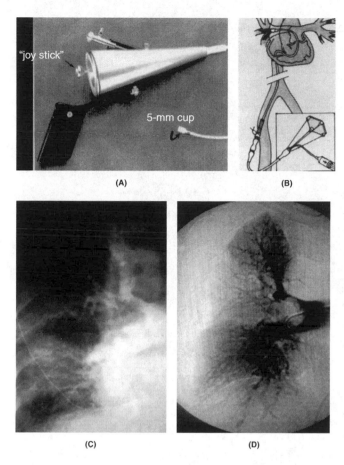

(A)

(B)

(C)

(D)

FIGURE 8 (**A**) Greenfield embolectomy device. The 10-French steerable catheter is seen with the 7-mm cup at the tip (*curved arrow*). The large metallic handle is used to attach the catheter and the "joy stick" is used to steer the tip of the catheter (*straight arrow*). The port at the top of the handle is for suction through the lumen of the catheter. (**B**) Schematic drawing of the embolectomy procedure showing the catheter inserted through the right femoral vein, passing through the right atrium and right ventricle into the pulmonary artery, sucking the thrombus with the catheter cup. (**C**) Right pulmonary artery arteriogram showed massive pulmonary embolism with occlusion of the main right pulmonary artery and multiple main peripheral branches of the pulmonary artery. (**D**) Post-embolectomy pulmonary angiogram showed significant improvement in right pulmonary perfusion but the major clot persisted. There was clinical improvement.

Rheolytic Thrombectomy Catheter (AngioJet Device)

The AngioJet (Possis, Minneapolis, Minnesota, U.S.A.) is similar to the Hydrolyser and Oasis catheters in concept. It also uses the Venturi effect to perform thrombectomy, but is different in design. It is a double-lumen system, with diameter ranging from 4- to 6-French. The smaller lumen is made of a fine, metal tubing that conducts a high-pressure stream of saline. The metal tubing makes a ring at the catheter tip, and the jet is oriented backwards in the direction of the main lumen of the catheter shaft, creating a low-pressure area promoting clot fragmentation and evacuation (Figs. 13 and 14). The catheter can be advanced over the wire, allowing for precise placement (52,55). The treatment of massive PE is a potential application for this device (66,67). The use of the AngioJet device in other vascular beds, such as coronary thrombectomy (68–70) portal vein and for transjugular intrahepatic portosystemic shunt recanalization (71) has led to incidences of severe bradyarrhythmia and type III heart block, possibly related to adenosine or other products liberated from the hemolyzed red cells acting on the atrio-ventricular node (71). Hyperkalemia causing ST segment elevations has also been described (72–74). The use of the AngioJet has been also linked to suspected pulmonary artery disruption after transvenous embolectomy, when used in arterial branches <6 mm in diameter (75). At least one case of unexpected pancreatitis was attributed to the hemolysis produced by the device (76). The AngioJet, however, has been used successfully and without complication in several small series of patients with massive PE (Fig. 15) (77–80).

Impeller Basket Device

The impeller basket device (Cook, Bjaeverskov, Denmark) is formed by a flexible wire shaft inside a 7-French catheter with a small impeller mounted on the wire in the center of a metallic

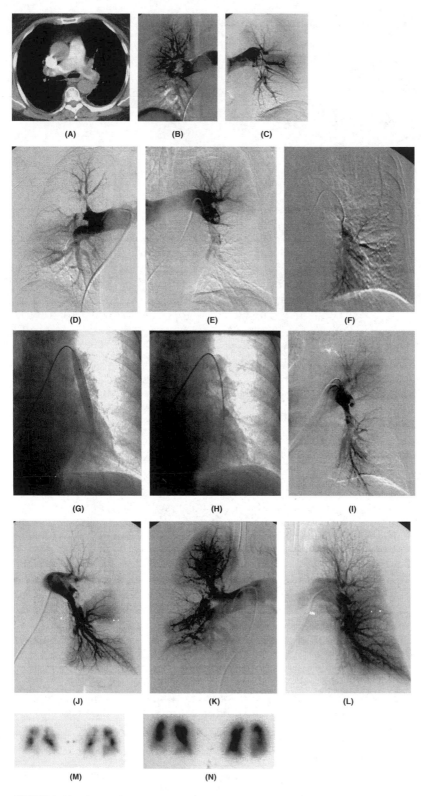

FIGURE 9 (*Caption on facing page*)

self-expandable basket. The impeller creates a vortex inside the vessel lumen and pulls the thrombus into the basket, causing clot fragmentation (Fig. 16). The basket protects the vessel wall from the rotational impeller (81). This device was designed for the treatment of PE and has been tested in animals and used in a limited number of unreported human cases, with relative success and without significant vessel wall damage. The device is limited in steerability and is relatively stiff. Multiple subsegmental occlusions were observed in the animal model after treating the thrombus in the main pulmonary artery (82).

Thrombolizer and Modified Impeller Catheter

The thrombolizer and the modified impeller catheter are similar devices in design and operation. The thrombolizer is an over-the-wire thrombectomy catheter consisting of an outer 8-French catheter with an inner 5-French catheter with longitudinal slits in the distal tip. The 5-French catheter is designed to rotate relative to the outer catheter. The centrifugal force created causes the flat segments of the catheter shaft, between the slits, to open into a basket shape, causing fragmentation of the clots (Fig. 17).

The impeller catheter consists of an over-the-wire outer 8-French Teflon catheter and an inner rotational 5-French catheter. The outer catheter has slits in the walls and is able to expand to 10 mm in diameter. The inner rotational catheter opens its basket to 5 mm in diameter, independent of the rotation/minute. This system rotates to high speeds of 100,000 rpm, creating a strong vortex and clot fragmentation (83). There are no reports of the use of these devices in humans, and it is unclear at this point if there will be a role for clinical application.

Rotatable Pigtail Catheter

The rotatable pigtail catheter is a modified high-torque 5-French pigtail catheter with a radiopaque tip, 115 cm in length, and with 10 side holes for contrast injection. A jugular version of the catheter is 105 cm long. There is an oval side hole in the outer aspect of the pigtail loop in straight projection with the axis of the catheter lumen, allowing direct passage

---

FIGURE 9 (*facing page*) A 78-year-old female patient with chronic obstructive pulmonary disease, on home oxygen, with a history of recent myocardial infarction, presented with symptoms of deep vein thrombosis, chest pain, shortness of breath and congestive heart failure. (**A**) Computed tomography scan of the chest showed large filling defects in both main pulmonary arteries. (**B**) Right pulmonary artery angiogram showed massive obstruction of the bifurcation of the right pulmonary artery. There is persistent, but reduced, perfusion of the right upper lobe and marked hypoperfusion of the right lower lobe. (**C**) Left pulmonary artery angiogram showed massive embolism in the left lower lobe segment, with marked reduction in peripheral perfusion. The pulmonary artery pressure was 39 mmHg. (**D**) Follow-up right pulmonary artery angiogram after 15 hours of treatment, with UK at 250,000 IU/hr through the pigtail catheter wedged into the thrombus on right side, showed marked improvement of the thrombus obstruction with some residual clots mainly occluding the right upper and middle lobe. There was improvement in the right lower lobe perfusion. (**E**) Follow-up arteriogram of the left pulmonary artery showed worsening of the occlusion of the left lower lobe, probably by distal migration of the thrombus from the main branch into the more peripheral circulation. Pulmonary artery pressure was 46 mmHg. (**F**) Selective catheterization of the lower lobe branch, through the clot, was performed and showed total occlusion of the lower lobe artery. (**G**) A 10-mm balloon catheter was used to break down the clot over a wire advanced into the lower lobe branches. (**H**) An occlusion balloon catheter was trawled back several times to thrombectomize the clots. (**I**) An angiogram following mechanical balloon thrombectomy showed improved patency of the lower lobe segment. The catheter was positioned within the partially occluded artery and U.K. infusion was performed at 100,000 IU/hr for eight hours. (**J**) Follow-up angiogram of the left pulmonary artery treatment showed significant improvement in the left lung perfusion. Infusion of U.K. at the same rate was performed for additional 15 hours. Upon arrival at the ICU the patient became tachypneic and lowered the O_2 saturation, requiring tracheal intubation. (**K**) Follow-up right pulmonary arteriogram at the end of the treatment showed significant improvement in the circulation of the right pulmonary artery. (**L**) Left pulmonary follow-up arteriogram at the end of the infusion showed almost complete patency of the left pulmonary artery and peripheral branches. Mean pulmonary artery pressure following treatment was 33 mmHg. After discontinuation of treatment the patient improved and was extubated. (**M**) Pretreatment perfusion scan showed a high-probability picture with multiple extensive areas of hypoperfusion, suggesting massive pulmonary embolism. (**N**) Perfusion scan three days following thrombolytic treatment showed remarkable improvement in bilateral pulmonary perfusion. The patient was discharged home five days later.

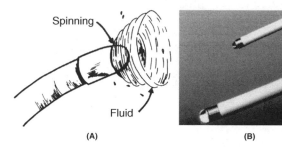

(A)

(B)

FIGURE 10 (**A**) Diagrammatic illustration and (**B**) picture of the Kensey catheter.

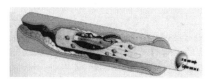

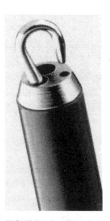

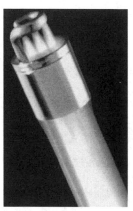

FIGURE 11 The Hydrolyser catheter.   **FIGURE 12** The Oasis catheter.   **FIGURE 13** The AngioJet system.

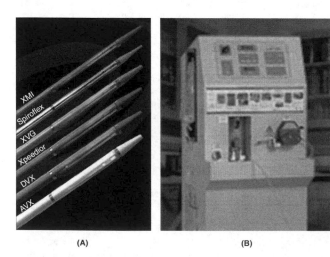

(A)

(B)

FIGURE 14 (**A**) Picture of the several AngioJet catheters available. The DVX and the AVX are the most powerful catheters for thrombectomy and aspiration. (**B**) Console of the AngioJet system. Note the pulsatile pump and the fluid pump with rollers.

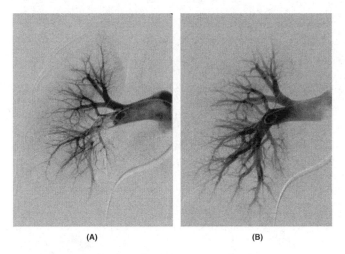

(A)   (B)

FIGURE 15 Significant pulmonary embolism affecting predominantly both lower lobe arteries. (**A**) Pretreatment right pulmonary angiogram showing the massive filling defect within the pulmonary artery. (**B**) Posttreatment angiogram showing patency of the right pulmonary artery. The AngioJet device was able to remove the clots and was followed by a few hours of thrombolytic infusion with urokinase.

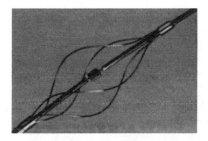

FIGURE 16 Impeller basket device depicted in a blown-up view of the self-expandable metal basket.

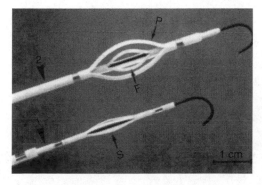

FIGURE 17 Thrombolizer and modified impeller device (MID) are all plastic rotational devices that create a vortex within the vessel pulling the clots and causing fragmentation. The MID is placed through a guiding catheter and the slitted catheter (*S*) expands like a basket due to the rotational movement of the catheter. Note that the basket is not protected and will scrape the vessel wall during activation. The thrombolizer is a coaxial catheter system with a plastic self-expandable basket (*P*), with a small rotational basket inside (*F*) that creates the vortex for thrombus fragmentation. Both systems work over the wire that increases the chances for correct positioning.

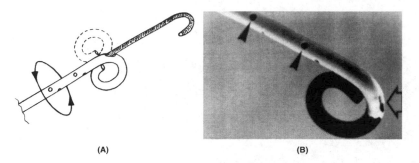

(A)   (B)

FIGURE 18   (**A**) Schematic drawing of the pigtail rotational catheter over the stationary guidewire, passed through the distal hole, and used as a directing axis of rotation. The clots are fragmented by the mechanical action of the rotating pigtail tip. The wire also allows the catheter to be advanced or withdrawn over the wire. (**B**) Tip of the rotational pigtail catheter, with a diameter of 7 mm. The oval shaped side hole (*arrow*) allows the wire to pass out through the outer curvature of the pigtail. The side holes (*arrowheads*) are used for contrast material injection as a regular angiographic catheter.

of a guidewire through the hole to act as a central axis around which the catheter rotates and disrupts the clot (Fig. 18). Extensive experimental work in animal models has been performed (84), though the clinical application is more recent, demonstrating a 70% success rate in 10 patients (85). A more recent unreported series of 20 patients showed a 33% recanalization rate by fragmentation alone, but a higher yield was obtained in association with thrombolysis.

Arrow-Trerotola Percutaneous Thrombolytic Device

The Arrow-Trerotola device (Arrow, Reading, Pennsylvania, U.S.A.) is a low-speed rotational basket (3000 rpm), used for thrombectomy in dialysis grafts (Fig. 19). It scrapes the walls of the vessel and fragments the thrombus. The device was adapted for the safe, successful treatment of PE in an animal model (86,87).

Amplatz Thrombectomy Device

The Amplatz thrombectomy device (Microvena/ev3, White Bear Lake, Minnesota, U.S.A.) is a 120-cm long, 8-French reinforced polyurethane catheter with a distal metal tip (can) housing an impeller mounted on a drive shaft. The metal can has three side ports, behind the impeller

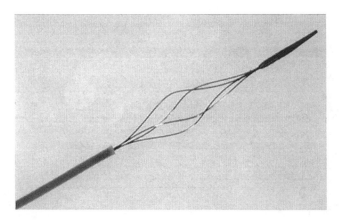

FIGURE 19   The Arrow-Trerotola percutaneous thrombolytic device.

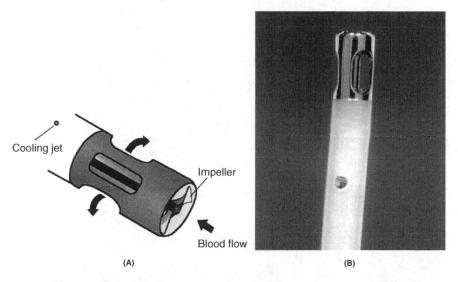

FIGURE 20 (**A**) Schematic drawing and (**B**) picture of the distal tip of the 8-French Amplatz thrombectomy device. *Source*: From Ref. 15.

used for recirculation of the particles. The high speed creates a vortex inside the vessel, pulling the clots toward the impeller, which re-circulates and pulverizes the fresh clots, creating a fluid with smaller particles (Fig. 20).

Access is achieved through a 10-French, 95-cm-long guiding catheter. The guiding catheter is advanced into the clot and the ATD is introduced through the catheter and activated at full speed. Initial experience with the ATD device showed clinical improvement in a limited group of patients, with reduction of respiratory symptoms and improvement of hypotension (Figs. 21 and 22) (15). The bleeding complication is probably related to reperfusion of infarcted pulmonary tissue (88). The ATD always causes some degree of hemolysis, which is mostly transient and is not associated with any incidences of renal failure (15,89–91). There is a more recent report of a young patient with large cell lymphoma and severe segmental PE (92). A number of unreported cases of massive PE had been treated by the ATD, the results of which are unknown. A 7-French, 27% more powerful device, became available recently, but has not been tested in the pulmonary circulation.

Lang Percutaneous Pulmonary Thrombectomy Device

The suction catheter system described by Lang et al. (93) is a homemade device which uses commercially available catheters of different sizes. A 14-French, 90-cm long Ultratane non-tapered catheter is used through a 16-French, 40-cm long stationary sheath. The 14-French catheter is advanced over a 6-French, 97-cm long multipurpose guiding catheter and a Rosen wire, to provide the stiffness and taper necessary for advancement of the system. A peel-away sheath is used for introduction of the system into the stationary sheath (Fig. 23). The suction catheter is used to compact, trap, and propel clot distally, and a 50-mL syringe is used to aspirate on the catheter as it is withdrawn. The peel-away sheath with the clots is carefully removed and flushed. The reported clinical experience with the technique, although successful, is small and included pretreatment of the clots with urokinase and fragmentation with a pigtail catheter or a large angioplasty balloon.

Amplatz Maceration Aspiration Thrombectomy Catheter

The Amplatz maceration aspiration thrombectomy catheter (AMATC) is an experimental double-lumen, 9-French aspiration catheter with a large side window close to the tip where there is an occlusion balloon. Inside, an electrically powered basket is rotated at 5000 rpm, at

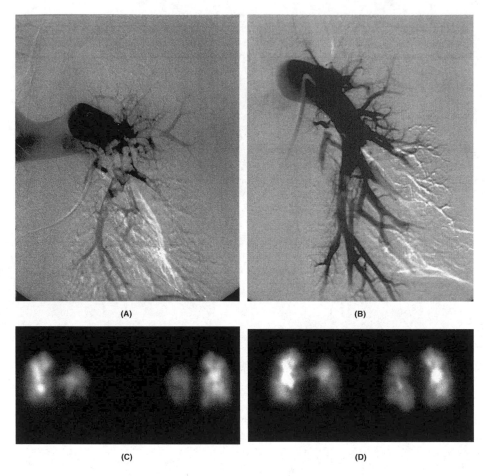

(A)   (B)

(C)   (D)

FIGURE 21   (**A**) Pulmonary angiogram showed massive pulmonary embolism (PE) occluding the left main pulmonary artery. Mechanical thrombectomy was indicated in this case due to recent neurologic surgery. The Amplatz thrombectomy device was used through a 10-French guiding catheter. (**B**) Post-thrombectomy pulmonary arteriogram showed improved patency in the main pulmonary artery and improved lung perfusion. (**C**) Initial positive perfusion scan shows bilateral PE that is massive on the left side. (**D**) Follow-up perfusion scan shows improved perfusion in the left lung, mostly appreciated in the posterior view. *Source*: From Ref. 15.

the level of the window, while manual suction is applied to the main lumen for aspiration of the clots macerated by the basket. The AMATC was used in the pulmonary circulation in an animal model and was effective in 60% of the cases, with minimal intimal injury. Difficulties in guidance of the device within the pulmonary artery and orientation of the side window were responsible for the rate of failure (53).

Aspirex Catheter

The Aspirex catheter is a new device for percutaneous mechanical removal of fresh and organized thrombi (Straub Medical, Wangs, Switzerland). The device has three components: the catheter, an electric motor drive and an electronic control unit. Inside the 11-French catheter, a stainless steel spiral rotates over the wire (Fig. 24). The high frequency of revolution creates a negative pressure at the catheter head in an L-shaped aspiration port. Thrombus is aspirated, macerated, caught in the slits and transported by the internal spiral to the proximal side port, from where it is discharged into a bag. This device has been tested in animal models (Fig. 25) (94), and more recently in humans (95), and data suggest that it may be effective.

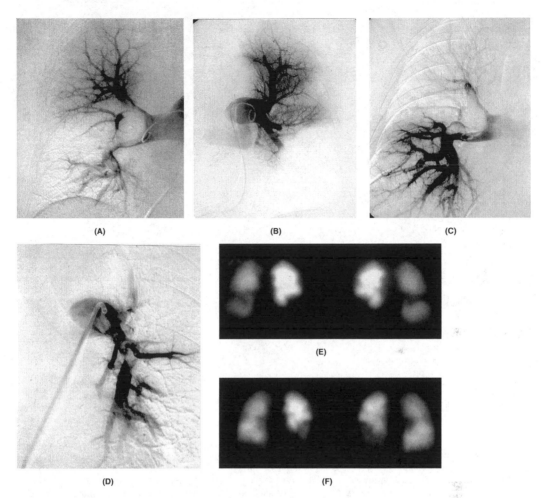

FIGURE 22 (**A**) Pulmonary arteriogram shows massive pulmonary embolism (PE) in the main right pulmonary artery with severely decreased perfusion of the whole right lung. (**B**) Pulmonary arteriogram shows complete obstruction of the descending left pulmonary artery and no substantial flow into the left lower lobe. The diagnostic catheter was exchanged for a 10-French guiding catheter, and the Amplatz thrombectomy device was used to debulk the PE on both sides. Activation time was 8 minutes 11 seconds. At the end of the procedure the patient experienced hemoptysis of about 900 mL. (**C**) Post-thrombectomy right pulmonary arteriogram shows improved perfusion of the right lower lobe, with a large filling defect within the bifurcation of the pulmonary artery. (**D**) Post-thrombectomy left pulmonary arteriogram shows improved perfusion of the left lower lobe and no extravasation of contrast medium. Large filling defects remain within the left main pulmonary artery. (**E**) Pre-thrombectomy perfusion scan shows signs of reduced perfusion in both lungs consistent with massive PE. (**F**) Follow-up perfusion scan obtained 12 hours after the procedure shows improved pulmonary perfusion on both sides. *Source*: From Ref. 15.

Pulmonary Artery Stent Placement

Recent reports described the use of metallic stents placed alongside organized, treatment-resistant PE. Both Wallstent (96) and Gianturco Z-stents (97) were used in critical situations where the patients presented with cor pulmonale, profound arterial hypoxemia and hypotension and did not respond to thrombolytic therapy and fragmentation.

OVERVIEW

Successful management of acute massive PE requires prompt risk stratification and decisive, early intervention (Table 1) (51). Typically, clinically undetected right heart failure

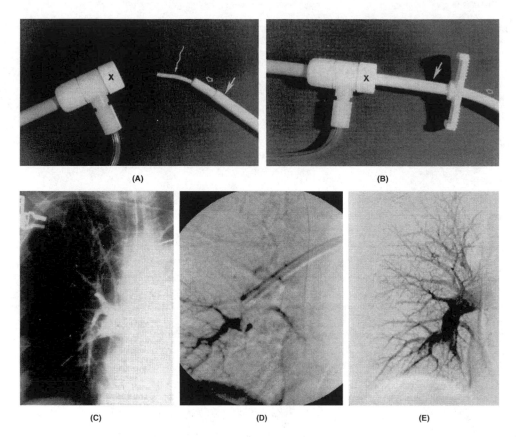

FIGURE 23 (**A**) Suction catheter system. The 6-French guiding catheter (*wavy arrow*) is coaxially loaded into the 14-French suction catheter (*open arrow*). The 14-French peel-away sheath is piggybacked onto the assembly (*closed arrow*). The assembly is advanced over a guidewire into the valve of the 16-French stationary sheath (*X*). (**B**) The assembly has been introduced into the stationary sheath (*X*) with advancement of the 14-French peel-away sheath (*closed arrow*). The suction catheter (*open arrow*) is loaded into the peel-away sheath. (**C**) Initial pulmonary arteriogram shows large clot in the right descending pulmonary artery. (**D**) Note distal migration of the clot, compacted by the tip of the suction catheter, as compared to (**C**). (**E**) Pulmonary arteriogram after clot suction. *Source*: From Ref. 93.

worsens with time, and may lead to unremitting cardiogenic shock. If thrombolysis or surgical embolectomy is considered at this stage, the outlook is poor (51). Despite adequate anti-coagulation, right ventricular dysfunction remains a life-threatening condition.

When high-risk patients are identified, adequate anticoagulation should be instituted and the patients should be considered for thrombolysis. Thrombolysis offers the potential for clot removal without the morbidity associated with surgical embolectomy, though incurs significant risks in itself. However, thrombolytic therapy also offers the opportunity of dissolution of more peripheral pulmonary clots. Despite the controversy regarding the efficacy of peripheral versus intrapulmonary thrombolytic therapy, recent experimental evidence (98) suggests that massive pulmonary occlusion causes a vortex adjacent to the embolus, and fluid infused proximal to the occlusion will make only evanescent contact with the thrombus edge. Fragmentation increases the distribution of infused fluid. This may explain why agents administered adjacent to the embolus may have similar effects to systemically infused thrombolytics (Fig. 26) (98). These results support the practice of direct intra-thrombotic injection or local infusion following embolus fragmentation techniques.

Catheter fragmentation followed by intrapulmonary thrombolytic infusion is an adequate but underused technique to achieve rapid thrombus resolution and hemodynamic improvement. The use of larger angioplasty balloons for clot fragmentation is also a simple

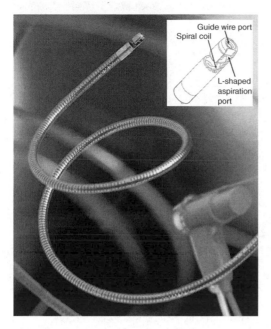

FIGURE 24 Picture and schematic drawing of the Aspirex 11-French thrombectomy device.

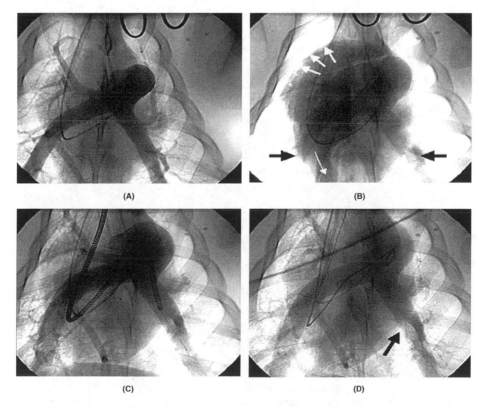

FIGURE 25 Animal experiment with artificially induced pulmonary embolism. (**A**) Pulmonary arteriogram. (**B**) Pulmonary arteriogram after injection of thrombus to create pulmonary embolism. (**C**) Aspirex device in action. (**D**) Post-thrombectomy pulmonary angiogram showing patency of the vessel.

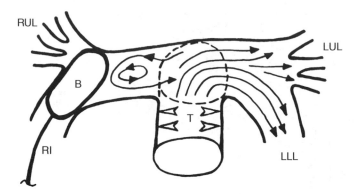

FIGURE 26 Schematic drawing of the flow model, showing vortex formation immediately proximal to the level of obstruction. Note that most of the fluid is washed into the non-occluded left pulmonary artery and the vortex close to the occlusion, with only minimal flow of fluid making evanescent contact with an occluding embolus (B). *Abbreviations*: B, balloon; LUL, left upper lobe; LLL, left lower lobe; RI, right intermediate artery; RUL, right upper lobe; T, pulmonary artery trunk. *Source*: From Ref. 98.

and cheap technique (46). The association of fragmentation, mechanical thrombectomy and thrombolytic therapy is desirable for potentially improving outcomes. For high-risk PE patients, unsuitable for thrombolysis or open embolectomy, mechanical thrombectomy technology may be used (Table 2). It is difficult to determine which is the best catheter intervention alternative. Catheter intervention, however, should be considered when heparin alone is insufficient, when thrombolysis is not feasible, while systemic arterial pressure is preserved and before pressor dependence ensues (51).

The advent of aggressive interventional regimes for the management of massive PE has tremendous potential. Nevertheless, the new technology requires an interdisciplinary team approach to the identification and treatment of these patients. The development and implementation of protocols for treatment of massive PE, tailored for each institution, is mandatory and may improve outcomes. No simple solution is currently available, and it is likely that new devices and thrombolytic techniques will be used in association, rather than in isolation.

REFERENCES

1. Dalen JE, Alper JS. Natural history of pulmonary embolism. Prog Cardiovasc Dis 1975; 17:259–70.
2. Uflacker R. Interventional therapy for pulmonary embolism. J Vasc Interv Radiol 2001; 12:147–64.
3. Olin JW. Pulmonary embolism. Rev Cardiovasc Med 2002; 3:S68–75.
4. Brotman DJ, Jaffer A. "Coach class thrombosis": is the risk real? What do we tell our patients? Cleve Clin J Med 2002; 69:832–7.
5. Lapostolle F, Surget V, Borron SW, et al. Severe pulmonary embolism associated with air travel. N Engl J Med 2001; 345:779–83.
6. Barrit DW, Jordan SE. Anticoagulant drugs in the treatment of pulmonary embolism: a controlled trial. Lancet 1960; 1:1309–12.
7. Elliot CG. Pulmonary physiology during pulmonary embolism. Chest 1992; 101(Suppl.):163S–71S.
8. Lilienfeld DE, Chan E, Ehland J, Landringan PJ, Marsh G. Mortality from pulmonary embolism. Prog Cardiovasc Dis 1975; 17:259–70.
9. Kearon C. Diagnosis of pulmonary embolism. CMAJ 2003; 168:183–94.
10. Mastora I, Remy-Jardin M, Masson P, et al. Severity of acute pulmonary embolism: evaluation of a new spiral CT angiographic score in correlation with echocardiographic data. Eur Radiol 2003; 13:29–35.
11. Haage P, Piroth W, Krombach G, et al. Pulmonary embolism: comparison of angiography with spiral CT, MRA and real-time MR imaging. Am J Respir Crit Care Med 2002; 167:729–34.
12. Pruszczyk P, Bochowicz A, Torbicki A, et al. Cardiac troponin T monitoring identifies high-risk group of normotensive patients with acute pulmonary embolism. Chest 2003; 123:1947–52.
13. De Gregorio MA, Gimeno MJ, Mainar A, et al. Mechanical and enzymatic thrombolysis for massive pulmonary embolism. J Vasc Interv Radiol 2002; 13:163–9.

14. Konstantinides S, Geibel A, Olschewski M, et al. Association between thrombolytic treatment and the prognosis of hemodynamically stable patients with major pulmonary embolism: results of a multicenter registry. Circulation 1997; 96:882–8.
15. Uflacker R, Strange C, Vujic I. Massive pulmonary embolism. Preliminary results of treatment with the Amplatz thrombectomy device. J Vasc Interv Radiol 1996; 7:519–28.
16. Moser KM. Pulmonary embolism. In: Braunwald E, Fauci A, Kasper D, Hauser S, Longo D, Jameson J, eds. Harrison's Principles of Internal Medicine. New York: McGraw-Hill, Inc., 2002:1214–20 (chap. 226).
17. Miller GAH, Sutton GC, Kerr IH, Gibson RV, Honey M. Comparison of streptokinase and heparin in treatment of isolated acute massive pulmonary embolism. Br Med J 1971; 2:681–4.
18. Jones TK, Barnes RW, Greenfield LJ. Greenfield vena cava filter: rationale and current indications. Ann Thorac Surg 1986; 42:S48–55.
19. Carson JL, Kelley MA, Duff A, et al. The clinical course of pulmonary embolism. N Engl J Med 1993; 326:1240–5.
20. Hull RD, Raskob GE, Hirsh J, et al. Continuous intravenous heparin compared with intermittent subcutaneous heparin in the initial treatment of proximal-vein thrombosis. N Engl J Med 1986; 315:1109–14.
21. Curry N, Bardana EJ, Pirofsky B. Enoxaparin: a low-molecular-weight heparin. Med Lett 1993; 35:75–6.
22. Aguilar D, Goldhager SZ. Clinical uses of low-molecular-weight heparins. Chest 1999; 115:1418–23.
23. Quader MA, Stump LS, Sumpio BE. Low molecular weight heparins: current use and indications. J Am Coll Surg 1998; 187:641–58.
24. Howard PA. Dalteparin: a low-molecular-weight heparin. Ann Pharmacoth 1997; 31:192–203.
25. Samama MM, Cohen AT, Darmon J-Y, et al. A comparison of enoxaparin with placebo for the prevention of venous thromboembolism in acutely ill medical patients. N Eng J Med 1999; 341:793–800.
26. Haas SK. Treatment of deep venous thrombosis and pulmonary embolism. Current recommendations. Med Clin North Am 1998; 82:495–510.
27. Levine M, Gent M, Hirsh J, et al. A comparison of low-molecular-weight heparin administered primarily at home with unfractionated heparin administered in the hospital for proximal deep-vein thrombosis. N Engl J Med 1996; 334:677–81.
28. Partsch H, Kechavarz B, Mostbeck A, Kohn H, Lipp C. Frequency of pulmonary embolism in patients who have iliofemoral deep vein thrombosis and are treated with once- or twice-daily low-molecular-weight heparin. J Vasc Surg 1996; 24:774–82.
29. Fiessinger JN, Lopez-Fernandez M, Gatterer E, et al. Once-daily subcutaneous dalteparin, a low-molecular-weight heparin, for the initial treatment of acute deep vein thrombosis. Thromb Haemost 1996; 76:195–9.
30. Ridker PM, Goldhaber SZ, Danielson E, et al. Long-term, low-intensity warfarin therapy for the prevention of recurrent venous thromboembolism. N Engl J Med 2003; 348:1425–34.
31. Konkle BA, Bauer TL, Arepally G, et al. Heparin-induced thrombocytopenia: bovine versus porcine heparin in cardiopulmonary bypass surgery. Ann Thorac Surg 2001; 71:1920–4.
32. Ranze O, Ranze P, Magnani HN, Greinacher A. Heparin-induced thrombocytopenia in paediatric patients- a review of the literature and a new case treated with danaparoid sodium. Eur J Pediatr 1999; 158:S130–3.
33. Ansell JE, Price JM, Shah S, Beckner RR. Heparin-induced thrombocytopenia. What is its real frequency. Chest 1985; 88:878–82.
34. Tow DE, Wagner HN. Urokinase pulmonary embolism trial: phase I results. JAMA 1970; 214:2163–72.
35. Urokinase-Streptokinase pulmonary embolism trial: phase II results. JAMA 1974; 229:1606–13.
36. Schwarz F, Stehr H, Zimmerman R, et al. Sustained improvement of pulmonary hemodynamics in patients at rest and during exercise after thrombolytic therapy of massive pulmonary embolism. Circulation 1985; 71:117–23.
37. Agnelli G, Becattini C, Kirschstein T. Thrombolysis vs heparin in the treatment of pulmonary embolism. A clinical outcome-based meta-analysis. Arch Intern Med 2002; 162:2537–41.
38. Konstantinides S, Geibel A, Heusel G, et al. Heparin plus alteplase compared with heparin alone in patients with submassive pulmonary embolism. N Engl J Med 2002; 347:1143–50.
39. Gunn NA, Tierney LM. Letter to the editor. N Engl J Med 2002; 348:357–8.
40. Goldhaber SZ. Thrombolytic therapy for pulmonary embolism. Semin Vasc Surg 1992; 5:69–75.
41. Verstraete M, Miller GAH, Bounameaux H, et al. Intravenous and intrapulmonary recombinant tissue-type plasminogen activator in the treatment of acute massive pulmonary embolism. Circulation 1988; 77:353–60.
42. Raschke RA, Reilly BM, Guidry JR, et al. The weight-based heparin dosing nomogram compared with a "standard of care" nomogram: a randomized controlled trial. Ann Intern Med 1993; 119:874–81.
43. Molina HE, Hunter DW, Yedlick JW, et al. Thrombolytic therapy for post operative pulmonary embolism. Am J Surg 1992; 163:375–81.

44. Gonzales-Juanatey JR, Valdes L, Amaro A, et al. Treatment of massive pulmonary thromboembolism with low intrapulmonary dosages of urokinase: short term angiographic and hemodynamic evolution. Chest 1992; 102:341–6.
45. Vujic I, Young JWR, Gobien RP, et al. Massive pulmonary embolism treatment with full heparinization and topical low-dose streptokinase. Radiology 1983; 148:671–5.
46. Fava M, Loyola S, Flores P, Huete I. Mechanical fragmentation and pharmacologic thrombolysis in massive pulmonary embolism. J Vasc Interv Radiol 1997; 8:261–6.
47. Goldhaber SZ, Markis JE, Meyrovitz MF, et al. Acute pulmonary embolism treated with tissue plasminogen activator. Lancet 1986; 2:886–9.
48. Jamieson SW, Auger WR, Fedullo PF, et al. Experience and results of 150 pulmonary thromboendarterectomy operations over a 29-month period. J Thorac Cardiovasc Surg 1993; 106:116–27.
49. Poletti GA, Actis Dato GM. Surgical treatment of massive pulmonary embolism. A case report. J Cardiovasc Surg 1999; 40:135–7.
50. Gulba DC, Schmid C, Borst HG, Lichtlen P, Dietz R, Luft FC. Medical compared with surgical treatment for massive pulmonary embolism. Lancet 1994; 343:576–7.
51. Goldhaber SZ. Integration of catheter thrombectomy into our armamentarium to treat acute pulmonary embolism. Chest 1998; 114:1237–8.
52. Sharafuddin MJA, Hicks ME. Current status of percutaneous mechanical thrombectomy. Part I. General principles. J Vasc Interv Radiol 1997; 8:911–21.
53. Sharafuddin MIA, Hicks ME. Current status of percutaneous mechanical thrombectomy. Part II. Devices and mechanisms of action. J Vasc Interv Radiol 1998; 9:15–31.
54. Brady AJ, Crake T, Oakley CM. Percutaneous catheter fragmentation and distal dispersion of proximal pulmonary embolus. Lancet 1991; 338:1186–9.
55. Handa K, Sasaki Y, Kiyonaga A, et al. Acute pulmonary thromboembolism treated successfully by balloon angioplasty: a case report. Angiology 1988; 8:775–8.
56. Girard P. Catheter fragmentation of pulmonary emboli. Chest 1999; 115:1759.
57. Timsit JF, Reynaud P, Meyer G, et al. Pulmonary embolectomy by catheter device in massive pulmonary embolism. Chest 1991; 100:655–8.
58. Oakley CM. Conservative management of pulmonary embolism. Br J Surg 1968; 55:801–5.
59. Greenfield LJ, Proctor MC, Williams DM, Wakefield TW. Long-term experience with transvenous catheter pulmonary embolectomy. J Vasc Surg 1993; 18:450–8.
60. Cela MC, Amplatz K. Nonsurgical pulmonary embolectomy. In: Cope C, ed. Current Techniques in Interventional Radiology., Vol. 12. Philadelphia, PA: Current Medicine, 1994:2–6.
61. Murphy JM, Mulvihill N, Mulcahy D, Foley B, Smiddy P, Molloy MP. Percutaneous catheter and guidewire fragmentation with local administration of recombinant tissue plasminogen activator as a treatment for massive pulmonary embolism. Eur Radiol 1999; 9:959–64.
62. Stock KW, Jacob AL, Schnabel KJ, Bongartz G, Steinbrich W. Massive pulmonary embolism: treatment with thrombus fragmentation and local fibrinolysis with recombinant human-tissue plasminogen activator. Cardiovasc Intervent Radiol 1997; 20:364–8.
63. Stein PD, Sabbah HN, Basha MA, et al. Mechanical disruption of pulmonary emboli in dogs with a flexible rotating-tip catheter (Kensey catheter). Chest 1990; 98:994–8.
64. Reekers J, Kromhout J, van der Wall K. Catheter for percutaneous thrombectomy: first clinical experience. Radiology 1993; 188:871–4.
65. Michalis LK, Tsetis DK, Rees MR. Case report: percutaneous removal of pulmonary artery thrombus in a patient with massive pulmonary embolism using the Hydrolyser catheter: the first human experience. Clin Radiol 1997; 52:158–61.
66. Koning R, Cribier A, Gerber L, et al. A new treatment for severe pulmonary embolism. Circulation 1997; 96:2498–500.
67. Voigtlander T, Rupprecht HJ, Nowak B, et al. Clinical application of a new rheolytic thrombectomy catheter system for massive pulmonary embolism. Catheter Cardiovasc Interv 1999; 47:91–6.
68. Mathie AG, Bell SD, Saibil EA. Mechanical thromboembolectomy in acute embolic peripheral arterial occlusions with use of the AngioJet rapid thrombectomy system. J Vasc Interv Radiol 1999; 10:583–90.
69. Nakagawa Y, Matsuo S, Kimura T, et al. Thrombectomy with AngioJet catheter in native coronary arteries for patients with acute or recent myocardial infarction. Am J Cardiol 1999; 83:994–9.
70. Whisenant BK, Baim DS, Kuntz RE, et al. Rheolytic thrombectomy with the Possis AngioJet: technical considerations and initial clinical experience. J Invasive Cardiol 1999; 11:421–6.
71. Fontaine AB, Borsa JJ, Hoffer EK, et al. Type III heart block with peripheral use of the Angiojet thrombectomy system. J Vasc Interv Radiol 2001; 12:1223–5.
72. Feldman JP, Feinstein JA, Lamberti JJ, Perry SB. Angiojet catheter-based thrombectomy in a neonate with postoperative pulmonary embolism. Catheter Cardiovasc Interv 2005; 66:442–5.
73. Murad B. Letter to the editor: intracoronary aminophylline for heart block with AngioJet thrombectomy. J Invasive Cardiol 2005; 17:1042–3.

74. Lee MS, Makkar R, Singh V, et al. Pre-procedural administration of aminophylline does not prevent AngioJet rheolytic thrombectomy-induced bradyarrhythmias. J Invasive Cardiol 2005; 17:19–22.
75. Biederer J, Schoene A, Reuter M, Heller M, Muller-Hulsbeck S. Suspected pulmonary artery disruption after transvenous pulmonary embolectomy using a hydrodynamic thrombectomy device: clinical case and experimental study of porcine lung explants. J Endovasc Ther 2003; 10:99–110.
76. Danetz JS, McLafferty RB, Ayerdi J, et al. Pancreatitis caused by rheolytic thrombolysis: an unexpected complication. J Vasc Interv Radiol 2004; 15:857–60.
77. Zeni PT, Jr., Blank BG, Peeler DW. Use of rheolytic thrombectomy in treatment of acute massive pulmonary embolism. J Vasc Interv Radiol 2003; 14:1511–5.
78. Chiam P, Kwok V, Johan BA, Chan C. Major pulmonary embolism treated with a rheolytic thrombectomy catheter. Singapore Med J 2005; 46:479–82.
79. Davidson B, Karmy-Jones R. When pulmonary embolism treatment isn't working. Chest 2006; 129:839–40.
80. Siablis D, Karnabatidis D, Katsanos K, Kagadis GC, Zabakis P, Hahalis G. AngioJet rheolytic thrombectomy versus local intrapulmonary thrombolysis in massive pulmonary embolism: a retrospective data analysis. J Endovasc Ther 2006; 12:206–14.
81. Schmitz-Rode T, Vorwerk D, Günther RW, et al. Percutaneous fragmentation of pulmonary emboli in dogs with the impeller basket catheter. Cardiovasc Intervent Radiol 1993; 16:234–42.
82. Schmitz-Rode T, Günther RW. New device for percutaneous fragmentation of pulmonary emboli. Radiology 1991; 180:135–7.
83. Schmitz-Rode T, Adam G, Kilbingr M, et al. Fragmentation of pulmonary emboli: in vivo experimental evaluation of 2 high-speed rotating catheters. Cardiovasc Intervent Radiol 1996; 19:165–9.
84. Schmitz-Rode T, Günther RW, Pjeffer JG, et al. Acute massive pulmonary embolism: use of a rotatable pigtail catheter for diagnosis and fragmentation therapy. Radiology 1995; 197:157–62.
85. Schmitz-Rode T, Janssens U, Schild HH, et al. Fragmentation of massive pulmonary embolism using a pigtail rotation catheter. Chest 1998; 114:1427–36.
86. Brown DB, Cardella JF, Wilson RP, Singh H, Waybill PN. Evaluation of a modified Arrow-Trerotola percutaneous thrombolytic device for treatment of acute pulmonary embolus in a canine model. J Vasc Interv Radiol 1999; 10:733–40.
87. Rocek M, Peregrin J, Velimsky T. Mechanical thrombectomy of massive pulmonary embolism using an Arrow-Trerotola percutaneous thrombolytic device. Eur Radiol 1998; 8:1683–5.
88. Levison RM, Shure D, Moser KM. Reperfusion pulmonary edema after pulmonary artery thromboendarterectomy. Am Rev Respir Dis 1986; 134:1241–5.
89. Uflacker R, Rajagopalan PR, Vujic I, Stutley JE. Treatment of thrombosed dialysis grafts: randomized trial of surgical thrombectomy versus mechanical thrombectomy with the Amplatz device. J Vasc Interv Radiol 1996; 7:185–92.
90. Houry D, Southall J, Manning M, Parsons D. Use of the Amplatz thrombectomy device for severe deep venous thrombosis. South Med J 1999; 92:915–7.
91. Uflacker R. Mechanical thrombectomy in acute and subacute thrombosis with use of the Amplatz device: arterial and venous applications. J Vasc Interv Radiol 1997; 8:923–32.
92. Peuster M, Bertram H, Windhagen-Mahnert B, Paul T, Hausdorf G. Mechanical recanalization of venous thrombosis and pulmonary embolism with the Clotbuster thrombectomy system in a 12-year-old boy. Z Kardiol 1998; 87:283–7.
93. Lang EV, Barnhart WH, Walton DL, Raab SS. Percutaneous pulmonary thrombectomy. J Vasc Interv Radiol 1997; 8:427–32.
94. Schmitt H-E, Jäger KA, Jacob AL, et al. A new rotational thrombectomy catheter: system design and first clinical experiences. Cardiovasc Intervent Radiol 1999; 22:504–9.
95. Kucher N, Eberli FR, Roffi M, et al. Compassionate use of catheter thrombectomy (Aspirex 11F) in patients with massive pulmonary embolism. Study Protocol submitted to the FDA. Sponsor: Straub Medical AG. August 29, 2005.
96. Haskal ZJ, Soulen MC, Huetti EA, Palevsky HI, Cope C. Life-threatening pulmonary emboli and cor pulmonale: treatment with percutaneous pulmonary artery stent placement. Radiology 1994; 191:473–5.
97. Koizumi J, Kusano S, Akima T, et al. Emergent Z stent placement for treatment of cor pulmonale due to pulmonary emboli after failed lytic treatment: technical considerations. Cardiovasc Intervent Radiol 1998; 21:254–5.
98. Schmitz-Rode T, Kilbinger M, Günther RW. Simulated flow pattern in massive pulmonary embolism: significance for selective intrapulmonary thrombolysis. Cardiosvasc Intervent Radiol 1998; 21:199–204.

56 | Endovascular Intervention (Principles and Practice)

Luc Turmel-Rodrigues
Department of Vascular Radiology, Clinique St-Gatien, Tours, and Department of Vascular Radiology, Centre Médico-chirurgical Ambroise Paré, Neuilly-sur-Seine, France

INTRODUCTION

The aim of this chapter is to discuss percutaneous techniques for arteriovenous access.

The best and most durable vascular access is autogenous direct AV fistula created in the forearm, of which there are a number of variations including radial-cephalic, ulnar-basilic, radial-basilic and ulnar-cephalic (1,2). Autogenous fistulae constructed at the elbow level are much less durable, and prosthetic grafts are the most prone to thrombosis and infection. The construction, maintenance and salvage of autogenous AV fistulae in the forearm should be a priority in the management of renal failure patients, especially in those with presumed long life expectancy.

VASCULAR ACCESS CREATION

Venous mapping is mandatory before creation of a fistula if clinical examination fails to identify a usable vein in the forearms (1,2). Venous mapping was historically obtained using iodine venography, replaced by CO_2 venography, and more recently Duplex ultrasound in experienced hands. Magnetic resonance imaging (MRI) and ultrasound provide excellent images of peripheral veins but can miss central vein problems. Venography is still the gold standard examination but is invasive.

ULTRASOUND SURVEILLANCE

For immature fistulae, ultrasound examination is probably the most desirable imaging technique because it is noninvasive, does not require iodine injection, and supports the triage between indications for open surgery or endovascular treatment. Deep location of the vein or an isolated stenosis close to the anastomosis in the lower forearm are indications for superficial surgical transposition or creation of a new anastomosis. On the other hand, stenoses located away from the anastomosis are indications for percutaneous dilatation (6).

Flow measurement in the brachial artery also helps to determine the risk of thrombosis.

In mature fistulae, systematic screening of fistulae by ultrasound imaging has little value, since fistula flow rates can be measured during dialysis. Asymptomatic stenoses must be treated only when patency of the fistula is threatened. The published literature suggests that flow rates below 350 mL/min in forearm fistulae, and below 600 mL/min in prosthetic grafts, reflect a high probability of stenosis and pose a threat to fistula patency (7,8).

ANGIOGRAPHY

Indications for Angiography

Now that flow rates can be accurately measured during dialysis and with ultrasound, angiography should be reserved for cases where concomitant therapeutic intervention is required. There are limited roles for diagnostic computed tomography or magnetic resonance angiography, since neither allows concomitant therapeutic intervention (9,10). The most common clinical abnormalities are repeated difficulties in cannulation, insufficient inflow during dialysis (usually associated with a flat vein), increased venous pressure (usually associated with a distended or pulsatile vein), and swelling of the upper limb. The development of collateral veins is not a problem in itself, but indicates either stenosis of the main outflow vein or excessively high flow. The appearance of enlarging black scars in cannulation areas indicates venous hypertension, usually secondary to stenosis in the main outflow vein. Unfortunately, ischemic complications are often recognized late and the causes of hand pain and ulceration are frequently investigated late and underdiagnosed.

Prevention of fistula thrombosis now relies on flow rate monitoring. Imaging and intervention should be reserved for when flow rates run below established thresholds or when consecutive measurements show a tendancy to flow reduction, indicating an underlying worsening stenosis. As mentioned previously, thresholds of 350 and 600 mL/min have been recommended for native fistulae and prosthetic grafts, respectively.

Ideally, flow rates should be measured at each dialysis session to detect stenoses and provide urgent treatment. Some publications question the value of systematic screening methods for the prevention of thrombosis in grafts.

Technique of Angiography

A complete evaluation from subclavian artery to hand, and wrist to superior vena cava is usually required. Good image quality and technical expertise are essential in the accurate assessment and intervention for fistulae problems. A good angiography can be performed only in an angio suite.

The angiography technique depends on the type of vascular access and indication for imaging. Iodine (at a dose of 300 g/L) is usually used, diluted to 90% in previously undialyzed patients. Gadolinium-based contrast media are used in patients with an established history of severe iodine allergy. CO_2 angiography is not recommended because of the risk of reflux to the vertebral or carotid artery.

In cases of insufficient inflow or cannulation problems in forearm fistulae (Figs. 1 and 2), angiography should be performed to image the forearm arteries, the anastomosis and the vasculature of the hand. Direct cannulation of the arterialized vein can be difficult, provides insufficient information regarding the arterial supply and confers a high risk of hematomas. The frequency of arterial abnormalities is high and the risk of hand ischemia following full reopening of a stenosed fistula is an increasing problem, particulary in the presence of significant ulnar artery disease (12). In addition, 20% of patients have a high radial artery origin and imaging of the brachial artery is only possible from a retrograde injection at the level of the elbow. Rarely, subclavian artery disease causes poor fistula flow.

The only contraindication for arterial cannulation at the elbow (usually brachial, though occasionally radial or ulnar-interosseous artery) is full anticoagulation. In our department, we perform a retrograde brachial puncture with an 18-G needle and a straight 0.035-in. Terumo™ wire, Tokyo, Japan over which the dilator of a 4-F introducer is passed. Five to ten millilitres of contrast is injected at a flow rate of 5 to 10 mL/sec for imaging of forearm vessels, increased to 20 mL at a flow rate of 10 mL/sec for proximal vessel imaging.

In cases of venous hypertension, the pulsatile segment of vein or graft can be cannulated directly for antegrade placement of a 6- to 8-F introducer, according to the presumed size of dilatation balloon required (Fig. 3). Imaging of the AV anastomosis and distal arterial tree is only necessary if there is a potential risk of secondary hand ischemia (particularly native elbow fistulae, elderly or diabetic patients and smokers). Retrograde opacification of the arterial

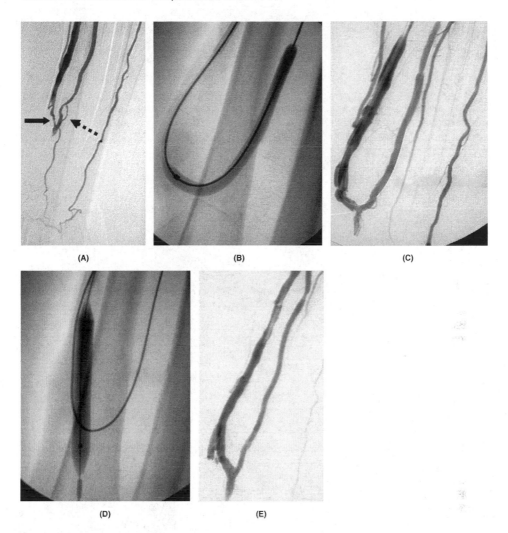

FIGURE 1 (**A**) This right radiocephalic fistula was created six months earlier. Indications for angiography were low flow and difficulties in cannulation. Angiography was performed by cannulation of the elbow artery since the patient was not anticoagulated and showed two stenoses of the radial artery (*dotted arrow*) and arterialized vein (*full arrow*). (**B**) Using a retrograde venous approach, a 0.035-in. hydrophilic guidewire was passed across the anastomosis into the proximal radial artery and a 4-mm wide and 60-mm long dilatation balloon (Powerflex-Extreme from Cordis, Miami, Florida, U.S.A.) was inflated across the anastomosis up to 25 atm. (**C**) Angiography after dilatation to 4 mm showed clear residual stenosis on the vein but it would have been dangerous to inflate a bigger balloon protruding into the artery. (**D**) The solution was to push the 7-mm ballon (Conquest from Bard) over another guidewire placed in the distal artery while leaving a safety wire through the anastomosis. (**E**) Final angiogram showed a satisfactory result with no residual stenosis after dilatation of the vein to 7 mm and of the proximal artery to 4 mm.

inflow can be performed with the balloon inflated to stop flow in the vascular access. If there are large collaterals between the AV anastomosis and the balloon, it may be necessary to perform retrograde cannulation of the vein in the direction of the anastomosis and to push a 4-F diagnostic catheter into the feeding artery.

In cases of hand ischemia, the entire arterial tree must be imaged, from subclavian to hand (12).

Similarly, for excessive high flow, full imaging is required to plan a flow reduction strategy. In addition, fistula flow rate can be measured during angiography by thermodilution (13).

(*Text continues on page 576.*)

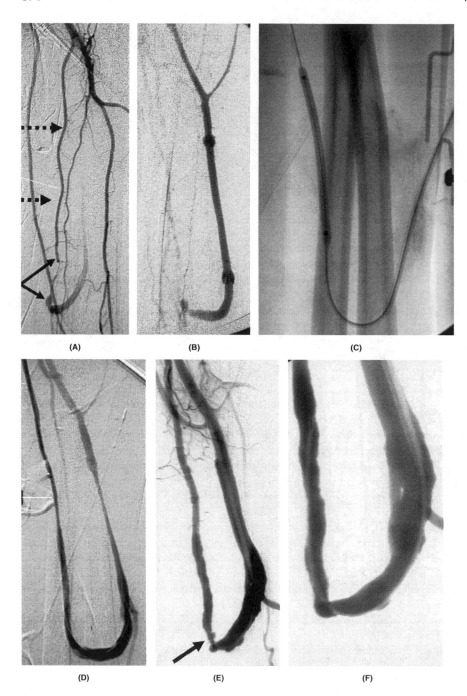

(A)   (B)   (C)

(D)   (E)   (F)

FIGURE 2 (**A**) This left radiocephalic fistula in a 74-year-old patient was created two months earlier and was referred for delayed maturation. Angiography was performed by cannulation of the elbow artery and revealed a small radial artery (*dotted arrows*) with a tight stenosis at the anastomosis (*full arrows*). (**B**) The arterialized vein was perfect. (**C**) From a venous retrograde approach after placement of a tourniquet in the upper arm, a 0.014-in. guidewire was placed across the anastomosis, a 4-F diagnostic catheter was then positioned over it and a 0.035-in. straight metallic wire then allowed placement of a 4-mm dilatation balloon (Powerflex-Extreme from Cordis). Low pressure was sufficient to abolish the waisting of the stenosis on the balloon. (**D**) Angiography after dilatation showed an excellent result, apart from transient spasms, and the fistula was immediately successfully used for dialysis. (**E**) This fistula was referred again four months later for recurrence of insufficient inflow. Restenosis was short and located at the anastomosis itself (*arrow*). (**F**) The final angiogram was satisfactory after focal redilatation to 5 mm.

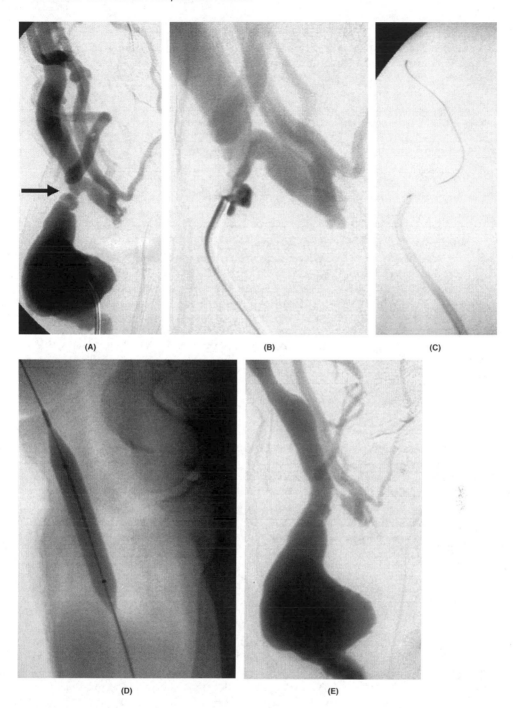

FIGURE 3 (**A**) This left radiocephalic fistula of more than three years was referred for venous hyperpressure and aneurysmal involution of dialysis sites. Angiography performed from an antegrade cannulation of the forearm vein showed an irregular tight stenosis at the junction of the cephalic with the basilic vein at the elbow (*arrow*). (**B**) Hydrophilic guidewires were unable to pass this stenosis which was relatively easily traversed using the combination of a 5-F vertebral-type Merit catheter and (**C**) a 0.014-in. Spartacore guidewire (Guidant). (**D**) After exchange of guidewires, an 8-mm dilatation balloon (Conquest from Bard) was inflated to 35 atm (**E**) with a good final result.

Interpretation of the Angiogram

A stenosis is a narrowing of the vessel, graded as the proportion of diameter reduction. The reference diameter is often difficult to determine in dialysis fistulae and the stenosis frequently involves the whole vein or artery (Fig. 2). The key is to determine whether the stenosis imaged is likely to explain the clinical abnormalities or flow reduction. Marked opacification of collateral indicates that outlow stenosis is significant.

DILATATION

Indications for and Technique of Dilatation

Although the brachial artery route, with placement of a 4-F catheter, is often necessary for accurate diagnosis, the arterial approach must be avoided for insertion of high-pressure dilatation balloons that require at least a 6-F introducer because of the risk of subsequent hematoma or pseudoaneurysm (14). The arterialized vein itself should be preferably cannulated, or recannulated in the direction of the stenosis at a distance sufficient to avoid direct contact of the introducer tip with the stenosis. A small subcutaneous tunnel should be made between the skin and vein entry points to facilitate compression or placement of a suture, while minimizing the risk of secondary bleeding or vessel wall necrosis (15).

Traversing the stenosis with a guidewire is usually simple in prosthetic grafts but can be challenging in native fistulae. Tight, long or irregular stenoses should not be approached in an antegrade fashion with a hydrophilic guidewire, which is prone to enter the venous wall and cause dissections. The retrograde approach and the combination of a 0.014-in. guidewire and a vertebral type catheter is the safest approach (e.g., Spartacore™, Guidant, Indianapolis, Indiana, U.S.A. and Vertebral, Merit Medical, South Jordan, Utah, U.S.A.). Soft stenoses (such as those encountered between aneurysms) are often passed by the 5-F catheter itself. Occasionally, when a retrograde approach fails, an antegrade approach is successful, and vice versa (Fig. 3).

Ideally, following dialatation, the stenosis will no longer be visible on angiography (Fig. 1). This is often easy to achieve at the venous anastomosis of prosthetic grafts. An 8-mm dilatation balloon is used for 6-mm grafts, inflated to a pressure which abolishes the waist of the stenosis. Dedicated balloons can now be inflated above 30 atm: stenoses resistant to such pressure are extremely rare (e.g., Conquest™, Bard Peripheral Vascular, Tempe, Arizona, U.S.A.). As long as "waisting" of the stenosis is abolished, there is no evidence to recommend prolonged inflation, so heparin is not required.

However, deliberate underdilatation with subsequent residual stenosis may be desirable in three clinical settings:

1. When circulation to the hand is poor, increased fistula flow rate after stenosis dilatation can disrupt the precarious balance between blood flow to the hand and the "steal" exerted by the fistula, particularly with native elbow fistulae and grafts. In such circumstances, we suggest limiting the balloon size for the first dilatation to 5 mm for stenoses close to the AV anastomosis and to 7 mm for stenoses located downstream from the venous return needle. Maintaining a flow rate below 800 mL/min in forearm fistulae and 1 L/min in elbow fistulae and grafts can be expected. A 1 mm larger balloon can then be used in cases of early recurrence if the previous dilatation was uncomplicated.
2. In cases where there is a history of cardiac ischemia or dyspnea, a high fistula flow is not desirable. Deliberate underdilatation, using the principles above, is recommended.
3. In cases of concomitant asymptomatic central vein stenosis, which is frequently encountered, full reopening of a fistula can increase the flow rate such that collaterals cannot divert the increased venous flow, resulting in pain or edema (Fig. 4). Central vein stenoses can be dilated, but the results are disappointing even with stent placement. Redilatation may be necessary every two to three months (16). It is preferable not to increase fistula flow above the capacity of collateral flow diversion, though this is difficult to quantify.

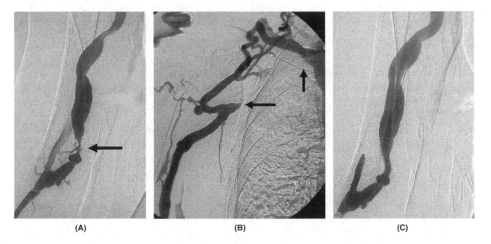

(A) (B) (C)

FIGURE 4 **(A)** This 2-year-old right transposed brachiobasilic fistula monitored using the Transonic flow rate measurement device was referred for low flow of 500 mL/min that did not impair dialysis. Angiography was performed via a retrograde catheterization of the arterialized vein and placement of a 4-F catheter down to the anastomosis. A tight stenosis was located relatively close to the anastomosis (*arrow*) and low flow of 550 mL/min was confirmed using a thermodilution catheter. **(B)** The other abnormality was a long occlusion of the axillary–subclavian vein (*arrows*) with flow diverted through relatively well-developed collaterals. Optimal dilatation of the juxta-anastomotic stenosis in such an elbow fistula risked secondary hand ischemia and/or arm edema. **(C)** The stenosis was dilated only to 6 mm, leaving this obvious residual stenosis but achieving a flow rate of 1.5 L/min. It was decided to end the procedure. The patient then developed moderate hand edema. He died 18 months later with no need for reintervention on this fistula that had been deliberately underdilated in view of the excellent flow rate achieved despite residual stenosis.

After dilatation, there are four potential angiographic results:

1. No residual stenosis
2. <30% residual stenosis. This is acceptable if nonrecurrent, though redilatation for two to three minutes, or dilatation with a 1-mm larger balloon should be considered
3. >30% residual stenosis. A 1-mm larger balloon should be used, unless under-dilatation is intentional. If despite this there is a residual stenosis, a stent should be considered.
4. Extravasation of contrast medium indicating rupture of the vessel wall. The ballon must be rapidly reinflated to 2 atm for intervals of five minutes. If the leak persists despite 15 minutes of balloon tamponade, a stent must be placed to seal the rupture (17,18)

Final compression of the introducer entry points can be shortened by purse-string suturing, and the fistula is immediately usable for dialysis (15).

Technical Refinements

Immature fistulae should be imaged from the fifth week using ultrasound or angiography. If delayed maturation is due to the deep location of the vein or to isolated stenosis of the anastomosis, surgical revision is indicated, with transposition of the vein beneath the skin or creation of a new anastomosis.

Stenoses located in the feeding artery or the vein should be dilated urgently to prevent acute fistula thrombosis (Fig. 2) (6), since it is usually impossible to declot an immature fistula. Even extensive stenoses of the feeding artery respond well to dilatation to at least 4 mm using flexible high-pressure balloons. Venous stenoses should be dilated to at least 5 mm. In our experience, stents have rarely been necessary in the feeding artery. In cases with main outflow vein stenosis, there is no indication for embolization or ligation of collaterals if the stenosis is sufficiently dilated.

Anastomotic venous stenoses in the forearm are often difficult to dilate because there is usually a discrepancy between the diameter of the feeding artery and the normal vein distally (Fig. 1). A dilatation balloon should be smaller than 5 mm to avoid rupture. We suggest placing an initial "safety" guidewire across the anastomosis from the vein into the proximal feeding artery using a retrograde venous approach and then a second guidewire to the distal artery. A 6 to 8 mm balloon can be inflated over the distal artery guidewire, preventing overdilatation of the proximal artery. This may cause spasm of the proximal artery, which can be reopened using a 4 mm balloon over the safety wire.

If there is an acute angle between the artery and the vein at the anastomosis, it may not be possible to pass a guidewire or balloon through the anastomosis using a retrograde venous approach. An arterial approach may be necessary, preferably using a retrograde distal radial artery cannulation at the wrist or antegrade brachial route.

Perforating and deep concomitant veins are sometimes the only remaining venous drainage because of previous repeated cannulation of basilic and cephalic veins (Fig. 5). Perforating vein stenoses can be passed with caution using a 0.014-in. guidewire but should then be deliberately overdilated to 7 or 8 mm to reestablish sufficient outflow from the fistula. A long covered stent can be placed across the elbow providing excellent results, though the development of further stenoses on the downstream vein is almost inevitable. However in obese patients, such stent placement is contraindicated because the upper arm concomitant veins often run too deep, leading to kinking of the stent at the elbow joint.

Stenosis of the final arch of the cephalic vein can be impossible to pass using a venous antegrade approach. The femoral route, with selective catheterization of the superior vena cava and subclavian vein, can be successful.

Stenoses resistant to dilatation are rare, since the advent of high pressure balloons, but cutting balloons may be useful in this situation.

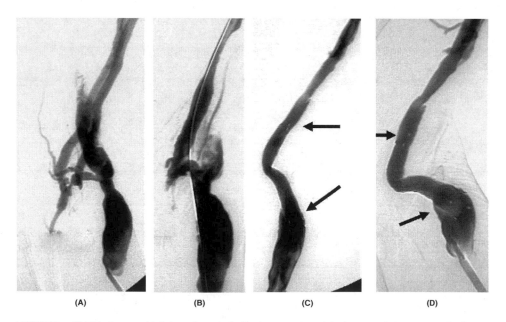

| (A) | (B) | (C) | (D) |

FIGURE 5   (**A**) This 2-year-old right radiocephalic fistula was referred for increased venous pressure and recirculation. Angiography was performed via an antegrade cannulation of the forearm vein and showed chronic occlusion of both basilic and cephalic veins in the upper arm, with elbow drainage relying only on a severely stenosed perforating vein connecting superficial veins and deep concomitant veins. (**B**) The stenosis was carefully passed using a 5-F vertebral catheter and a 0.014-in. guidewire, with subsequent exchange of guidewires and dilatation to 8 mm using a Conquest balloon. (**C**) A stent (8×80 mm Fluency from Bard) was eventually placed in order to avoid significant recoil (*arrows*) (**D**) especially in the flexed elbow position. The residual stenosis visible on the deep brachial vein downstream from the stent then worsened and was dilated four months later.

STENTS

Only self-expandable stents should be used in dialysis fistulae (16–19), but sometimes have disappointing results and can be detrimental if they overlap major side branches (Figs. 6 and 7). Their placement should be limited to the treatment of complications and failures of dilatation.

Indications for stents include rupture, major stenosis recoil after dilatation, early repeated stenosis recurrence and trapping of thrombus during thrombectomy.

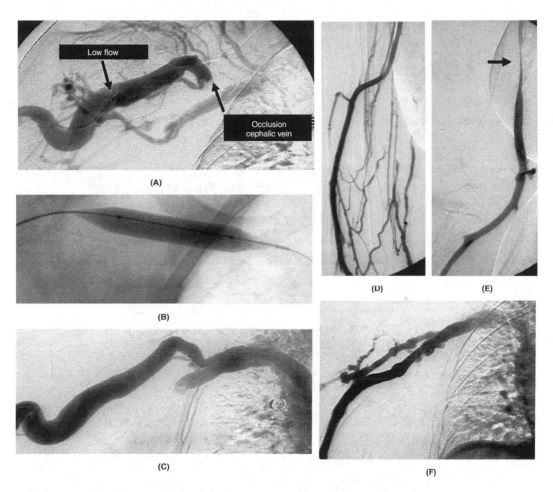

FIGURE 6 (**A**) This 7-year-old right brachiocephalic fistula was referred for very low flow and dramatically increased venous pressure only six weeks after previous dilatation of a stenosis located in the final arch at the confluence with the subclavian vein. Angiography was performed from an antegrade cannulation of the cephalic vein and showed a short complete reocclusion of the final part of the cephalic vein (*arrow*). (**B**) This short occlusion was easily recanalized using a straight 0.035-in. Terumo hydrophilic guidewire and was dilated to 10 mm using a Conquest balloon. (**C**) Angiography after redilatation to 10 mm with no residual waisting showed evidence of major recoil, for which it was tempting to place a stent. However, stent placement in this location would automatically overlap the subclavian vein and preclude any further construction of any type of vascular access on this right upper limb. (**D**) It was therefore decided to perform an upper limb venography immediately from cannulation of a vein of the dorsum of the hand. This venography showed that there was a cephalic vein of more than 3 mm in the forearm, with excellent radial pulse at clinical examination. (**E**) The upper arm basilic vein was also patent apart from extrinsic compression of the chest (*arrow*). (**F**) The axillary and subclavian veins were also perfect. It was therefore decided not to place a stent but to refer the patient immediately to a surgeon for creation of a radiocephalic fistula. Creation of this brachiocephalic fistula seven years earlier was obviously the result of lack of preoperative venous mapping.

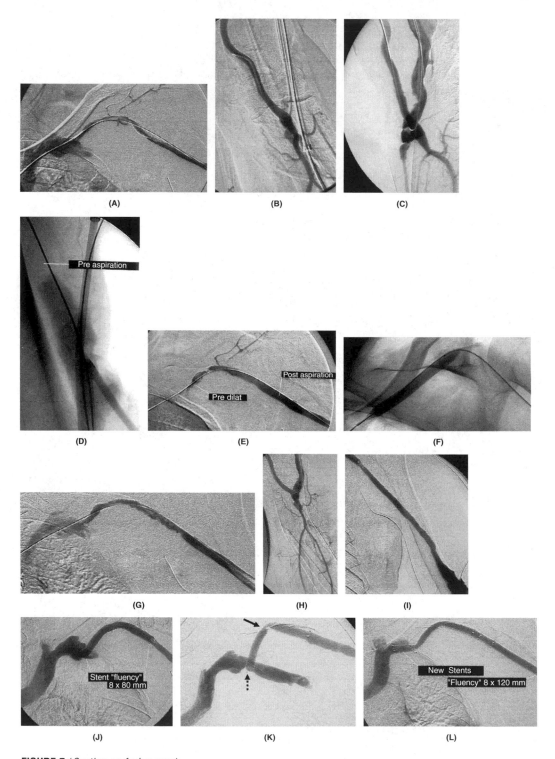

FIGURE 7 (*Caption on facing page*)

THROMBOSIS

Background

Acute access thrombosis is usually diagnosed at the time of dialysis. Hyperkalemia or fluid overload may require urgent dialysis using a temporary central line, preferably using the femoral vein. Otherwise, the fistula should be declotted prior to dialysis where possible.

This can be difficult logistically and technically, and significant efforts should be made to prevent fistula thrombosis.

The results of endovascular treatment are significantly better than conventional surgery in thrombosed native fistulae (2). For prosthetic grafts, conventional surgery might be more effective than endovascular treatment, but is clearly more invasive.

A thrombosed fistula or graft can be declotted for up to four weeks using endovascular techniques. Delayed treatment can occur in patients in intensive care units after major surgery where early transfer to an angiography suite would be unsafe, and nondialyzed patients in whom the fistula is not currently used.

Technique

Declotting a polytetrafluoroethylene graft is similar in most cases, thrombosis usually caused by a stenosis at the venous anastomosis, but native fistulae are more complex for a variety of reasons (20):

1. a thin wall and small diameter can make it difficult gain endovascular access
2. it can be difficult to traverse the anastomosis because of collaterals
3. the site of underlying stenosis is variable and often difficult to localize
4. the underlying stenosis is often severe, irregular and difficult to traverse
5. the volume of thrombus can be high
6. aneurysms are frequently encountered, often with adherent thrombi
7. concomitant thrombosis of the feeding artery is common in cases of end-to-end anastomosis

The treatment of a thrombosed access involves firstly the removal of all thrombus and secondly treatment of the underlying cause. Percutaneous declotting a fistula is an outpatient procedure. Anticoagulation (at least 3000 U of heparin) is essential and antistaphylococcal antibiotics should be administered. Firstly, the thrombosed vessel is punctured under local anesthesia and two introducer sheaths placed in opposite directions to gain access to the venous outflow and arterial inflow.

FIGURE 7 (*facing page*) (**A**) This 8-month-old left brachiocephalic fistula was referred for acute thrombosis. The thrombosed vein was first cannulated in an antegrade fashion. A safety guidewire was placed in central veins and a short 5-F catheter was pushed parallel to the safety wire. A small injection of iodine showed thrombi and probable stenosis of the final arch of the cephalic vein. (**B**) The vein was then cannulated in a retrograde fashion and a catheter was pushed through the anastomosis into the brachial artery. Local injection showed complete occlusion of the fistula and widely patent forearm arteries, and a safety wire was then left across the anastomosis. (**C**) A residual thrombus close to the anastomosis can be seen after the first range of aspiration maneuvers. (**D**) This residual thrombus was detached by additional aspirations and was stopped by a narrowing of the cephalic vein where it was eventually aspirated. (**E**) Once the vein was freed from any residual thrombus, angiography confirmed a severe stenosis of the final arch of the cephalic vein which explained why the fistula became thrombosed. (**F**) Dilatation to 8 mm was performed using a Conquest balloon. (**G**) Angiography after dilatation showed a heterogeneous result, making it essential to place a stent. There was little room for discussion, although we were aware of the risk of damage to the subclavian vein. (**H**) Final angiogram ruled out any iatrogenic embolism in the forearm arteries. (**I**) There was no residual stenosis and no residual clots in the cephalic vein. (**J**) Here the stent (8×80 mm Fluency from Bard) protrudes as little as possible into the subclavian vein. (**K**) Acute thrombosis recurred five months later and showed evidence of kinking (*full arrow*) and displacement (*dotted arrow*) of the stent. It was then obvious that this subclavian vein overlapped by a stent would never allow creation of a new vascular access in the left upper limb. (**L**) Two new stents were eventually necessary to reopen the fistula.

The site for initial catheterization is variable. If the stenosis in forearm fistulae is thought to be close to the wrist anastomosis, a single retrograde approach from the vein at the elbow is sufficient. If the first few centimeters of the fistula are still patent, a single antegrade approach from the patent segment is appropriate. In native fistulae, we recommend the systematic use of safety wires, particularly in the presence of tortuousity, angulations and aneurysms, or when blind predilatation is necessary to allow the passage of the thrombectomy device.

Typically an initial introducer sheath is placed a few centimeters from the anastomosis using an antegrade approach to treat the venous outflow. A 5-F catheter is then pushed over a wire up to the superior vena cava and then slowly pulled back, while contrast medium is injected under fluoroscopy in order to localize the downstream extension of the thrombosis. The fistula is abandoned at this stage if the venous outflow cannot be traversed. A regular metallic 0.035-in. safety guidewire is then positioned through the 5-F catheter, which is subsequently removed. A hydrophilic wire is positioned in the superior vena cava, parallel to the safety wire, through a sheath. Thrombectomy and dilatation are performed through the sheath, while the safety guidewire represents a fluoroscopic landmark of the anatomy of the fistula and can be used for the passage of a dilatation balloon or stent in the event of complications (Fig. 7).

A second ("arterial") introducer is placed with a retrograde approach some distance downstream from the "venous" introducer in the direction of the arterial inflow and a further safety wire is placed as before. Once access to both the arterial inflow and venous outflow is guaranteed with safety guidewires in place, the thrombus can be removed starting at the venous side.

We recommend the use of manual catheter-directed thromboaspiration. A slightly angulated 6- to 9-F firm catheter with a wide inner lumen and soft atraumatic tip is passed through the introducer sheath in contact with the thrombus. Strong manual aspiration is performed through a regular Luer-Lok™ 50-mL syringe while pulling back the catheter. The syringe and the aspiration catheter are flushed through a gauze and the maneuver repeated until clear of thrombus. We use 9-F catheters in mature native fistulae, 8-F catheters in prosthetic grafts, and 6- or 7-F catheters when an arterial approach is unavoidable.

Once the thrombus has been cleared, the underlying stenoses must be dilated using high pressure balloons. The use of stents is limited to the treatment of acute ruptures not controlled by balloon tamponade, acute pseudoaneurysms, major stenosis recoil (>50%) after dilatation, and occlusive residual clots not detached by the thrombectomy device.

Finally, the whole fistula must be checked from the feeding artery to the superior vena cava to rule out residual thrombi and stenoses. Minor residual thrombi or residual stenoses of less than 50% are acceptable if excellent flow is restored. In contrast, they must be treated more aggressively if flow is insufficient. Incidental arterial embolism must be treated by thromboaspiration or backbleeding, even when asymptomatic (21).

Specific Cases and Technical Refinements

Recent forearm fistulae, which are immature are frequently impossible to cannulate. The solution is to place a tourniquet on the upper arm to increase venous pressure. The cephalic or basilic vein at the elbow is then easily punctured and catheterized with a retrograde approach back into the fistula.

When the anastomosis cannot be reached by retrograde approach from the fistula, either because of stenoses or collaterals, it is helpful to perform angiography from the brachial artery to delineate the anastomosis and aid catheterization by mapping. If there is a tight anastomotic stenosis which cannot be traversed in the retrograde fashion, antegrade cannulation of the brachial artery at the elbow and selective catheterization of the feeding artery should be considered, or a retrograde approach from the distal radial artery. The combination of an angled (4 or 5 F) catheter and a (0.035 in.) hydrophilic guidewire usually enable crossing of the stenosis.

In cases of concomitant thrombosis of the feeding artery, retrograde catheterization of the thrombosed artery from the fistula is usually possible and thromboaspiration can be performed with a flexible 6-F catheter. If not, aspiration can be performed after antegrade cannulation of the feeding artery and placement of a 6- or 7-F introducer sheath in the brachial artery.

Thrombus within aneurysms, if fresh, is usually relatively easy to aspirate. If the aneurysm is large, external compression of the aneurysm facilitates contact between thrombus and catheter. In contrast, wall-adherent thrombi are usually resistant to lysis or aspiration. Such old thrombi frequently detach during unblocking maneuvres and can impede flow and embolize to the lungs, so must be trapped with stent placement across the aneurysm. A wide mesh puncturable stent is preferred to enable further cannulation of adjacent segments if early surgical correction of the aneurysm is not feasible.

Concomitant acute thrombosis of central veins is a problem common to native fistulae and grafts. Catheter-directed thromboaspiration proves to be very effective in thrombosed subclavian and brachiocephalic veins though involves large thrombus volume with risk of embolization.

RESULTS OF INTERVENTIONAL PROCEDURES

Reports on the success and patency rates of fistulae are extremely variable (2,22). The location and nature of access (forearm/upper arm, native/prosthetic), the location of stenoses (artery or vein, peripheral or central vein), the age of access and patient, and the presence of comorbidity (diabetes, smoking, hypertension, cardiovascular disease) significantly affect the outcome of percutaneous interventions.

The immediate success rates for thrombectomy are best for prosthetic grafts (approaching 100%), but there is a high rate of early rethrombosis (ranging from 16–70% at one month), largely influenced by the presence of residual clot (2). In contrast, immediate failure is not uncommon in native fistulae (5–30%) but with a low rate of early rethrombosis. Including early failures, one-year patency rates are approxiamately 50% for forearm fistulae, 35% for upper arm fistulae and 25% for prosthetic grafts in the largest comparative series.

Patency rates after dilatation of failing but nonthrombosed vascular access are slightly better than those achieved in thrombosed fistulae and grafts. Results after stent placement also tend to be slightly better compared with the results of simple dilatation, but this is controversial. As a result of repeated interventions, secondary patency rates are better, reaching 80% at one year.

Conventional surgery is more invasive and has not been shown to improve patency rates.

COMPLICATIONS

Hyperkalemia and fluid overload are common causes of mortality in dialyzed patients and can occur during interventions. Problems specific to percutaneous interventions include bacteremia and pulmonary embolism. Dilatation-induced rupture can lead to the loss of the access if the guidewire is inadvertently removed. It can also cause significant hematoma, blood loss or pseudoaneurysm in high-flow fistulae, even after stent placement. Hematomas and pseudoaneurysms can occur at puncture sites.

Hand ischemia can complicate excessive dilatation of a peripheral stenosis in cases of poor arterial supply to the hand, mainly in elbow fistulae. Ischemia can also result from an iatrogenic embolism in the forearm arteries during a thrombectomy procedure.

Arm edema can unmask concomitant central vein stenosis after dilatation of a peripheral vein.

Stents can migrate into central veins, right heart or pulmonary arteries if the diameter of the vein was underestimated. They are also prone to infection or ulceration if superficial. Stents can also be destroyed by inadvertent cannulations and create obstruction to the flow.

CONCLUSION

The creation and maintenance of AV vascular access for hemodialysis is challenging. Endovascular techniques are essential for the treatment of stenoses and thrombosis, to achieve reasonable patency rates.

REFERENCES

1. National Kidney Foundation-Dialysis Outcomes Quality Initiative. NKF-DOQI clinical practice guidelines for vascular access. Am J Kidney Dis 1997; 30(Suppl. 3):S150–91.
2. Turmel-Rodrigues L, Pengloan J, Bourquelot P. Interventional radiology in hemodialysis fistulae and grafts: a multidisciplinary approach. Cardiovasc Intervent Radiol 2002; 25:3–16.
3. Brown P. Preoperative radiological assessment of vascular access. Eur J Vasc Endovasc Surg 2006; 31:64–9.
4. Grobner T, Prischl F. Gadolinium and nephrogenic systemic fibrosis. Kidney Int 2007; 72:260–4.
5. Turmel-Rodrigues L, Bourquelot P, Raynaud A, Beyssen B. Hemodialysis fistula: preoperative MR venography. A promising but partial view. Radiology 2000; 211:302.
6. Turmel-Rodrigues L, Mouton A, Birmelé B, et al. Salvage of immature forearm fistulas for haemodialysis by interventional radiology. Nephrol Dial Transplant 2001; 16:2365–71.
7. McCarley P, Wingard RL, Shyr Y, Pettus W, Hakim RM, Ikizler TA. Vascular access blood flow monitoring reduces access morbidity and costs. Kidney Int 2001; 60:1164–72.
8. Tessitore N, Mansucto G, Bedogna V, et al. A prospective controlled trial on effect of percutaneous transluminal angioplasty on functioning arteriovenous fistulae survival. J Am Soc Nephrol 2003; 14:1623–7.
9. Ko S, Huang C, Ng S, et al. MDCT angiography for evaluation of the complete vascular tree of hemodialysis fistulas. Am J Radiol 2005; 185:1268–74.
10. Doelman C, Duijm L, Liem Y, et al. Stenosis detection in failing hemodialysis access fistulas and grafts: comparison of color Doppler ultrasonography, contrast-enhanced magnetic resonance angiography, and digital subtraction angiography. J Vasc Surg 2005; 42:739–46.
11. Turmel-Rodrigues L, Pengloan J, Baudin S, et al. Treatment of stenosis and thrombosis in haemodialysis fistulas and grafts by interventional radiology. Nephrol Dial Transplant 2000; 15:2029–36.
12. Guerra A, Raynaud A, Beyssen B, Pagny JY, Sapoval M, Angel C. Arterial percutaneous angioplasty in upper limbs with vascular access devices for haemodialysis. Nephrol Dial Transplant 2002; 17:843–51.
13. Vesely T, Gherardini D, Gleed R, Kislukhin V, Krivitski N. Use of a catheter-based system to emasure blood flow in hemodialysis grafts during angioplasty procedures. J Vasc Interv Radiol 2002; 13:371–9.
14. Trerotola S, Turmel-Rodrigues L. Off the beaten path: transbrachial approach for native fistula interventions. Radiology 2001; 218:617–9.
15. Zaleski G, Funaki B, Gentile L, Garofalo R. Purse-string sutures and miniature tourniquet to achieve immediate hemostasis of percutaneous grafts and fistulas. Am J Radiol 2000; 175:1643–5.
16. Haage P, Vorwerk D, Piroth W, Schuermann K, Guenther R. Treatment of hemodialysis-related central venous stenosis or occlusion: results of primary Wallstent placement and follow-up in 50 patients. Radiology 1999; 212:175–80.
17. Sapoval M, Turmel-Rodrigues L, Raynaud A, Bourquelot P, Rodrigue H, Gaux JC. Cragg covered stents in hemodialysis access: initial and mid-term results. J Vasc Interv Radiol 1996; 7:335–42.
18. Raynaud A, Angel C, Sapoval M, Beyssen B, Pagny J, Auguste M. Treatment of hemodialysis access rupture during PTA with Wallstent implantation. J Vasc Interv Radiol 1998; 9:437–42.
19. Turmel-Rodrigues L, Blanchard D, Pengloan J, et al. Wallstents and Craggstents in hemodialysis grafts and fistulae: results for selective indications. J Vasc Interv Radiol 1997; 8:975–82.
20. Turmel-Rodrigues L, Raynaud A, Louail B, Beyssen B, Sapoval M. Manual catheter-directed aspiration and other thrombectomy techniques for declotting native fistulas for hemodialysis. J Vasc Interv Radiol 2001; 12:1365–71.
21. Trerotola S, Johnson M, Shah H, Namylowski J, Filo R. Incidence and management of arterial emboli from hemodialysis graft surgical thrombectomy. J Vasc Interv Radiol 1997; 8:557–62.
22. Sidawy A, Gray R, Besarab A, et al. Recommended standards for reports dealing with arteriovenous hemodialysis accesses. J Vasc Surg 2002; 35:603–10.

Index